MW00575265

Pulmonary Pathology:

An Atlas and Text

Third Edition

Pulmonary Pathology:

An Atlas and Text

Third Edition

► Editor-in-Chief

Philip T. Cagle, MD
Professor
Department of Pathology and Genomic Medicine
Houston Methodist Hospital
Houston, Texas

► Associate Editors

Timothy C. Allen, MD, JD
Professor and Chair
Department of Pathology
University of Mississippi Medical Center
Jackson, Mississippi

Mary Beth Beasley, MD
Professor
Department of Pathology
Icahn School of Medicine at Mount Sinai
New York, New York

Alain Borczuk, MD
Professor of Pathology
Department of Pathology
NewYork-Presbyterian Hospital/Weill Cornell Medical Center
New York, New York

Yasmeen M. Butt, MD
Assistant Professor
Department of Pathology
University of Texas Southwestern Medical Center
Dallas, Texas

Sanja Dacic, MD, PhD
Professor of Pathology
Department of Pathology
University of Pittsburgh
Staff Pathologist
Department of Pathology
University of Pittsburgh Medical Center
Pittsburgh, Pennsylvania

Aliya N. Husain, MD
Professor
Department of Pathology
University of Chicago
Chicago, Illinois

Brandon T. Larsen, MD, PhD
Assistant Professor
Department of Laboratory Medicine and Pathology
Mayo Clinic School of Medicine
Senior Associate Consultant
Department of Laboratory Medicine and Pathology
Mayo Clinic Arizona
Scottsdale, Arizona

Ross A. Miller, MD
Assistant Professor
Pathologist
Department of Pathology and Genomic Medicine
Houston Methodist Hospital
Houston, Texas

Mari Mino-Kenudson, MD
Associate Professor
Department of Pathology
Harvard Medical School
Director, Pulmonary Pathology Service
Department of Pathology
Massachusetts General Hospital
Boston, Massachusetts

Sergio Pina-Oviedo, MD
Assistant Professor
Department of Pathology
University of Arkansas for Medical Sciences
Little Rock, Arkansas

Kirtee Raparia, MD
Associate Pathologist
Department of Pathology
Kaiser Permanente Santa Clara Medical Center
Santa Clara, California

Natasha Rekhtman, MD, PhD
Associate Attending Pathologist
Department of Pathology
Memorial Sloan Kettering Cancer Center
New York, New York

Anja C. Roden, MD
Associate Professor
Consultant
Department of Laboratory Medicine and Pathology
Mayo Clinic
Rochester, Minnesota

Sinchita Roy-Chowdhuri, MD, PhD
Assistant Professor
Department of Pathology
University of Texas MD Anderson Cancer Center
Houston, Texas

Lynette M. Sholl, MD
Associate Pathologist
Department of Pathology
Brigham and Women's Faulkner Hospital
Boston, Massachusetts

Maxwell L. Smith, MD
Associate Professor
Department of Laboratory Medicine and Pathology
Mayo Clinic School of Medicine
Consultant
Department of Laboratory Medicine and Pathology
Mayo Clinic Arizona
Scottsdale, Arizona

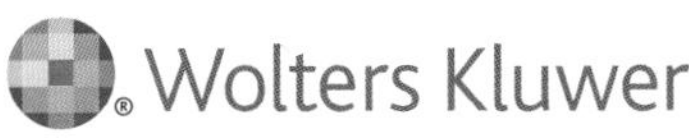

Philadelphia • Baltimore • New York • London
Buenos Aires • Hong Kong • Sydney • Tokyo

Senior Acquisitions Editor: Ryan Shaw
Development Editor: Sean McGuire
Editorial Coordinator: Jennifer DiRicco
Marketing Manager: Rachel Mante Leung
Production Project Manager: Joan Sinclair
Design Coordinator: Holly McLaughlin
Manufacturing Coordinator: Beth Welsh
Prepress Vendor: TNQ Books and Journals

Third edition

9 8 7 6 5 4 3 2 1

Printed in China

Library of Congress Cataloging-in-Publication Data

Names: Cagle, Philip T., editor.
Title: Pulmonary pathology : an atlas and text/editor-in-chief, Philip T. Cagle ; associate editors, Timothy Craig Allen [and 15 others].
Other titles: Color atlas and text of pulmonary pathology.
Description: Third edition. | Philadelphia : Wolters Kluwer, [2019] | Preceded by Color atlas and text of pulmonary pathology / editor-in-chief, Philip T. Cagle ; associate editors, Timothy C. Allen ... [et al.]. c2008. | Includes bibliographical references and index.
Identifiers: LCCN 2017058337 | ISBN 9781496346094 (hardback)
Subjects: | MESH: Lung Diseases–pathology | Atlases
Classification: LCC RC756 | NLM WF 17 | DDC 616.2/407–dc23 LC record available at https://lccn.loc.gov/2017058337

LWW.com

CCS0218

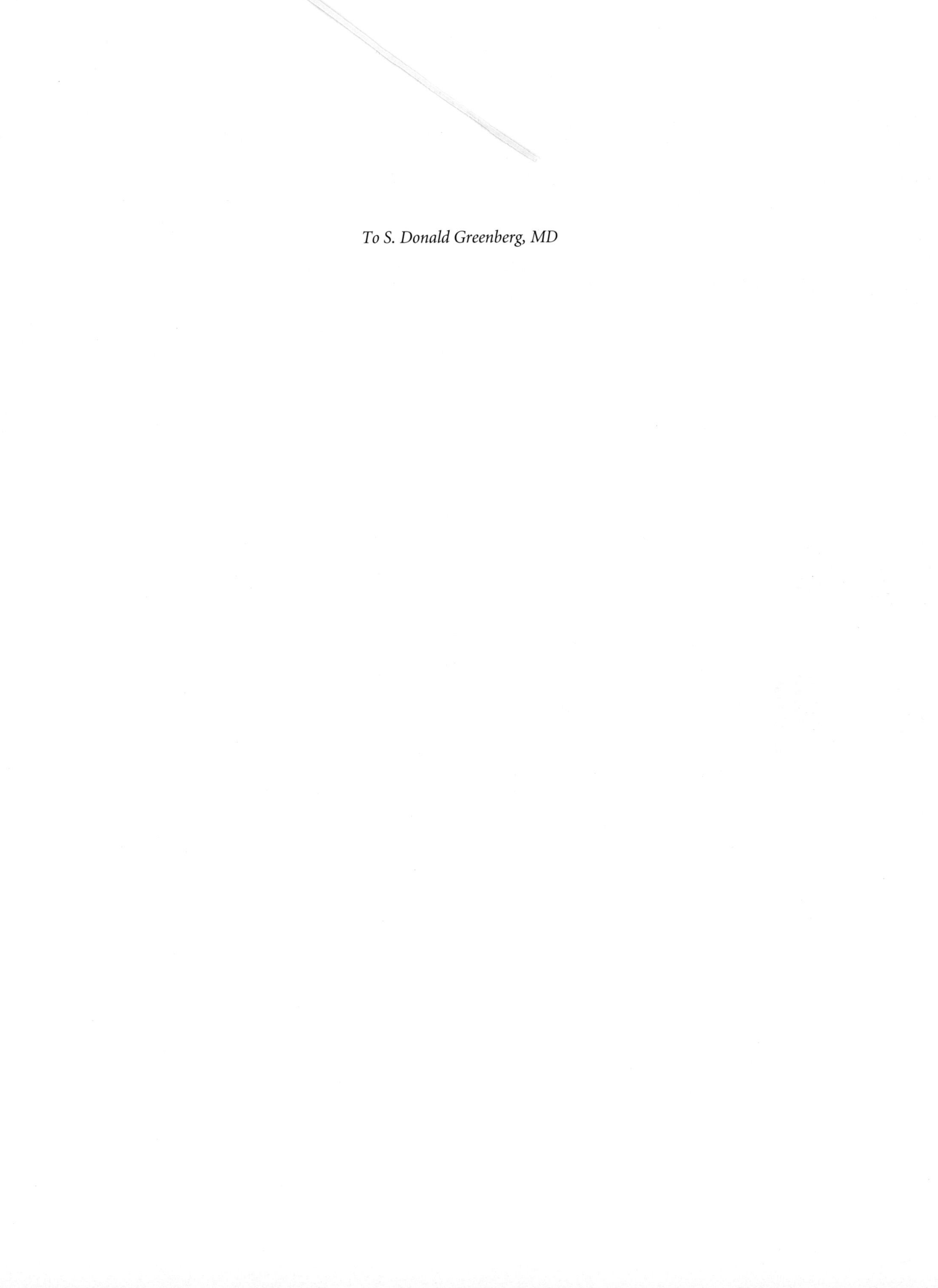

To S. Donald Greenberg, MD

Contributing Authors

Timothy C. Allen, MD, JD
Professor and Chair
Department of Pathology
University of Mississippi Medical Center
Jackson, Mississippi

Richard Attanoos, MD
Consultant Pathologist
Department of Cellular Pathology
University Hospital of Wales
Cardiff, Wales, United Kingdom

Marcelo L. Balancin, MD, PhD(c)
Consulting Pathologist
Department of Surgical Pathology
Diagnostika-Institute Hermes Pardini
São Paulo, Brazil

Roberto Barrios, MD
Professor of Pathology
Department of Pathology and Genomic Medicine
Weill Cornell Medical College of Cornell University
Houston Methodist Hospital
Houston, Texas

Mary Beth Beasley, MD
Professor
Department of Pathology
Icahn School of Medicine at Mount Sinai
New York, New York

Carlos Bedrossian, MD, PhD(Hon)
Professor of Pathology
Rush Medical College
Consulting Pathologist
Norwegian American Hospital
Chicago, Illinois

Debra Beneck, MD
Professor
Department of Pathology
Weill Cornell Medicine
New York, New York

Melanie C. Bois, MD
Assistant Professor
Department of Laboratory Medicine and Pathology
Fellow
Department of Laboratory Medicine and Pathology
Mayo Clinic
Rochester, Minnesota

Alain Borczuk, MD
Professor of Pathology
Department of Pathology
NewYork-Presbyterian Hospital/Weill Cornell Medical Center
New York, New York

Darren Buonocore, MD
Assistant Attending
Department of Pathology
Memorial Sloan Kettering Cancer Center
New York, New York

Yasmeen M. Butt, MD
Assistant Professor
Department of Pathology
University of Texas Southwestern Medical Center
Dallas, Texas

Philip T. Cagle, MD
Professor
Department of Pathology and Genomic Medicine
Houston Methodist Hospital
Houston, Texas

Vera Capelozzi, MD
Associate Professor
Department of Pathology
University of São Paulo School of Medicine
São Paulo, Brazil

Ivan Chebib, MD, FRCPC
Assistant Professor
James Homer Wright Pathology Laboratories
Harvard Medical School
Assistant Pathologist
James Homer Wright Pathology Laboratories
Massachusetts General Hospital
Boston, Massachusetts

Sanja Dacic, MD, PhD
Professor of Pathology
Department of Pathology
University of Pittsburgh
Staff Pathologist
Department of Pathology
University of Pittsburgh Medical Center
Pittsburgh, Pennsylvania

John C. English, MD, FRCPC
Professor
Department of Pathology
Vancouver General Hospital
Vancouver, British Columbia, Canada

Armando E. Fraire, MD
Professor Emeritus
University of Massachusetts Medical School
Worcester, Massachusetts

Allen R. Gibbs, MBBS, FRCPath
Consultant Histopathologist
Department of Cellular Pathology
University Hospital of Wales
Cardiff, Wales, United Kingdom

Krzysztof Glomski, MD, PhD
Resident
Department of Pathology
Massachusetts General Hospital
Boston, Massachusetts

Jason K. Graham, MD
First Deputy Chief Medical Examiner
The New York City Office of Chief Medical Examiner
New York, New York

Jeannette Guarner, MD
Professor
Department of Pathology and Laboratory Medicine
Emory University
Medical Director of Laboratories
Laboratory Department
Emory University Hospital Midtown
Atlanta, Georgia

Ying-Han (Roger) Hsu, MD, FRCPC
Clinical Lecturer
Department of Laboratory Medicine and Pathology
University of Alberta
Staff Pathologist
Department of Laboratory Medicine and Pathology
Royal Alexandra Hospital
Edmonton, Alberta, Canada

Aliya N. Husain, MD
Professor
Department of Pathology
University of Chicago
Chicago, Illinois

Deepali Jain, MD, FIAC
Associate Professor
Department of Pathology
All India Institute of Medical Sciences
New Delhi, India

Keith M. Kerr, FRCPath
Professor
Department of Pathology
Aberdeen University Medical School
Consultant
Department of Pathology
Aberdeen Royal Infirmary
Aberdeen, Scotland, United Kingdom

Stacey A. Kim, MD
Assistant Professor
Department of Pathology and Laboratory Medicine
Cedars-Sinai Medical Center
Los Angeles, California

Brandon T. Larsen, MD, PhD
Assistant Professor
Department of Laboratory Medicine and Pathology
Mayo Clinic School of Medicine
Senior Associate Consultant
Department of Laboratory Medicine and Pathology
Mayo Clinic Arizona
Scottsdale, Arizona

Rodolfo Laucirica, MD
Vice Chair and Professor of Pathology
Department of Pathology and Laboratory Medicine
University of Tennessee Health Science Center
Director of Anatomic Pathology
Methodist Hospital System
Memphis, Tennessee

Charles Leduc, MD, MSc
Assistant Professor
Department of Pathology and Cell Biology
University of Montreal
Thoracic Pathologist
Department of Pathology
University of Montreal Health Center
Montreal, Quebec, Canada

Yen-Wen Lu, MD
Chief Resident
Department of Pathology and Laboratory Medicine
Taipai Veterans General Hospital
Taipai, Taiwan

Maria Cecilia Mengoli, MD
Department of Surgical Pathology
Arcispedale Santa Maria Nuova-Azienda Sanitaria Locale-IRCCS
Reggio Emilia, Italy

Ross A. Miller, MD
Assistant Professor
Pathologist
Department of Pathology and Genomic Medicine
Houston Methodist Hospital
Houston, Texas

Mari Mino-Kenudson, MD
Associate Professor
Department of Pathology
Harvard Medical School
Director, Pulmonary Pathology Service
Department of Pathology
Massachusetts General Hospital
Boston, Massachusetts

Paloma del C. Monroig-Bosque, MD, PhD
Physician Resident PGY2
Department of Pathology and Genomic Medicine
Houston Methodist Hospital
Houston, Texas

Cesar Moran, MD
Tenured Professor of Pathology
Department of Pathology
University of Texas MD Anderson Cancer Center
Houston, Texas

Bruno Murer, MD
Pathologist
Department of Pathology
Regional Hospital
Venezia, Italy

Raghavendra Pillappa, MD
Pulmonary Pathology Fellow
Department of Laboratory Medicine and Pathology
Mayo Clinic
Rochester, Minnesota

Sergio Pina-Oviedo, MD
Assistant Professor
Department of Pathology
University of Arkansas for Medical Sciences
Little Rock, Arkansas

Jennifer Pogoriler, MD, PhD
Assistant Professor
Department of Pathology and Laboratory Medicine
Children's Hospital of Philadelphia
Philadelphia, Pennsylvania

Theodore J. Pysher, MD
Professor (clinical)
Department of Pathology
University of Utah School of Medicine
Salt Lake City, Utah

Kirtee Raparia, MD
Associate Pathologist
Department of Pathology
Kaiser Permanente Santa Clara Medical Center
Santa Clara, California

Natasha Rekhtman, MD, PhD
Associate Attending Pathologist
Department of Pathology
Memorial Sloan Kettering Cancer Center
New York, New York

Robert W. Ricciotti, MD
Acting Assistant Professor
Department of Anatomic Pathology
University of Washington
Attending Pathologist
Department of Anatomic Pathology
University of Washington Medical Center
Seattle, Washington

Anja C. Roden, MD
Associate Professor
Consultant
Department of Laboratory Medicine and Pathology
Mayo Clinic
Rochester, Minnesota

Philippe Romeo, MD
Assistant Professor
Department of Pathology
Université de Montréal
Attending Pathologist
Department of Pathology
Centre Hospitalier de l'Université de Montréal
Montreal, Quebec, Canada

Matthew W. Rosenbaum, MD
Resident
Department of Pathology
Massachusetts General Hospital
Boston, Massachusetts

Sinchita Roy-Chowdhuri, MD, PhD
Assistant Professor
Department of Pathology
University of Texas MD Anderson Cancer Center
Houston, Texas

Anjali Saqi, MD, MBA
Professor
Department of Pathology and Cell Biology
Columbia University Medical Center
New York-Presbyterian
New York, New York

Lynette M. Sholl, MD
Associate Pathologist
Department of Pathology
Brigham and Women's Faulkner Hospital
Boston, Massachusetts

Anna Sienko, MD
Full Clinical Professor
Department of Pathology
College of Medicine
University of Calgary
Pathologist
Calgary Lab Services
Department of Pathology
Peter Lougheed Centre
Calgary, Alberta, Canada

Maxwell L. Smith, MD
Associate Professor
Department of Laboratory Medicine and Pathology
Mayo Clinic School of Medicine
Consultant
Department of Laboratory Medicine and Pathology
Mayo Clinic Arizona
Scottsdale, Arizona

Paul A. VanderLaan, MD, PhD
Assistant Professor
Department of Pathology
Harvard Medical School
Director of Cytopathology
Director of Thoracic Pathology
Department of Pathology
Beth Israel Deaconess Medical Center
Boston, Massachusetts

Sara O. Vargas, MD
Associate Professor
Department of Pathology
Harvard Medical School
Staff Pathologist
Department of Pathology
Boston Children's Hospital
Boston, Massachusetts

Paul Wawryko, MD, FRCPC
Assistant Professor
Department of Pathology
University of Manitoba, Max Rady College of Medicine
Pathologist
Department of Pathology
St. Boniface Hospital
Winnipeg, Manitoba, Canada

Hui-Min Yang, MD
Assistant Clinical Professor
Department of Pathology and Laboratory Medicine
University of British Columbia
Consultant Pathologist
Department of Pathology and Laboratory Medicine
Vancouver General Hospital
Vancouver, British Columbia, Canada

Yi-Chen Yeh, MD
Attending Pathologist
Department of Pathology and Laboratory Medicine
Taipai Veterans General Hospital
Taipai, Taiwan

Fang Zhou, MD
Assistant Professor
Department of Pathology
New York University School of Medicine
New York University Langone Health: Tisch Hospital
New York, New York

Preface to the Third Edition

New technologies at the time the first edition of *Color Atlas and Text of Pulmonary Pathology* was published allowed us to create a unique textbook of digital age conciseness with all figures printed in color. Subsequently, those technologies have become widespread, but the distinctive virtues of the original work have not been duplicated. In the decade since the publication of the second edition of this book, diagnosis in pulmonary pathology has undergone a number of modifications. New entities have been described, older entities redefined, and several major classifications revised: An update of the 2002 American Thoracic Society/European Respiratory Society (ATS/ERS) classification of idiopathic interstitial pneumonias was published in 2013; the Fifth World Symposium on Pulmonary Hypertension was held in Nice, France, in 2013; the fourth edition of the *World Health Organization Classification of Tumours of the Lung, Pleura, Thymus and Heart* was published in 2015. Since the second edition, the introduction of testing for molecular targeted therapies and other advances has forever altered the role of the pathologist in the diagnosis and treatment of pulmonary diseases.

We elected to produce a third edition that is not merely an adjustment of the previous text based on new developments in pulmonary pathology, but one predominantly constructed by new editors and largely written by new contributors. Even the title of the book is modified to reflect this progress: *Pulmonary Pathology: An Atlas and Text, third edition.* While it is a newly composed book, the general format of a user-friendly atlas that is highly illustrated, divided into readily accessible individual entities, and offering brief handy text with bullet points to expedite use is retained. Conciseness and efficiency are the continuing legacy of this book. Its guiding spirit is still the late Dr S. Donald Greenberg.

Philip T. Cagle, MD
September, 2017

Preface to the First Edition

We have attempted to compile a comprehensive atlas covering common, rare, and newly described lung diseases, both neoplastic and nonneoplastic, in one volume. Topics are organized into sections, chapters, parts, and subparts for ready accessibility. Although diseases are designated according to the most current classification schemes, topics are divided into chapters, parts, and subparts based on their histopathologic distinctiveness, a more intuitive approach for the practicing pathologist. Our objective is to provide a format of color figures and handy lists of diagnostic features that provide clear-cut essentials for diagnosis undiluted by other types of information that can be obtained from other sources when necessary. Our goal for the practicing pathologist is to expedite timely and accurate diagnosis when signing out cases. For students, residents, fellows, and specialty board applicants, this same format facilitates rapid, comprehensible study of all topics in lung pathology. The use of gross pathology, cytopathology, and histopathology figures and tables in this book allows a multidimensional approach to pathologic diagnoses. We have attempted to illustrate common nonspecific findings, false-positive features, and potential diagnostic traps that the practicing pathologist may encounter so that these can be distinguished from specific diseases.

This book was conceived as a tribute to our mentor, one of the outstanding pioneers of modern lung pathology in the 1960s, 1970s, and 1980s, Dr. S. Donald Greenberg. He spent most of his career at Baylor College of Medicine in the Texas Medical Center in Houston and worked closely with community and academic physicians throughout Texas. Above all else, Dr. Greenberg was highly respected as an inspiring teacher to students, house staff, and practicing pathologists and clinicians, both in the community and in the university, and he received many teaching awards during his career. Therefore, a practical atlas of lung pathology that would be useful to students, house staff, and practicing pathologists and clinicians, both community based and university based, was felt to be the best tribute to Dr. Greenberg's legacy.

Because of the logistics, it was not possible to include all of Dr. Greenberg's many protégés and students as contributors to this book, so an editorial staff composed of lung pathologists of the Houston-Galveston area plus one of Dr. Greenberg's first protégés, Dr. Carlos Bedrossian, was organized. In addition to the editors, other faculty from the Houston-Galveston area contributed to this book, as did those lung pathologists who came as visiting professors to the Texas Medical Center during the time when the book was in preparation.

Our hope is that this book represents a culmination of Dr. Greenberg's work through those who learned from him.

Philip T. Cagle, MD
February 17, 2004

Acknowledgments

I would like to acknowledge our Editorial Coordinator, Jennifer DiRicco, for her assistance with this book.

Contents

Section 6

Benign and Borderline Lymphoid Proliferations *Kirtee Raparia* 231

Section 7

Focal Lesions *Ross A. Miller* 239

Section 8

Granulomatous Diseases *Yasmeen M. Butt* 251

Section 9

Diffuse Pulmonary Hemorrhage *Lynette M. Sholl* 277

Section 10

Pulmonary Hypertension and Embolic Disease *Alain Borczuk* 295

Section 11

Large Airways *Ross A. Miller* 317

Section 15

Diffuse Interstitial Lung Diseases *Maxwell L. Smith* 375

Section 16

Idiopathic Interstitial Pneumonias *Kirtee Raparia* 411

Section 17

Specific Infectious Agents *Alain Borczuk* 423

Section 23

Section 24

Section 1

Normal Cytology and Histology

▶ Sinchita Roy-Chowdhuri

Bronchus

1

Deepali Jain
Sinchita Roy-Chowdhuri
Paul A. VanderLaan

The conducting system of the respiratory tract is responsible for transporting inspired and expired gas to and from the alveolar spaces where gas exchange occurs. It begins as a single semirigid tube (the trachea), which progressively ramifies with reducing airway diameters. The airways begin from the trachea in the upper neck, which branches into two mainstem bronchi (right and left, one for each lung in the thorax) at approximately the level of the fifth thoracic vertebra. The extrapulmonary portion of the right bronchus is shorter (half the length of the left bronchus), wider, and has a more vertical orientation than the left mainstem bronchus. The mainstem bronchi enter each lung along with a pulmonary artery at the hilum. Airways course with paired pulmonary arteries up to the level of the terminal bronchiole. As the mainstem bronchi progress peripherally, they divide into lobar and segmental branches. Lobar bronchi supply each of the two left lobes and three right lobes. Each of these 5 lobar bronchi branches into segmental bronchi that deliver air to the 19 total lung segments. The pattern of airway branching is asymmetrical and dichotomous as each airway has two branches of different diameter and length. All large proximal airways up to the subsegmental level are called bronchi and are defined histologically as airways containing cartilage and seromucinous glands in their walls. Bronchi progress to small airways of <1 mm diameter called bronchioles, which are thin membranous structures and lack cartilage and seromucinous glands in their walls.

The larger tubular airways include an epithelial layer lining the airway lumen; a submucosal layer containing connective tissue, blood vessels, lymphatics, and seromucinous salivary-type glands; a smooth muscle muscularis layer; and discontinuous cartilaginous rings providing structural integrity to the airways. The bronchial epithelium is composed of pseudostratified ciliated columnar epithelial cells (which comprise the majority of surface epithelial cells), mucin-secreting goblet cells, basal cells, and scattered neuroendocrine (Kulchitsky) cells. Goblet cells are more abundant in the mainstem and lobar bronchi. Neuroendocrine cells are located on the basement membrane, scattered among ciliated cells, and present in higher numbers in smaller bronchi.

The submucosal layer lies beneath the epithelial layer and is formed by mesenchymal stroma containing variable amounts of fibrocollagenous tissue, elastic fibers, and seromucinous glands. The submucosal glands connect to the airway lumen through short and long ducts. These seromucinous salivary-type glands have a serous component with eosinophilic granular cytoplasm containing lysozyme and glycoproteins, as well as a mucinous component with more clear vacuolated cytoplasm containing mucin. The mucus secreted provides protection to the lower respiratory tract as part of the mucociliary escalator system. Bronchus-associated lymphoid tissues are lymphoid aggregates that are present within the submucosal tissue. In the larger airways, the smooth muscle is arranged in two sets of fibers in an opposing spiral orientation. The smooth muscle bundles become less contiguous as the airways progress to the peripheral bronchioles.

The C-shaped discontinuous cartilaginous rings of the mainstem bronchi are connected posteriorly by a smooth muscle and elastic fiber–rich posterior membrane. Progressing more peripherally, the intrapulmonary bronchi have segmented into irregularly circumferential cartilage plates. As the bronchi branch further, the cartilage plates diminish and eventually remain only at the bifurcation point.

HISTOLOGIC FEATURES

- The bronchus consists of a central lumen lined by respiratory epithelium mostly comprising pseudostratified ciliated columnar cells, goblet cells containing mucin, basal cells, and neuroendocrine (Kulchitsky) cells.
- The submucosal layer consists of fibrocollagenous loose connective tissue and elastic fibers with seromucinous glands that secrete mucus into the bronchial lumen.
- Smooth muscle bundles and cartilaginous plates lie beneath the submucosal layer.

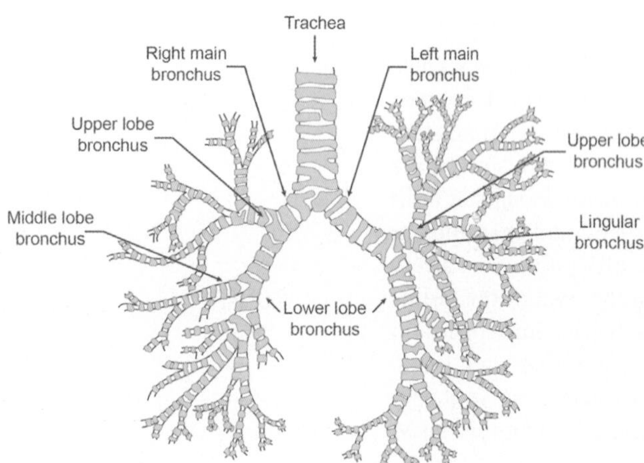

Figure 1.1 Schematic of the tracheobronchial tree showing the left and right mainstem bronchi branching into the lobar bronchi.

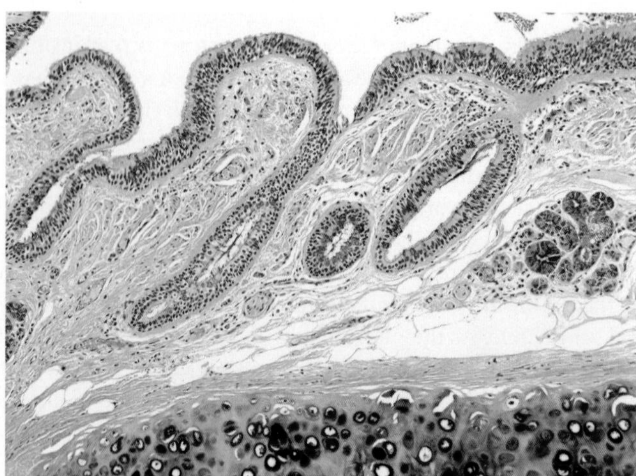

Figure 1.2 Bronchial wall lined by respiratory epithelium and the underlying submucosal stroma containing fibrocollagenous connective tissue, seromucinous glands, smooth muscle, and cartilage.

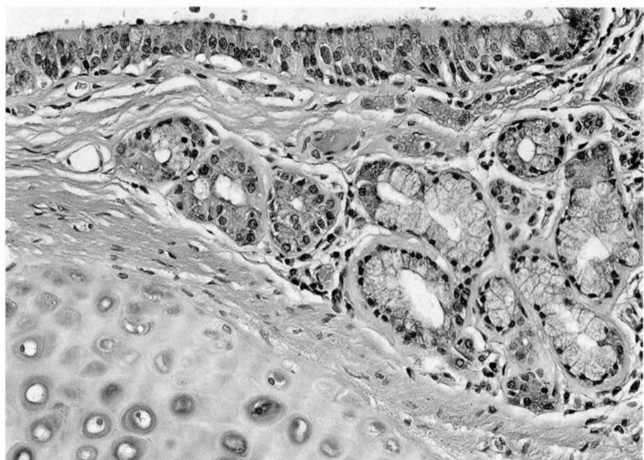

Figure 1.3 Pseudostratified ciliated columnar epithelium with interspersed goblet cells and underlying seromucinous glands and cartilage.

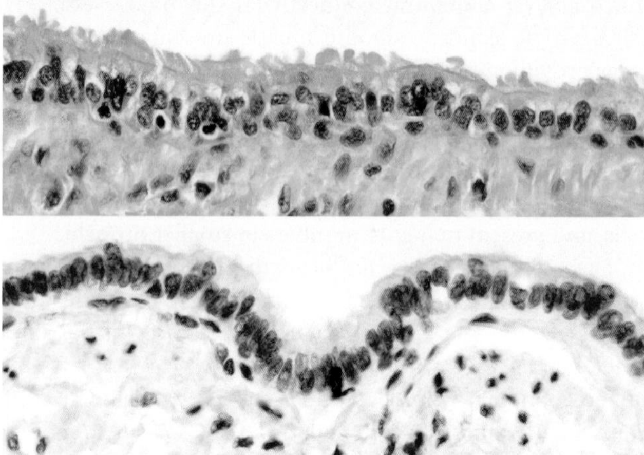

Figure 1.4 Bronchial epithelium with ciliated columnar cells and scattered hyperchromatic neuroendocrine (Kulchitsky) cells located at the basement membrane of the epithelium (**upper panel**); an immunoperoxidase stain for chromogranin highlights the neuroendocrine cells (**lower panel**).

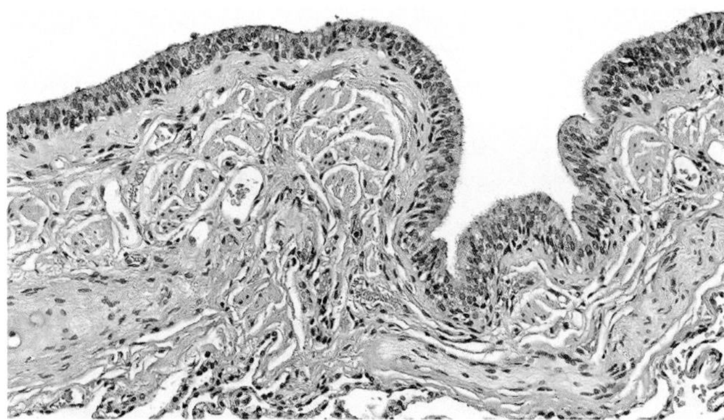

Figure 1.5 Submucosal connective tissue underlying the bronchial epithelium showing smooth muscle and nerve bundles.

2 Bronchioles and Alveolar Ducts

Sinchita Roy-Chowdhuri
Paul A. VanderLaan

Bronchioles are the final conductors of air that branch off from the bronchi. Bronchioles by definition are airways less than 1 mm in diameter that lack cartilage and submucosal glands within their walls. Bronchioles branch into terminal (membranous) bronchioles that are lined completely by ciliated columnar cells and nonciliated cuboidal Club cells. Terminal bronchioles further branch into respiratory bronchioles, which are lined by simple columnar to cuboidal epithelia that conduct air and participate in gas exchange via alveoli in their walls. The lungs contain approximately 30,000 terminal bronchioles, each of which directs air to approximately 10,000 alveoli. Bronchioles are accompanied by pulmonary artery branches of similar caliber.

The functional unit of the lung distal to the terminal bronchiole is called the acinus, which consists of the respiratory bronchiole, alveolar ducts, and grape-like clusters of alveoli. A cluster of 3 to 10 terminal bronchioles, each with its corresponding acinus, is referred to as a lobule, bound together by an interlobular septum. The respiratory bronchiole typically gives rise to two or three generations of respiratory bronchioles, with increasing numbers of alveoli budding from their walls. These bronchioles then form alveolar ducts, tubular spaces bound entirely by alveoli, which terminate in alveolar sacs, the blind ends of the respiratory unit. As the airways of the acinus progressively branch out and diminish in caliber, the cuboidal epithelium transitions to more flattened epithelial cells.

HISTOLOGIC FEATURES

- Terminal (membranous) bronchioles branch off bronchi and are lined by ciliated columnar cells and nonciliated cuboidal Club cells.
- Respiratory bronchioles branch off terminal bronchioles and are lined by simple columnar to cuboidal epithelia and alveoli.
- Respiratory bronchioles form alveolar ducts that are lined entirely by alveoli and terminate in alveolar sacs.
- The acinus is the functional unit distal to the terminal bronchiole and is composed of the respiratory bronchiole, alveolar ducts, and associated alveoli.

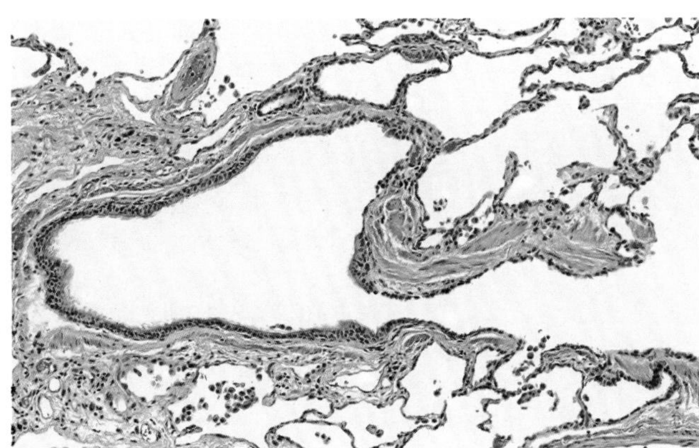

Figure 2.1 Longitudinal section of a terminal (membranous) bronchiole lined by simple ciliated columnar cells.

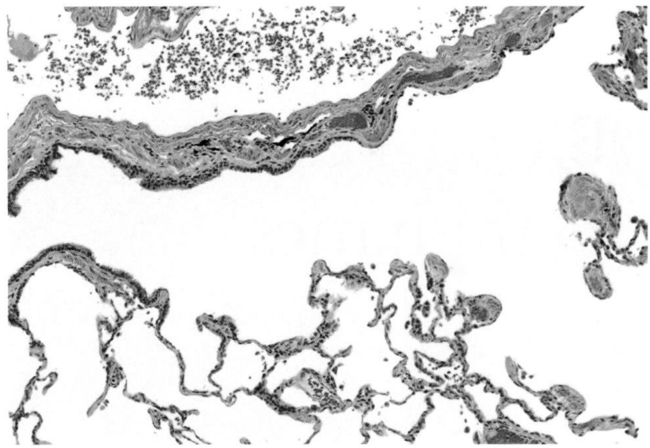

Figure 2.2 Longitudinal section of a terminal (membranous) bronchiole branching into a respiratory bronchiole lined by simple columnar epithelium and with alveoli budding from its wall.

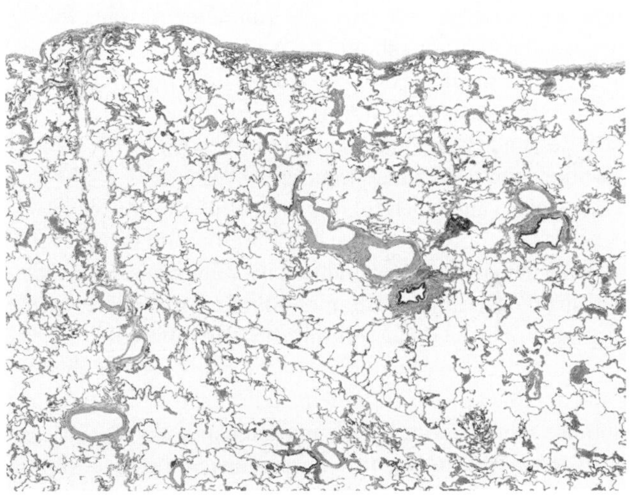

Figure 2.3 Low-magnification view of a lobule containing the terminal bronchiole with an accompanying pulmonary artery, leading into respiratory bronchioles, alveolar ducts, and associated alveoli.

Blood Vessels and Lymphatics

3

▶ Paul A. VanderLaan
▶ Sinchita Roy-Chowdhuri

The lungs have a dual blood supply, comprising the pulmonary circulation (carrying deoxygenated blood from the right ventricle) and the bronchial circulation (carrying oxygenated blood from the left ventricle). The pulmonary circulation delivers blood from the right side of the heart through progressively smaller branches of pulmonary arteries and arterioles to the small capillaries of the alveolar walls where gas exchange occurs. The oxygenated blood is returned to the left atrium via pulmonary venules and veins. The bronchial circulation is part of the high-pressure systemic circulation and provides oxygen and nutrients to the bronchi and lung parenchyma.

Pulmonary arteries and arterioles run along airways (bronchi and bronchioles) and, under normal conditions, should have equivalent cross-sectional luminal diameters at any given level. The inconspicuous capillaries have no muscular wall and run in the alveolar walls. The pulmonary veins normally have thinner muscular walls compared with pulmonary arteries, and often their draining relationship to the interlobular septa and pleura can be identified with serial tissue sections.

Elastic stains can be helpful in highlighting the concentric elastic lamina of pulmonary arteries (the larger of which have both internal and external elastic laminae). Smaller arterioles, bronchial arteries, and pulmonary veins often have only one (internal) elastic lamina. The histologic differentiation of pulmonary arterioles from pulmonary venules can be challenging, but serial tissue sections can help differentiate the two.

The lymphatics are generally inconspicuous vascular channels without muscular vessel walls and are lined by flat endothelial cells. Lymphatic vessels run along the airways, in the interlobular septa, and in the pleura; alveolar walls do not contain lymphatics. The lymphatic distribution can become conspicuous in instances of pulmonary edema, lymphangitic carcinomatosis, or when examining lung parenchyma involved by sarcoid.

HISTOLOGIC FEATURES

- Larger muscular pulmonary arteries have a tunica media layer comprising circularly oriented smooth muscle cells bounded by internal and external elastic laminae.
- Smaller pulmonary artery branches and pulmonary arterioles have a thinner tunica media compared with bronchial arteries because of differences in pressure between the two circulations.
- Pulmonary veins have relatively thin muscular walls and have a single (internal) elastic lamina; however, morphologic arterialization can occur in circumstances of chronic pulmonary venous hypertension.
- Lymphatic vessels are indistinct, but the channels can be found running along bronchovascular bundles, in the interlobular septa, and in the pleura.

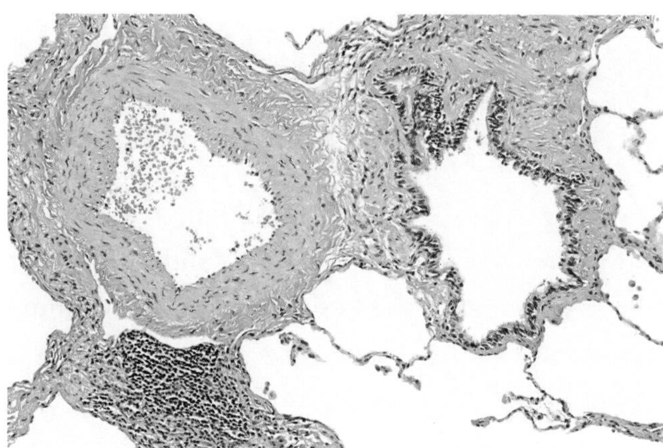

Figure 3.1 Cross section of a pulmonary bronchovascular bundle containing a small muscular pulmonary artery (**left**) and the paired terminal (membranous) bronchiole (**right**) of roughly equivalent diameter.

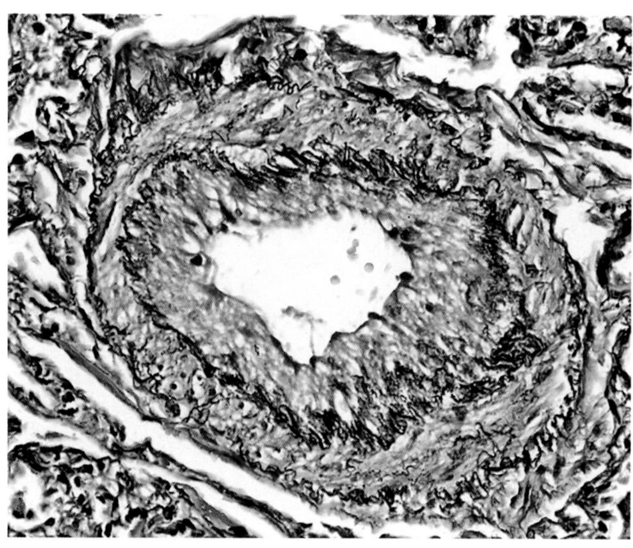

Figure 3.2 Elastic stain highlighting the concentric internal and external elastic laminae of this small muscular pulmonary artery branch. Note the mild intimal hypertrophy present in this vessel.

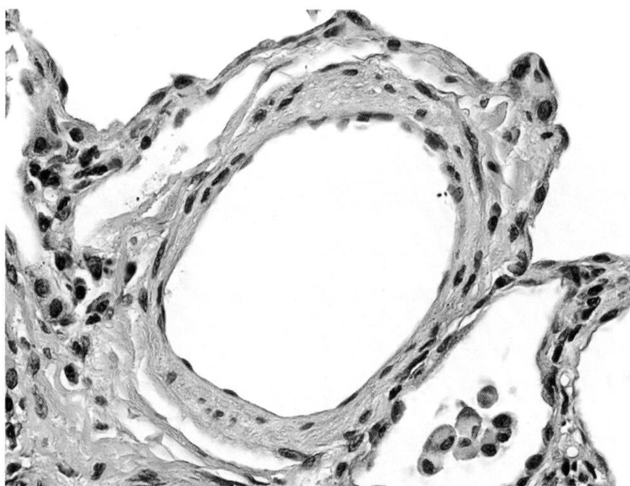

Figure 3.3 Cross section of a small, thin-walled pulmonary vein.

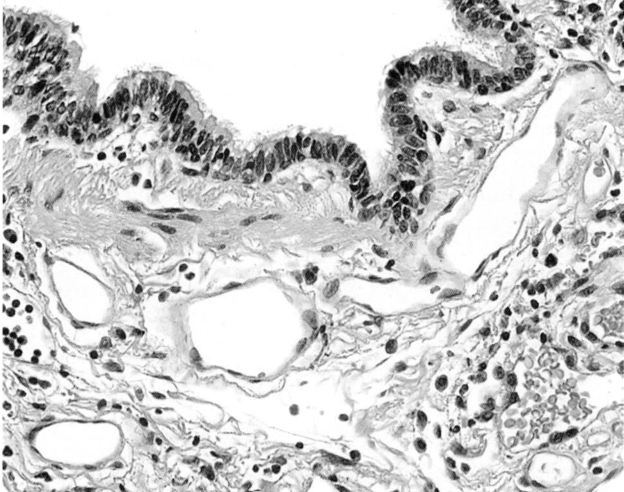

Figure 3.4 Lymphatic vessels lined by inconspicuous thin endothelial cells, running along an adjacent bronchus.

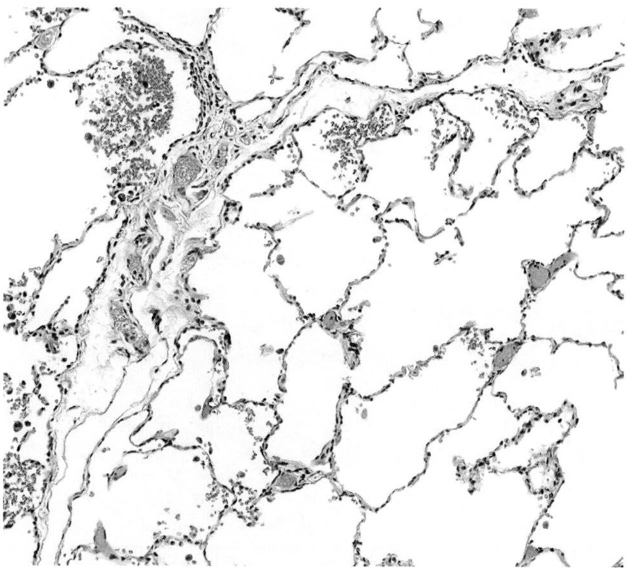

Figure 3.5 Lymphatic vessel present in an interlobular septum.

Alveoli

4

Deepali Jain
Paul A. VanderLaan
Sinchita Roy-Chowdhuri

Alveoli are part of the terminal respiratory unit that consists of alveolar ducts and accompanying sac-like alveoli emanating from the respiratory bronchioles. Although each generation of airway is shorter and narrower than its precursor, the summed-up cross-sectional surface area beyond the segmental bronchi is significantly high because of numerous tiny alveoli that allow for gas exchange. In addition, the presence of Lambert's canals and pores of Kohn allow for collateral ventilation. Lambert's canals are tubular connections that connect the terminal and respiratory bronchioles with adjacent alveoli and serve as accessory air channels of the distant alveoli by bypassing the main conductive airways. The pores of Kohn, on the other hand, are small holes found in the alveolar walls.

The cuboidal epithelium of the respiratory bronchiole abruptly transitions to the alveolar epithelium, which extends throughout the alveoli. The alveolar lining epithelium consists of flattened type I pneumocytes, comprising greater than 90% of the alveolar surface lumen, and cuboidal alveolar type II pneumocytes, which produce surfactant, act as a progenitor for type I pneumocytes, and are involved in alveolar repair (Table 4.1).

Table 4.1. **Comparison of Type I and Type II Pneumocytes**

Features	Type I	Type II
Morphology	Thin flat cells	Cuboidal cells
Number and size	Each cell can line more than one alveolus due to attenuated cytoplasm, no more than 0.2 μm in thickness	Greater in number than type I cells although covers less alveolar surface area
Surface area covered	Approximately 90%–95% of the alveolar surface area of the peripheral lung	Less than 10% of the alveolar surface
Ultrastructure	Few cytoplasmic organelles	Rich in mitochondria, endoplasmic reticulum, Golgi apparatus, and lamellar structures of surfactant
Location	Attenuated cytoplasm provides complete thin covering	Occupy corners of alveoli
Function	Facilitate rapid gas exchange and increased efficiency of air–blood barrier	Source of surfactant and acts as a progenitor for type I cells
Cell injury response	Most vulnerable to damage, incapable of division	Cells can divide, respond to chronic injury, and may serve as a progenitor for type I cells

The wall of each alveolus is typically very thin to allow for efficient gas exchange. The alveolar wall is composed of pneumocytes and endothelial cells of the alveolar capillaries where gas exchange occurs between the inhaled air and the blood in the capillaries. The basement membranes of the pneumocytes and endothelial cells are typically fused. The alveolar interstitium is the connective tissue framework, which is composed of collagen and elastin fibers, fibroblasts, myofibroblasts, pericytes, histiocytes, dendritic cells, Langerhans cells, mast cells, nerves, and nerve terminals. The alveolar epithelium, interstitium, and capillary endothelium make the air–blood barrier. The elastic fibers are interconnected and form an integrated network that has an immense capacity of stretch and recoil, thus helping in uniform expansion and contraction of the lung during respiration and preventing bronchiolar and alveolar collapse during exhalation.

HISTOLOGIC FEATURES

- The alveolar wall is very thin to allow for gas exchange and is composed of pneumocytes (type I and type II) and endothelial cells of the alveolar capillaries.
- Type I pneumocytes are inconspicuous flat squamous epithelial cells that cover greater than 90% of the alveolar surface.
- Type II pneumocytes are cuboidal cells that secrete surfactant, give rise to type I pneumocytes, and can show reactive hyperplasia in response to alveolar damage.

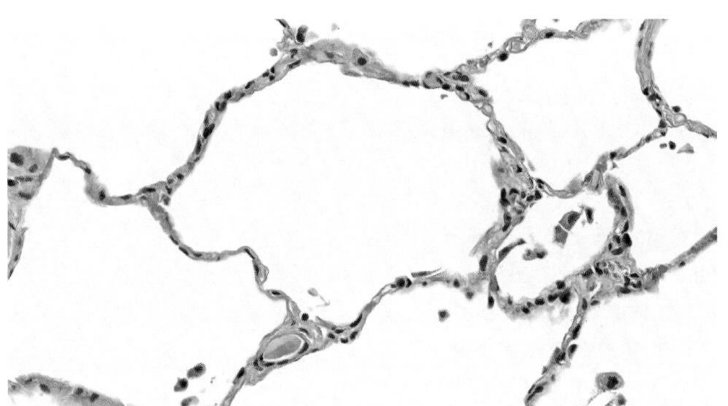

Figure 4.1 The thin delicate alveolar walls are rich in blood-filled capillaries that are lined by endothelial cells. The open alveolar spaces contain occasional pulmonary macrophages, characterized by moderate amounts of variably foamy, vacuolated cytoplasm.

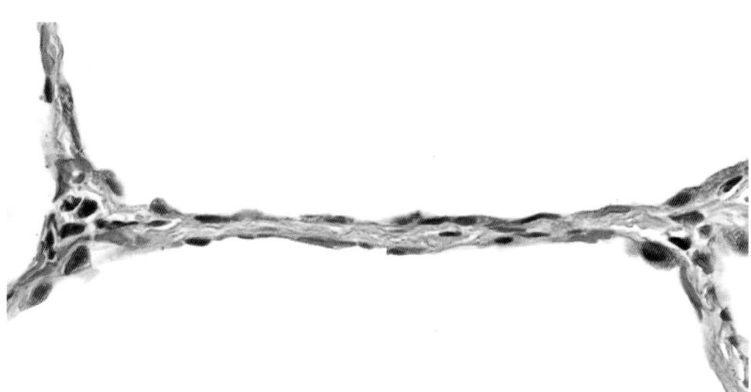

Figure 4.2 High-power magnification of the alveolar wall showing flattened type I pneumocytes and occasional, more prominent, cuboidal type II pneumocytes, found in the corners of the alveolar walls.

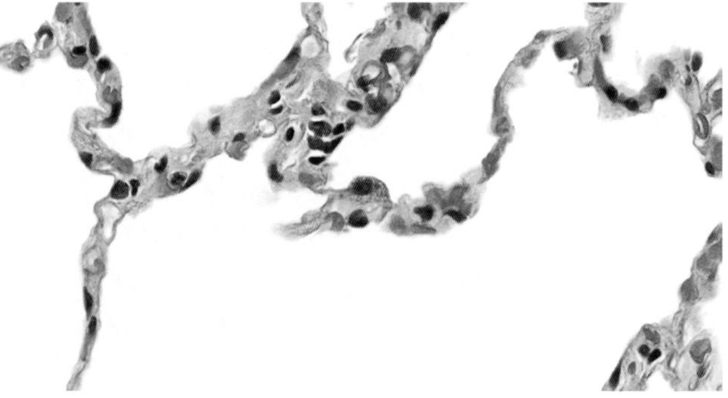

Figure 4.3 Scattered cuboidal type II pneumocytes seen along the alveolar wall together with capillaries and interstitial connective tissue cells.

Pleura

5

Paul A. VanderLaan
Anjali Saqi
Sinchita Roy-Chowdhuri

The thin serous membrane lining the lungs and thoracic cavity is termed the pleura, which is anatomically divided into the visceral pleura (covering the surface of the lung parenchyma including the interlobular fissures) and the parietal pleura (covering the inner surface of the thoracic cage, mediastinum, and diaphragm). Usually the visceral and parietal pleurae are directly opposed with only a thin layer of clear colorless fluid between them, serving as a lubricating layer, as the surfaces move against each other during respiration. Under pathologic conditions, fluid and cellular elements may accumulate in this pleural space, representing a pleural effusion.

The pleural surface is lined by mesothelial cells, which are present as a single flat monolayer of inconspicuous cells under normal conditions. Apparent on ultrastructural examination, mesothelial cells are characterized by long surface microvilli (up to 0.1 μm in length), which account for the spaces (the so-called windows) between adjacent mesothelial cells observed on light microscopy. The connective tissue underlying the visceral pleural surface is composed of collagen and elastic laminae (the fibers of the latter can be highlighted by an elastic stain), along with lymphatics and blood vessels. The blood supply of the visceral pleura arises from the bronchial arteries, whereas the parietal pleura is supplied by branches of the intercostal and internal mammary arteries. The visceral pleura contains branches of the vagus nerve and the sympathetic trunk but does not contain pain nerve fibers. Therefore, pleuritic chest pain always originates from the parietal pleura.

HISTOLOGIC FEATURES

- The pleural membranes are composed of a single monolayer of inconspicuous flat mesothelial cells overlying a connective tissue layer that is composed of collagen and elastic fibers.
- Mesothelial cells under normal conditions are flat to polygonal cells with low to moderate amounts of cytoplasm, round to oval nuclei, and small nucleoli.
- Ultrastructurally, mesothelial cells have long surface microvilli covered by a film of hyaluronic acid–rich glycoprotein.
- The visceral and parietal pleurae contain lymphatics and blood vessels; however, pain nerve fibers are present only in the parietal pleura.

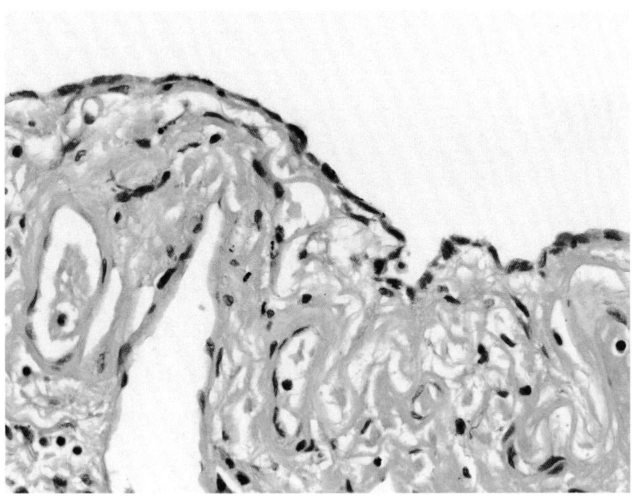

Figure 5.1 Section of the visceral pleura highlighting the flat surface mesothelial cells and an underlying connective tissue with wavy elastic fibers, small blood vessels, and lymphatics.

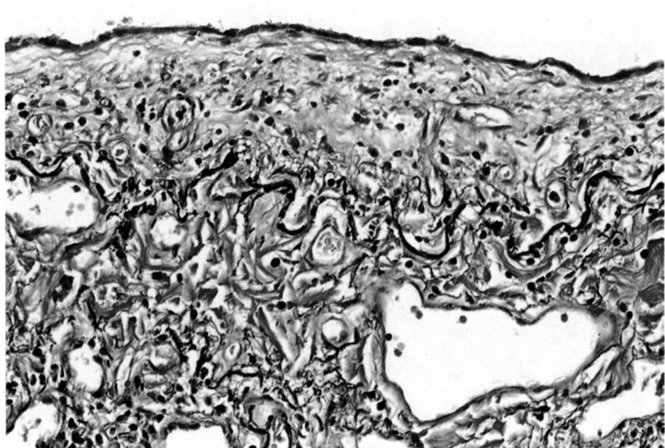

Figure 5.2 Elastic tissue stain highlighting the wavy elastic lamina *(black)* under the mesothelial-lined surface.

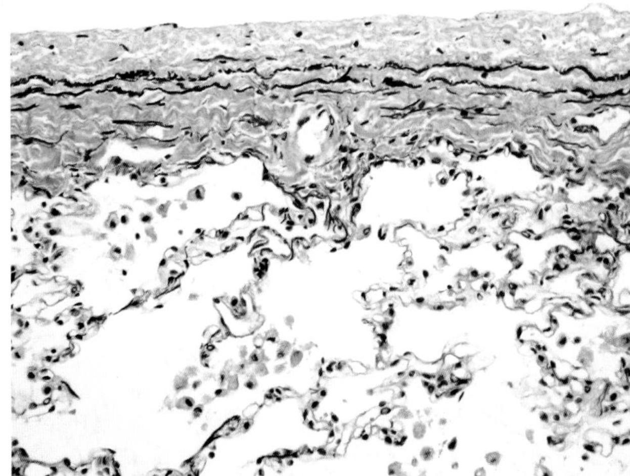

Figure 5.3 Elastic stain demonstrating the more intact superficial elastic layer with duplication of the underlying less-conspicuous and interrupted deep elastic layers that extend into the adjacent alveolar septal walls.

Normal Cytology of the Lung and Pleura

6

- Anjali Saqi
- Hui-Min Yang
- Deepali Jain
- Paul A. VanderLaan
- Sinchita Roy-Chowdhuri

Cytology specimens from the respiratory tract are typically divided into two groups: fine needle aspiration (FNA) and exfoliative specimens.

Generally, an FNA represents sampling of a targeted lesion in the thorax and mediastinum. FNA samples of the lung and mediastinum are usually obtained under image guidance using a variety of sampling modalities. These include transthoracic FNAs, most commonly using computerized tomography guidance, and bronchoscopic FNAs, typically using radial or curvilinear endobronchial ultrasound (EBUS) guidance or electromagnetic navigation. The modality used depends on various factors, including location of the lesion (e.g., curvilinear EBUS-FNAs can access central but not peripheral lesions), expertise of the proceduralist, and the infrastructure available at institution, among others. The cells seen on cytology are reflective of the type of procedure. In EBUS-FNA procedures, because the needle traverses the bronchus to reach the targeted lesion, incidentally sampled ciliated columnar cells, goblet cells, and cartilage may be present. In contrast, a transthoracic FNA, especially when sampling a pleural-based lesion, may show incidental mesothelial cells in sheets. FNA specimens may also have alveolar macrophages, reactive pneumocytes, and inflammatory cells.

Exfoliative specimens include sputum, bronchial washing (aspiration of small aliquots of saline injections into the more proximal airways), bronchial brushing (sampling of the tracheobronchial tree), bronchoalveolar lavage (BAL) (aspiration of larger amounts of saline injected into the distal airways and alveolar spaces), and pleural effusions. Adequacy of a sputum sample is determined by the presence of pulmonary alveolar macrophages (evidence of lower respiratory tract sampling), and a sample is deemed unsatisfactory when it demonstrates only squamous cells, indicative of oropharyngeal or upper respiratory tract sampling only. Ciliated columnar cells and goblet cells are often seen in bronchial brushing specimens, whereas the adequacy of BAL specimens is based on the presence of alveolar macrophages. Benign pleural effusions typically contain mesothelial cells, most often singly dispersed along with histiocytes and lymphocytes. In reactive conditions, the mesothelial cells that shed into the effusion may demonstrate cytologic atypia within cell clusters that can mimic a neoplastic process.

CYTOLOGIC FEATURES

- Ciliated columnar bronchial epithelial cells are characterized by fine hair-like projections anchored on the terminal bar on the apical surface of the cells. The base of these cells terminates in slender tails rooted on the basement membrane. Sometimes, the cilia may be lost, e.g., secondary to bronchial irritation. The presence of cilia nearly always indicates a benign process, a rare exception being ciliated pulmonary muconodular papillary tumor. Multinucleation of bronchial cells can be seen as a reactive/reparative change.

- Goblet cells are nonciliated cells with basally located nuclei and abundant cytoplasmic mucin. Normally, these are fewer in number compared to the ciliated columnar cells and the number of cells decreases progressively from proximal to distal airways.
- Reserve cells, also known as basal cells, often occur as tightly cohesive clusters in cytology preparations (see Chapter 8). They have small round uniform cells, scant cytoplasm, hyperchromatic nuclei, and high nuclear to cytoplasmic ratios. These may mimic small-cell carcinoma; however, they lack necrosis and mitoses and are more cohesive. Sprinkling of occasional ciliated columnar cells among reserve cell clusters may serve as a clue to their origin.
- Type II pneumocytes are round cells with granular/foamy/finely vacuolated cytoplasm. Reactive type II pneumocytes may have conspicuous nucleoli.
- Alveolar macrophages may be mononucleated or multinucleated with round/oval to reniform nuclei and foamy to finely granular cytoplasm.
- Siderophages are hemosiderin-laden macrophages. The refractile pigment appears golden brown on hematoxylin and eosin and Papanicolaou stains but is basophilic on Diff-Quik stain.
- Carbon histiocytes ("dust cells") are macrophages containing fine darkly pigmented carbon particles that accumulate secondary to various sources, including smoking and air pollution.
- Lipophages are lipid-containing macrophages. Exogenous lipoid pneumonia has mostly larger cytoplasmic vacuoles, whereas endogenous lipoid pneumonia has smaller vacuoles.
- Ciliocytophthoria represents detached cilia from ciliated bronchial cells, often secondary to injury, and can also be seen in cysts.
- Creola bodies are three-dimensional cohesive clusters of ciliated columnar cells with smooth or knobby borders and cilia on the surface (see Chapter 8).
- In pulmonary cytology specimens, mesothelial cells may be incidentally aspirated, especially when sampling pleural-based lesions. These generally occur as flat sheets and can mimic low-grade adenocarcinoma (lepidic pattern). Generally, the presence of "windows" between cells and the absence of nuclear atypia are clues to their mesothelial origin.
- Benign-appearing squamous cells in respiratory specimens often represent oral or upper airway contaminant. A predominance of mature superficial cells and occasional intermediate cells with admixed bacteria and/or yeast forms is frequently seen.

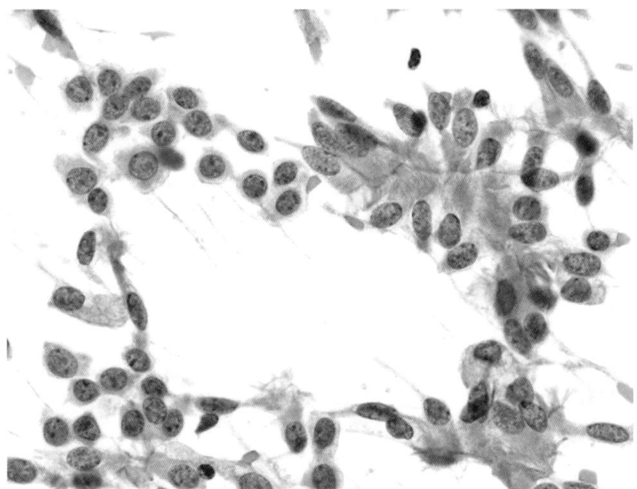

Figure 6.1 Flask-shaped ciliated columnar bronchial epithelial cells (Papanicolaou stain) with prominent apical cilia and terminal bars, basally located nuclei, and evenly distributed finely granular chromatin.

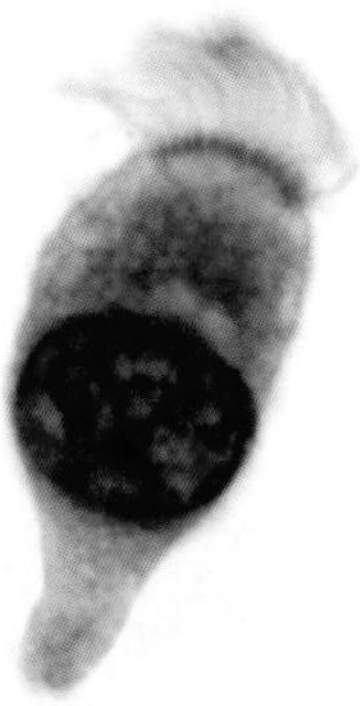

Figure 6.2 Higher magnification of a bronchial cell (Papanicolaou stain) demonstrating the terminal bar and apical cilia.

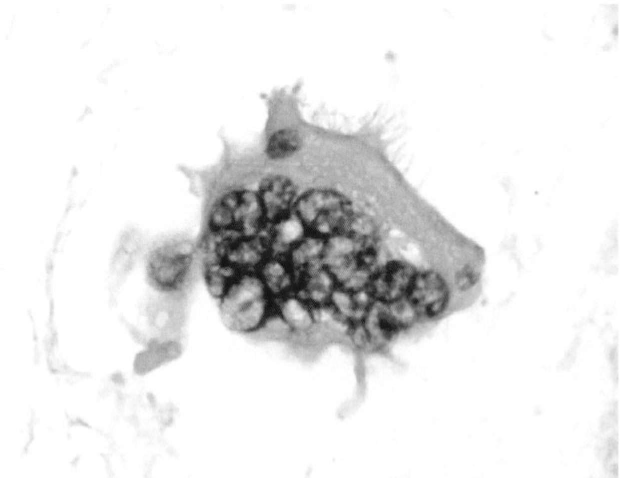

Figure 6.3 Reactive giant (bronchial) cell (hematoxylin and eosin stain) with multinucleation, terminal bar, and cilia.

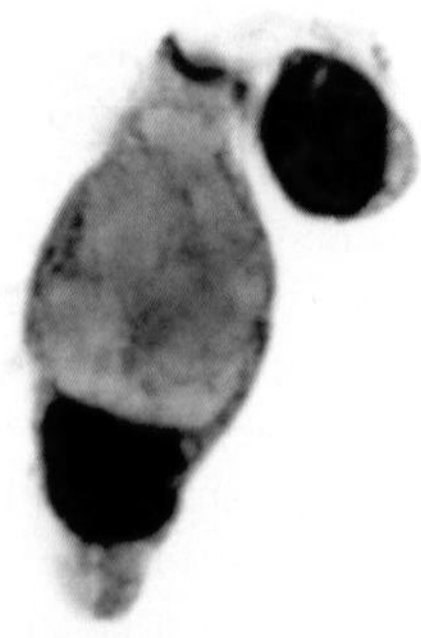

Figure 6.4 Goblet cell (Papanicolaou stain) showing basally located nucleus and prominent apical mucin.

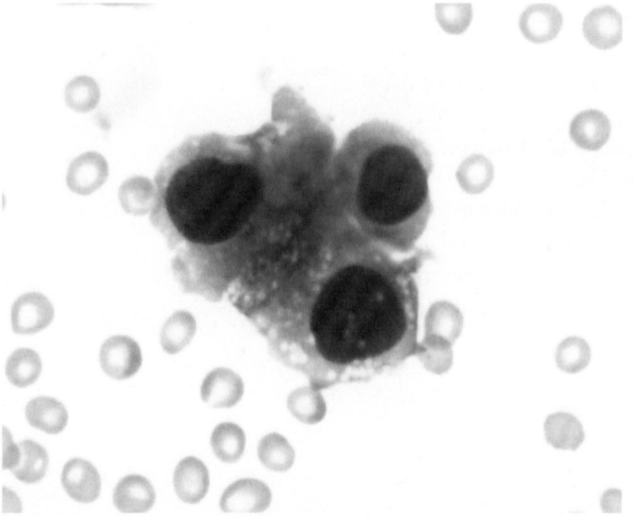

Figure 6.5 Type II pneumocytes (Diff-Quik stain) seen in flat sheets, with round to oval nuclei, and moderate amounts of granular/finely vacuolated cytoplasm.

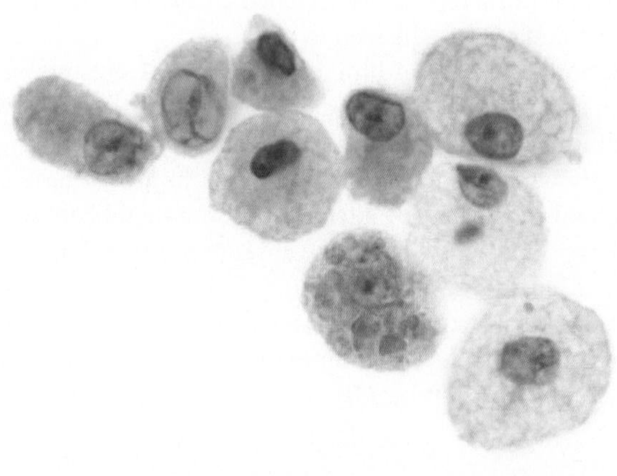

Figure 6.6 Pulmonary macrophages (Papanicolaou stain) demonstrating round to oval nuclei and abundant foamy cytoplasm. Note a siderophage with coarse and variably sized clumps of refractile golden-brown hemosiderin pigment within the cytoplasm.

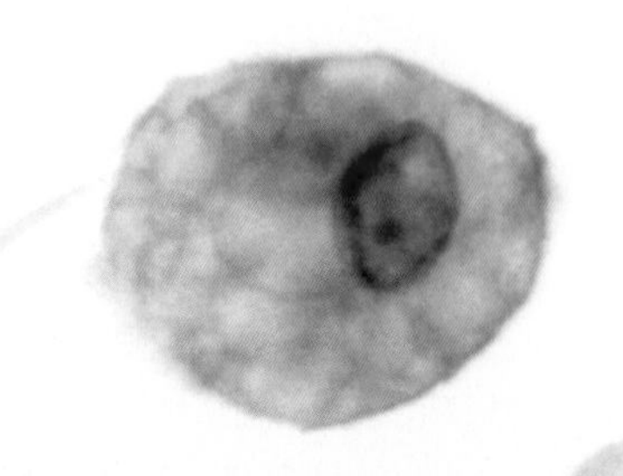

Figure 6.7 Lipophage (Papanicolaou stain) with multiple enlarged optically clear cytoplasmic vacuoles.

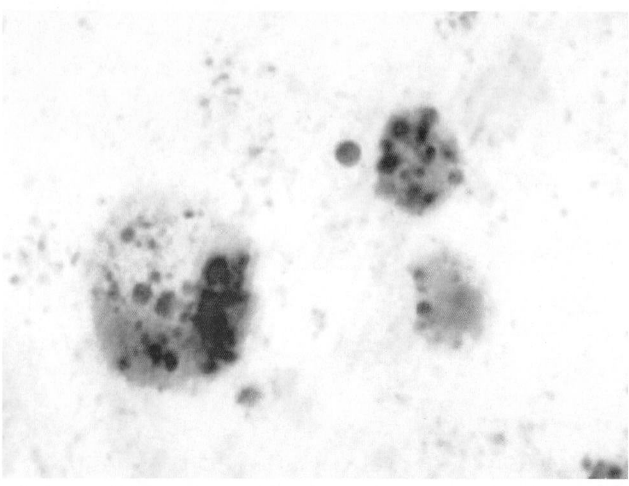

Figure 6.8 Oil red O stain highlights the lipid contained within the cytoplasmic vacuoles of lipophages.

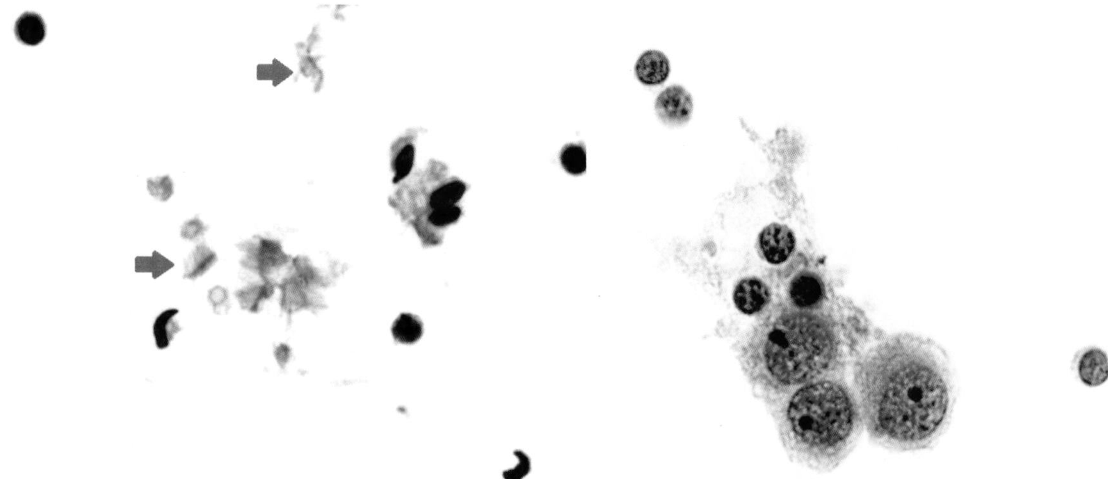

Figure 6.9 Ciliocytophthoria, seen as tufts of detached cilia *(arrows)*.

Figure 6.10 Mesothelial cells (Papanicolaou stain) seen in an exfoliative cytology specimen with round to oval nuclei, two-toned cytoplasm, and "windows" between the cells. Note the lymphocytes in the background.

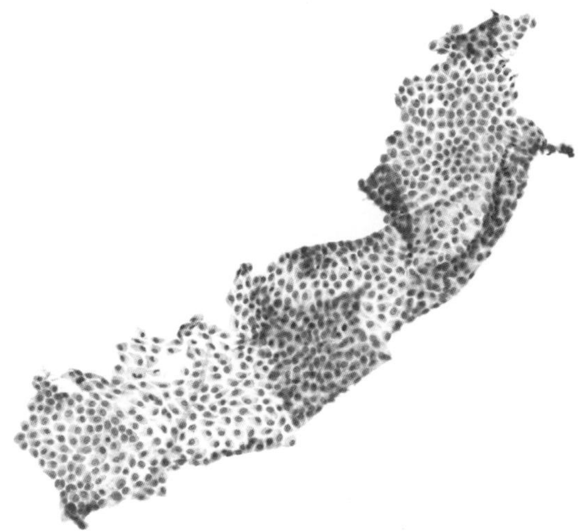

Figure 6.11 Sheets of mesothelial cells (Papanicolaou stain) seen in transthoracic fine needle aspiration with uniform polygonal cells with round to oval nuclei and spaces or "windows" between the cells.

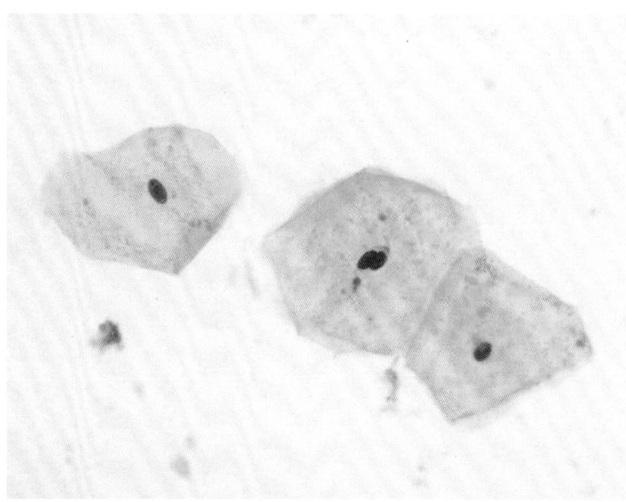

Figure 6.12 Superficial squamous cells (Papanicolaou stain) with abundant pink and cyanophilic cytoplasm, frequently seen as an oral contaminant in exfoliative cytology specimens.

Section 2

Artifacts and Age-Related Changes

Sinchita Roy-Chowdhuri

7 Procedural and Laboratory Artifacts

Sinchita Roy-Chowdhuri
Anjali Saqi
Paul A. VanderLaan

Numerous artifacts may arise during specimen collection and from subsequent tissue handling that should not be misinterpreted for specific pathologic changes. Some commonly encountered artifactual changes seen in lung biopsies and cytology specimens are listed here.

HISTOLOGIC AND CYTOLOGIC FEATURES

- Crush artifact in endobronchial or transbronchial biopsy and wedge biopsy specimens occurs during the procedure when the jaws of the forceps clamp down on tissue, when trying to remove the tissue from the forceps after the procedure, or when cutting into unfixed lung tissue (e.g., during frozen section). Crush artifact can include (1) compression of alveolar parenchyma causing atelectasis artifact; (2) compression of alveolar parenchyma creating artificial spaces between alveoli giving the impression of lipid vacuoles; (3) compression of peribronchial lymphoid tissue mimicking small-cell carcinoma; and (4) compression of airway and airway glands that may be confused as interstitial fibrosis or cellular infiltrates.
- Bleeding caused by the procedure may be misinterpreted as intra-alveolar hemorrhage; true pulmonary hemorrhage should be accompanied by hemosiderin deposition (if older than 2 to 3 days).
- Artifactual lymphatic dilatation due to clamping of the tissue during the procedure can lead to changes within the tissue seen with pulmonary edema.
- Endobronchial or transbronchial biopsy procedures may result in mechanical denudation of the bronchial epithelial cells leading to loss of cilia and should not be mistaken for malignancy.
- Artifactual hyperinflation of specimens can give an impression of emphysema.
- Foreign objects introduced during the procedure or during processing (including starch or talc from surgical gloves, sutures, fibers from cotton gauze pads, dust particles, and pollen) may be seen on special stains and appear birefringent on polarized light and should not be mistaken for organisms or foreign material present within the lung.
- Fixation artifacts: biopsy and cytology samples that are not fixed immediately may have air-drying artifact, altering cytomorphology and causing difficulty in interpretation.
- Insufficiently dehydrated tissue that is infiltrated with paraffin wax causes tearing and fragmentation artifacts in tissue sections when preparing slides.
- Presence of formalin–heme pigment is seen as a fine black precipitate on slides, frequently adjacent to tissue or within vessels. Formalin–heme pigment is formed when the formalin buffer is exhausted, promoting the complex of heme and unbuffered formalin in an acidic pH; this formalin–heme pigment is birefringent when viewed under polarized light and should not be confused for silicate or crystalline material.

- Drying up of sections between the last xylene step and coverslipping can result in entrapment of minute bubbles over the nuclei, leading to cornflake artifact with the nuclei lacking visible details.
- Mounting medium, when too dilute, can pull in air under the coverslip while drying, leading to air bubbles under the coverslip.

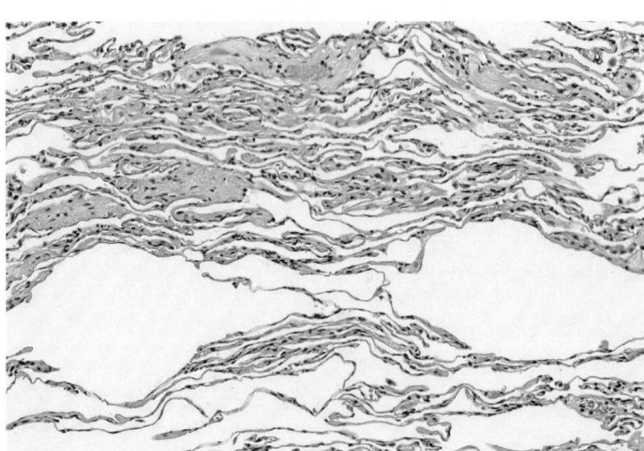

Figure 7.1 Transbronchial biopsy showing compression of alveolar parenchyma causing a false impression of increased interstitial cellularity and atelectasis artifact.

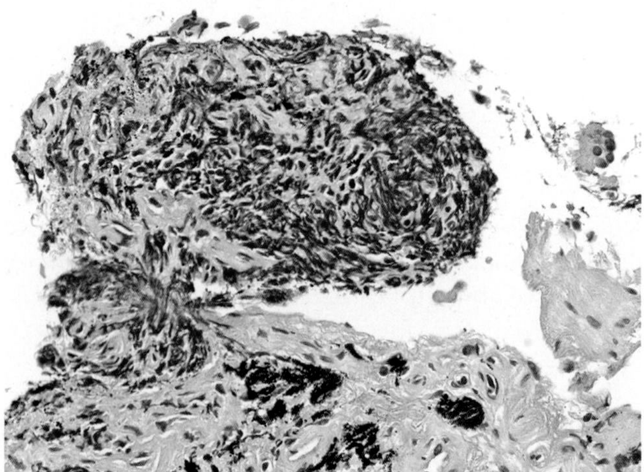

Figure 7.2 Transbronchial biopsy with crushed lymphoid tissue that can be confused for small-cell carcinoma.

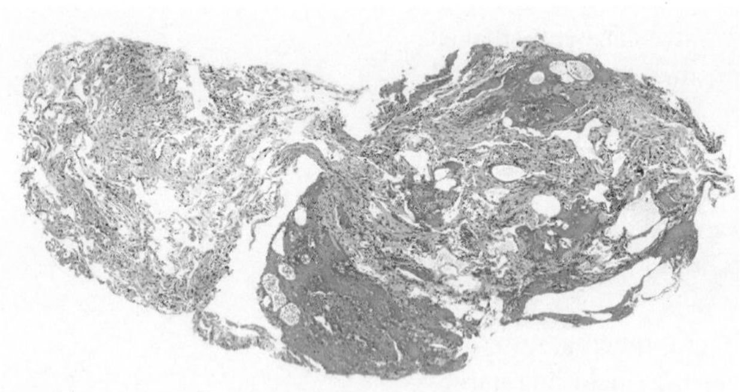

Figure 7.3 Low-power view of a transbronchial biopsy showing intra-alveolar hemorrhage resulting from the procedure. Note areas of crush artifact and artifactual "holes" within the alveolar parenchyma.

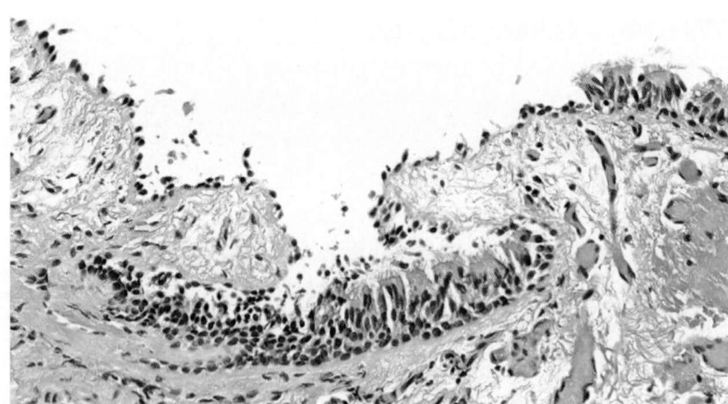

Figure 7.4 Denuded bronchial epithelium with few basal cells still clinging to the basement membrane. The clusters of detached bronchial epithelial cells may be mistaken for malignant cells, but the presence of terminal bars and cilia are important clues to their benign nature.

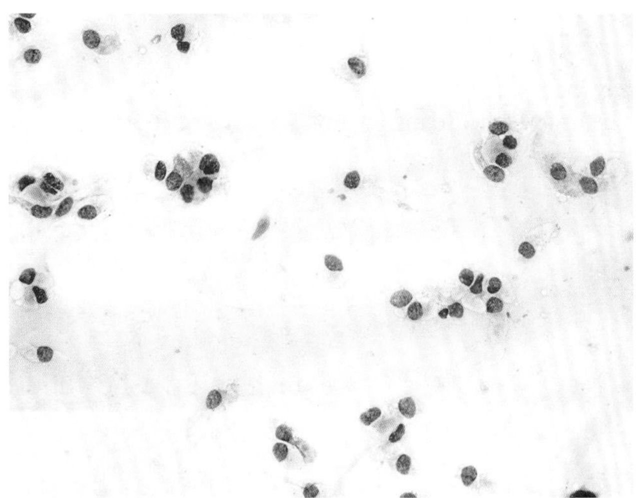

Figure 7.5 Cytology specimen with air-drying artifact showing bronchial epithelial cells with overall enlargement, pale-stained nuclei with loss of chromatin details, and obscuration of the terminal bars and cilia (Papanicolaou stain).

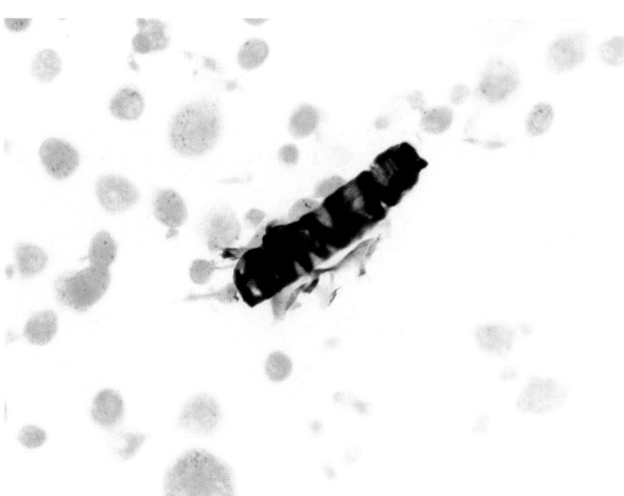

Figure 7.6 Gomori methenamine silver stain, a special stain, highlights a cotton fiber that can be misinterpreted as a fungal organism.

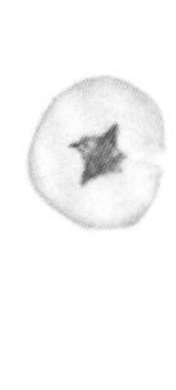

Figure 7.7 Starch granule from surgical gloves showing characteristic central cross-like dimple.

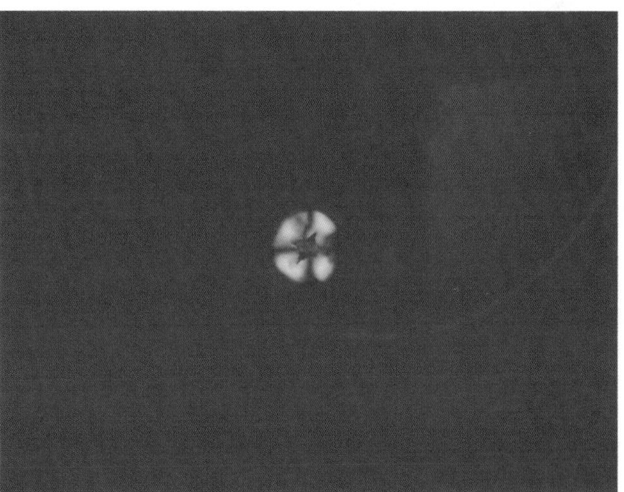

Figure 7.8 The Maltese cross configuration of a starch granule as seen under plane polarized light.

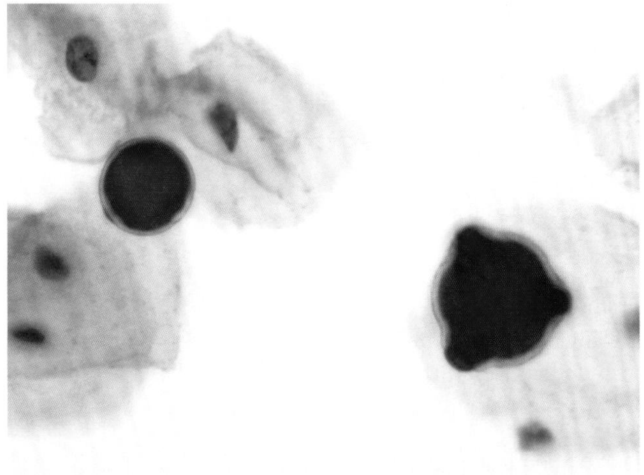

Figure 7.9 Pollen can have variable morphology with refractile walls and can show a smooth round surface or a surface with distinct protrusions (Papanicolaou stain).

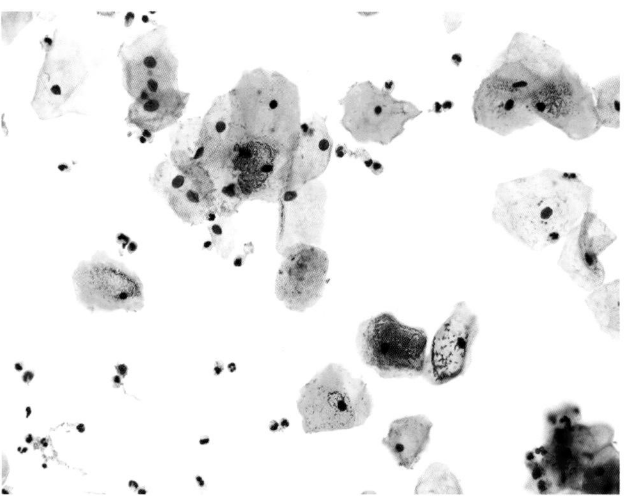

Figure 7.10 Cornflake artifact seen as minute entrapped bubbles causing obscuring of cellular details (Papanicolaou stain).

Reactive Changes, Nonspecific Findings, and Age-Related Changes

8

Sinchita Roy-Chowdhuri
Anjali Saqi
Deepali Jain
Paul A. VanderLaan

The respiratory tract responds to injury in a variety of ways, including metaplasia, hyperplasia, inflammation, degeneration, and repair. Recognizing these reactive changes is important, as some of these can be misinterpreted as neoplastic in nature. Reactive and reparative changes can occur in response to a variety of etiologies, including infection; an exposure to toxic agents, including chemoradiation or inhalation of noxious chemicals; or may be associated with chronic pulmonary conditions, such as asthma and chronic obstructive pulmonary disorder. Certain changes may point to specific infectious agents, such as bacterial, viral, fungal, mycobacterial, or parasitic infections (see Section 17: Specific Infectious Agents). Other changes may be nonspecific and need to be considered in context of the clinical and radiologic findings to exclude a malignant process.

Reactive changes of bronchial epithelial cells can include a spectrum of atypia encompassing nuclear enlargement, anisonucleosis, prominent nucleoli, and mitoses, all features that may suggest malignancy. The lack of overt malignant features and the presence of fine uniformly distributed chromatin and smooth nuclear membranes, together with the presence of cilia and/or terminal bars, can often help distinguish reactive bronchial cells from their malignant counterparts. Multinucleated bronchial epithelial giant cells may also be seen in reactive processes that demonstrate oval uniform nuclei, thin nuclear membranes, and small nucleoli.

In cytology specimens, reactive pneumocytes and reserve cell hyperplasia may pose some cytologic challenges. Reactive pneumocytes may form three-dimensional or papillary clusters with cytoplasmic vacuoles that can be mistaken for a well-differentiated adenocarcinoma. The distinction can be challenging, although the overall cellularity of a specimen and the lack of hyperchromasia in reactive pneumocytes compared with the thick irregular nuclear membranes and intranuclear cytoplasmic inclusions that are frequently seen in adenocarcinoma can be helpful clues. Reserve cell hyperplasia, seen in exfoliative cytology specimens, forms tight cohesive clusters of small cells with round to oval small nuclei, bland uniform chromatin, and scant cyanophilic cytoplasm and should not be mistaken for small-cell carcinoma cells (which would display tumor necrosis, nuclear molding, and increased mitotic activity).

Creola bodies seen in exfoliative cytology are papillary fragments of reactive bronchial cells covered by ciliated epithelium, often seen in inflammatory conditions, which can mimic adenocarcinoma because of the three-dimensional tight clustering of cells. The presence of bland nuclei with smooth nuclear membranes, evenly distributed chromatin, and small nucleoli, together with the presence of cilia along the edge of the cluster, can indicate the benign nature of the cells.

Goblet cell hyperplasia is a common airway reactive change. The ciliated bronchial epithelium demonstrates greatly increased numbers of interspersed goblet cells, morphologically characterized by cytoplasmic hyperdistention with a single large mucinous vacuole or less frequently with multiple smaller vacuoles that push the nuclei to the base of the cell. Excess mucus production from goblet cell hyperplasia can lead to mucostasis with mucus distending the alveolar ducts. Goblet cell hyperplasia should not be confused with a well-differentiated mucinous carcinoma.

Other reactive changes include squamous metaplasia of the bronchial and bronchiolar epithelium. Anthracosis, seen as collections of anthracotic pigment deposited along lymphatics and bronchovascular sheaths, within macrophages, and around areas of fibrosis, is commonly seen in smokers and urban dwellers. Smokers and patients with reactive airway disease/asthma can have increased numbers of eosinophils in the bronchial mucosa.

Cytologic changes due to chemotherapy or radiation may be reflected in bronchial epithelial cells as cytomegaly and karyomegaly with multinucleation and cytoplasmic vacuoles and should not be mistaken for malignancy. Nuclear to cytoplasmic ratios are typically maintained despite the nuclear enlargement and degenerative changes.

Nonspecific findings may include smooth muscle hyperplasia present at the tips of the alveoli opening into the alveolar ducts sometimes seen in smokers or as a consequence of chronic irritation. Fibrotic lung processes are commonly associated with osseous metaplasia. Occasionally circulating megakaryocytes may be seen within the alveolar capillaries and should not be mistaken for tumor cells. Chronic vascular congestion or hemorrhage can cause hemosiderin to accumulate within macrophages and even encrust elastic fibers along pulmonary veins. Other nonspecific findings include thickening of the bronchial mucosal basement membrane, in smokers and patients with asthma.

Age-related changes can be seen in pulmonary arteries as vessel tortuosity. Pulmonary arteries may also demonstrate medial thickening, sclerosis, and calcification. Rarely senile amyloid deposition may be encountered. Nonspecific muscular hyperplasia of veins traversing the pleura can also be associated with age. Other age-related changes include calcification and ossification of bronchial cartilage and oncocytic changes of the bronchial seromucinous glands.

HISTOLOGIC FEATURES

- Reactive changes include cytologic atypia with nuclear enlargement, anisonucleosis, prominent nucleoli, multinucleation, and mitoses; goblet cell and type II pneumocyte hyperplasia; squamous metaplasia; anthracosis and increased numbers of eosinophils.
- Reactive changes in exfoliative cytology include the presence of Creola bodies, reserve cell hyperplasia, and reactive bronchial cells and type II pneumocytes.
- Treatment or therapy-related changes include cytomegaly, karyomegaly, multinucleation, and degenerative changes such as cytoplasmic vacuolization.
- Nonspecific changes include smooth muscle hyperplasia at the tips of alveoli, thickening of the bronchial mucosal basement membrane, accumulation of hemosiderin within alveolar macrophages, osseous metaplasia within fibrotic areas, and the presence of megakaryocytes within capillaries.
- Age-related changes include vessel tortuosity, arterial thickening and calcification, amyloid deposition, calcification and ossification of bronchial cartilage, and oncocytic changes of the bronchial seromucinous glands.

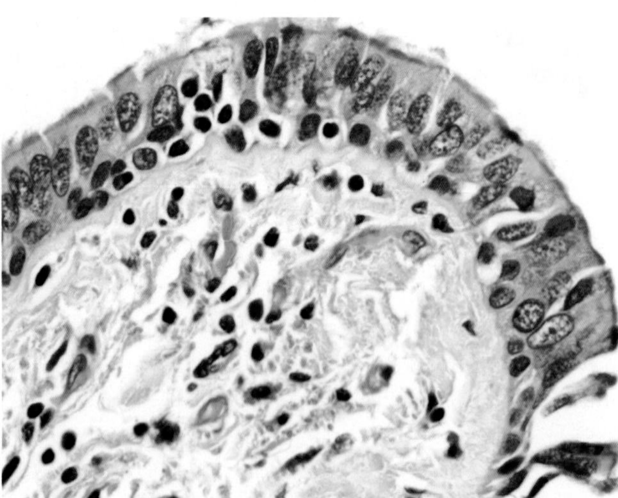

Figure 8.1 Reactive bronchial cells can display atypia, including nuclear enlargement, anisonucleosis, and prominent nucleoli.

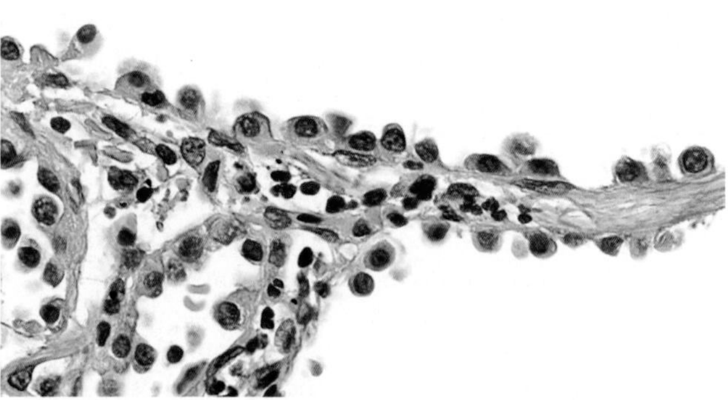

Figure 8.2 Reactive type II pneumocytes prominently stand out in a hobnail fashion from the alveolar wall, showing enlarged nuclei and prominent nucleoli, although usually space exists between adjacent reactive pneumocytes.

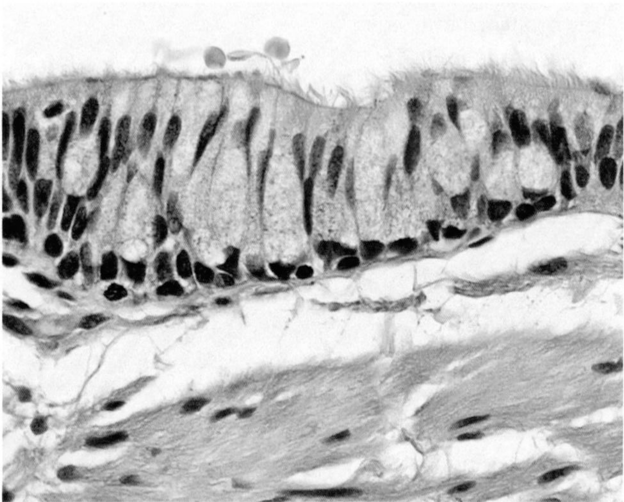

Figure 8.3 Goblet cell hyperplasia is seen as increased numbers of goblet cells relative to ciliated bronchial epithelial cells. The goblet cells are hyperdistended with a mucinous vacuole or multiple smaller vacuoles that push the nucleus to the base of the cell.

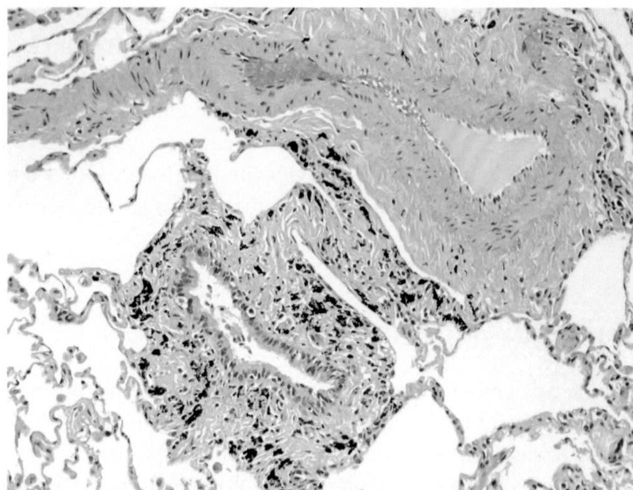

Figure 8.4 Collections of anthracotic pigment deposited along lymphatics and bronchovascular sheaths and within macrophages can be commonly seen in smokers and urban dwellers.

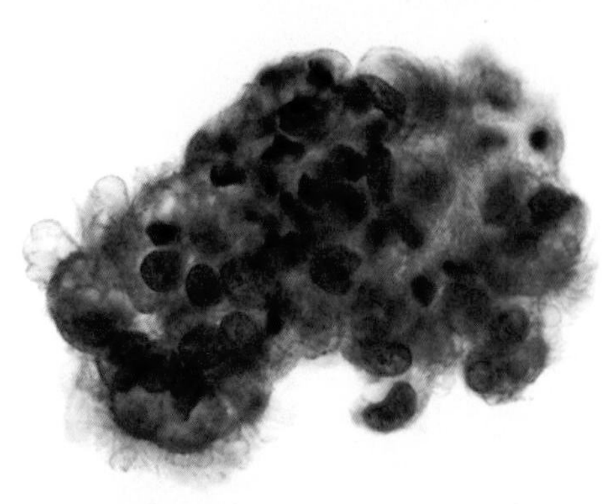

Figure 8.5 Creola bodies are clusters of reactive bronchial cells covered by ciliated epithelium sometimes seen in exfoliative cytology specimens (Papanicolaou stain).

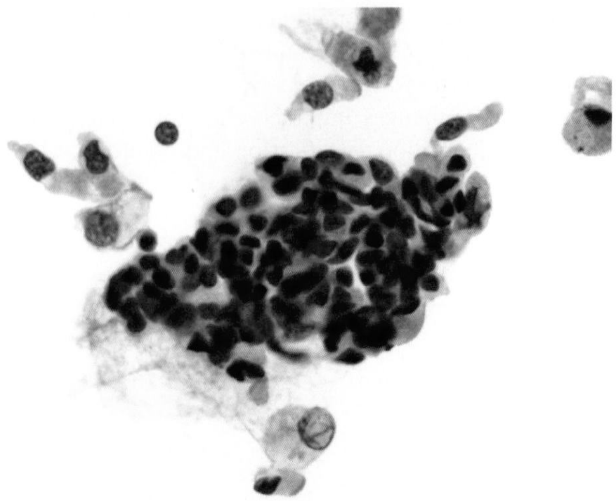

Figure 8.6 Reserve cell hyperplasia (*center*) seen in exfoliative cytology specimens form cohesive clusters of small cells with round to oval small nuclei, bland uniform chromatin, and scant cyanophilic cytoplasm. Note benign bronchial cells and macrophages for comparison (Papanicolaou stain).

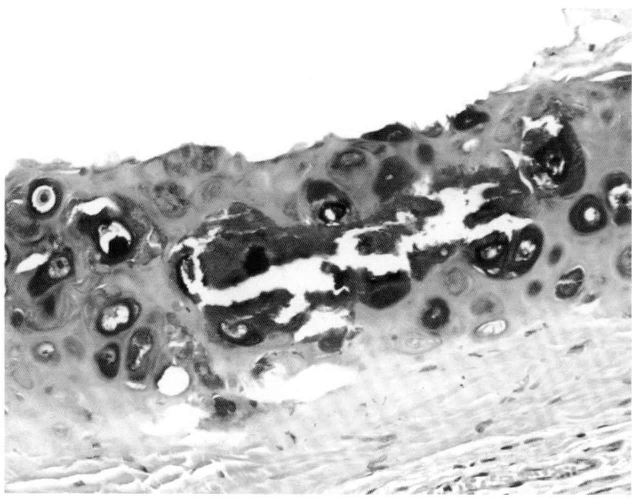

Figure 8.7 Age-related changes can include calcification and even frank ossification of bronchial cartilage.

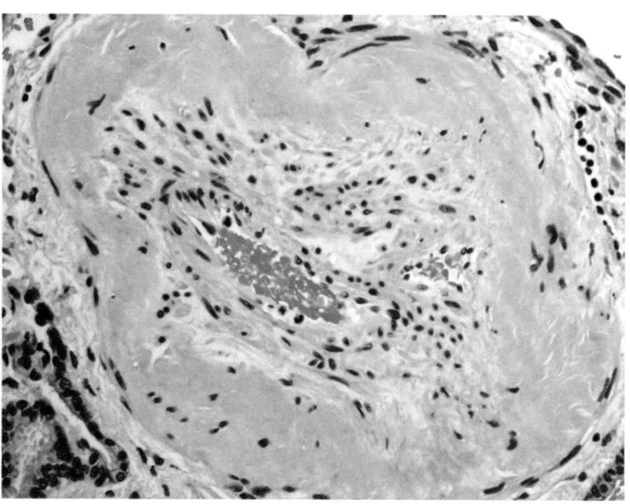

Figure 8.8 Amyloid can be seen as a waxy, pink, amorphous deposit within the vessel wall in this example of senile amyloidosis.

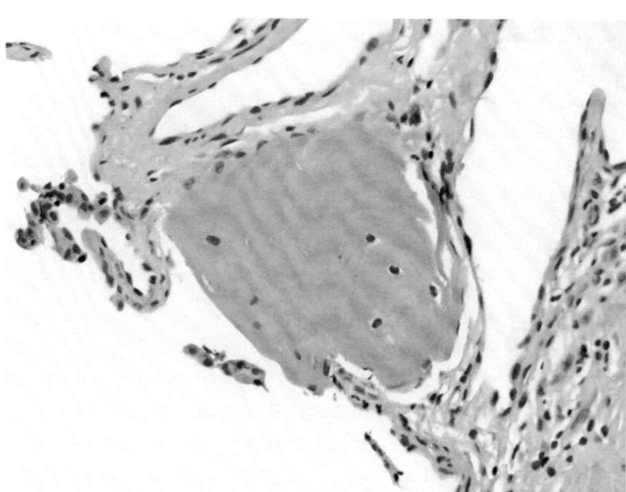

Figure 8.9 Osseous metaplasia may be seen as a nonspecific finding in fibrotic lung processes.

9 Noncellular Structures

▶ Hui-Min Yang
▶ Anjali Saqi
▶ Deepali Jain
▶ Sinchita Roy-Chowdhuri
▶ Paul A. VanderLaan

Noncellular structures are sometimes encountered in pulmonary specimens. These may be endogenous or formed within the lung, arise from an extrapulmonary source (e.g., aspiration, inhalation, and embolization), or represent a combination of the two. Some structures can suggest underlying pathology (e.g., psammoma bodies), whereas others are nonspecific findings. As certain structures demonstrate birefringence under polarized light or are highlighted with silver/acid-fast stains, they may potentially mimic pneumoconiosis and microorganisms, respectively. Some of the commonly encountered noncellular structures are listed.

HISTOLOGIC FEATURES

- Mucus may be an incidental finding or part of a neoplasm (e.g., mucinous adenocarcinoma or colloid carcinoma). Lubricant or ultrasound gel is an incidental finding in cytology specimens and can resemble mucus; however, the overall texture and relatively discrete boundaries compared with the more stringy edges of mucin can help distinguish the two.
- Curschmann's spirals are wiry coiled structures formed from inspissated and often excess mucus production, sometimes seen in patients with asthma and chronic bronchitis. The staining is more intense in the center than the periphery.
- Charcot–Leyden crystals are eosinophilic bipyramidal, rhomboid, or needle-shaped refractile crystals derived from cytoplasmic granules of eosinophils.
- Pulmonary alveolar proteinosis (PAP) is a condition in which coarsely granular proteinaceous material fills predominantly alveolar spaces. The proteinaceous material may also form small dense globules. There may be peripheral retraction artifact separating the proteinaceous material from the adjacent alveolar wall. Punched out clear spaces, cholesterol clefts, and foamy macrophages are also seen in this material within the alveolar spaces.
- Amyloid deposits appear as amorphous eosinophilic material on hematoxylin and eosin (H&E) stain, dark blue to purple on Diff-Quik stain, and cyanophilic to orangeophilic on Papanicolaou stain. Their presence can be confirmed with congo red and crystal violet special stains.
- Hematoidin, a yellow-orange pigment formed as a breakdown product of heme in the setting of hemorrhage, can be found in histiocytes or extracellularly. The shape may resemble an asteroid body or microorganisms; however, the bright yellow-orange coloration is a clue to its identity.
- Endogenous pneumoconiosis results from iron and calcium deposition on elastic fibers around blood vessels, which may result in degradation of the fibers and elicit a foreign-body giant cell reaction. These are often seen in states of chronic hemorrhage.

- Corpora amylacea (30 to 200 μm) are round to oval concentrically laminated structures with delicate radiating spokes that are birefringent under plane-polarized light. Corpora amylacea are formed from glycoprotein casts of alveolar spaces and may be surrounded by macrophages in some instances. A central Maltese cross pattern can be observed under polarized light. Although the presence of corpora amylacea has no known significance, they may be formed around inhaled foreign material or from excess secretions. Corpora amylacea are noncalcified structures as opposed to psammoma bodies and microliths, which are calcified. Relative to microliths, these occur in fewer numbers, are smaller, may have a central nidus comprising dark fragments/rings, and show a smaller number of concentric rings.
- Asteroid bodies (5 to 30 μm) are eosinophilic stellate inclusions within multinucleated giant cells frequently seen in granulomatous diseases.
- Schaumann bodies (25 to 200 μm) are calcified basophilic usually nonbirefringent laminated bodies within histiocytic multinucleated giant cells. These commonly occur in granulomatous diseases, such as sarcoidosis, but may also be seen in other conditions.
- Blue bodies (15 to 40 μm) are round to oval basophilic calcified laminated bodies formed by histiocytes. Blue bodies are smaller than Schaumann bodies, corpora amylacea, and microliths.
- Hamazaki-Wesenberg bodies are orange-to-yellow/brown spherical to ovoid structures that may be intracellular or extracellular. They may appear to form "buds" and their size is similar to some yeast forms. Hamazaki-Wesenberg bodies are often seen in lymph nodes in sarcoidosis and/or infection and are postulated to form from an inability to process certain bacteria, resulting in intralysosomal accumulation of partly digested material. These structures are highlighted with silver and acid-fast stains and therefore can mimic microorganisms. Staining with Fontana-Masson distinguishes them from most fungal and mycobacterial organisms.
- Microliths (250 to 1000 μm) are calcified round to elongated concentrically laminated bodies within alveolar spaces and may be seen in pulmonary alveolar microlithiasis, a rare autosomal recessive disease occurring with increased incidence in individuals of Turkish ancestry.
- Psammoma bodies are calcified round basophilic concentrically laminate concretions, often seen in neoplasms with papillary architecture but can also occur in benign conditions.
- Ferruginous bodies are formed as a result of iron encrustation of inhaled foreign materials, including asbestos (asbestos bodies) and nonasbestos materials ("pseudoasbestos" bodies), such as silicates, iron oxide, and carbon, among others. These take on the shape of the underlying material.
- Elastin fibers are slender, elongated, and curved fibers seen in specimens with underlying pathology or as an artifact of brisk sampling.
- Aspirated material: polystyrene sulfonate (Kayexalate), microcrystalline cellulose, crospovidone, and other pill fragment/filler material may be seen in alveolar spaces with aspiration. Some of these structures may be birefringent under polarized light. Food particles aspirated may have a variety of appearance, depending on the type of food aspirated. Vegetable matter will demonstrate cell walls, whereas meat or animal protein may display skeletal muscle fragments.
- Starch appears as transparent particles with a Maltese cross configuration under plane-polarized light, which may occur as a result of glove powder contamination (see Chapter 7).
- Pollen can be seen as a contaminant with refractile walls and may be morphologically variable with a round surface to a surface with distinct protrusions (see Chapter 7).

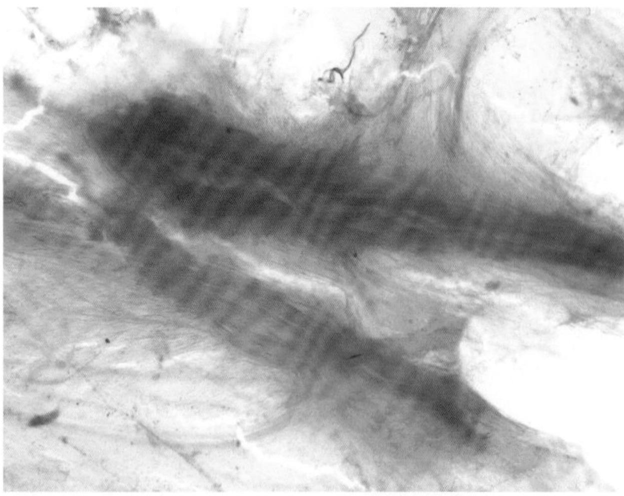

Figure 9.1 Cytology preparation (Papanicolaou stain) demonstrating mucus with edges that are delicate, stringy, and ill defined.

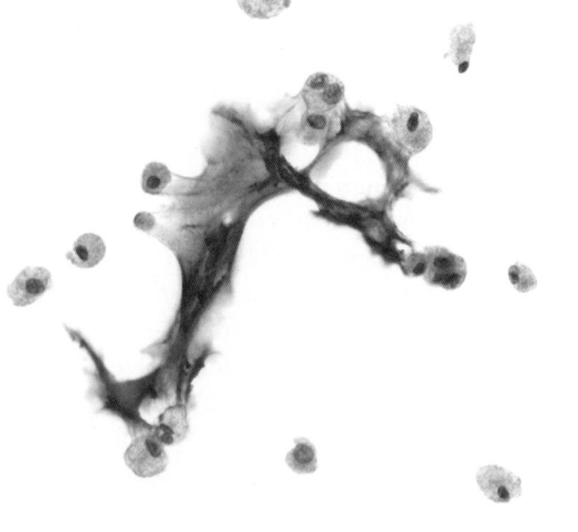

Figure 9.2 Lubricant (Papanicolaou stain), in contrast to mucus, shows more well-defined borders.

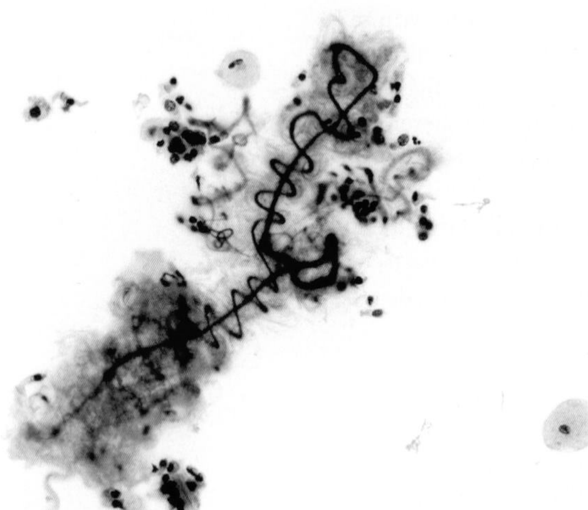

Figure 9.3 Curschmann's spirals are mucus-forming coil-like structures in an exfoliative cytology preparation (Papanicolaou stain). Ciliated columnar cells and alveolar macrophages are seen in the background.

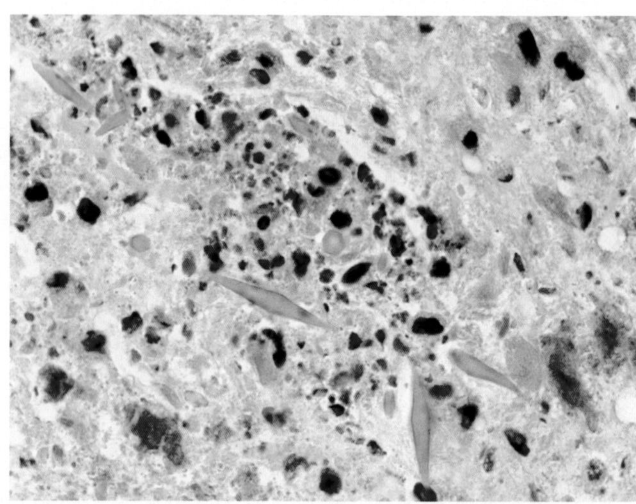

Figure 9.4 Charcot–Leyden crystals are bipyramidal and hexagonal, red on H&E stain, similar to the eosinophil cytoplasmic granules from which they are derived.

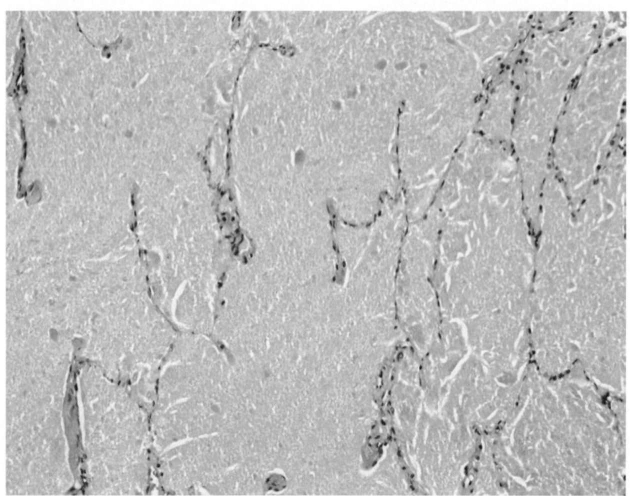

Figure 9.5 Pulmonary alveolar proteinosis seen within the alveolar spaces as an eosinophilic granular material with retraction artifact and small globules.

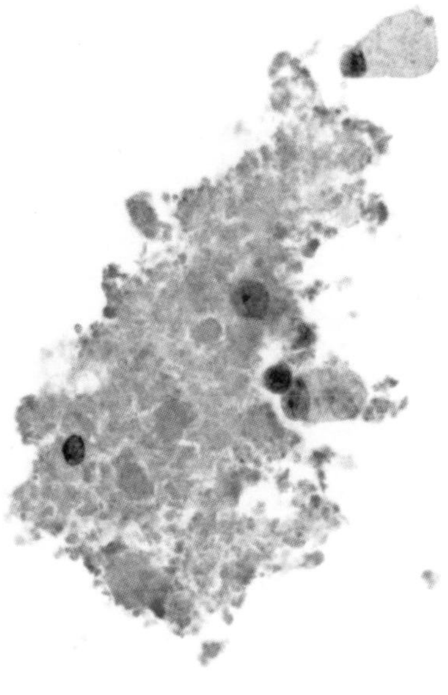

Figure 9.6 The granular proteinaceous material of pulmonary alveolar proteinosis as seen on a Papanicolaou-stained cytology preparation.

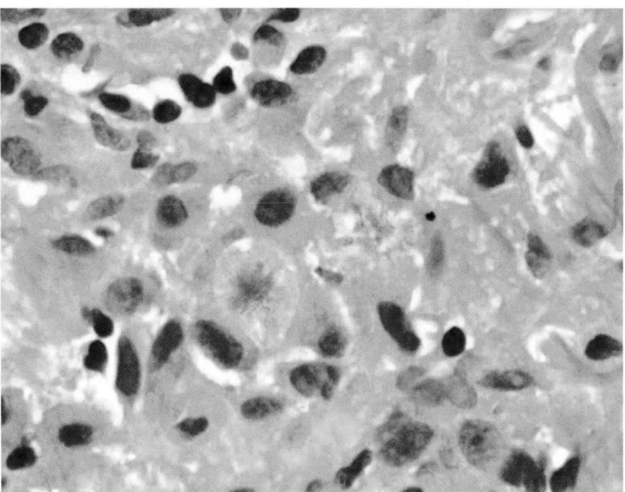

Figure 9.7 The yellow hematoidin pigment within histiocytes may resemble an asteroid body (which in contrast is red-pink).

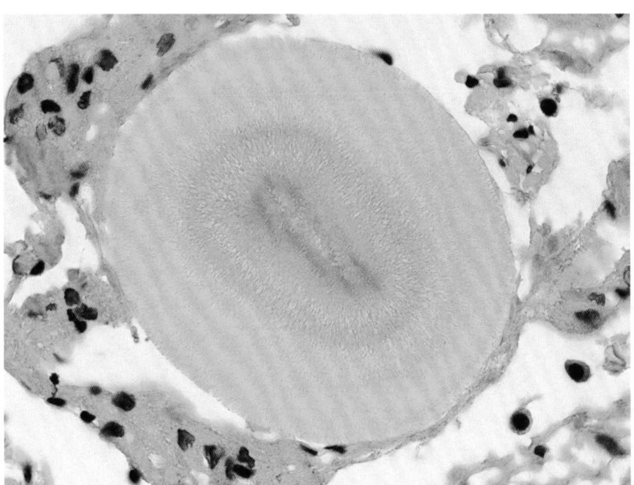

Figure 9.8 Corpora amylacea are round to oval concentrically laminated structures with delicate radiating spokes.

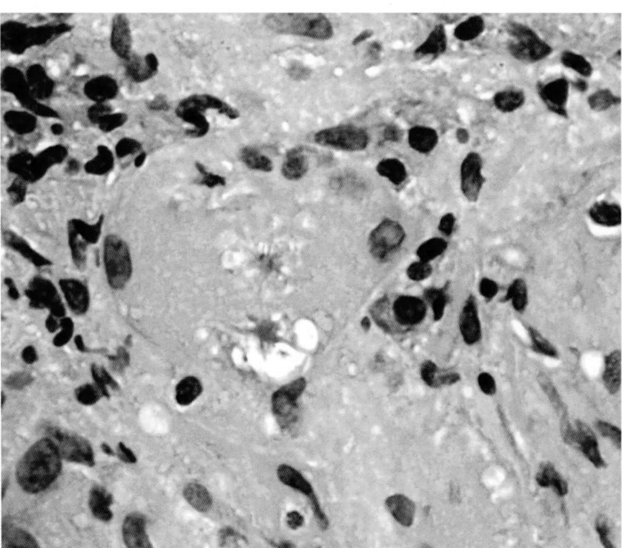

Figure 9.9 Multinucleated giant cell with intracytoplasmic asteroid bodies demonstrating multiple eosinophilic radiating spine-like projections often seen in granulomatous diseases.

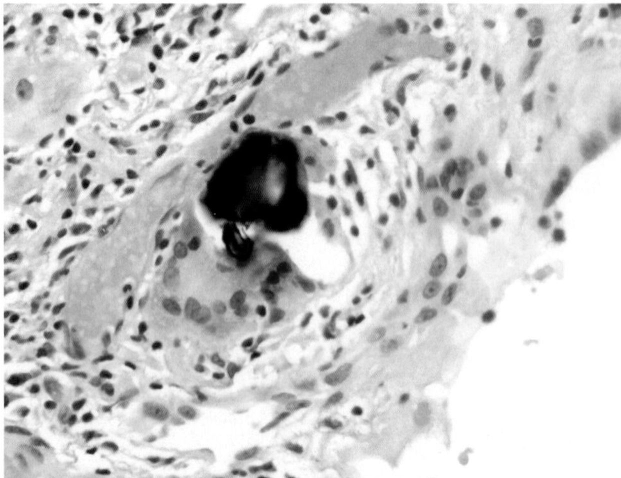

Figure 9.10 Multinucleated giant cell containing laminated calcified Schaumann bodies.

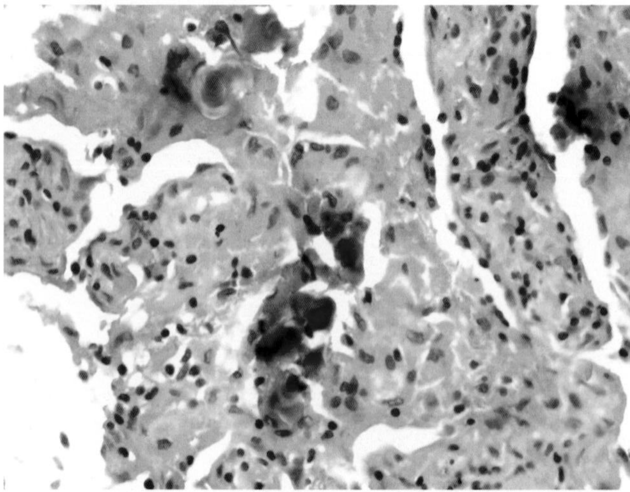

Figure 9.11 Calcified laminated blue bodies within alveolar spaces seen here in association with giant cells.

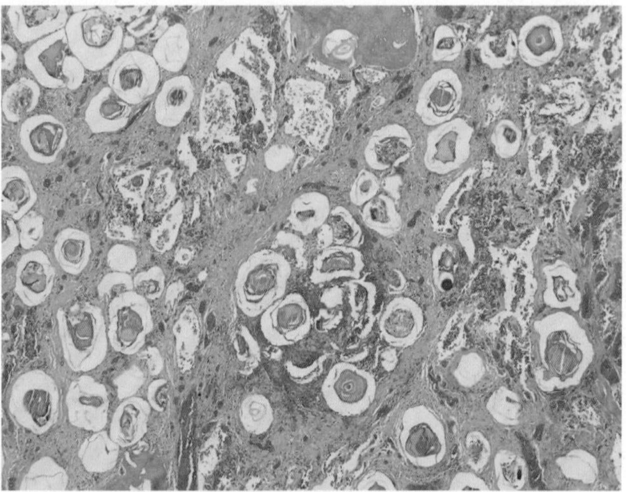

Figure 9.12 Pulmonary alveolar microlithiasis with numerous microliths seen within alveolar spaces.

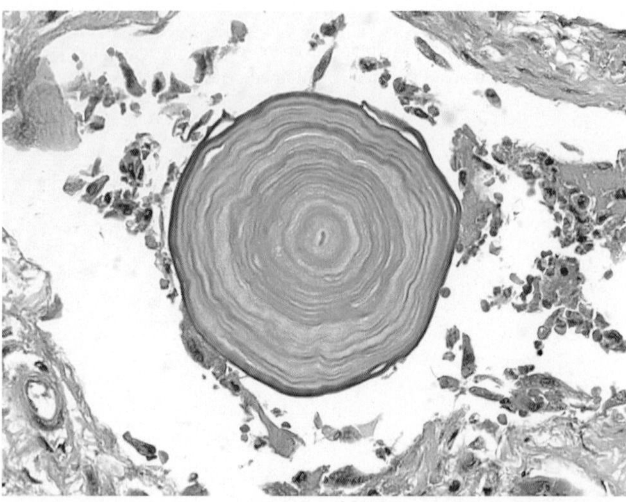

Figure 9.13 Higher magnification of a microlith with laminated concentric rings.

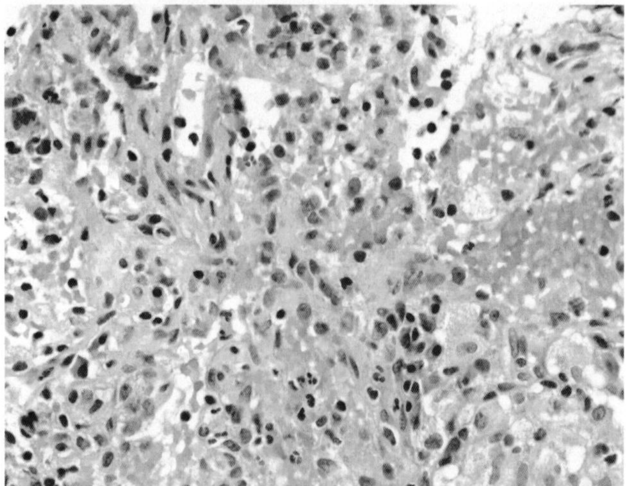

Figure 9.14 Hamazaki-Wesenberg bodies are seen as small round to oval intracellularly and extracellular yellow-brown structures.

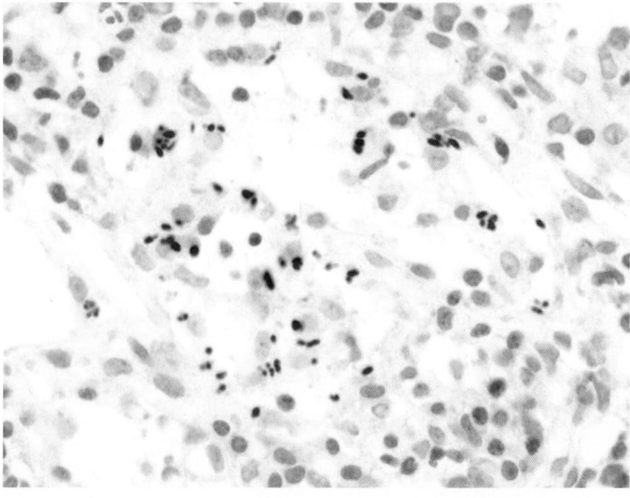

Figure 9.15 Hamazaki-Wesenberg bodies are intensely positive on the acid-fast stain.

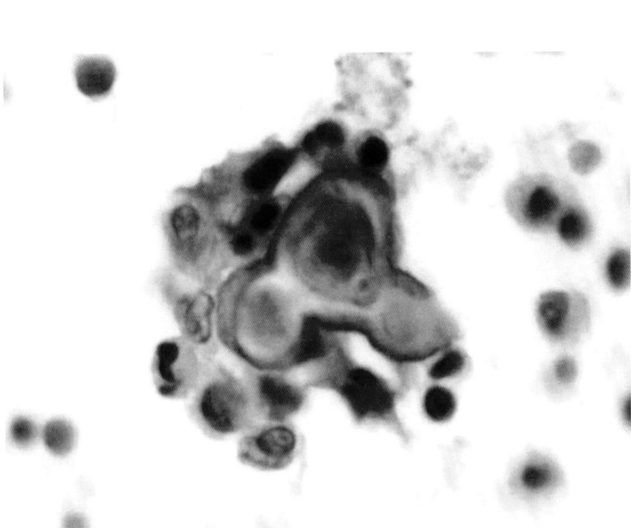

Figure 9.16 Concentrically laminated psammoma bodies can be seen in both benign and malignant conditions.

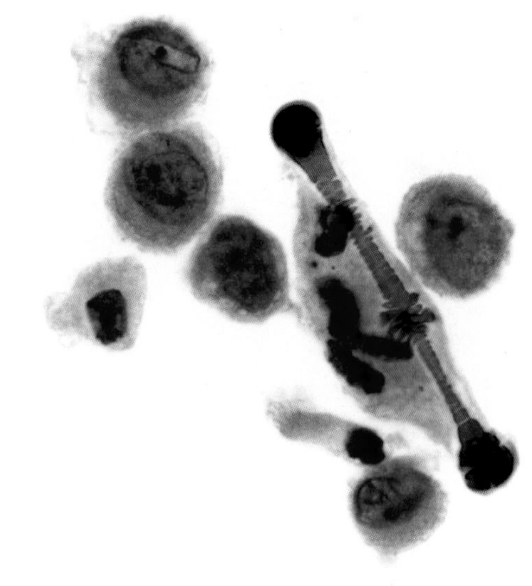

Figure 9.17 Ferruginous body formed as a result of iron encrustation of inhaled foreign material may have a dumbbell-shaped appearance.

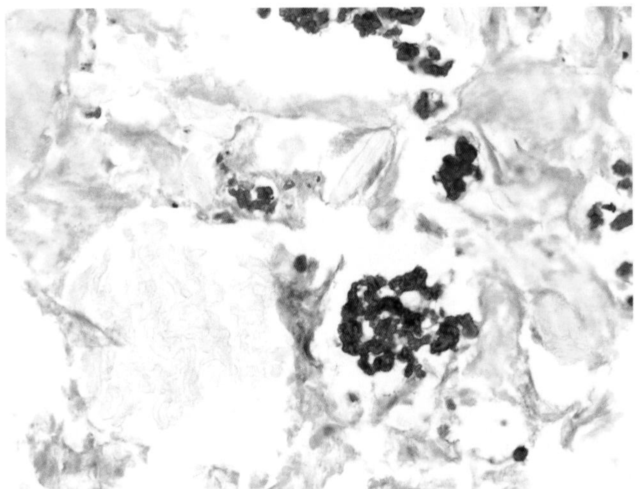

Figure 9.18 Aspirated pill fragment/filler material seen in alveolar spaces, with the colorless microcrystalline cellulose seen on the *left* and the amorphous, coral-like magenta-colored crospovidone material on the *right*.

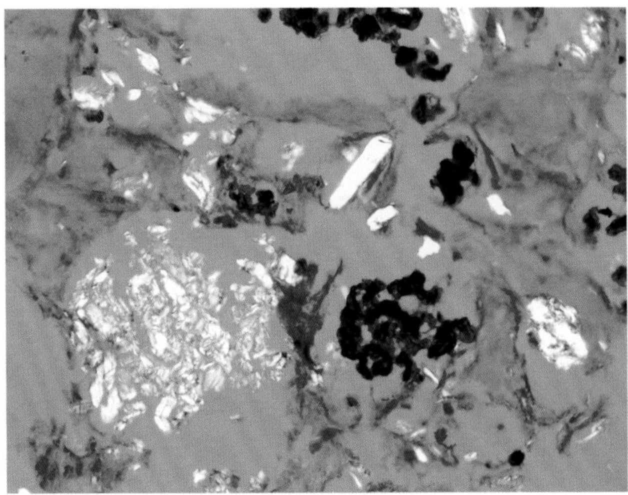

Figure 9.19 Microcrystalline cellulose but not crospovidone appears birefringent when viewed under polarized light.

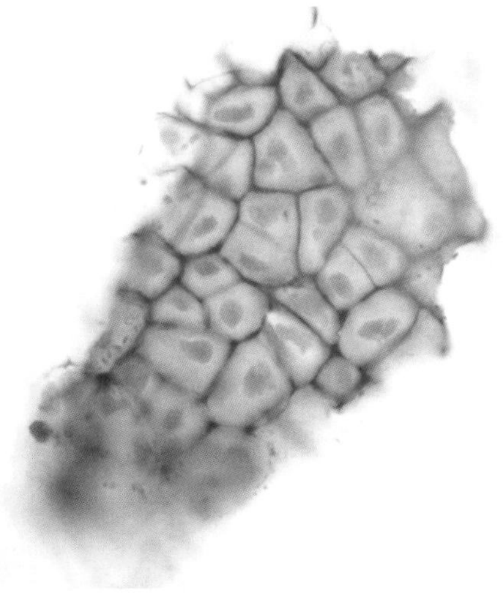

Figure 9.20 Aspirated vegetable matter can show prominent cell walls and intracellular starch.

Section 3

Malignant Neoplasms

- Mari Mino-Kenudson
- Sergio Pina-Oviedo
- Sanja Dacic
- Timothy C. Allen
- Ross A. Miller
- Philip T. Cagle

10 Adenocarcinoma

Paloma del C. Monroig-Bosque
Ross A. Miller
Philip T. Cagle

The majority of lung cancers are invasive adenocarcinomas, accounting for more than 40% of lung cancers by cell type. Adenocarcinoma in situ is covered in Chapter 28, Part 2. Only about 30% of invasive adenocarcinomas are seen by the pathologist as early-stage resection specimens and the majority, about 70%, are seen only as small biopsies and cytology specimens because of the advanced stage of disease at diagnosis. Most invasive adenocarcinomas are solid nodules or masses on CT scan, most often peripheral, and ground glass opacity around the periphery suggests a lepidic (in situ) component.

The 2015 World Health Organization classification recognizes several histologic subtypes of invasive adenocarcinomas: lepidic, acinar, papillary, micropapillary, and solid. There are also several histologic variants: invasive mucinous, colloid, fetal, and enteric. More than 90% of invasive adenocarcinomas are histologically heterogeneous with mixtures of these subtypes and variants on microscopic examination with one subtype predominant.

Invasive adenocarcinomas may be positive for any of a number of actionable mutations or rearrangements on molecular testing. These include primarily EGFR and ALK followed by ROS1, BRAF, RET, MET, ERBB2/HER2, and a few others less frequently. KRAS is the most common mutation in invasive adenocarcinoma but is not yet the target of molecular therapy. Although there is some variation in frequency of mutations/rearrangements in differing subtypes, any of the subtypes of invasive adenocarcinoma may potentially have one of these mutations/rearrangements and, therefore, almost all invasive adenocarcinomas have the potential to be positive for one of these actionable mutations/rearrangements on molecular testing.

CYTOLOGIC FEATURES

- Abundant malignant cells in sheets, clusters, gland-like structures, or single cells.
- Eccentric large nuclei with finely granular chromatin.
- Prominent nucleoli.
- Foamy or vacuolated, usually cyanophilic cytoplasm.
- May have large intracytoplasmic mucin vacuoles.

HISTOLOGIC FEATURES

- See Parts 1 through 10 below.

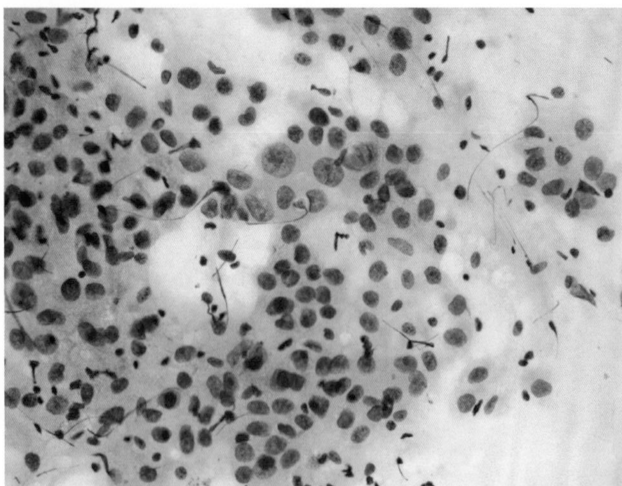

Figure 10.1 Low-power view of cytology specimen shows large numbers of adenocarcinoma cells with abundant cytoplasm, large pleomorphic nuclei, and occasional cytoplasmic mucin vacuoles (Papanicolaou stain).

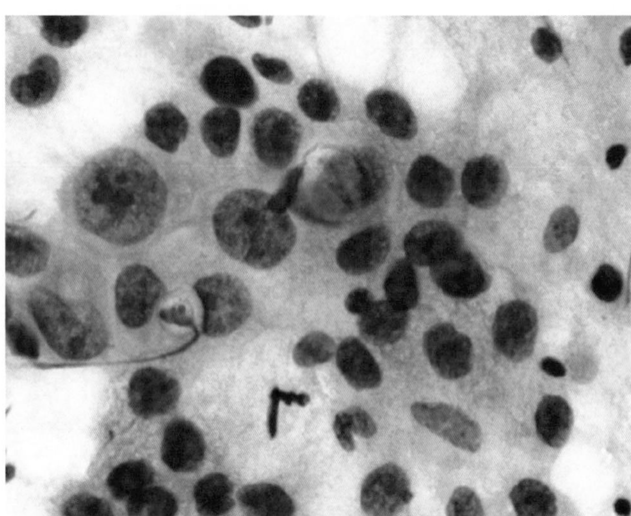

Figure 10.2 Higher power of same specimen displays prominent nucleoli within the large nuclei. Cytoplasmic mucin vacuoles are also seen (Papanicolaou stain).

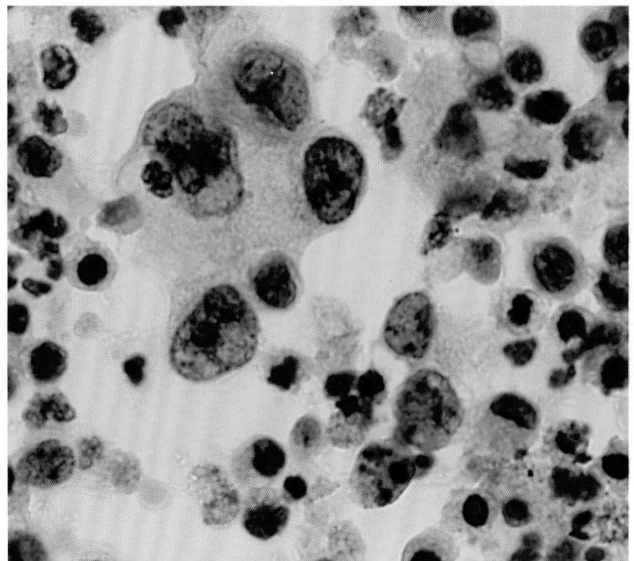

Figure 10.3 High-power view of cytology shows adenocarcinoma cells with large pleomorphic nuclei and prominent nucleoli arranged in clusters (Papanicolaou stain).

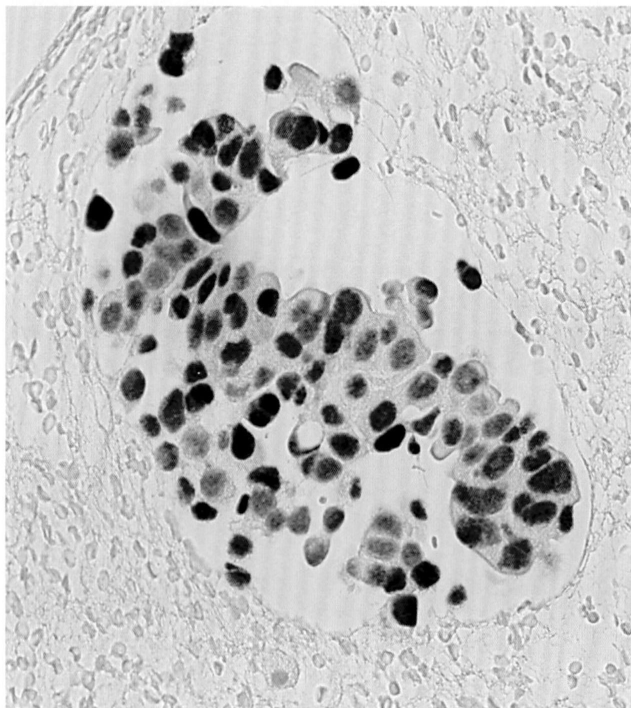

Figure 10.4 TTF-1 immunostain performed on cytology specimen shows strong nuclear staining in the malignant cells confirming the diagnosis of adenocarcinoma.

Part 1

Lepidic Adenocarcinoma

Paloma del C. Monroig-Bosque, Ross A. Miller, and Philip T. Cagle

Growth of adenocarcinoma cells along the luminal surface of intact alveoli without invasion into the underlying septa or other structures is referred to as lepidic growth. Lepidic growth is noninvasive or in situ growth. Pure adenocarcinomas in situ and minimally invasive adenocarcinomas exist and are described in detail under those headings in Chapter 28 "Premalignant and Preinvasive Lesions." Lepidic adenocarcinomas are a subtype consisting of a predominantly lepidic pattern with at least one focus of invasive adenocarcinoma that is greater than 5 mm, which may consist of any of the other histologic patterns observed in invasive adenocarcinoma. The lepidic cells are nonmucinous and ordinarily cytologically bland and uniform.

Stage I lepidic adenocarcinoma has a favorable prognosis with a 90% 5-year survival rate and is sometimes considered grade I adenocarcinoma.

HISTOLOGIC FEATURES

- A majority of tumor consists of a nonmucinous noninvasive lepidic pattern growing along intact alveolar septa plus one or more of the invasive criteria below.
- Invasive criteria include (1) stromal invasive component that is more than 5 mm in one discrete focus or as sum of multiple foci (exceeds the definition of minimally invasive adenocarcinoma); (2) invasion of the lymphatics, blood vessels, and/or pleura; (3) tumor necrosis; and (4) aerogenous spread or spread through the airways.
- A stromal invasive component may consist (1) of tumor cells infiltrating desmoplastic stroma or (2) one of the other histologic patterns (acinar, papillary, micropapillary, solid, colloid, fetal, enteric).
- The neoplastic cells of the noninvasive lepidic pattern growing along intact alveolar septa may (1) resemble the bland cells of adenocarcinoma in situ described in Chapter 28, Part 2, or (2) display the same cytologic atypia as the invasive component.
- Tumors that have a predominantly mucinous lepidic component should not be classified as lepidic invasive adenocarcinomas and are separately classified as invasive mucinous adenocarcinoma. Invasive mucinous adenocarcinomas are described in Part 6 of this chapter.

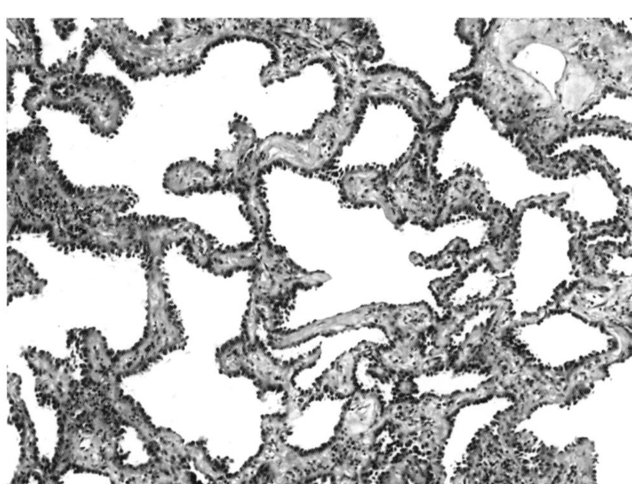

Figure 10.5 Medium power shows adenocarcinoma cells growing in a lepidic pattern on intact alveolar septa.

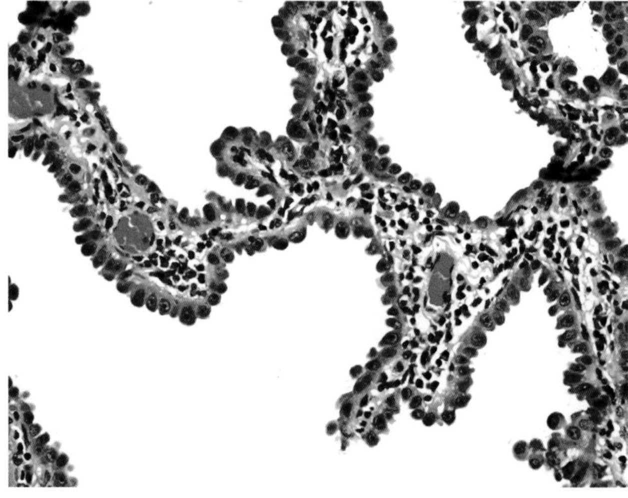

Figure 10.6 Higher power demonstrates the adenocarcinoma cells lined up uniformly along intact alveolar septa.

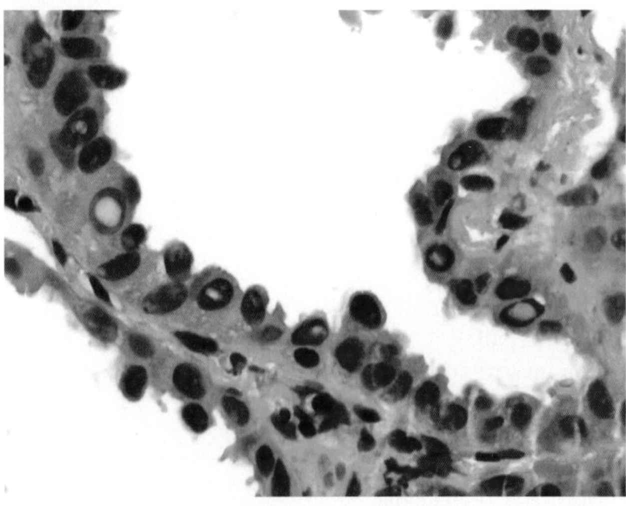

Figure 10.7 High-power view of lepidic carcinoma shows malignant cells with intranuclear inclusions.

Part 2

Acinar Adenocarcinoma

▶ Paloma del C. Monroig-Bosque, Ross A. Miller, and Philip T. Cagle

Acinar adenocarcinomas are an adenocarcinoma subtype characterized by invasive glands lined as a majority component of the tumor.

HISTOLOGIC FEATURES

- Invasive glands have different sizes and shapes, varying from small round glands to glands with larger oval lumens to glands with more complex patterns, for example, cribriform.
- Malignant cells lining glands may be oval, cuboidal, or columnar.
- Cells and/or the lumens of glands may contain mucin.
- Presence of mucin can be confirmed on histochemical stains, including mucicarmine, Alcian blue, and periodic acid–Schiff with digestion.

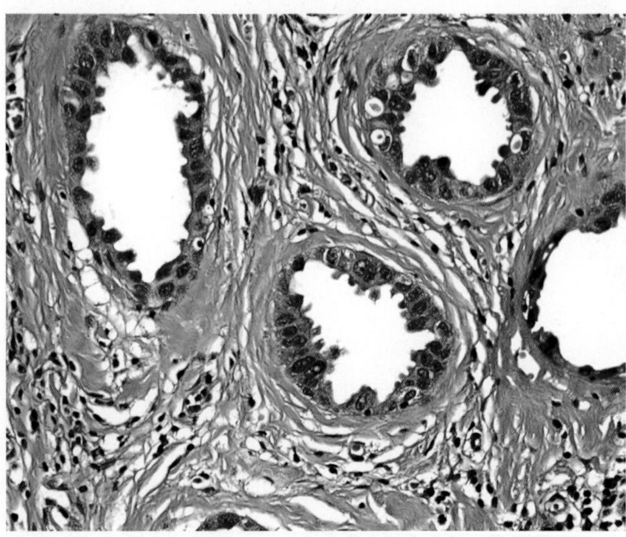

Figure 10.8 Acinar adenocarcinoma consists of invasive glands with lumens lined by malignant cells.

Part 3

Papillary Adenocarcinoma

Paloma del C. Monroig-Bosque, Ross A. Miller, and Philip T. Cagle

Papillary adenocarcinomas are a subtype consisting of malignant cells growing along the surface of papillary fibrovascular cores in a majority of the tumor.

HISTOLOGIC FEATURES

- Malignant adenocarcinoma cells grow along the surface of papillary fibrovascular cores.
- Presence of fibrovascular cores distinguishes papillary adenocarcinoma from micropapillary adenocarcinoma.
- Documentation of stromal invasion is not necessary to make the diagnosis of invasive papillary adenocarcinoma.

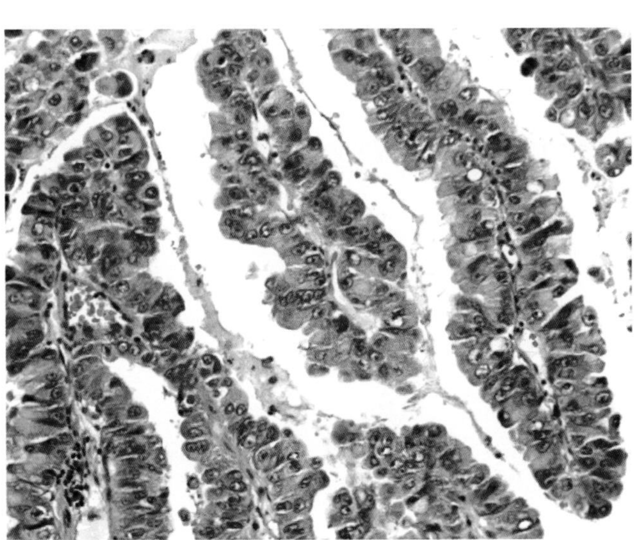

Figure 10.9 Papillary adenocarcinoma has fibrovascular cores with malignant cells on the surface.

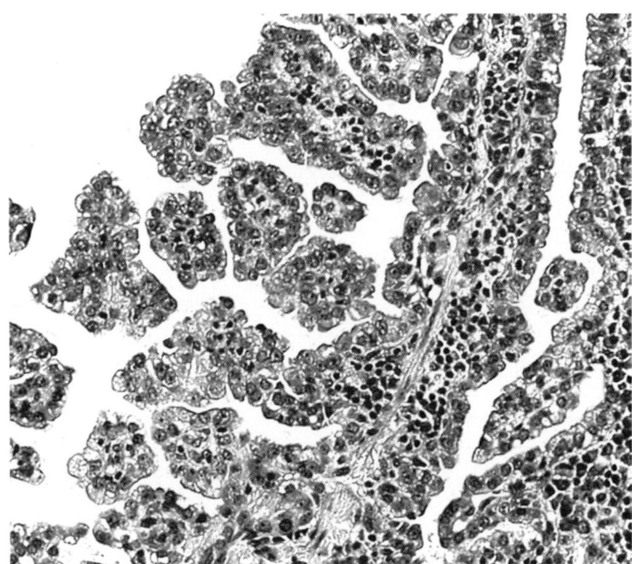

Figure 10.10 Papillary adenocarcinoma shows fronds cut in cross section. The fibrovascular cores distinguish papillary adenocarcinoma from micropapillary adenocarcinoma.

Part 4

Micropapillary Adenocarcinoma

Paloma del C. Monroig-Bosque, Ross A. Miller, and Philip T. Cagle

Micropapillary adenocarcinomas are a subtype of invasive adenocarcinoma in which a majority of the tumor is composed of small cuboidal malignant cells arranged in papillary tufts or florets without fibrovascular cores. Micropapillary adenocarcinoma is associated with a poorer prognosis than other adenocarcinoma subtypes.

HISTOLOGIC FEATURES

- A majority of the tumor consists of small cuboidal malignant cells clustered in small papillary tufts or florets lacking fibrovascular cores.
- Papillary tufts may be attached to alveolar walls and may "float" in the alveolar spaces detached from the alveolar walls.
- Small ring-like glands may be formed.
- Psammoma bodies may be present.
- Vascular and stromal invasion may often be present.

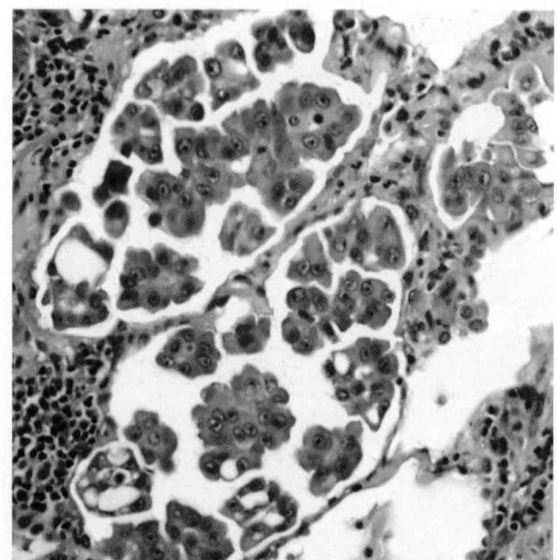

Figure 10.11 Small clusters or papillary tufts of micropapillary adenocarcinoma float in adjacent alveolar spaces.

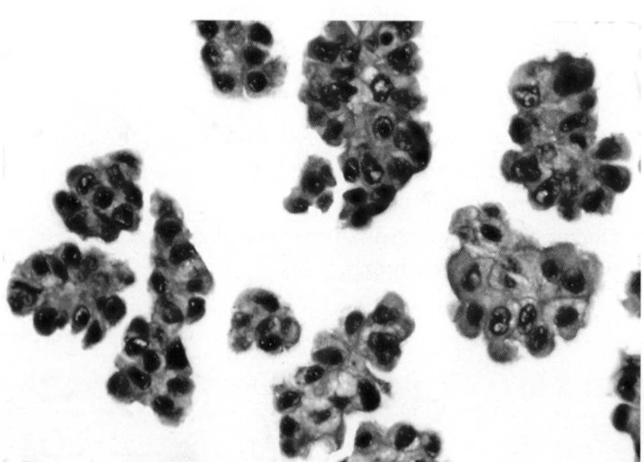

Figure 10.12 Higher power shows that the papillary tufts of micropapillary adenocarcinoma lack fibrovascular cores.

Part 5

Solid Adenocarcinoma

Paloma del C. Monroig-Bosque, Ross A. Miller, and Philip T. Cagle

Solid adenocarcinomas are a subtype composed of solid sheets or nests of polygonal malignant cells in a majority of the neoplasm. Solid adenocarcinomas have a poorer prognosis than most other subtypes of adenocarcinomas.

HISTOLOGIC FEATURES

- Solid adenocarcinomas are solid sheets or nests of polygonal malignant cells.
- Differential on hematoxylin and eosin includes nonkeratinizing squamous-cell carcinoma and large-cell carcinoma.
- These may be diagnosed if intracellular mucin is demonstrated by histochemical stains (see Part 2: Acinar Adenocarcinoma) consisting of intracellular mucin in five or more tumor cells in each of two high-power fields.
- These may be diagnosed if positive for adenocarcinoma immunohistochemical markers such as TTF-1.

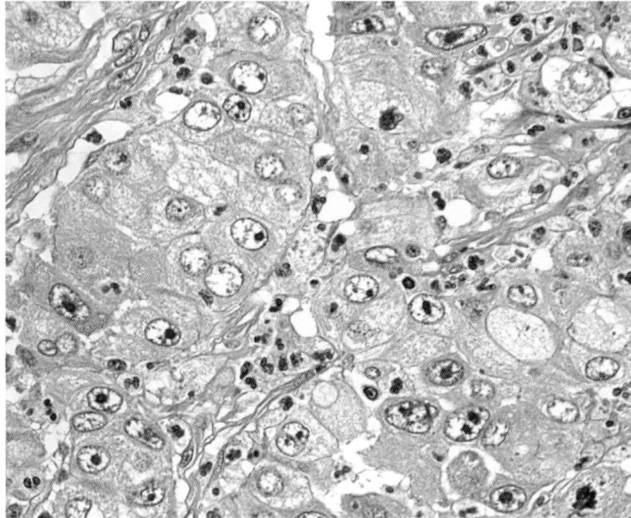

Figure 10.13 Solid adenocarcinoma consists of sheets of polygonal malignant cells.

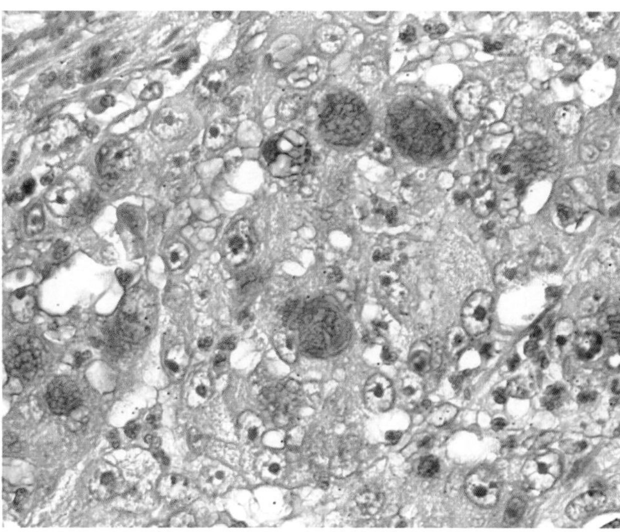

Figure 10.14 This solid adenocarcinoma stains for intracytoplasmic mucin on mucicarmine stain confirming the diagnosis.

Part 6

Invasive Mucinous Adenocarcinoma

Paloma del C. Monroig-Bosque, Ross A. Miller, and Philip T. Cagle

Invasive mucinous adenocarcinomas are a variant of adenocarcinoma in which neoplastic goblet cells containing apical mucin often grow in a lepidic pattern and are often associated with intra-alveolar mucin. They are much more likely than other lung cancers to present as disseminated multifocal lesions or pneumonia-like consolidation.

HISTOLOGIC FEATURES

- Homogenous goblet cells with abundant apical mucin and small, bland basal nuclei often growing in a lepidic pattern on intact alveolar septa.
- Alveolar spaces often filled with mucin with strips or clusters of goblet cells floating in the mucin.
- Invasive mucinous adenocarcinomas may also grow in acinar, papillary, or micropapillary patterns but do not grow in solid patterns.
- Invasive component is present, but because of prominence of lepidic pattern, it may be difficult to recognize and require additional sections to confirm invasion.
- In contrast to other adenocarcinomas, mucinous adenocarcinomas are typically immunopositive for CK7 and CK20 and immunonegative for adenocarcinoma markers such as TTF-1 and napsin A.
- Rarely, no invasive component may be present in a small solitary mucinous tumor growing only in a lepidic pattern consistent with a mucinous adenocarcinoma in situ (see Chapter 28).

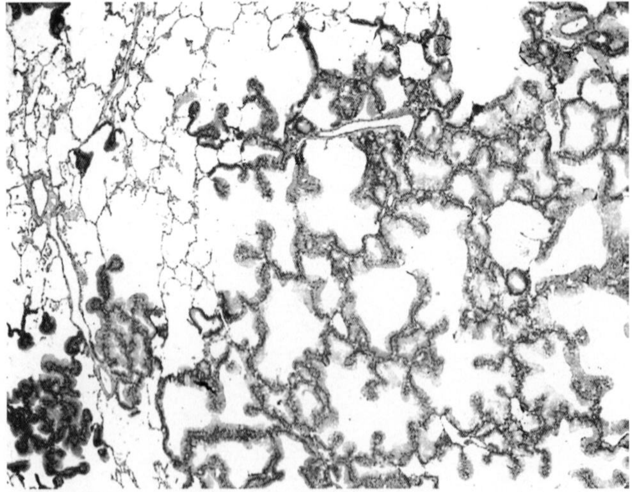

Figure 10.15 Low-power view of an invasive mucinous adenocarcinoma demonstrates that most of the tumor is growing in a lepidic pattern on intact alveolar septa.

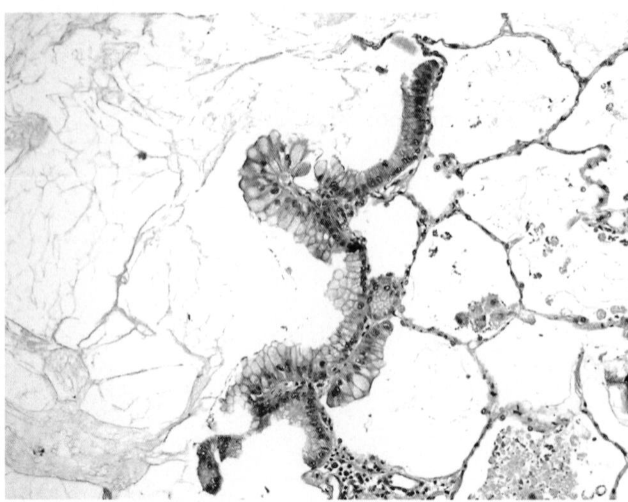

Figure 10.16 Malignant goblet cells with apical mucin and bland basal nuclei line an intact alveolar septum.

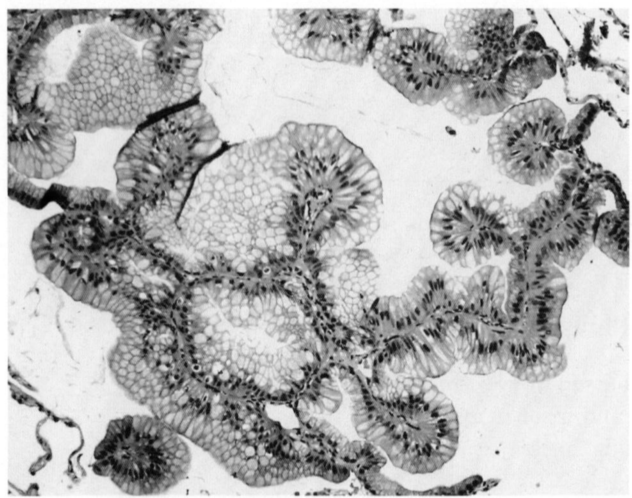

Figure 10.17 Invasive mucinous adenocarcinoma demonstrates mostly lepidic pattern with focal invasion in this field.

Part 7

Colloid Adenocarcinoma

Paloma del C. Monroig-Bosque, Ross A. Miller, and Philip T. Cagle

Colloid adenocarcinomas are a rare variant of invasive adenocarcinoma characterized by mucin pools. Grossly, colloid adenocarcinomas are well-demarcated peripheral mucinous masses, which may be loculated or sometimes cystic.

HISTOLOGIC FEATURES

- Pools of mucin distend alveolar tissue and rupture alveolar walls.
- Well-differentiated columnar cells with apical mucin line the pools of mucin.

- Pool lining is intermittent with extensive gaps without lining cells between strips of lining cells.
- Columnar mucinous cells may also "float" in the mucin pools as strips or glands.
- Cells may be immunopositive for CDX2 and CK20 and only weakly or focally positive for TTF-1 and CK7.

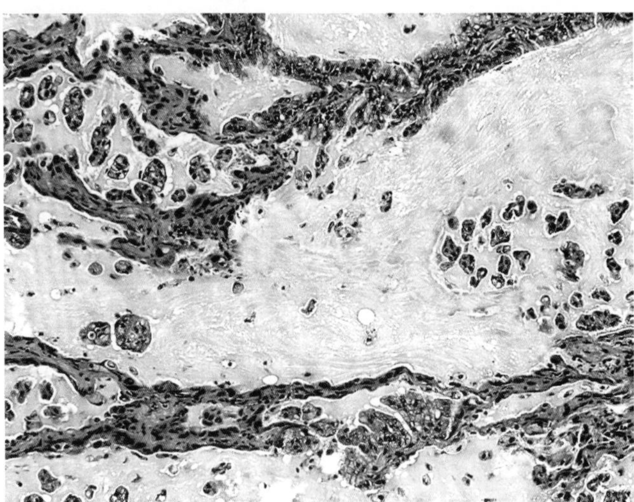

Figure 10.18 Colloid adenocarcinoma with pools of mucin within alveolar spaces. Columnar mucinous cells line alveolar septa and float in the pools of mucin.

Part 8

Fetal Adenocarcinoma

Paloma del C. Monroig-Bosque, Ross A. Miller, and Philip T. Cagle

Fetal adenocarcinomas are an uncommon variant of invasive adenocarcinoma characterized by their histologic resemblance to the pseudoglandular phase of fetal lung development. Grossly, they are usually well-circumscribed peripheral nodules or masses.

HISTOLOGIC FEATURES

- Histologic pattern reminiscent of low-grade endometrioid carcinoma.
- Complex glands, tubules, and papillae lined by columnar cells with supranuclear and subnuclear glycogen clearing.
- Myxoid stroma.
- Formation of squamous morules.
- High-grade form shows greater cytologic atypia and necrosis, lacks squamous morules, and is typically associated with more conventional patterns of invasive adenocarcinoma.

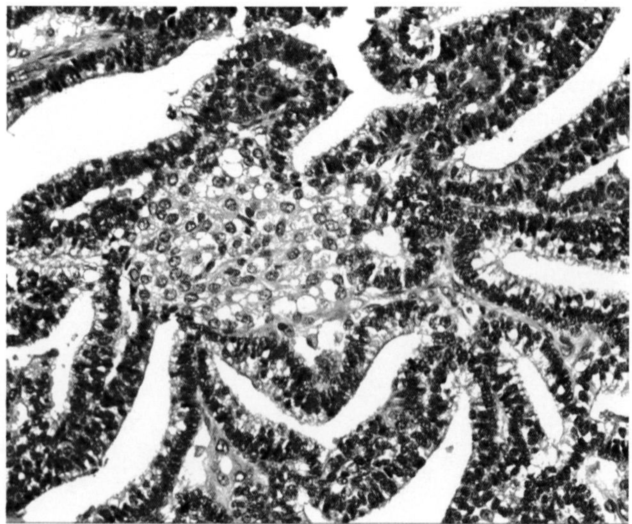

Figure 10.19 Fetal adenocarcinoma shows papillae lined by columnar cells with subnuclear glycogen clearing and a squamous morule.

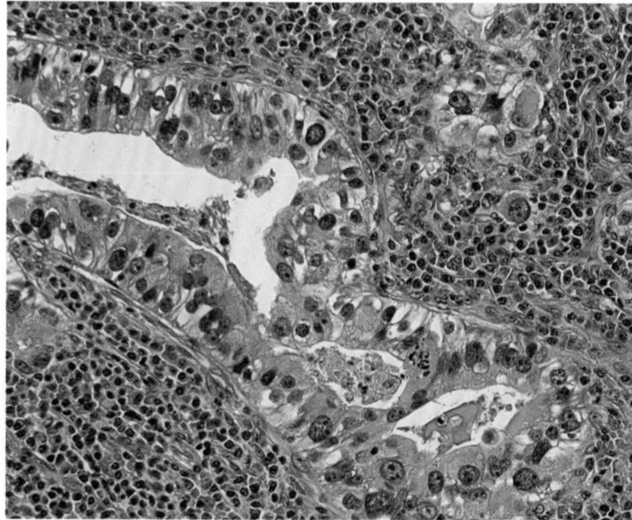

Figure 10.20 High-grade fetal adenocarcinoma demonstrates greater cytologic atypia in columnar cells with subnuclear glycogen.

Part 9

Enteric Adenocarcinoma

▸ Paloma del C. Monroig-Bosque, Ross A. Miller, and Philip T. Cagle

Enteric adenocarcinomas are a rare variant of invasive adenocarcinoma that histologically resembles colorectal adenocarcinoma. A primary colorectal adenocarcinoma must be excluded before a diagnosis of an enteric adenocarcinoma of the lung is made.

HISTOLOGIC FEATURES

- Cribriform glandular pattern of columnar cells resembling colorectal adenocarcinoma.
- Dirty necrosis may be present similar to colorectal adenocarcinoma.
- Some cases positive for CDX2 and CK20 and negative for CK7 similar to colorectal adenocarcinoma.

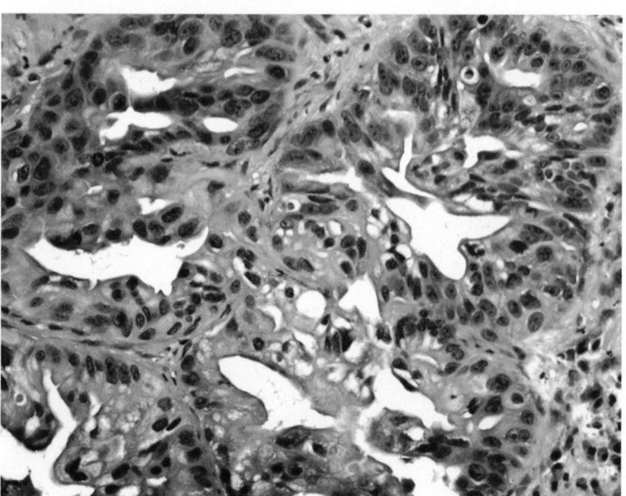

Figure 10.21 Enteric adenocarcinoma resembles colonic adenocarcinoma with cribriform glands lined by malignant columnar cells.

Part 10

Signet Ring and Clear Cell Features

▶ Paloma del C. Monroig-Bosque, Ross A. Miller, and Philip T. Cagle

Signet ring features and clear cell features are no longer considered separate variants or subtypes of adenocarcinoma. Most adenocarcinomas with signet ring or clear cell features are solid adenocarcinomas, although these features may be seen in other subtypes as well.

HISTOLOGIC FEATURES

- Signet ring features consist of intracytoplasmic vacuoles, which push the nucleus to one side.
- Clear cell features consist of cancer cells with clear cytoplasm.

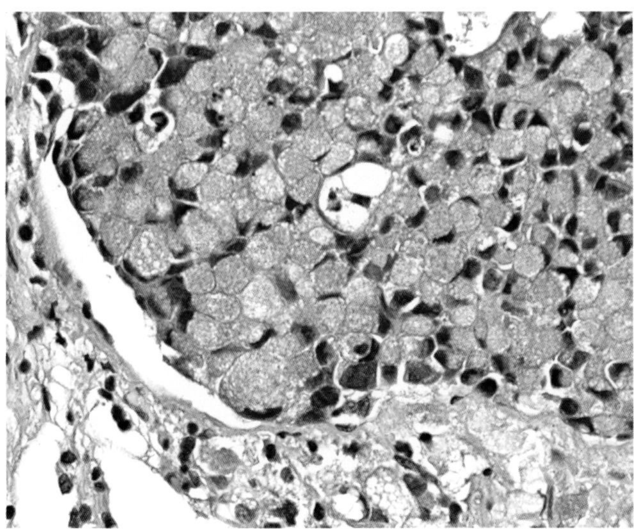

Figure 10.22 This solid adenocarcinoma has signet ring features with the nuclei of malignant cells pushed to one side by intracytoplasmic vacuoles.

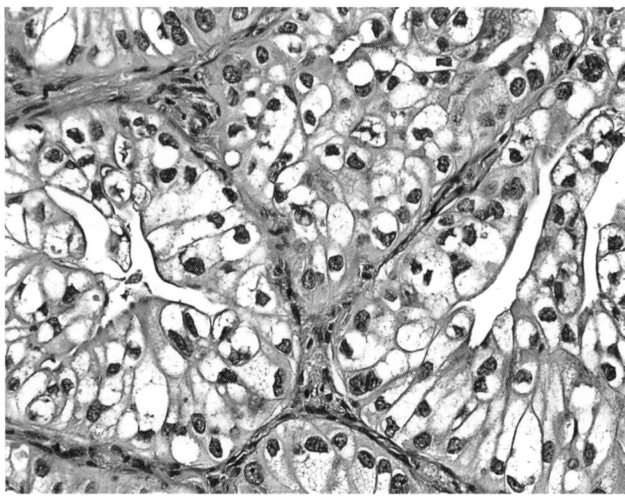

Figure 10.23 This adenocarcinoma has malignant cells with clear cytoplasm.

Squamous-Cell Carcinoma

11

Paloma del C. Monroig-Bosque
Ross A. Miller
Philip T. Cagle

Squamous-cell carcinoma is currently the second most common cell type of lung cancer after adenocarcinoma. Until the 1970s, squamous-cell carcinoma was the most common cell type of lung cancer. Squamous-cell carcinoma is a non–small cell carcinoma that has cytologic, histologic, or immunohistochemical features that demonstrate squamous differentiation.

Squamous-cell carcinoma is strongly associated with tobacco smoking. It frequently metastasizes to lymph nodes and distant organs and has a poor prognosis related to its stage. Squamous-cell carcinomas are traditionally considered to be centrally located tumors often arising in main stem bronchi or lobar bronchi. Owing to this central location, they may be associated with hemoptysis and may obstruct the bronchial lumens causing postobstructive atelectasis, acute pneumonia, organizing pneumonia, or lipid pneumonia. A large bulky tumor with central cavitary necrosis is a classic presentation for squamous-cell carcinoma. However, squamous-cell carcinoma may also arise in the periphery of the lung.

Prior to the 2015 World Health Organization (WHO) classification, previous WHO classifications required strict histologic criteria for squamous-cell carcinoma consisting of features that are seen with better differentiated tumors: keratinization, keratin pearl formation, and/or intercellular bridges on routine histologic stains. The 2015 WHO classification follows the practice that began a decade previously and includes as squamous-cell carcinomas those less well-differentiated tumors that are nonkeratinizing but are immunopositive for squamous-cell carcinoma markers such as p40. In addition, basaloid carcinomas were classified as a subtype of large-cell carcinoma and a subtype of squamous-cell carcinoma in the 2004 WHO classification, but basaloid carcinomas are p40 positive and all are now classified as basaloid squamous-cell carcinomas. Previously classified as separate variants, features such as clear cell cytoplasm, small-cell characteristics, and exophytic papilloma growth are now considered to be no more than patterns of squamous-cell carcinomas.

Therefore, in summary, based on the 2015 WHO classification, squamous-cell carcinomas may be (1) keratinizing squamous-cell carcinomas, (2) nonkeratinizing squamous-cell carcinomas, or (3) basaloid squamous-cell carcinomas. These have some differences in their histology, but all are immunopositive for p40.

Part 1

Keratinizing Squamous-Cell Carcinoma

▸ Paloma del C. Monroig-Bosque, Ross A. Miller, and Philip T. Cagle

The degree of keratinization in a squamous-cell carcinoma is associated with the degree of differentiation. Keratinization is most prominent and widespread in well-differentiated tumors. Most keratinizing squamous-cell carcinomas are moderately differentiated with foci of conspicuous keratinization admixed within the nests of polygonal tumor cells. In less-differentiated tumors, one may have to search to find foci of keratinization.

CYTOLOGIC FEATURES

- Sheets of pleomorphic cells with hyperchromatic nuclei.
- Bizarre cytoplasmic shapes may be present (tadpole or caudate cells, spindle or fiber cells).
- Cytoplasm ranges from dense and orangeophilic ("hard" cytoplasm) to deeply cyanophilic (Papanicolaou stain) due to keratin; prominent cell borders.

HISTOLOGIC FEATURES

- Sheets or nests of polygonal cells with abundant to moderately abundant pink to clear cytoplasm.
- Generally, sharp distinct cell borders.
- Vesicular nuclei with prominent nucleoli or hyperchromatic nuclei.
- Foci or areas of conspicuous keratinization of tumor cells interspersed within the nests of polygonal cells.
- Keratinizing tumor cells have dense pink cytoplasm with small hyperchromatic nuclei.
- Keratin pearls consist of whorls of cells with keratinized cytoplasm without nuclei.
- Intercellular bridges are thin lines in the spaces between cells best observed under high power.

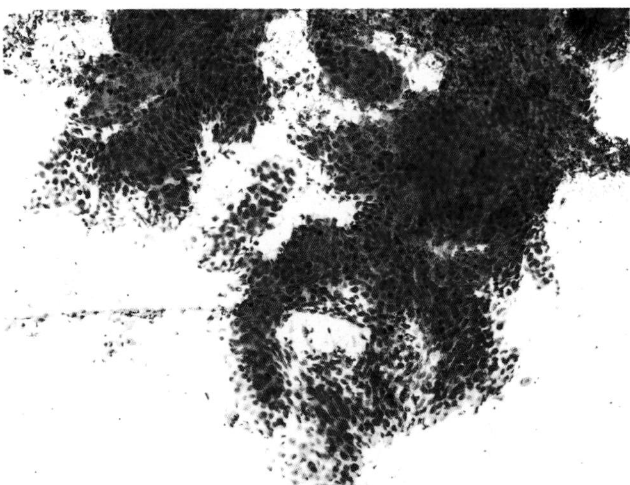

Figure 11.1 Highly cellular cytology specimen (Papanicolaou stain) showing sheets of cells with pleomorphic, hyperchromatic nuclei, and mostly orangeophilic cytoplasm.

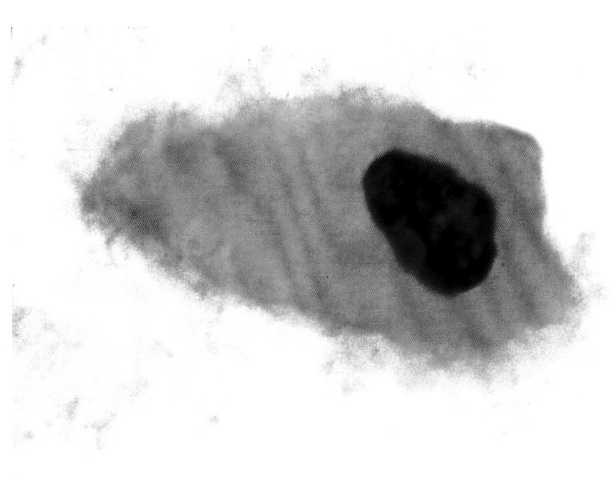

Figure 11.2 Cytology of squamous-cell carcinoma displays keratinized cytoplasm (orangeophilic or "hard" cytoplasm) and hyperchromatic nucleus on Papanicolaou stain.

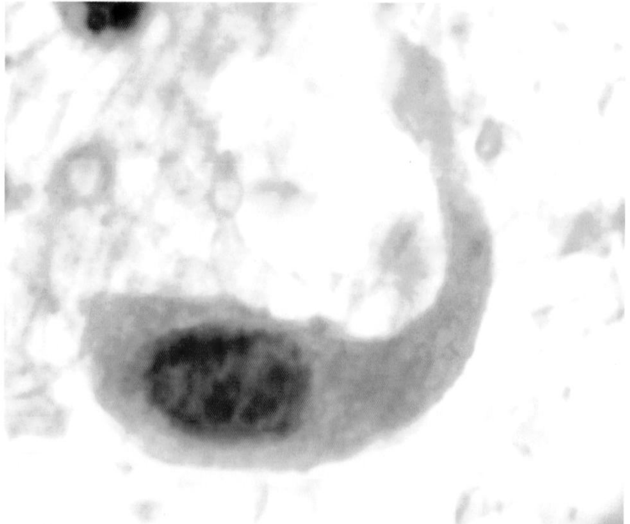

Figure 11.3 Papanicolaou-stained cytology specimen includes tadpole-shaped cell with orangeophilic or "hard" cytoplasm and hyperchromatic nucleus.

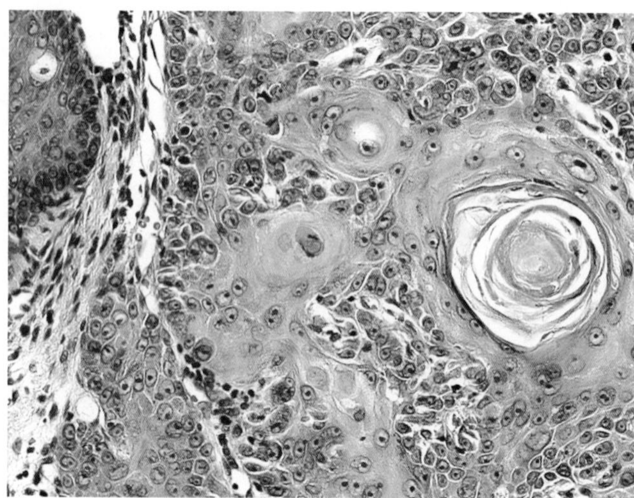

Figure 11.4 Keratinizing squamous-cell carcinoma with keratin pearl.

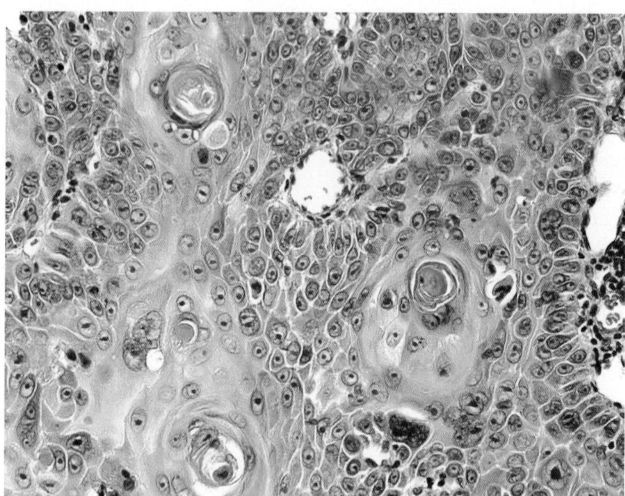

Figure 11.5 Keratinizing squamous-cell carcinoma with scattered apoptotic cells with pyknotic nuclei and bright eosinophilic cytoplasm and several small keratin pearls.

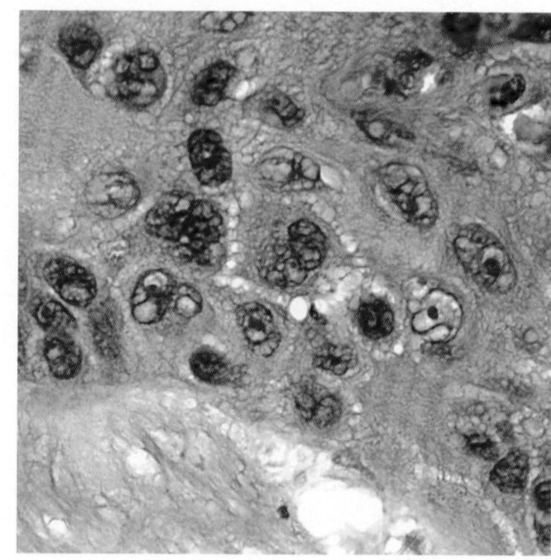

Figure 11.6 High-power view of keratinizing squamous-cell carcinoma showing intercellular bridges as thin lines in the space between tumor cells.

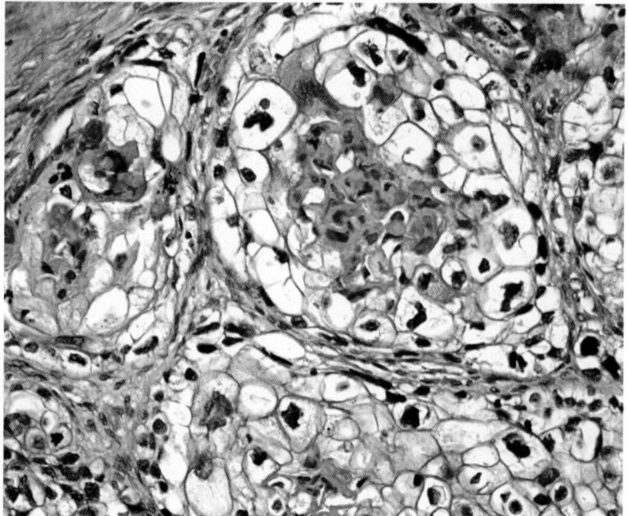

Figure 11.7 Some squamous-cell carcinomas may exhibit clear cytoplasm.

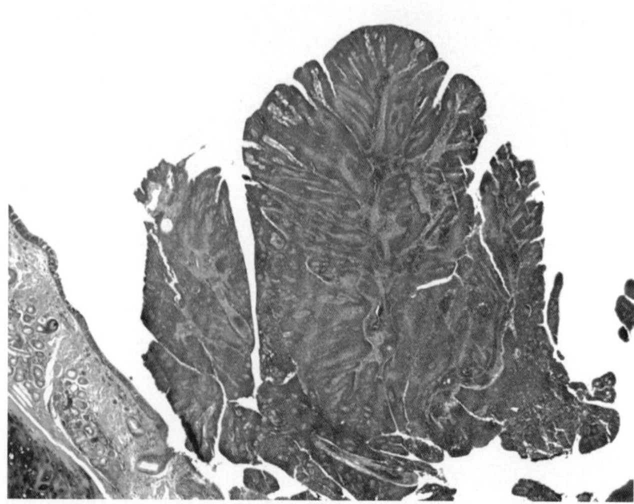

Figure 11.8 Occasional squamous-cell carcinomas may present primarily in the form of an exophytic papilloma.

Part 2

Nonkeratinizing Squamous-Cell Carcinoma

Paloma del C. Monroig-Bosque, Ross A. Miller, and Philip T. Cagle

More poorly differentiated squamous-cell carcinomas may lack histologic features of keratinization. Nevertheless, the tumor cells are immunopositive for p40 or other squamous-cell carcinoma immunohistochemical markers. Prior to the use of p40 or other markers to confirm their squamous differentiation, these tumors were previously classified as large-cell carcinomas based on their non–small cell histology lacking histologic features of squamous or other differentiation.

CYTOLOGIC FEATURES

- Sheets of pleomorphic cells lacking features of keratinization.
- Nucleoli may be present.

HISTOLOGIC FEATURES

- Poorly differentiated non–small cell carcinomas consisting of nests or sheets of polygonal cells that lack any findings of keratinization.
- Nests of cells may sometimes suggest the nonkeratinizing cells of a keratinizing squamous-cell carcinoma creating a "squamoid" appearance.
- Diagnosis depends on immunopositivity for squamous-cell markers, such as p40, p63, and CK 5/6. If only one stain is to be used, p40 is preferred.

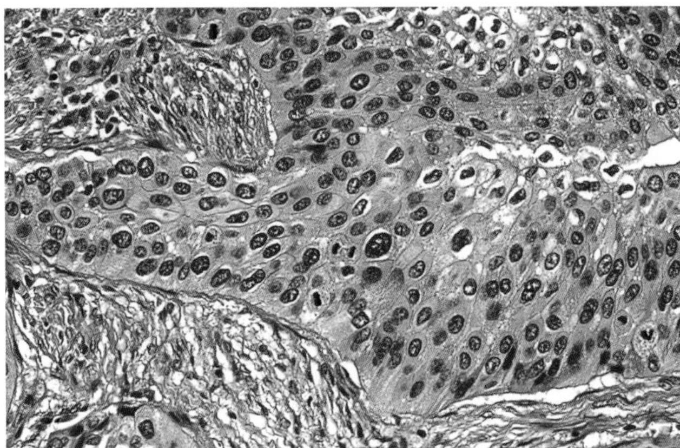

Figure 11.9 Moderately differentiated nonkeratinizing squamous-cell carcinoma consists of nests of polygonal cells with crisp cell borders reminiscent of keratinizing squamous-cell carcinoma but lacking features of keratinization. Immunostains of squamous-cell carcinoma markers are necessary to confirm the diagnosis.

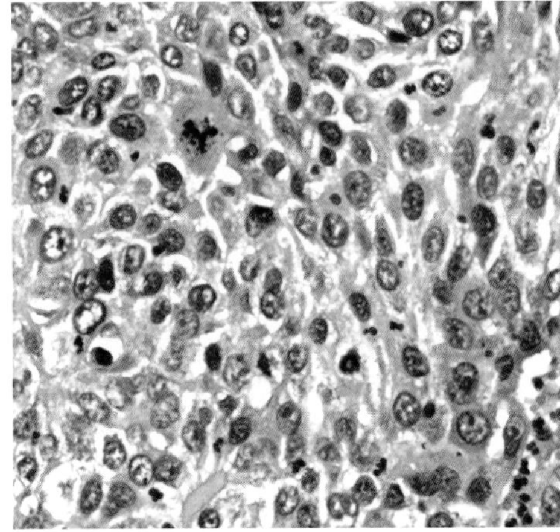

Figure 11.10 Poorly differentiated nonkeratinizing squamous-cell carcinoma is composed of sheets of pleomorphic polygonal cells. An abnormal mitotic figure is present. Immunostains of squamous-cell carcinoma markers are necessary to confirm the diagnosis.

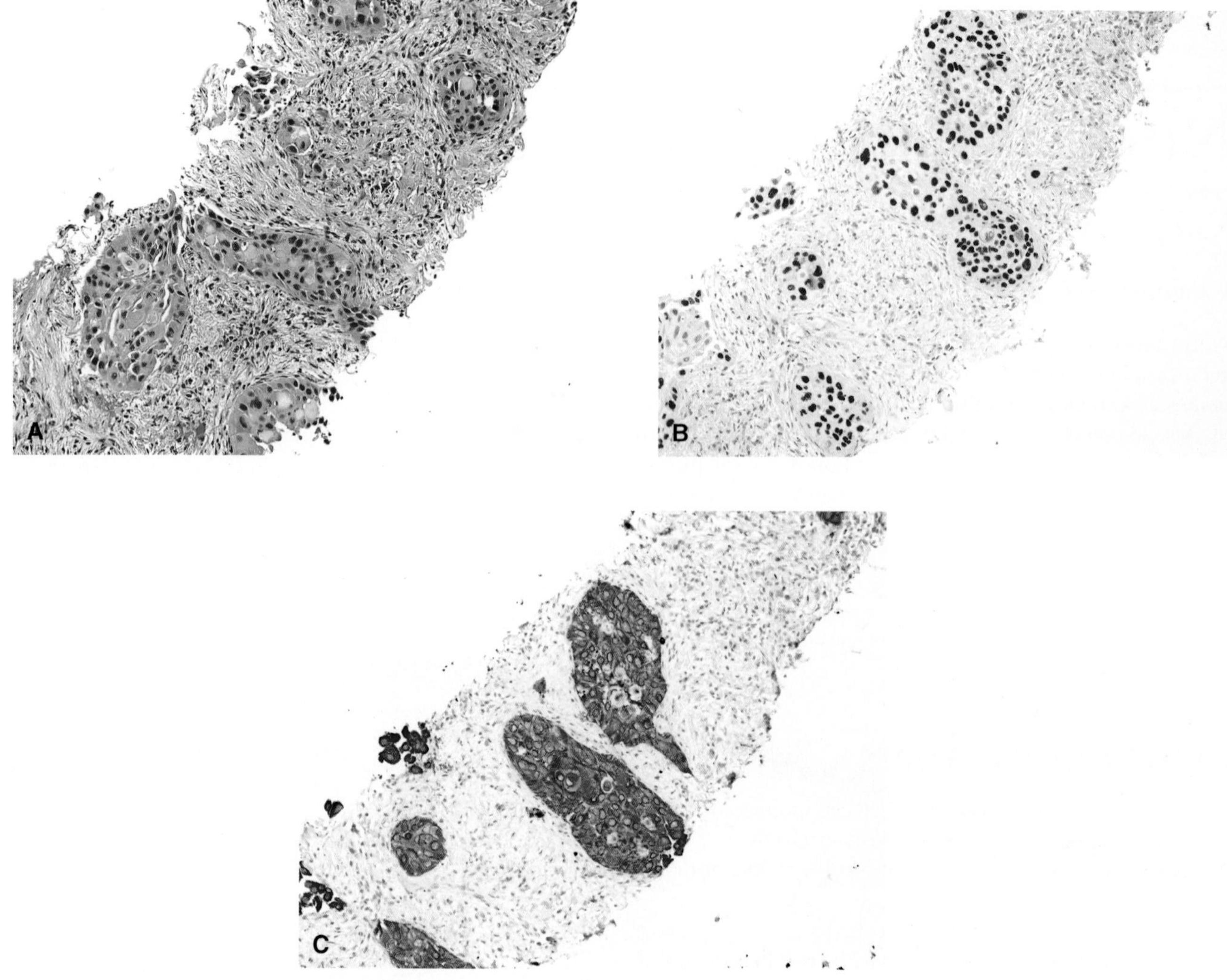

Figure 11.11 **A:** Needle biopsy of non–small cell carcinoma suggestive of nonkeratinizing squamous-cell carcinoma. **B:** Immunostain for p40 shows strong nuclear staining consistent with squamous-cell carcinoma. **C:** Immunostain for CK 5/6 shows strong cytoplasmic staining consistent with squamous-cell carcinoma.

Part 3

Basaloid Squamous-Cell Carcinoma

▸ Paloma del C. Monroig-Bosque, Ross A. Miller, and Philip T. Cagle

Basaloid squamous-cell carcinomas are rare. Histologically, these tumors have features that resemble basal cell carcinoma of the skin, may sometimes have keratin pearls, and are immunopositive for squamous-cell carcinoma markers such as p40. They are similar to other squamous-cell carcinomas in terms of clinical and imaging findings but are thought to potentially have a worse prognosis than other non–small cell carcinomas.

CYTOLOGIC FEATURES

- Small cells with high nuclear to cytoplasmic ratios.
- Hyperchromatic nuclei, chromatin often finely granular.
- Inconspicuous nucleoli, mitotic figures can be seen.
- Given the cytologic features, small-cell carcinoma is often a diagnostic consideration.

HISTOLOGIC FEATURES

- Relatively small cells with hyperchromatic nuclei and relatively scant cytoplasm (high nucleus to cytoplasm ratio).
- Tumor cells in lobules, trabeculae, or rosettes with peripheral palisading and hyaline or mucoid stroma.
- Keratin pearls may be present.
- Mitoses usually numerous.
- Comedo-type necrosis may be present.
- Keratinizing or nonkeratinizing squamous-cell carcinoma is considered a basaloid squamous-cell carcinoma if more than half of the tumor is basaloid histology.
- Positive for squamous-cell carcinoma immunohistochemical markers such as p40.
- Negative for neuroendocrine immunohistochemical markers, but rare cases can be positive.

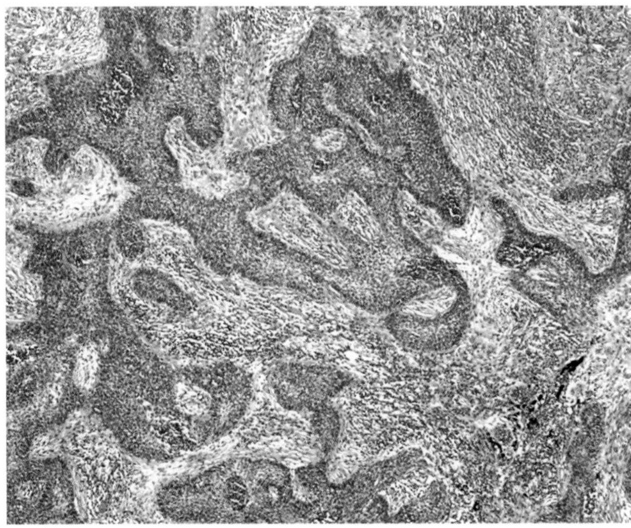

Figure 11.12 Low-power view of basaloid squamous-cell carcinoma has irregular nests of cells with relatively small cells with hyperchromatic nuclei and relatively scant cytoplasm and peripheral palisading.

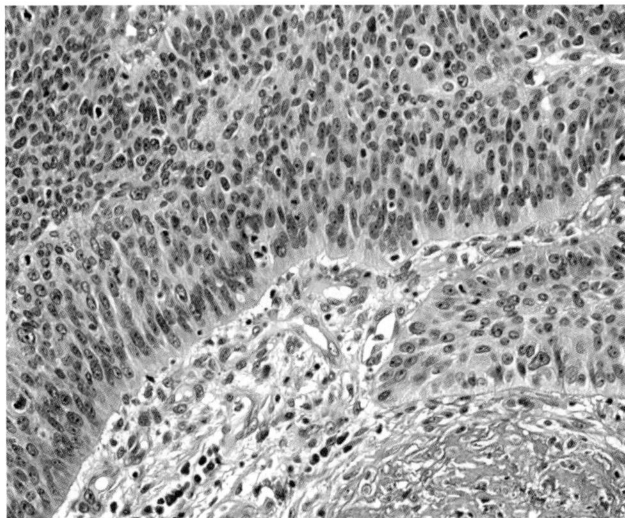

Figure 11.13 High-power view of basaloid squamous-cell carcinoma emphasizes the peripheral palisading.

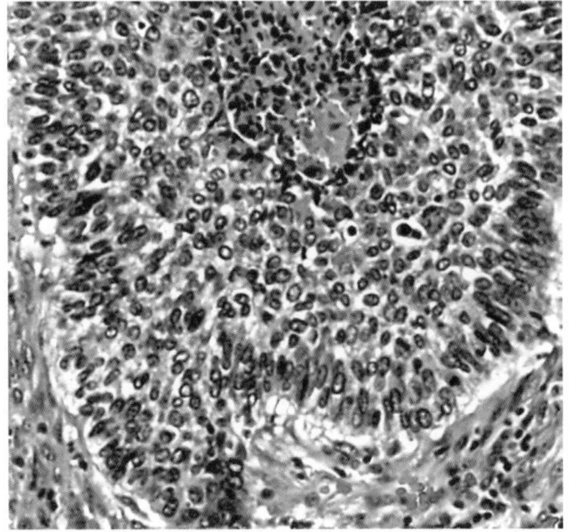

Figure 11.14 Focus of comedo-type necrosis is present in this high-power view of basaloid squamous-cell carcinoma.

Adenosquamous Carcinoma

12

Paloma del C. Monroig-Bosque
Ross A. Miller
Philip T. Cagle

Adenosquamous carcinoma is an uncommon form of non–small cell carcinoma associated with poor prognosis, smoking history, and generally the same clinical and imaging features found with other non–small cell carcinomas. Adenosquamous carcinoma has an adenocarcinoma histologic component distinct from a squamous-cell carcinoma histologic component consisting of at least 10% of each cell type within the same tumor.

CYTOLOGIC FEATURES

- Cytologic features of both adenocarcinoma and squamous-cell carcinoma may be present.
- Owing to sampling, cytologic features of only one of the histologic components may be present.

HISTOLOGIC FEATURES

- Combined adenocarcinoma and squamous-cell carcinoma histology in the same tumor consisting of at least 10% adenocarcinoma mixed with at least 10% squamous-cell carcinoma.
- The adenocarcinoma component can consist of any of the histologic subtypes of adenocarcinoma.
- The squamous-cell carcinoma component can consist of any of the histologic subtypes of squamous-cell carcinoma.
- The adenocarcinoma and squamous-cell carcinoma components may exist side by side in the same tumor or be intermixed within the same tumor.
- Adenocarcinoma component is positive for adenocarcinoma immunostain markers such as TTF-1.
- Squamous-cell carcinoma component is positive for squamous-cell carcinoma immunostain markers such as p40.
- Adenocarcinoma component may be positive for adenocarcinoma predictive biomarkers such as *EGFR*.

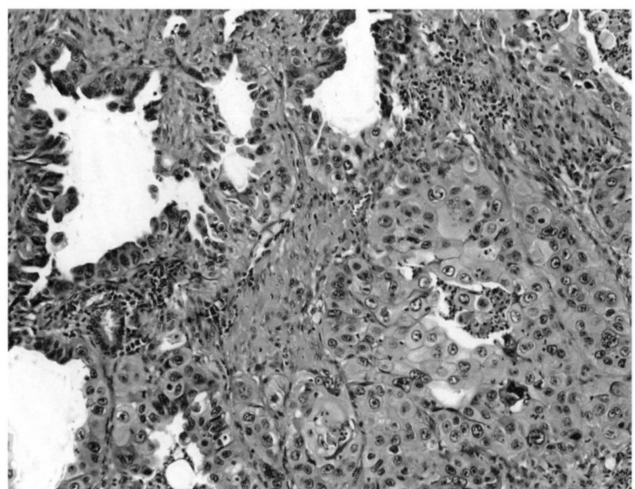

Figure 12.1 Adenosquamous carcinoma shows adenocarcinoma component with cuboidal cells lining lumens in the upper left and squamous-cell carcinoma with nests of cells with abundant eosinophilic cytoplasm and sharp cell borders in the *lower right*.

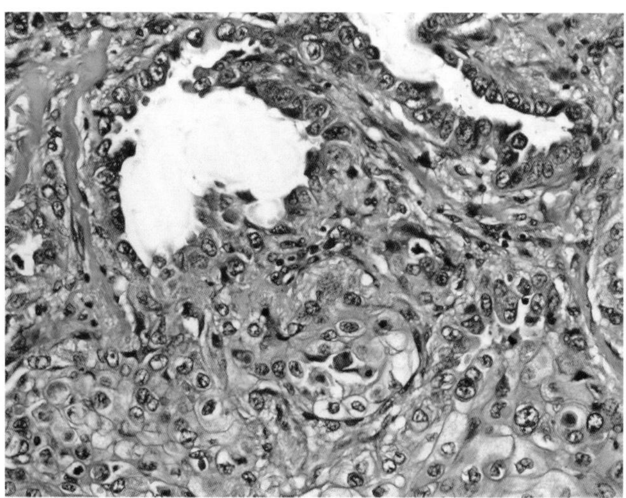

Figure 12.2 Adenosquamous carcinoma at slightly higher power view consists of a glandular adenocarcinoma component in the upper part of the field and nests of cells with abundant cytoplasm and sharp cell borders in the lower part of the field representing squamous-cell carcinoma.

13 Large-Cell Carcinoma

▶ Paloma del C. Monroig-Bosque
▶ Ross A. Miller
▶ Philip T. Cagle

Large-cell carcinomas lack histologic, histochemical, and immunohistochemical features diagnostic of other specific lung cancer cell types, such as adenocarcinoma, squamous-cell carcinoma, small-cell carcinoma, and large-cell neuroendocrine carcinoma. Therefore, the diagnosis of large-cell carcinoma is a diagnosis of exclusion. Most large-cell carcinomas are associated with a positive smoking history and generally share the same clinical and imaging features seen in other non–small cell carcinomas.

By criteria of the 2015 World Health Organization (WHO) Classification of Tumors of the Lung, large-cell carcinomas are non–small cell carcinomas that are negative for histologic criteria of adenocarcinoma, squamous-cell carcinoma, or other specific cell types; negative for mucin (histochemical marker of adenocarcinoma); and negative for immunohistochemical markers of adenocarcinoma (such as TTF-1), squamous-cell carcinoma (such as p40), and neuroendocrine cancers (if performance of neuroendocrine immunostains is warranted by the histology).

The 2015 WHO classification caused many tumors previously classified as large-cell carcinoma to be reclassified as solid adenocarcinoma or nonkeratinizing squamous-cell carcinoma based on the finding of a positive TTF-1 or p40 or other cell type–specific immunostain. These criteria are consistent with changes in the practice of pathology that had already been occurring for a decade. Besides reclassification of cell types on the basis of immunohistochemical features, large-cell neuroendocrine carcinoma, basaloid carcinoma, and lymphoepithelioma-like carcinoma were removed as subtypes of large-cell carcinoma and reclassified elsewhere in the 2015 WHO classification. In addition, clear cell features and rhabdoid features are no longer considered histologic variants of large-cell carcinoma. As a result, 10% to 25% of lung cancers in the past series were classified as large-cell carcinoma, whereas the 2015 WHO criteria have reduced large-cell carcinomas to only 1% to 2% of lung cancers.

A resection specimen must be thoroughly sampled to completely exclude a diagnosis of a specific lung cancer cell type and make a diagnosis of large-cell carcinoma. A small biopsy or cytology specimen does not provide a sufficient sample to exclude an adenocarcinoma, squamous-cell carcinoma, or other specific lung cancer cell types. Therefore, the diagnosis of "non–small cell carcinoma not otherwise specified" is used for small biopsy and cytology specimens, which lack clear cytologic, histochemical, and immunohistochemical diagnostic features of adenocarcinoma, squamous-cell carcinoma, small-cell carcinoma, or other neuroendocrine carcinomas.

Based on the 2015 World Health Organization Classification of Tumors of the Lung, a diagnosis of large-cell carcinoma may be made in one of several circumstances. All are non–small cell carcinomas that lack the histologic features of a specific cell type, but the reason for inability to further classify by immunostains varies. Most fulfill the current criteria for large-cell carcinoma and are "large-cell carcinoma with null immunohistochemical features," which are found to be negative for adenocarcinoma and squamous-cell carcinoma immunostain markers, such as TTF-1 and p40, respectively, after immunohistochemistry has been performed (mucin stains are also negative). Less often, when the results of the immunostains are ambiguous or equivocal (and mucin stains are negative), a diagnosis of "large-cell carcinoma with unclear immunohistochemical features" can be made. When no immunostains and no mucin stains are available for review, a diagnosis of "large-cell carcinoma with no stains available" is recommended.

CYTOLOGIC FEATURES

- Diagnosis of large-cell carcinoma cannot be made on small biopsy or cytology specimens because of insufficient sampling to rule out a specific cell type.
- Diagnosis of "non–small cell carcinoma not otherwise specified" is used for small biopsy and cytology specimens, which lack clear cytologic, histochemical, and immunohistochemical diagnostic features of a specific cell type.

HISTOLOGIC FEATURES

- Undifferentiated non–small cell carcinoma diagnosed on resection specimen.
- Sheets or nests of polygonal cells with moderately abundant cytoplasm and vesicular nuclei with prominent nucleoli.
- Large-cell carcinomas lack histologic features of adenocarcinoma, squamous-cell carcinoma, small-cell carcinoma, or other specific cell types.
- These lack mucin staining diagnostic of adenocarcinoma.
- Positive immunohistochemical staining for cytokeratins.
- Negative immunohistochemical staining for adenocarcinoma markers (TTF-1, napsin A), squamous-cell carcinomas markers (p40, p63, CK5/6), and neuroendocrine markers (synaptophysin, chromogranin, CD56).

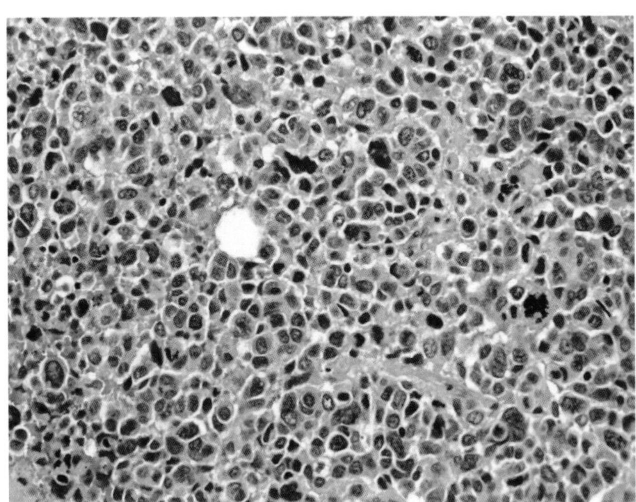

Figure 13.1 Low-power view of large-cell carcinoma consisting of sheets of pleomorphic cells with moderate cytoplasm. Tumor is negative for mucin and negative for immunohistochemical markers of specific cell types.

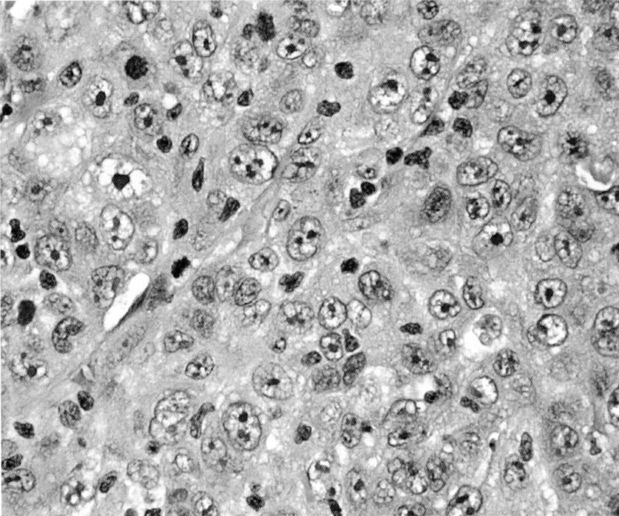

Figure 13.2 Higher power view of large-cell carcinoma shows pleomorphic cells with vesicular nuclei, prominent nucleoli, and moderate amounts of cytoplasm. Tumor is negative for mucin and negative for immunohistochemical markers of specific cell types.

Neuroendocrine Carcinomas

14

Part 1

Small-Cell Carcinoma

▸ Timothy C. Allen

Pulmonary small-cell carcinoma is a high-grade neuroendocrine carcinoma that makes up approximately 15% of primary lung cancers. Patients are typically smokers. Most tumors are central, and patients often present due to rapid tumor growth, extrapulmonary disease, and paraneoplastic syndromes. Malignant pleural and pericardial effusions are often seen. Small-cell carcinoma most commonly metastasizes to intrathoracic and supraclavicular lymph nodes, as well as bone, brain, liver, adrenal glands, and lung. Radiographically, patients often show bulky mediastinal lymphadenopathy. Because small-cell carcinoma is often diagnosed at the late clinical stage, surgical excision is usually not a therapeutic option. Grossly, small-cell carcinoma is a large central mass, with nodal involvement, that compresses or obstructs peribronchial structures. Tumor frequently spreads along bronchi and involves lymphatics. Differential diagnosis includes lymphoma and large-cell neuroendocrine carcinoma, as well as typical carcinoid tumor and atypical carcinoid tumor, small-cell squamous-cell carcinoma, Ewing sarcoma, and metastatic carcinoma. Prognosis is extremely poor, with a median overall survival of approximately 12 months.

CYTOLOGIC FEATURES

- Nests of cells and single tumor cells with bare nuclei or scant cytoplasm, with occasional rosettes.
- Small tumor cells are round, oval, or spindle-shaped, with dense finely granular "salt and pepper" chromatin, inconspicuous nucleoli, and nuclear molding.
- Tumor cells are usually two to three times as large as normal lymphocytes.
- Background of necrotic debris.

HISTOLOGIC FEATURES

- Sheets and nests of small tumor cells, with nesting, trabecular, and pseudopapillary patterns and organoid pattern with rosettes and peripheral palisading.
- Peripheral palisading may be seen.
- Tumor cells are round, oval, or spindle-shaped, and crush artifact may be prominent.
- Nuclei have dense finely granular "salt and pepper" chromatin with inconspicuous nucleoli.
- Nuclear molding is a characteristic of small-cell carcinoma.

- Cytoplasm is scant, and cell margins are inapparent.
- Tumor cells are approximately three times the size of a normal lymphocyte.
- Necrosis is frequently present and may be prominent.
- Mitotic figures are abundant, at least 10 mitoses per 2 mm^2.
- Transbronchial biopsies frequently have conspicuous crush artifact; however, larger, better preserved specimens often show better preserved tumor cells.
- Tumor cells are typically immunopositive with TTF-1; keratin stains such as CK7 and CAM5.2, with a characteristic punctate cytoplasmic staining pattern; and one or more neuroendocrine markers, including chromogranin, synaptophysin, and CD56 (NCAM).
- Tumor cells are typically immunonegative with CK20.

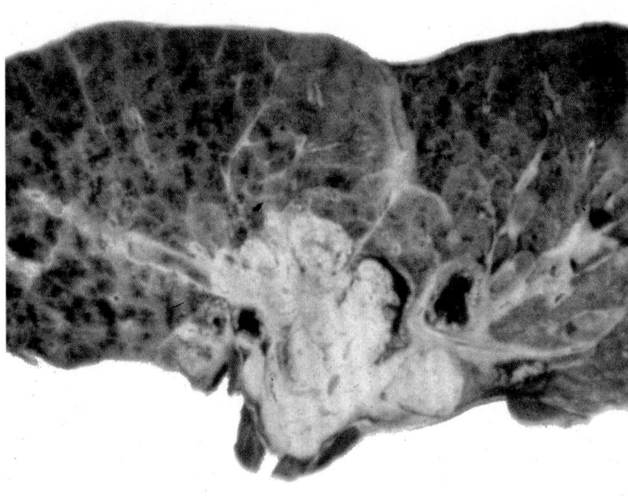

Figure 14.1 Gross image of small-cell carcinoma showing central tumor mass.

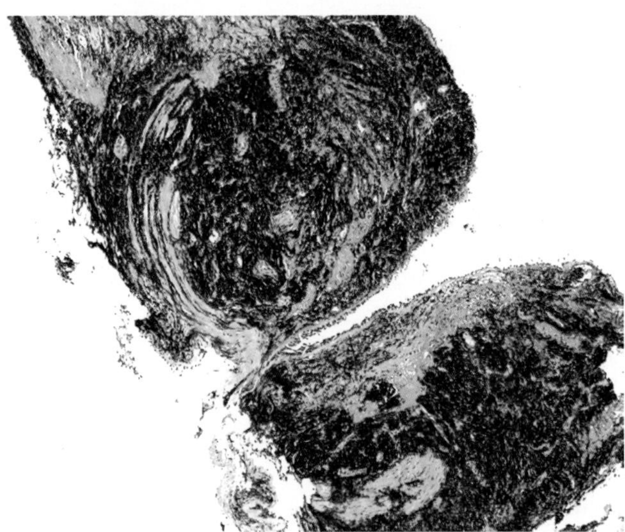

Figure 14.2 Small transbronchial biopsies often show significant crush artifact and should be interpreted cautiously.

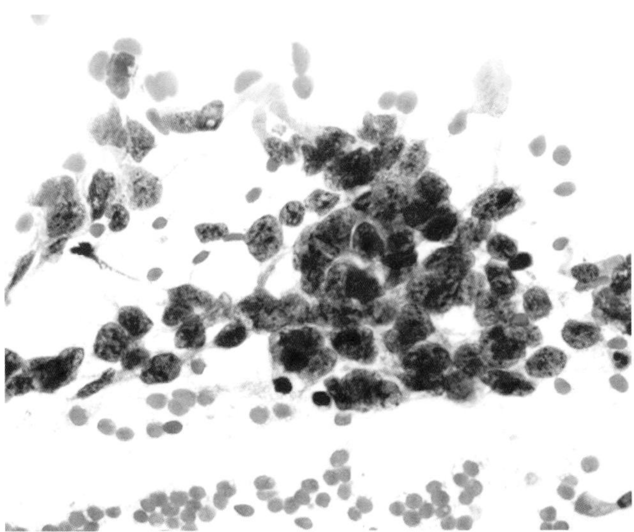

Figure 14.3 Cytologically, there is a cluster of small tumor cells with nuclear molding; tumor cells have round to oval nuclei containing finely granular "salt and pepper" chromatin and little to no cytoplasm.

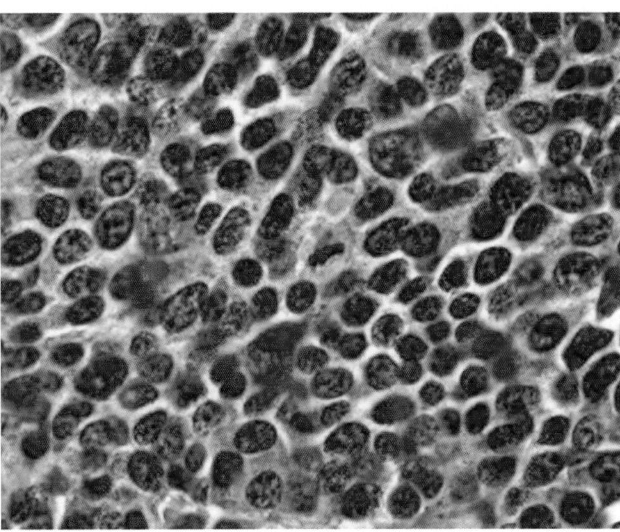

Figure 14.4 Mitoses are frequent in small-cell carcinoma.

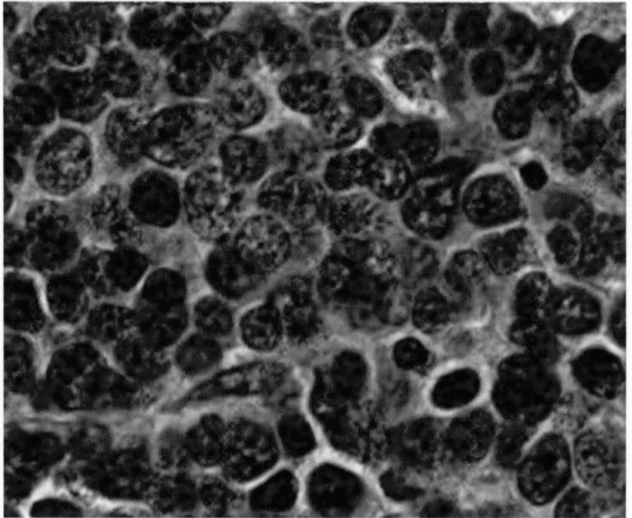

Figure 14.5 Small-cell carcinoma shows dense finely granular "salt and pepper" chromatin with occasional inconspicuous nucleoli, nuclear molding, and scant cytoplasm with inapparent cell margins.

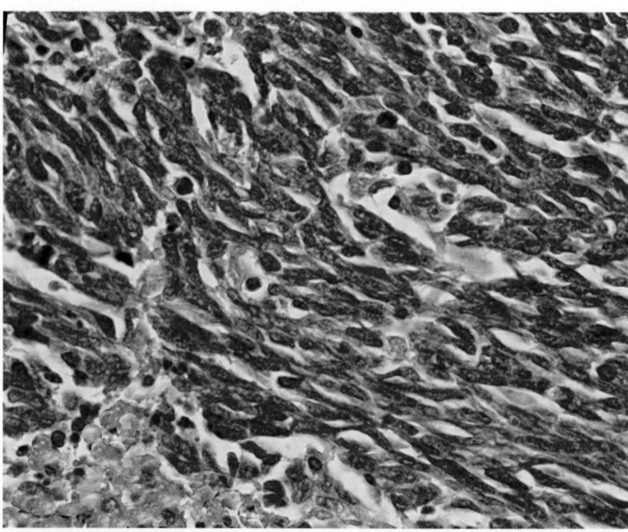

Figure 14.6 Small-cell carcinoma may have a spindled pattern; note tumor necrosis at the *bottom left*.

Part 2

Carcinoid Tumor

Timothy C. Allen

Pulmonary carcinoid tumor is a low-grade neuroendocrine carcinoma, characterized by having less than 2 mitotic figures per 2 mm^2 and without necrosis. They are uncommon, accounting for less than 1% of lung cancers, and are not smoking-related. Approximately two-thirds of carcinoid tumors arise in the central airways, and those patients may present with obstructive symptoms. Carcinoid tumors are usually indolent; however, they may spread, metastasize, and be fatal. Carcinoid tumors usually spread via lymphatics or blood vessels, and metastases often involve bone, liver, and mediastinal and hilar lymph nodes. Grossly, central carcinoid tumors are well-circumscribed tumors lying within the large airways or trachea, either pedunculated or sessile, and may fill the lumen and cause resultant postobstructive pneumonia. Differential diagnosis includes atypical carcinoid tumor, large-cell neuroendocrine carcinoma, small-cell carcinoma, metastatic carcinoid tumor from another primary location, and metastatic lobular breast carcinoma. Prognosis is good, with a 5-year survival of approximately 90%.

CYTOLOGIC FEATURES

- Single cells and small clusters of tumor cells, with uniform round nuclei and abundant cytoplasm.
- Some tumor cells may be plasmacytoid, and some may have little or no cytoplasm.
- No mitotic figures and no necrosis are seen.

HISTOLOGIC FEATURES

- Carcinoid tumor may be arranged in trabecular, spindle-cell, and organoid patterns and may show papillary, follicular, pseudoglandular, and rosette formations.
- Tumor cells are generally uniform with eosinophilic cytoplasm; however, cytoplasm may be clear, granular, or oncocytic.

- Carcinoid tumor may show areas of atypia, but it is not a criterion for distinguishing typical carcinoid from atypical carcinoid.
- Nuclei show finely granular chromatin with small or no nucleoli; however, prominent nucleoli may occur.
- Stroma is usually vascular; with dense hyaline collagen, metaplastic cartilage, bone, or amyloid-like stroma is seen.
- Tumors typically are immunopositive with cytokeratins and neuroendocrine markers, including chromogranin, synaptophysin, and CD56 (NCAM).
- TTF-1 stain is typically negative; however, some peripheral carcinoid tumors may show positivity.
- Ki-67 immunostain is not currently suggested for differentiating carcinoid tumor from atypical carcinoid tumor.

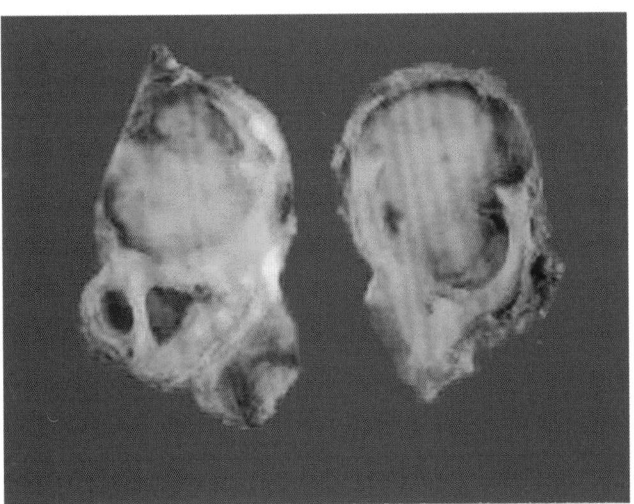

Figure 14.7 Gross image of typical carcinoid tumor showing tumor occluding a large bronchus.

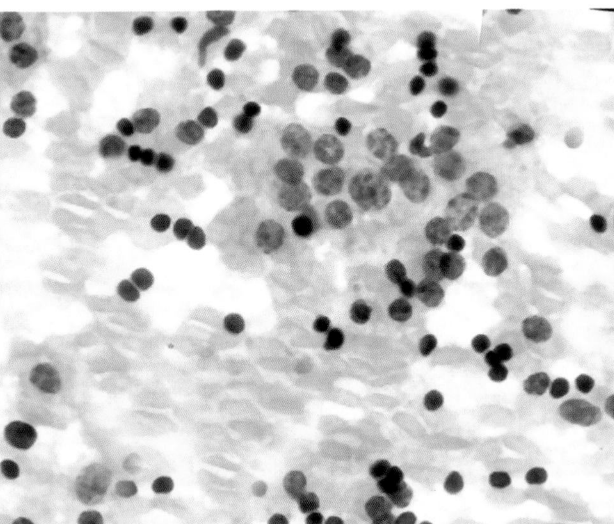

Figure 14.8 Cytology of typical carcinoid tumor showing single tumor cells and a small cluster of tumor cells, with uniform round nuclei, as well as scattered lymphocytes; no necrosis or mitoses are present.

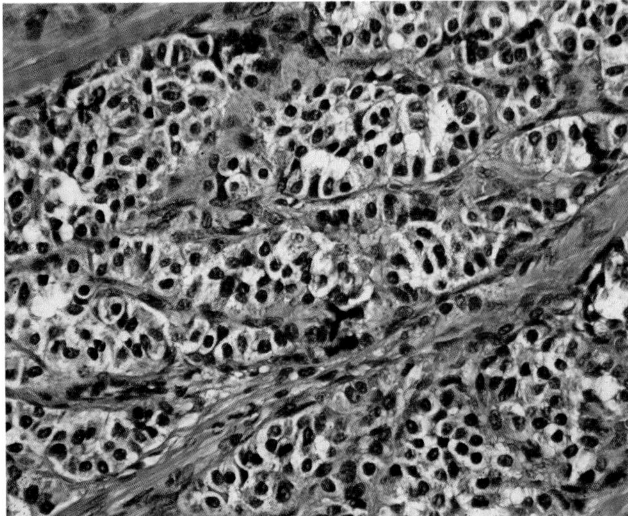

Figure 14.9 Typical carcinoid tumor displaying its classic organoid pattern.

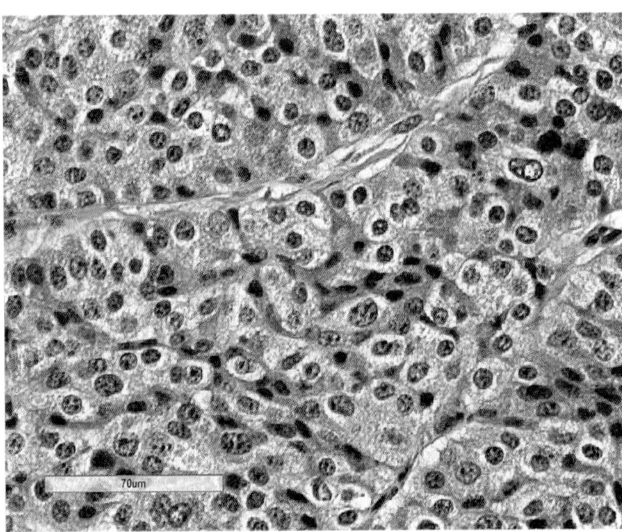

Figure 14.10 Typical carcinoid tumor cells with intervening delicate fibrous stroma.

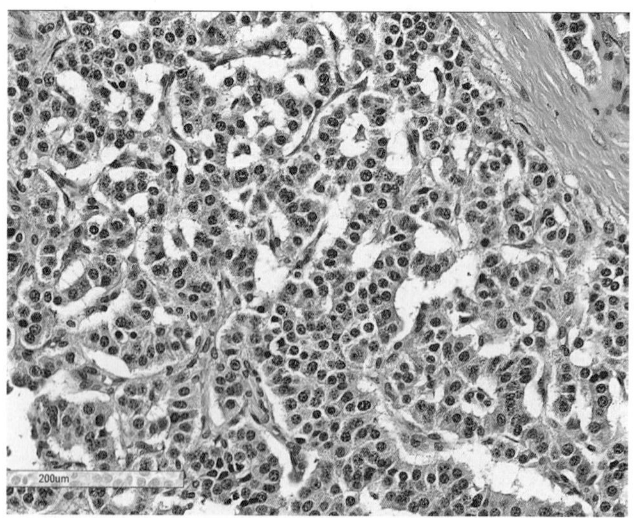

Figure 14.11 Typical carcinoid tumor displaying a trabecular pattern.

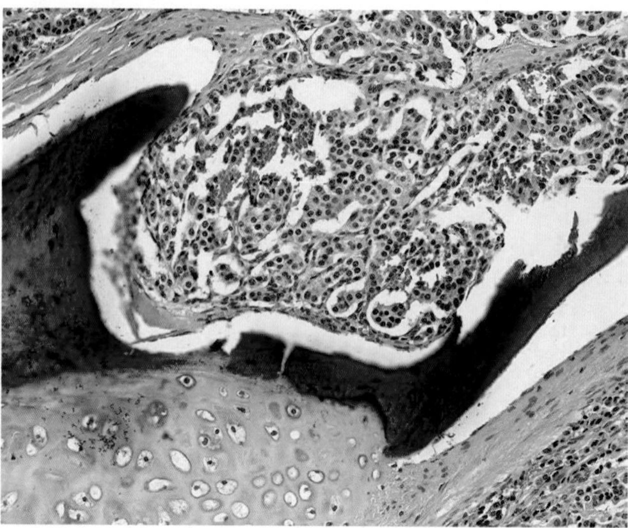

Figure 14.12 Typical carcinoid tumor invading bronchial cartilage.

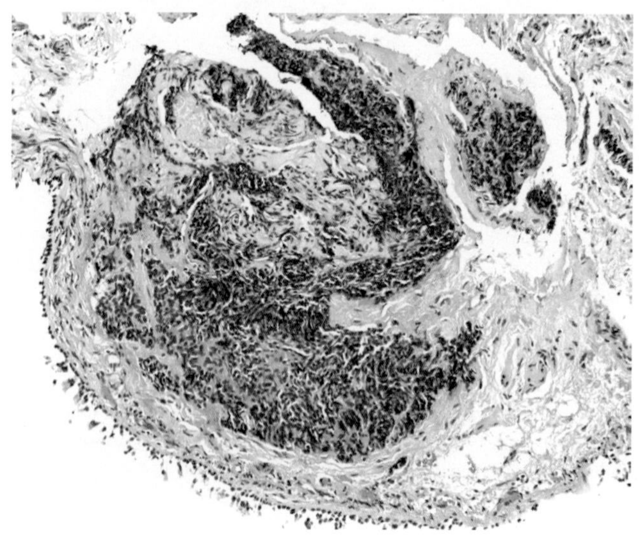

Figure 14.13 Care must be taken in diagnosing typical carcinoid tumor, as biopsy crush artifact can mimic small-cell carcinoma.

Part 3

Atypical Carcinoid Tumor

Timothy C. Allen

Atypical carcinoid tumor is an intermediate-grade neuroendocrine carcinoma characterized by 2 to 10 mitotic figures per 2 mm^2, with or without necrotic foci. Atypical carcinoid tumors are clinically similar to carcinoid tumors; however, atypical carcinoid tumors are often larger and are more often peripheral lesions. Also, metastatic disease is more common with atypical carcinoid tumors than carcinoid tumors. Prognosis is poorer with atypical carcinoid tumor than with carcinoid tumor; 5 year survival is approximately 60%. Differential diagnosis is similar to carcinoid tumor.

CYTOLOGIC FEATURES

- Atypical carcinoid tumors are cytologically similar to carcinoid tumors.
- Necrosis may be seen.

HISTOLOGIC FEATURES

- Atypical carcinoid tumors are histologically similar to carcinoid tumors, except that necrosis may be seen and the mitotic rate is 2 to 10 mitoses per 2 mm^2.
- Mitotic count is based on the average of three groups of 10 high-power fields from the most mitotically active areas.
- Necrosis may involve a few cells or the central area of an organoid nest; it may occasionally be widespread and infarct-like.
- Atypical carcinoid tumor shows an immunostaining pattern similar to carcinoid tumor, except that atypical carcinoid tumor is more likely to be positive with TTF-1.

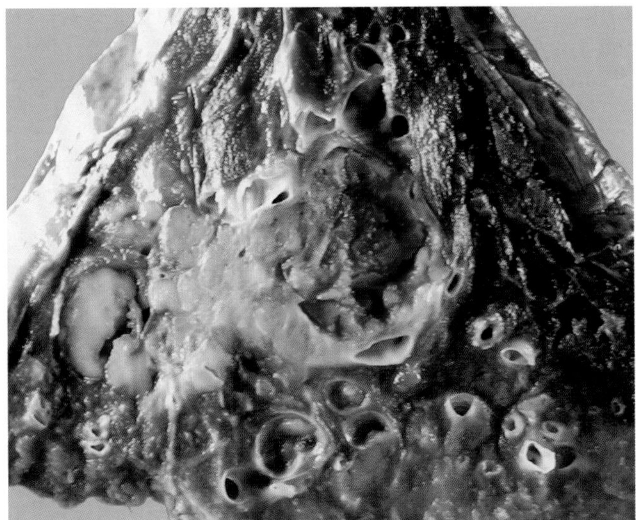

Figure 14.14 Gross image of atypical carcinoid tumor with tumor obstructing and extending from a bronchus, with postobstructive pneumonia and bronchiectasis.

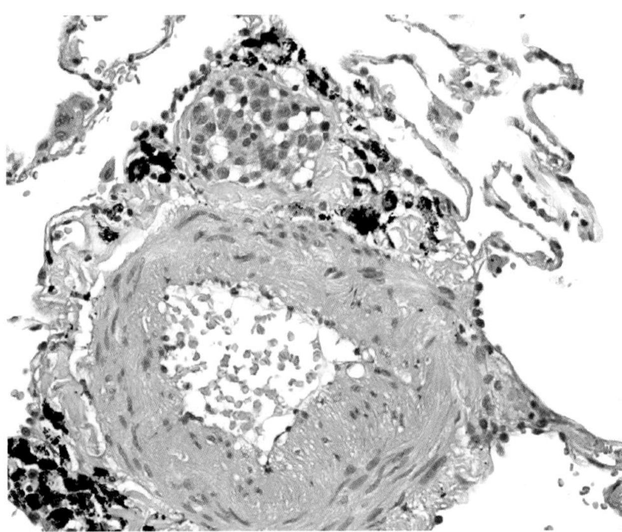

Figure 14.15 Metastatic atypical carcinoid tumor expanding a lymphatic space.

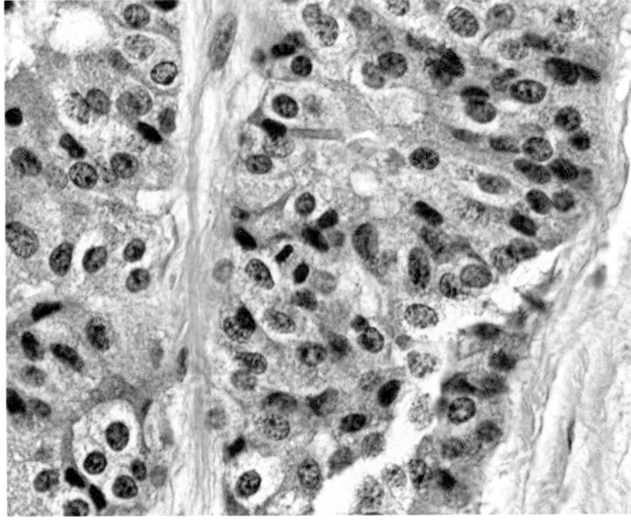

Figure 14.16 Atypical carcinoid tumor with mitosis.

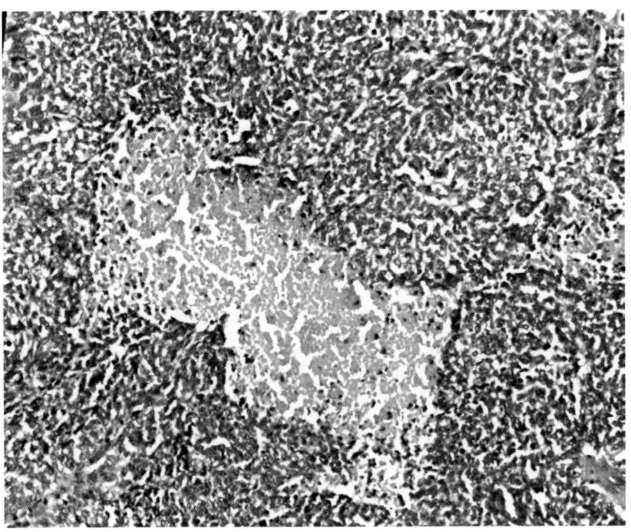

Figure 14.17 Atypical carcinoid tumor with an area of necrosis.

Part 4

Large-Cell Neuroendocrine Carcinoma

▶ Timothy C. Allen

Pulmonary large-cell neuroendocrine carcinoma is a high-grade neuroendocrine carcinoma, which is characterized by a non–small cell carcinoma, which shows neuroendocrine features, such as peripheral palisading and rosette formation, and shows immunopositivity with neuroendocrine markers. Patients are smokers who often present with dyspnea, cough, and chest pain. Patients may present with late-stage disease and may have weight loss and fatigue. Patients also may have mediastinal disease and exhibit superior vena cava syndrome or vocal cord paralysis. Most are peripheral, but approximately 20% are central and may present with postobstructive pneumonia. Large-cell neuroendocrine carcinoma patients usually do not develop paraneoplastic syndromes. Grossly, tumors are typically well-circumscribed large peripheral upper lobe masses with hemorrhage and necrosis on cut section. Cytologic features are those of a non–small cell carcinoma and are often nonspecific. Prognosis is generally poor and similar to that of small-cell carcinoma.

HISTOLOGIC FEATURES

- Non–small cell lung carcinoma with neuroendocrine features including organoid or trabecular patterns, rosette formation, and peripheral palisading.
- Tumor cells are typically large and polygonal, with vesicular nuclei, prominent nucleoli, and abundant cytoplasm.
- Mitoses are frequent, greater than 10 mitoses per 2 mm^2, and are typically much greater, averaging 70 mitoses per 10 high-power fields.
- Necrosis may be seen within the tumor cell nests.
- By definition, tumor cells are immunopositive with neuroendocrine markers, such as chromogranin, synaptophysin, and CD56 (NCAM).
- Tumor cells are typically immunopositive with CK7 and pankeratin.
- Approximately 50% of cases show TTF-1 immunopositivity.
- Tumors may show combined large-cell neuroendocrine carcinoma and adenocarcinoma or squamous-cell carcinoma.

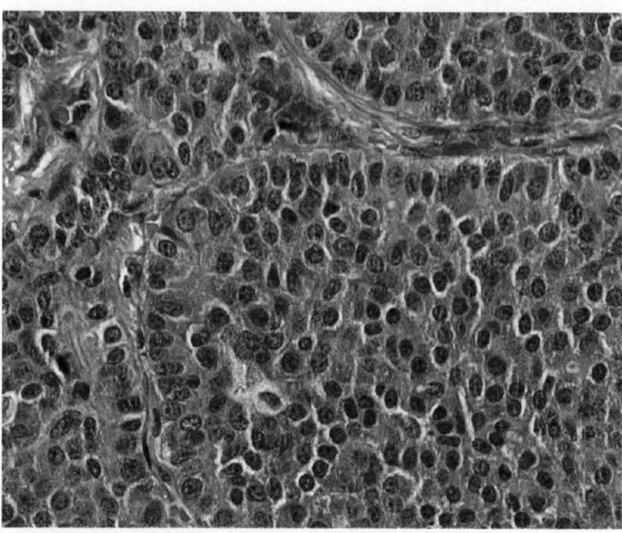

Figure 14.18 Large-cell neuroendocrine carcinoma with organoid pattern and peripheral palisading.

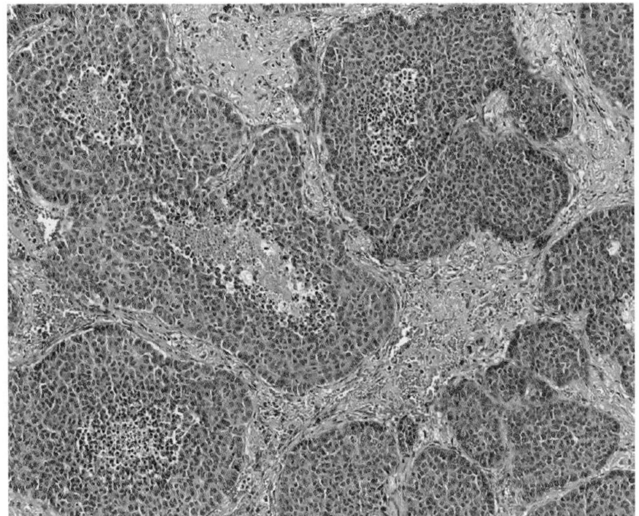

Figure 14.19 Tumor nests show areas of central necrosis.

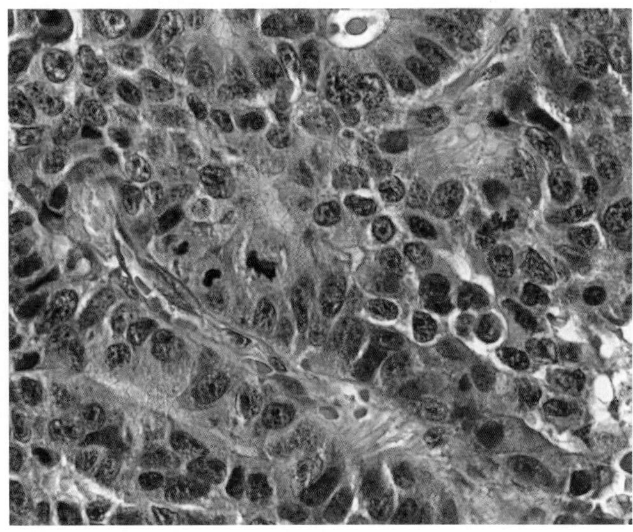

Figure 14.20 Mitotic figures are frequent in large-cell neuroendocrine carcinoma.

Sarcomatoid Carcinomas

15

Part 1

Carcinosarcoma

▶ Timothy C. Allen

Carcinosarcoma is a rare, aggressive lung cancer, predominantly occurring in men with a smoking history. It has a poor prognosis. Carcinosarcoma is made up of a combination of a non–small cell lung carcinoma component, usually adenocarcinoma or squamous-cell carcinoma, and sarcoma, including osteosarcomatous, chondrosarcomatous, or rhabdomyosarcomatous components. Carcinosarcoma is typically a central tumor, which shows necrosis and hemorrhage grossly. Cytology is typically nondiagnostic; rarely, cytology specimens contain both components. Metastatic carcinosarcoma may be made up of the carcinomatous component, the sarcomatous component, or both components.

HISTOLOGIC FEATURES

- A combination of non–small cell carcinoma and sarcoma containing heterologous elements.
- The non–small cell lung carcinoma component is usually adenocarcinoma or squamous-cell carcinoma.
- Approximately one-fifth may contain clear cell adenocarcinoma or high-grade fetal adenocarcinoma.
- Heterologous sarcomatous elements include rhabdomyosarcoma, chondrosarcoma, and osteosarcoma; combinations of these may occur.
- Rarely, angiosarcoma and liposarcoma may make up the sarcomatous component.
- Immunostains highlight carcinomatous and sarcomatous differentiation.
- The non–small cell component is typically positive with CK7, TTF-1, napsin A in adenocarcinoma, and CK5/6, p63, p40 in squamous-cell carcinoma.
- The sarcomatous component is typically positive with desmin in the chondrosarcomatous component and myosin in the rhabdomyosarcomatous component.

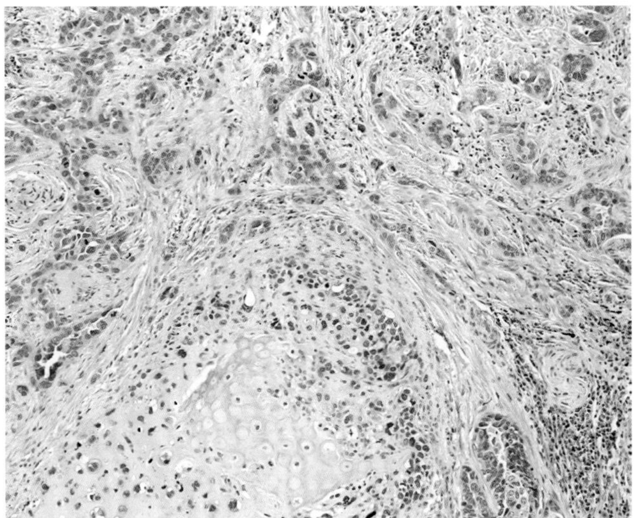

Figure 15.1 Carcinosarcoma with a combination of adenocarcinoma and chondrosarcoma.

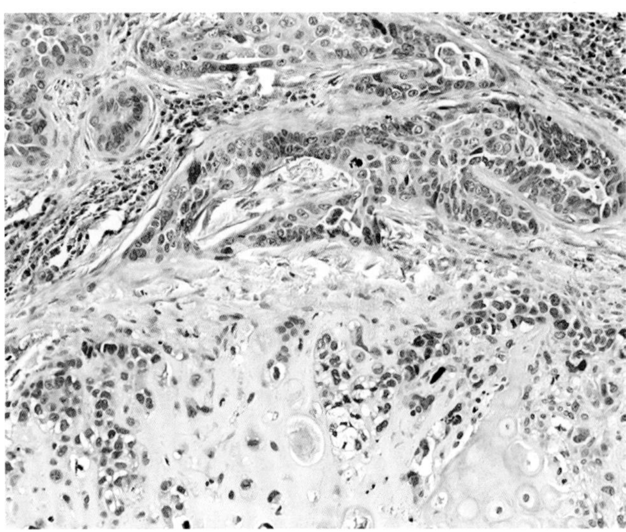

Figure 15.2 Higher power showing adenocarcinoma abutting chondrosarcoma.

Part 2

Pulmonary Blastoma

Timothy C. Allen and Yasmeen M. Butt

Pulmonary blastoma, a rare, clinically aggressive, biphasic lung carcinoma, has no sex predilection and most commonly arises in adult smokers in the fifth decade. It has a poor prognosis and typically spreads in a manner similar to other non–small cell lung cancers. It is made up of fetal adenocarcinoma and primitive mesenchymal stroma, with primitive epithelial and mesenchymal components resembling embryonic lung. Both the epithelial and mesenchymal components are malignant. Blastomas usually arise as large, well-circumscribed, unencapsulated, peripheral masses, often with satellite lesions. Approximately half of cases have associated pleural effusions. On cut section, necrosis and hemorrhage can be seen frequently. Differential diagnosis includes metastasis, fetal adenocarcinoma, pleuropulmonary blastoma, biphasic synovial sarcoma, and malignant mixed Mullerian tumor. Differentiating pulmonary blastoma from fetal adenocarcinoma is important, as pulmonary blastoma is generally worse than fetal adenocarcinoma.

CYTOLOGIC FEATURES

- Small, uniform columnar cells with supranuclear and subnuclear vacuolization and small nuclei representing fetal adenocarcinoma are intermixed with small, elongated to oval stromal cells. There may be a "tigroid background" or bubbly glycogen due to vacuole rupture.

HISTOPATHOLOGIC FEATURES

- Pulmonary blastomas are biphasic and contain both a malignant epithelial component and a malignant mesenchymal component.
- The epithelial component is made up of branching glands lined by columnar cells with small uniform nuclei, containing glycogen-filled vacuoles, reminiscent of low-grade fetal adenocarcinoma.

- Approximately half to two-thirds of pulmonary blastomas contain squamous morules.
- Pleomorphic areas with high-grade fetal adenocarcinoma or conventional adenocarcinoma may occur.
- The mesenchymal component of pulmonary blastoma consists of histologically primitive, blastema-like spindle to oval cells with a high nuclear to cytoplasmic ratio and occasional bizarre giant cells, lying within a myxoid stroma.
- Foci of adult-type sarcoma may occur, with up to one-fourth of pulmonary blastomas showing heterologous (differentiated) elements, such as osteosarcomatous, rhabdomyosarcomatous, or chondrosarcomatous elements.
- The epithelial component is typically immunopositive with AE1/AE3, CK7, TTF-1, and CEA and may show focal staining with neuroendocrine markers.
- The mesenchymal component is typically immunopositive with muscle specific actin and vimentin and may be focally immunopositive with AE1/AE3.

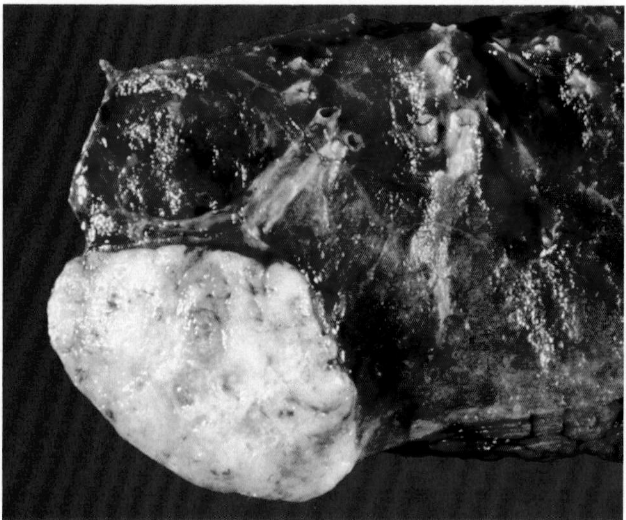

Figure 15.3 Pulmonary blastoma grossly showing a large peripheral unencapsulated fleshy mass.

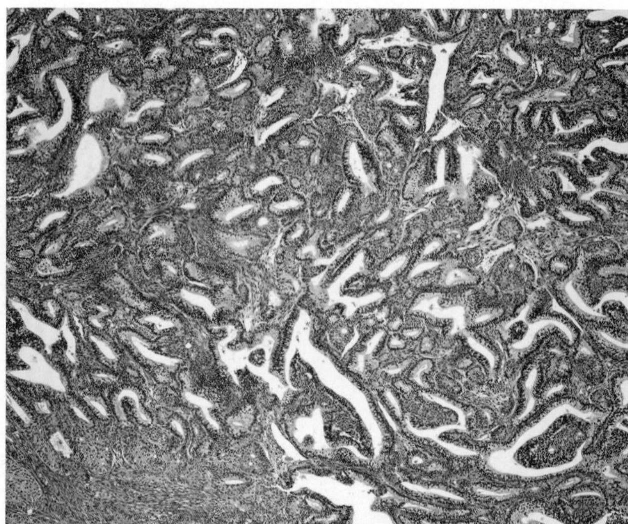

Figure 15.4 Pulmonary blastoma showing branching glands within a mesenchymal stroma.

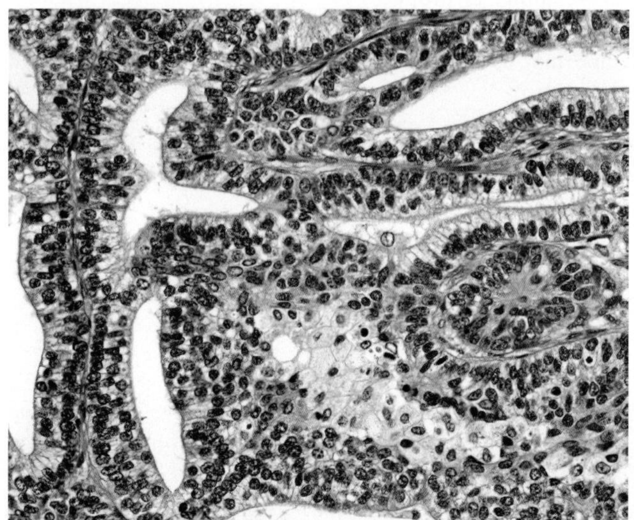

Figure 15.5 Epithelial component contains glands with supranuclear and subnuclear vacuoles, reminiscent of fetal adenocarcinoma.

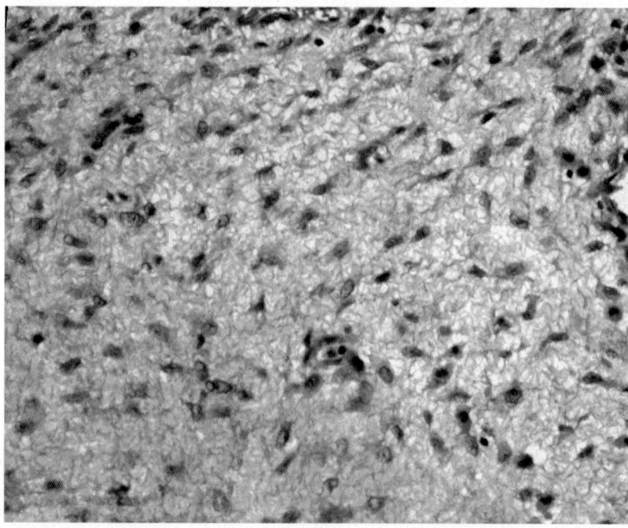

Figure 15.6 Primitive spindle-cell mesenchymal component with myxoid stroma and a malignant glandular component.

Part 3

Pleomorphic Carcinoma

▸ Timothy C. Allen

Pleomorphic carcinoma is a rare, aggressive lung cancer, defined as a poorly differentiated adenocarcinoma or squamous-cell carcinoma, or undifferentiated non–small cell carcinoma, for which 10% or more of the tumor is made up of spindle cells or giant cells; or it is defined as a carcinoma composed entirely of spindle cells and giant cells, without an observable carcinomatous element. Because of the need for complete examination of the tumor to meet the criteria for this diagnosis, pleomorphic carcinoma can only be diagnosed on a resected lung cancer. Most patients have a smoking history. Grossly, pleomorphic adenocarcinoma is typically a large, peripheral, often upper lobe neoplasm, which often shows pleural invasion. Pleomorphic carcinoma is, by definition, not diagnosable by cytology. Metastatic and primary melanoma and sarcoma must be considered as differential diagnoses.

HISTOLOGIC FEATURES

- Pleomorphic carcinoma consists of adenocarcinoma, squamous-cell carcinoma, or undifferentiated carcinoma within which there is a component composed of spindle cell or giant cells, comprising at least 10% of the tumor; or it is a carcinoma composed entirely of spindle cells and giant cells, without an observable carcinomatous element.
- The giant-cell or spindle-cell component may be admixed within the carcinomatous component.
- Pleomorphic carcinomas may be made up of purely a spindle-cell component or a giant-cell component, termed *spindle-cell carcinoma* and *giant-cell carcinoma*, respectively.
- Spindle-cell carcinoma consists of malignant spindle cells with storiform or fascicular patterns, without a differentiated carcinomatous component.
- Giant-cell carcinoma consists of typically discohesive malignant pleomorphic giant cells, which may include multinucleated giant cells.
- Giant cells have abundant eosinophilic cytoplasm, may have bizarre nuclei, and may exhibit emperipolesis.
- Immunostains assist in highlighting the different components; the spindle-cell and giant-cell components are typically positive with fascin and vimentin and show variable positivity with carcinoma markers, such as CK5/6, TTF-1, and napsin A .

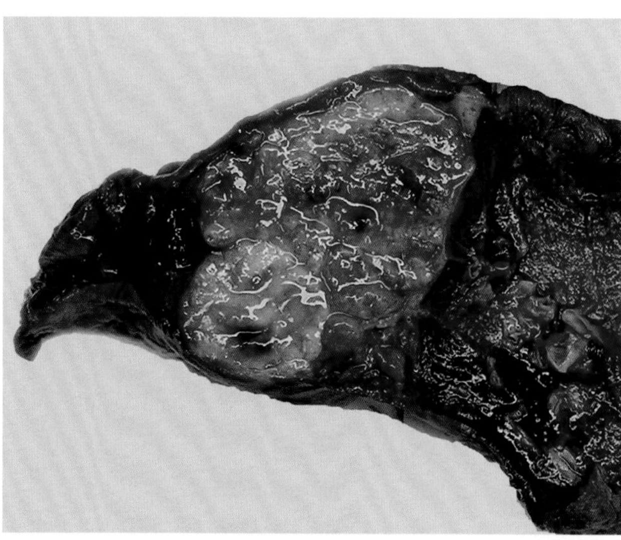

Figure 15.7 Gross image of pleomorphic carcinoma showing a large, well-circumscribed peripheral mass.

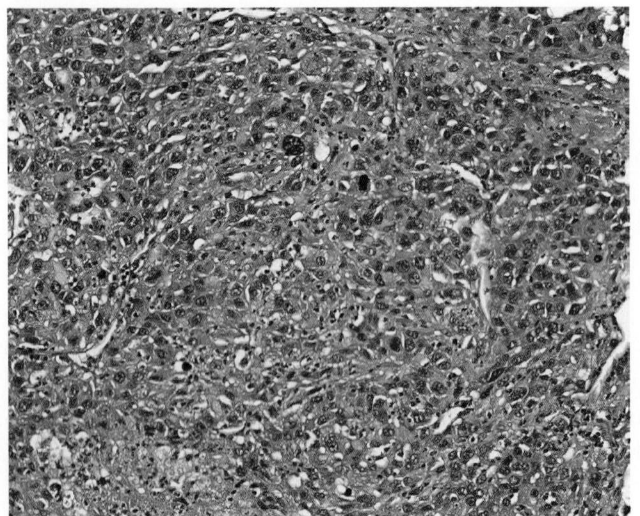

Figure 15.8 Pleomorphic carcinoma showing a sheet of tumor cells composed entirely of spindle cells and giant cells, without an observable carcinomatous element.

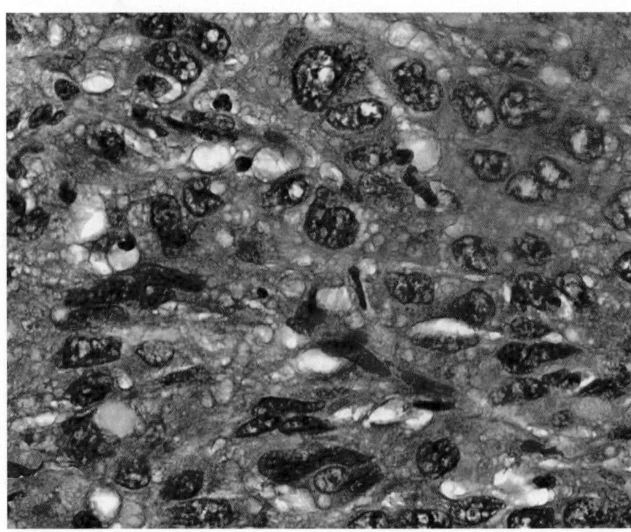

Figure 15.9 Higher power of pleomorphic carcinoma showing spindle cells admixed with giant cells.

Salivary Gland–Type Cancers

16

Part 1

Adenoid Cystic Carcinoma

Timothy C. Allen

Pulmonary adenoid cystic carcinoma (ACC) is a rare, endobronchial, exophytic (polypoid or intraluminal), or endophytic, epithelial tumor that is histologically similar to ACC of the salivary glands. ACC is generally a well-circumscribed endobronchial mass that histologically demonstrates most commonly cribriform pattern, as well as tubular and solid growth patterns. As a slow-growing tumor, ACC often contains no necrosis, mitotic figures, or angiolymphatic invasion. ACC generally infiltrates along the tracheobronchial wall and shows perineural invasion. ACC is characteristically immunopositive for S-100, actin, calponin, and CAM5.2.

CYTOLOGIC FEATURES

- ACC contains epithelial cells, generally uniform small cells with a high nuclear to cytoplasm ratio, oval regular nuclei, and characteristic hyaline eosinophilic or myxoid stroma.

HISTOLOGIC FEATURES

- Exophytic (polypoid or intraluminal) or endophytic, soft, tan, well-circumscribed mass, typically approximately 1 to 4 cm.
- Cribriform, tubular, and solid growth patterns.
- Hyalinized, sclerotic, or myxoid basement membrane-like material is deposited in the lumens of cribriform cylinders or tubules.
- ACC often infiltrates tracheobronchial wall and shows perineural invasion. Generally immunopositive for S-100, actin, calponin, and CAM5.2.

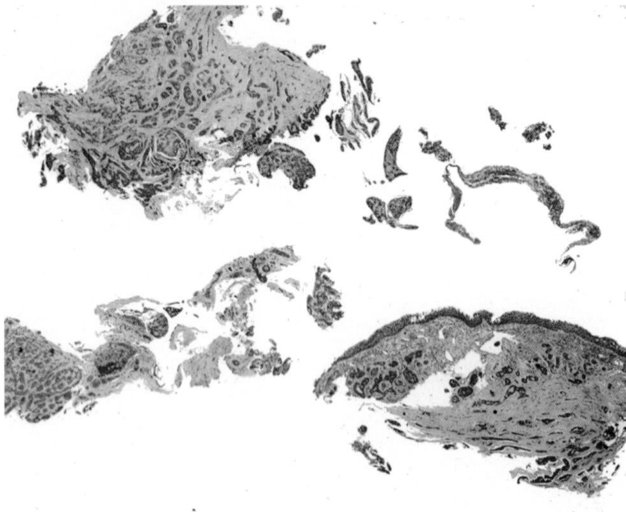

Figure 16.1 Biopsy specimen containing pulmonary ACC; the central tumor is frequently amenable to biopsy diagnosis.

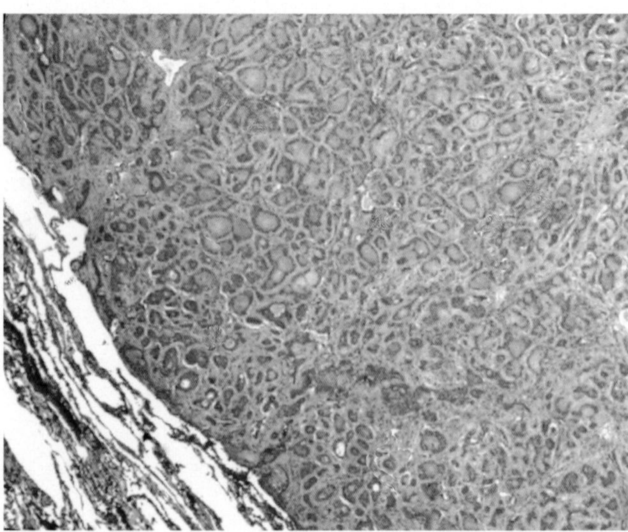

Figure 16.2 Low-power view of ACC with predominantly cribriform and tubular pattern, and loose myxoid stroma; this tumor mass compresses surrounding lung parenchyma.

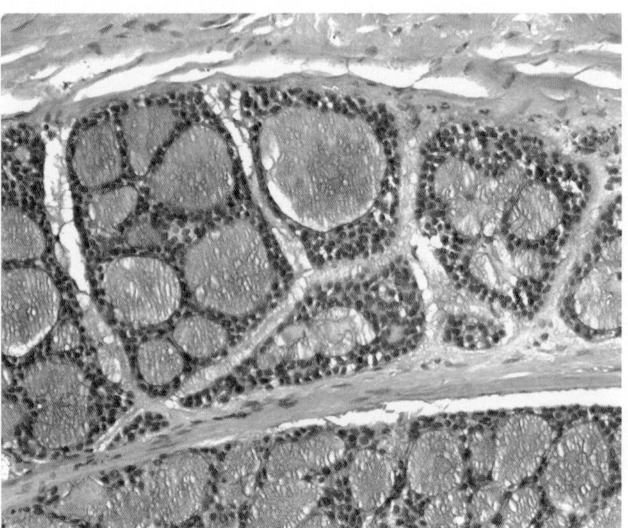

Figure 16.3 Higher power of ACC showing cylindrical hyalinized matrix surrounded by small oval cells with scant cytoplasm.

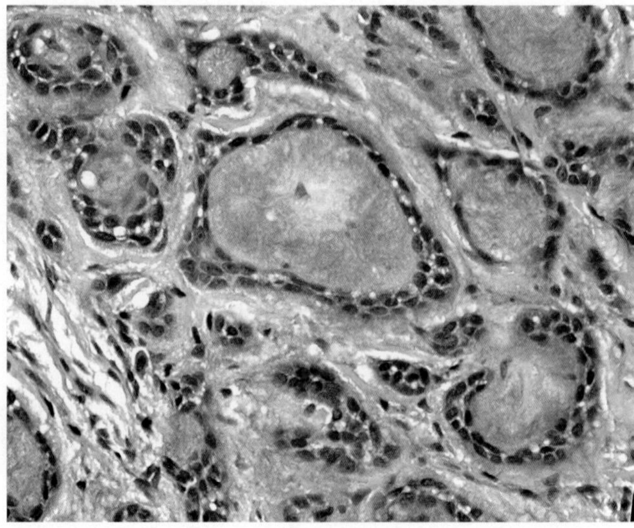

Figure 16.4 High-power view of ACC highlighting the cylindrical mucinous matrix surrounded by small hyperchromatic oval cells with scant cytoplasm.

Part 2

Mucoepidermoid Carcinoma

▸ Timothy C. Allen

Morphologically similar to mucoepidermoid carcinoma of salivary gland origin, mucoepidermoid carcinoma of the lung is uncommon, accounting for fewer than 1% of primary lung cancers, and arises from the submucosal bronchial glands. Mucoepidermoid carcinoma is composed of varying mixtures of mucinous glandular cells, squamoid cells, and intermediate cells. It is classified as either high-grade or low-grade mucoepidermoid carcinoma based on its histologic appearance.

Low-grade mucoepidermoid carcinomas typically have prominent cystic areas. Solid areas are composed of glands and small cysts lined by mucinous cells and columnar cells. In low-grade tumors, the mucinous cells have mild cytologic atypia and rare mitoses. Typically intermixed with the mucinous cells are sheets of nonkeratinizing squamoid cells and oval intermediate cells with eosinophilic cytoplasm. The stroma tends to be myxoid with focal hyalinization.

High-grade mucoepidermoid carcinoma generally shows areas of solid growth composed mostly of squamoid and intermediate cells with a lesser glandular component. The cells show increased cytologic atypia and mitotic figures, and tumor necrosis is more prominent. Despite some resemblance to adenosquamous carcinoma, keratinization and squamous pearl formation are not expected in high-grade mucoepidermoid carcinomas.

HISTOLOGIC FEATURES

- Exophytic mass, with smooth or papillary contours, soft, cystic, solid, and mucoid, approximately 0.5 to 6 cm.
- Low-grade mucoepidermoid carcinomas have abundant mucinous cysts and predominantly bland glandular components with sheets of squamoid cells, rare mitoses, and mild cytologic atypia.
- High-grade mucoepidermoid carcinomas have sheets of squamoid and intermediate cells with fewer glandular components, frequent mitotic figures, moderate cytologic atypia, and necrosis.

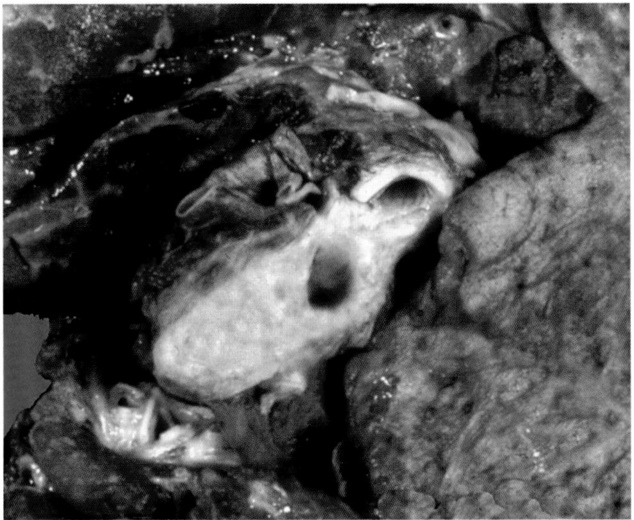

Figure 16.5 Gross image of pulmonary mucoepidermoid carcinoma involving a large airway.

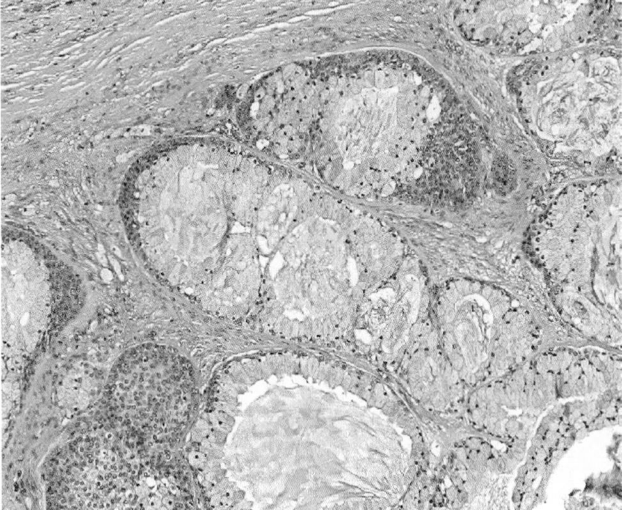

Figure 16.6 Low-grade mucoepidermoid carcinoma showing mucinous epithelium with prominent cystic changes and associated nonkeratinizing squamous cells.

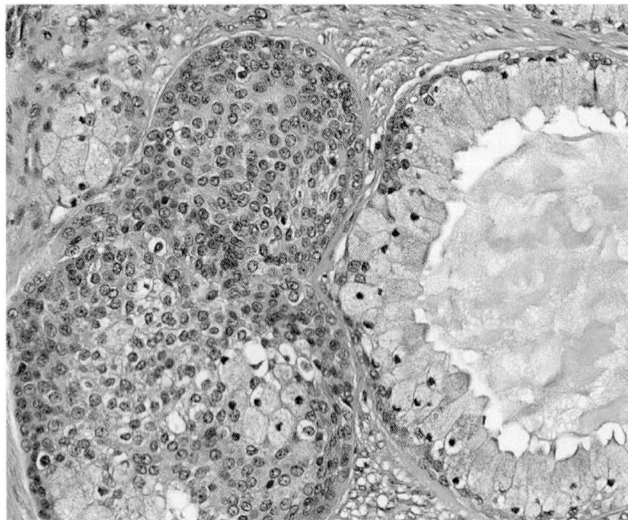

Figure 16.7 Higher power of low-grade mucoepidermoid carcinoma showing bland glandular components with sheets of squamoid cell with little cytologic atypia and no mitoses.

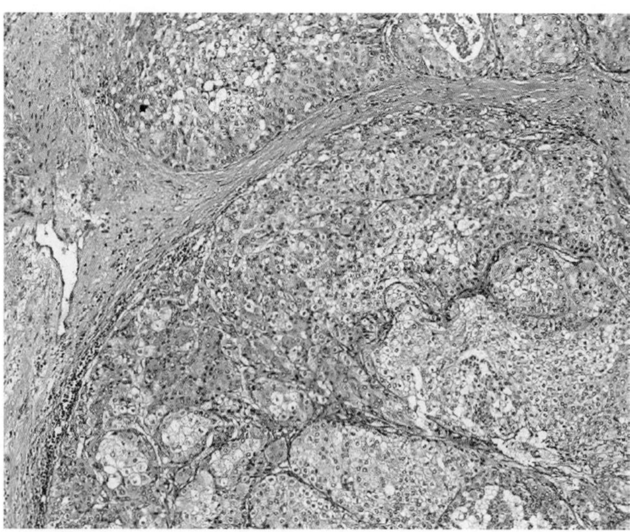

Figure 16.8 High-grade mucoepidermoid carcinoma with less mucinous epithelium and fewer cystic structures.

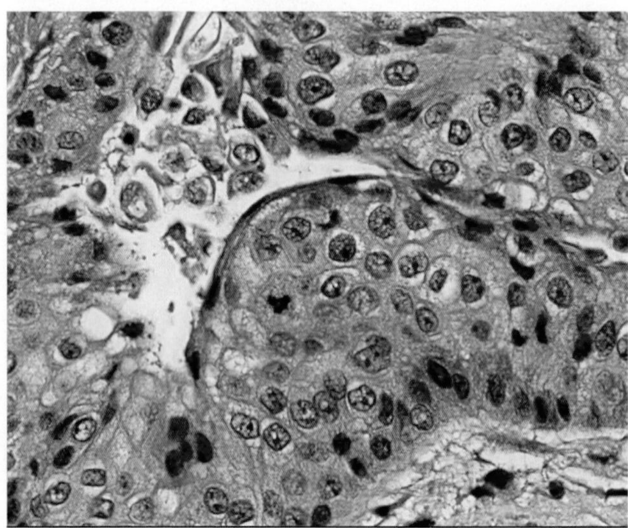

Figure 16.9 The squamous epithelial component of high-grade mucoepidermoid carcinoma shows increased nuclear pleomorphism and hyperchromasia; there is a mitosis identified centrally.

Part 3

Epithelial–Myoepithelial Carcinoma

▸ Timothy C. Allen and Yasmeen M. Butt

Epithelial–myoepithelial carcinoma is a rare primary low-grade lung cancer characterized by biphasic morphology, specifically a layer of spindle cells, clear cells, or plasmacytoid myoepithelial cells surrounding a layer of glandular structures. It occurs in adults and has no association with smoking. Patients typically present with dyspnea, cough, and fever. Grossly, epithelial–myoepithelial carcinoma is a solid, well-circumscribed endobronchial mass with a tan to gray-white cut surface. Differential diagnosis includes metastatic renal-cell carcinoma, pleomorphic adenoma, ACC, PEComa (perivascular epitheliod cell tumor), and mucoepidermoid carcinoma. Tumors are typically indolent, and surgery is usually curative.

HISTOLOGIC FEATURES

- Epithelial–myoepithelial carcinoma is biphasic, with a glandular structure surrounded by a layer of myoepithelial cells.
- The glandular cells are cuboidal with generally bland nuclei.
- The myoepithelial cells are spindled, clear, or plasmacytoid and may form solid nests.
- Necrosis and mitoses are not characteristic of epithelial–myoepithelial carcinoma.
- Immunostains show tumor cell positivity in epithelial cells with keratins; show myoepithelial cell positivity with S100 and actin; and may show weak keratin positivity.

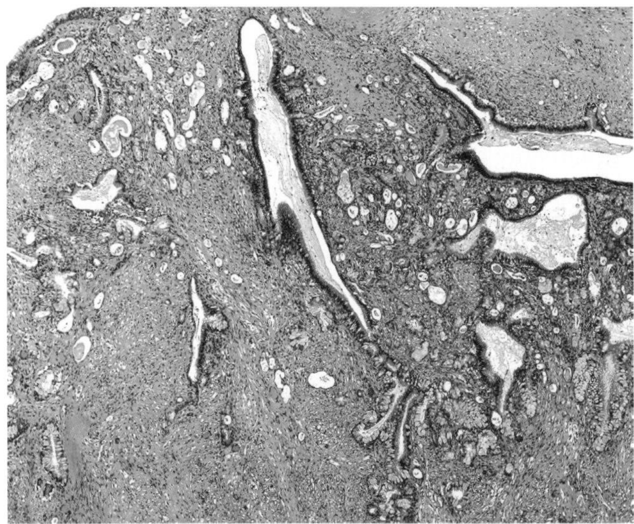

Figure 16.10 Endobronchial epithelial–myoepithelial carcinoma showing a well-circumscribed tumor with surface mucosa at the upper left.

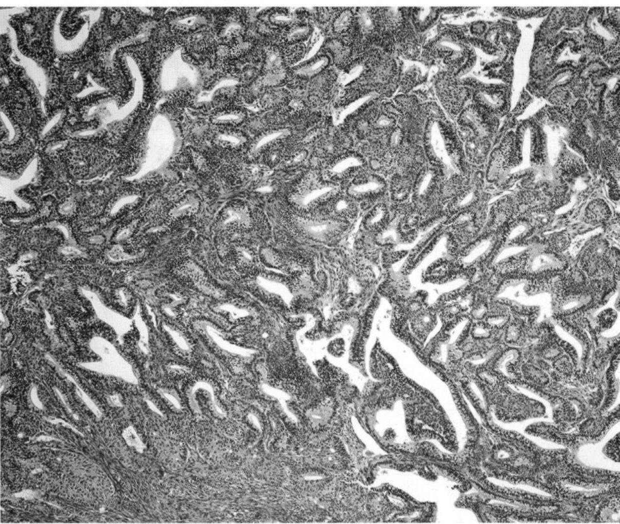

Figure 16.11 Epithelial–myoepithelial carcinoma showing epithelial glandular component and surrounding layer of myoepithelial cells.

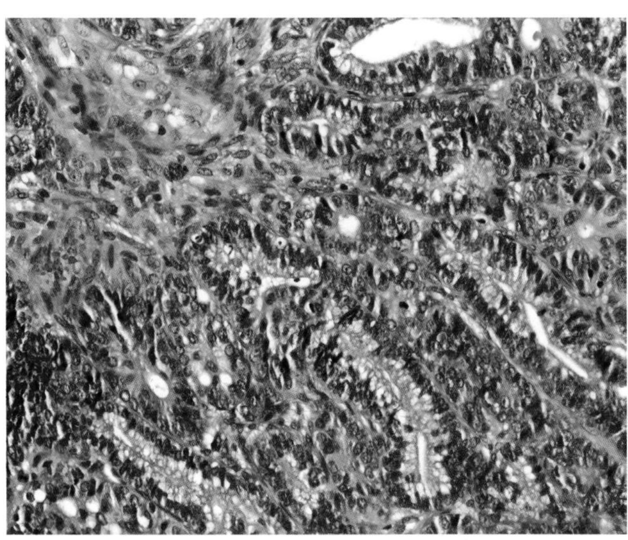

Figure 16.12 The ductal component has cuboidal cells with bland nuclei and eosinophilic cytoplasm, with surrounding somewhat spindled myoepithelial cells.

17 Lymphoepithelioma-Like Carcinoma

Timothy C. Allen

Lymphoepithelioma-like carcinoma is a rare lung carcinoma, most commonly found in young, nonsmoking, Southeast Asian women, characterized by the presence of admixed lymphocytes within poorly differentiated carcinoma. Tumor cell nuclei contain Epstein–Barr virus. Most patients present with cough; however, a significant minority of patients are asymptomatic at diagnosis. Patients are often found to have a discrete peripheral mass; pleural effusions are not characteristically present. Grossly, lymphoepithelioma-like carcinoma shows a rubbery mass with a fleshy cut surface. Differential diagnosis includes metastatic nasopharyngeal carcinoma and non-Hodgkin lymphoma. Prognosis is better than typical lung cancers.

CYTOLOGIC FEATURES

- Clusters and sheets of cohesive undifferentiated tumor cells showing oval to round vesicular nuclei and prominent nucleoli, with an associated infiltration of lymphocytes.

HISTOLOGIC FEATURES

- Lymphoepithelioma-like carcinoma is characterized by a syncytial arrangement of tumor cells with an infiltrate of lymphocytes.
- The tumor frequently exhibits a pushing border, with a permeative interface with lung parenchyma.
- Tumor cells exhibit large vesicular nuclei with prominent nucleoli and abundant cytoplasm.
- Mitotic figures are frequent.
- Spindle and squamous cell differentiation may occur focally.
- Areas of necrosis may occur.
- Immunostains show tumor cell positivity with cytokeratins, such as p40, p64, AE1/AE3, and CK5/6, suggesting squamous origin.
- The lymphoid infiltrate is made up of a mixed population of CD3 positive T cells and CD20 positive B cells.

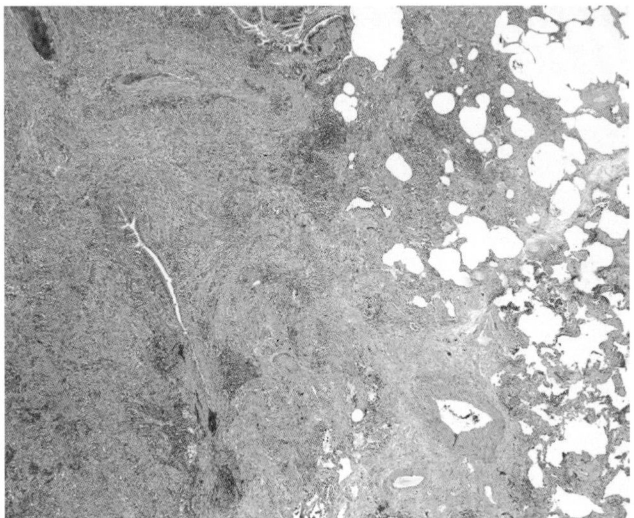

Figure 17.1 Lymphoepithelioma-like carcinoma showing a pushing, permeative border.

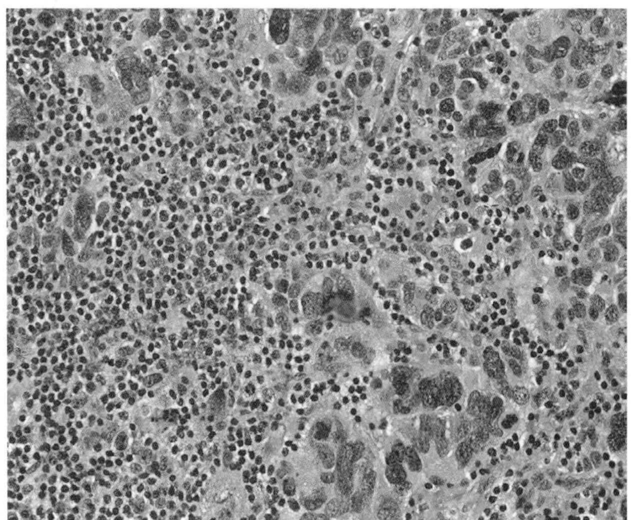

Figure 17.2 Islands of large tumor cells with a surrounding lymphoid infiltrate.

18 NUT Carcinoma

Timothy C. Allen
Mari Mino-Kenudson

NUT carcinoma is a rare, poorly differentiated lung carcinoma characterized by the presence of nuclear protein in testis (NUT) gene rearrangement. It is an aggressive lung cancer that is often diagnosed in advanced stage in patients with dyspnea, weight loss, pleuritic chest pain, and pleural effusion. NUT carcinoma is not associated with smoking. It has no sex predilection and may occur at any age. Prognosis is poor. NUT carcinoma is usually identified radiographically as a large mass extending to mediastinum or chest wall. Grossly, it is a large fleshy white tumor, often with necrosis. Differential diagnosis includes primarily squamous-cell carcinoma; however, acute leukemia, Ewing sarcoma, and metastatic germ cell tumors must also be considered in the appropriate age group.

CYTOLOGIC FEATURES

- Fine needle aspiration is nonspecific and shows discohesive tumor cell nests and single tumor cells characterized by irregular nuclei with granular chromatin, necrosis, and crush artifact.

HISTOLOGIC FEATURES

- NUT carcinoma is characterized by groups and sheets of small, monomorphic, undifferentiated tumor cells with irregular nuclei containing granular chromatin, nucleoli, and a moderate amount of cytoplasm.
- Tumor may abruptly show foci of keratinization.
- Clear spaces between tumor cells are a frequent finding.
- Immunostains are important for accurate diagnosis; NUT antibody shows greater than 50% of tumor cells with speckled nuclear positivity, and most cases show p63 and p40 positivity, suggesting squamous origin.
- CD34 is typically positive in tumor cells; care must be taken not to misdiagnose NUT carcinoma as acute leukemia.
- Cytokeratin stains are typically positive in NUT carcinoma, and neuroendocrine markers and TTF-1 may occasionally be positive in tumor cells.

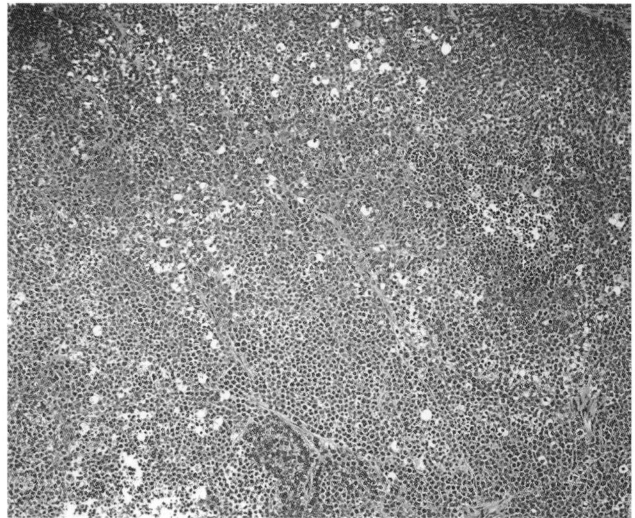

Figure 18.1 Somewhat discohesive sheets and nests of small, monomorphic NUT carcinoma tumor cells.

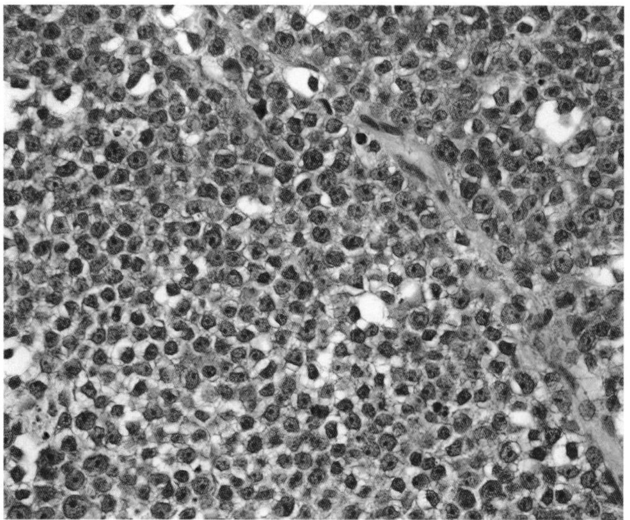

Figure 18.2 NUT carcinoma tumor cells with granular chromatin, nucleoli, and spaces between some tumor cells.

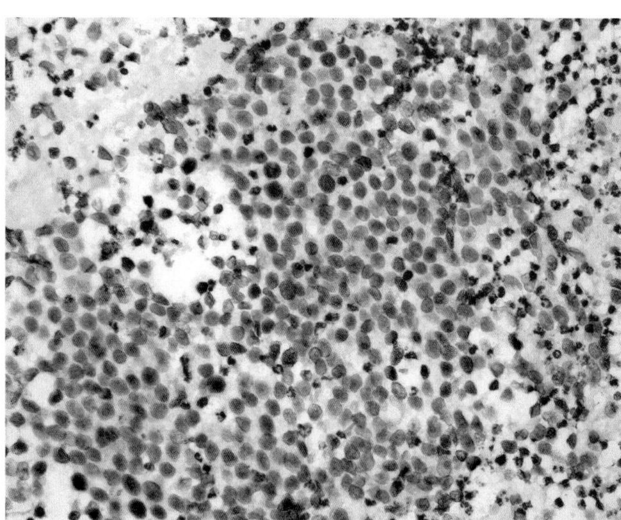

Figure 18.3 NUT antibody immunopositivity within NUT carcinoma tumor cells.

Primary Pulmonary Sarcomas

19

Krzysztof Glomski
Matthew W. Rosenbaum
Ivan Chebib
Mari Mino-Kenudson

Part 1

Inflammatory Myofibroblastic Tumor

Inflammatory myofibroblastic tumor (IMT) is a mesenchymal neoplasm of intermediate (rarely metastasizing) malignant potential composed of myofibroblastic spindled cells and an associated inflammatory infiltrate that usually consists of lymphocytes and plasma cells. IMT is most commonly diagnosed in children and adolescents, although it may occur at any age. The clinical manifestations of pulmonary IMT may include dyspnea, chest pain, fatigue, weight loss, and malaise with associated elevation of serum inflammatory markers. Macroscopically, IMTs are nodular/multinodular, well circumscribed, and nonencapsulated and have a white-tan fleshy to myxoid cut surface with variable calcification, necrosis, and hemorrhage.

CYTOLOGIC FEATURES

- Most commonly low-grade spindle cells with oval nuclei, small nucleoli, and background lymphocytes, neutrophils, and plasma cells.

HISTOLOGIC FEATURES

- Nodular growth of myofibroblasts and admixed lymphocytes, plasma cells, and eosinophils in any of the three microscopic patterns:
  - Spindled to plump cells within a loose, myxoid background containing blood vessels, plasma cells, lymphocytes, and eosinophils.
  - Compact, fascicular growth of spindled myofibroblasts with small aggregates of plasma cells, lymphocytes, and eosinophils.
  - Collagen-rich, sclerosing/scar-like growth that is sparsely cellular with interspersed eosinophils and plasma cells.
- Calcifications, osseous metaplasia, and hemorrhage are uncommon; mitotic rate is generally low, and necrosis is rare.

ANCILLARY TESTING

- Immunohistochemistry (IHC) is variably positive for smooth muscle actin (SMA) and muscle-specific actin and desmin, and a subset is keratin-positive. Myogenin and S100 are negative.
- ALK IHC is positive in ~50% of cases.
- Rearrangements of *ALK* (50% to 60%) are the most common. *ROS1* (~10%) and *RET* (<5%) may also be identified.
- Gene rearrangements are more commonly seen in pediatric tumors than in adult-onset IMT.

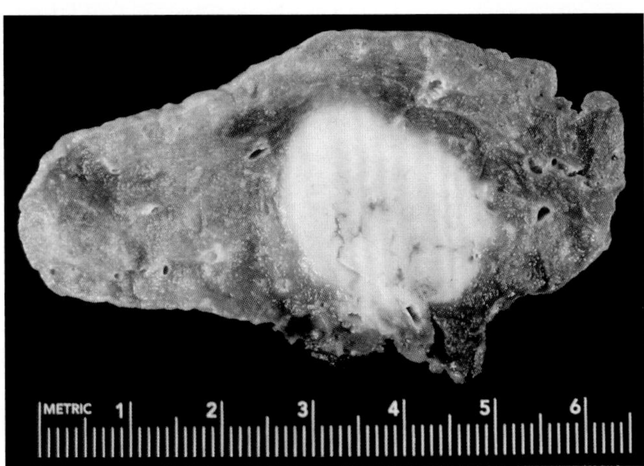

Figure 19.1 A gross image showing a well-circumscribed, nonencapsulated white-tan fleshy mass in a lung resection specimen.

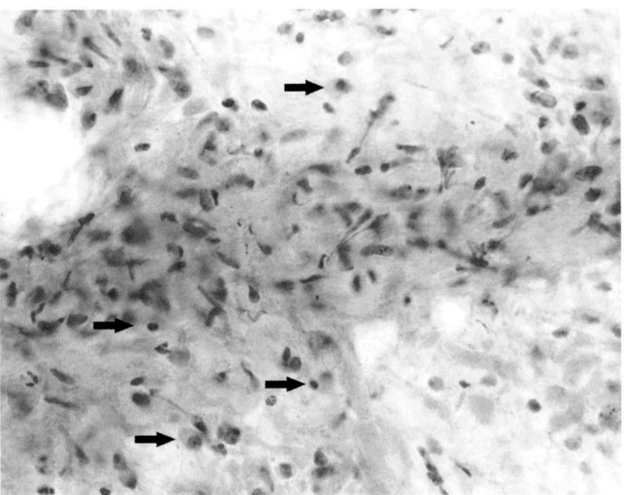

Figure 19.2 Cytology smear demonstrating low-grade spindle-cell neoplasm with fibrillar cytoplasm, fibrous stroma, and abundant infiltrating lymphoplasmacytic inflammation *(arrows)*.

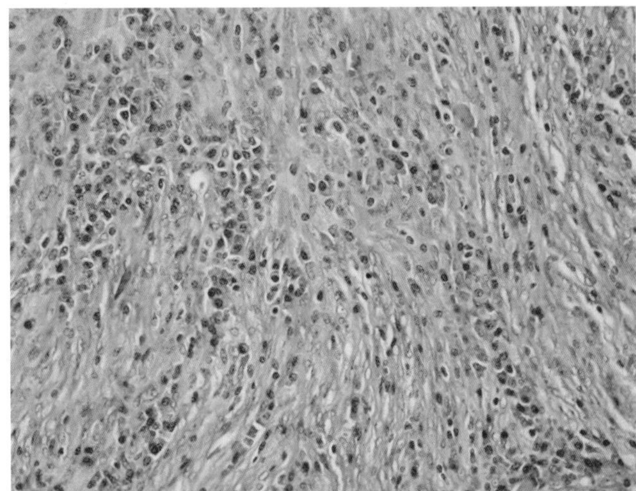

Figure 19.3 Low-grade spindled to plump myofibroblastic proliferation with admixed plasma cells and histiocytes.

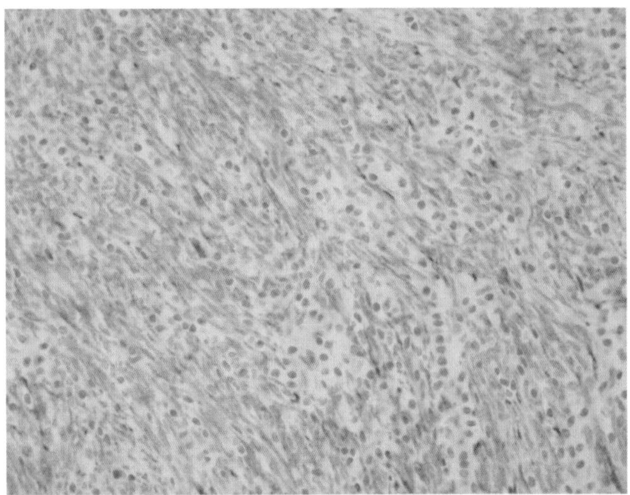

Figure 19.4 Immunohistochemical staining for ALK shows strong cytoplasmic staining within the spindle-cell population, whereas admixed inflammatory cells are negative.

Part 2

Pleuropulmonary Blastoma

Pleuropulmonary blastoma (PPB) is the most common malignant pulmonary tumor of early childhood (<7 years), consisting of primitive neoplastic cells with a histopathologic spectrum of cystic (type I), mixed (type II), and solid (type III) growth. There is a strong association with germ line heterozygous *DICER1* mutation. When symptomatic, PPB presents with respiratory distress with or without pneumothorax, recurrent pneumonia, cough, and shortness of breath. Symptoms, epidemiology, histomorphology, therapy, and prognosis all correlate with subtype: type I PPB carries the best prognosis, whereas type III PPB carries a poor prognosis.

CYTOLOGIC FEATURES

- Variable and based on type (see morphologic features below). Tumor cells may show primitive, small, round cells with scant cytoplasm, while cystic lining consists of ciliated, respiratory epithelium.

MORPHOLOGIC FEATURES

- Type I:
  - Exclusively cystic (unilocular or multilocular), thin-walled, and without a solid component.
  - Microscopically, cysts are typically lined by benign respiratory epithelium and underlined multifocally by small, round, primitive tumor (blastematous) cells and variably admixed rhabdoid cells with eccentric, round nuclei and abundant eosinophilic cytoplasm and/or immature cartilage.
  - Complete specimen submission is necessary to render accurate diagnosis.
- Type II:
  - Mixed solid/nodular/plaque-like and cystic components, and this type of PPB may arise intrapulmonary or along visceral pleura.
  - Cystic areas resemble type I PPB.
  - Solid/nodular/plaque-like component shows an overgrowth of blastematous, spindle-cell sarcomatous, and/or rhabdomyosarcomatous tumor cells.
- Type III:
  - Exclusively solid, grossly tan-white, fleshy to myxoid, and friable with hemorrhage and necrosis.
  - This type of PPB often replaces the hemithorax and involves adjacent structures.
  - Microscopically, blastematous, spindle-cell sarcomatous, and rhabdomyosarcomatous tumor cells with high mitotic activity.
  - Necrosis is common, and cartilaginous differentiation may occur.

ANCILLARY TESTING

- Blastematous elements stain variably for muscle-specific actin and desmin and neuron-specific enolase; rhabdomyosarcomatous components are positive for SMA, desmin, and myogenin. Keratins and TTF-1 highlight native respiratory epithelial cells, both entrapped and lining the cystic lesions, and S100 highlights cartilaginous components when present.

- Most common tumor seen in DICER1 PPB familial tumor predisposition syndrome, an autosomal dominant condition also associated with pediatric cystic nephroma and Sertoli–Leydig cell tumor. Association with nasal chondromesenchymal hamartoma, multinodular goiter of the thyroid, embryonal rhabdomyosarcoma of the cervix, and ciliary body medulloepithelioma is also reported.

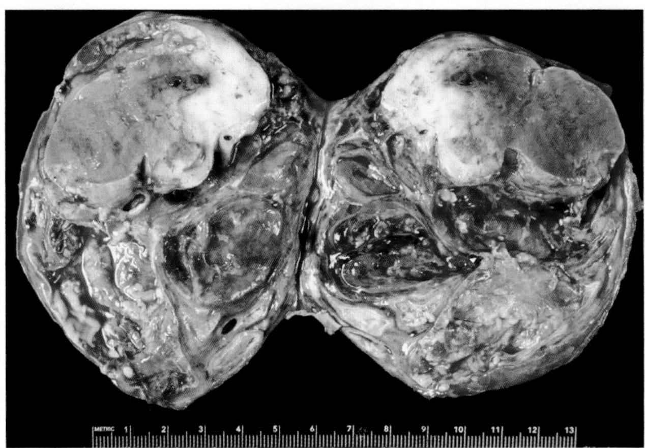

Figure 19.5 A gross image of a type II PPB with tan-white solid and prominent cystic components. Hemorrhage and necrosis are present within the solid component.

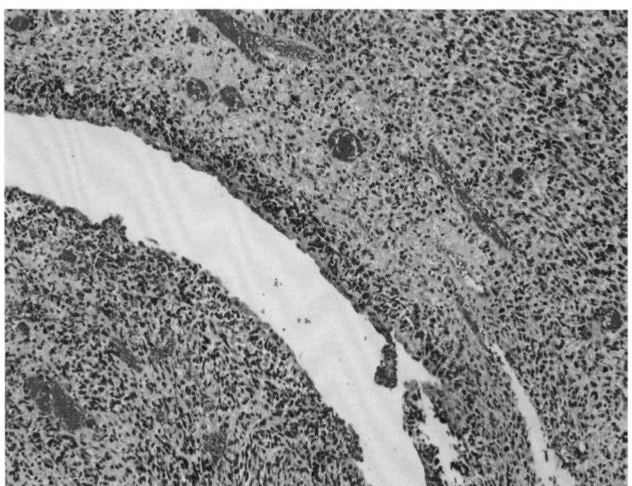

Figure 19.6 Cystic areas are lined by a benign respiratory epithelium with subjacent small, round, primitive blastematous cells. Away from the cyst wall, a dense, hyperchromatic population of tumor cells is present.

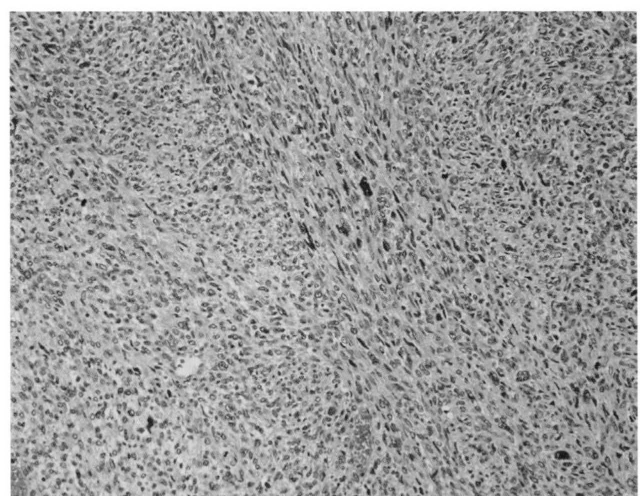

Figure 19.7 The solid component of a type II PPB shows a fascicular growth of pleomorphic spindled cells.

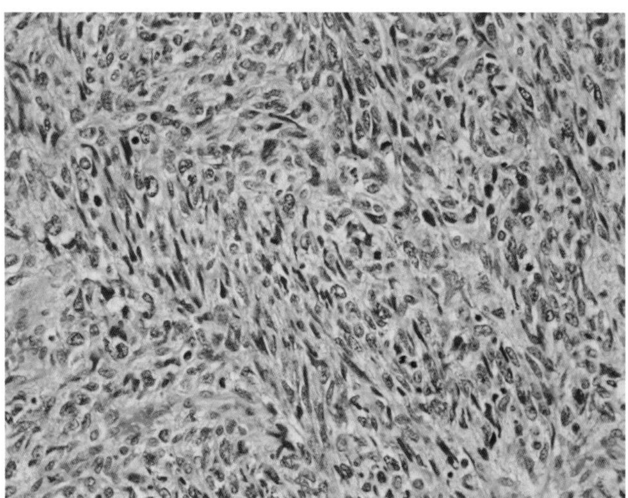

Figure 19.8 The sarcomatous areas contain spindled cells with angulated, pleomorphic, hyperchromatic cells with mitotic activity and apoptosis.

Part 3

Epithelioid Hemangioendothelioma

Epithelioid hemangioendothelioma (EHE) is a low-grade to intermediate-grade malignant vascular tumor, commonly arising in the liver, lung, and bones of adults. EHE is often multifocal at presentation and may involve multiple organs; discerning primary versus metastatic versus multifocal primary tumors is often difficult. Although typically asymptomatic at presentation, EHE may induce pain, cough, dyspnea, hemoptysis, and systemic symptoms. Pleural thickening with effusions, grossly mimicking malignant mesothelioma, may be seen. Imaging studies reveal multiple bilateral perivascular nodules in most cases.

CYTOLOGIC FEATURES

- Large, polygonal, eosinophilic, epithelioid cells, often vacuolated.

HISTOLOGIC FEATURES

- Epithelioid endothelial cells with abundant distinctive myxohyaline stroma.
- Endothelial cells grow in corded, nested, or tubulopapillary patterns; have pale eosinophilic cytoplasm, vesicular nuclei, and inconspicuous nucleoli; and may possess large intracytoplasmic vacuoles ("blister" cells) that may contain fragmented red blood cells (RBCs).
- Most EHEs show low-grade nuclear features and rare mitoses.
- High-grade tumors contain necrosis, solid sheets of cells with marked nuclear atypia, and increased mitotic activity (2 per 2 mm^2) and have broad differential diagnoses including epithelioid angiosarcoma, other sarcomas, mesothelioma, and adenocarcinoma.

ANCILLARY TESTING

- Vascular markers (FLI1, ERG, CD31, and CD34) are positive in epithelioid endothelial cells. Focal keratin positivity may be seen in some cases. Immunohistochemical staining for CAMTA1 shows nuclear expression with high specificity.
- Rearrangement of WWTR1-CAMTA1 is commonly seen (>90%), and YAP1-TFE3 fusions have been reported in a subset of EHEs from young adults without WWTR1-CAMTA1 rearrangement.

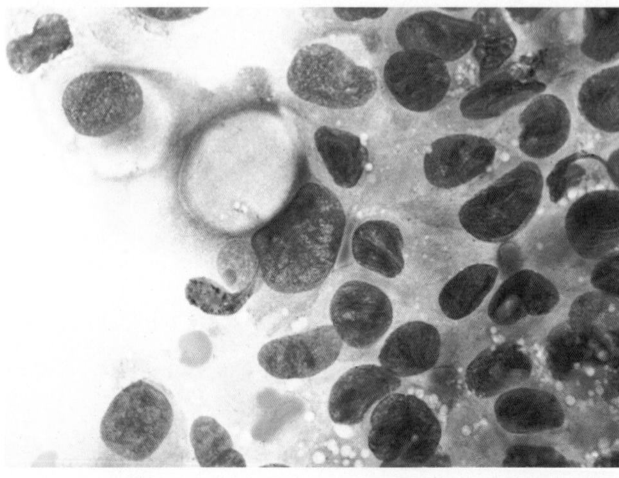

Figure 19.9 A cytology smear demonstrating round and polygonal cells with a prominent cytoplasmic vacuole.

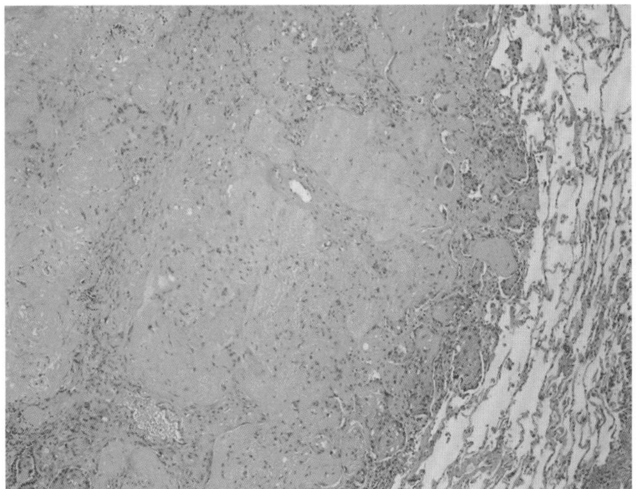

Figure 19.10 Low-power magnification showing a lobulated growth with nodules of epithelioid cells embedded in a myxoid stroma. Fibrosis is present in the central portion of the lesion *(left side of the image)*.

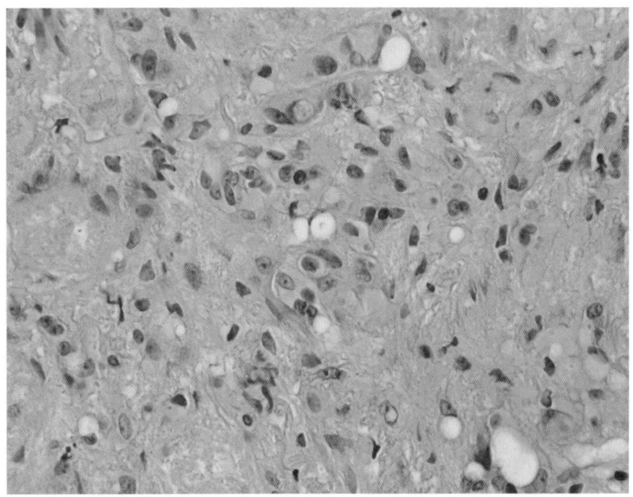

Figure 19.11 Low-grade EHE contains epithelioid cells with "glassy" pale eosinophilic cytoplasm; round, uniform nuclei; and small nucleoli admixed with a gray-blue myxoid stroma. Intracytoplasmic lumina are present in some lesional cells.

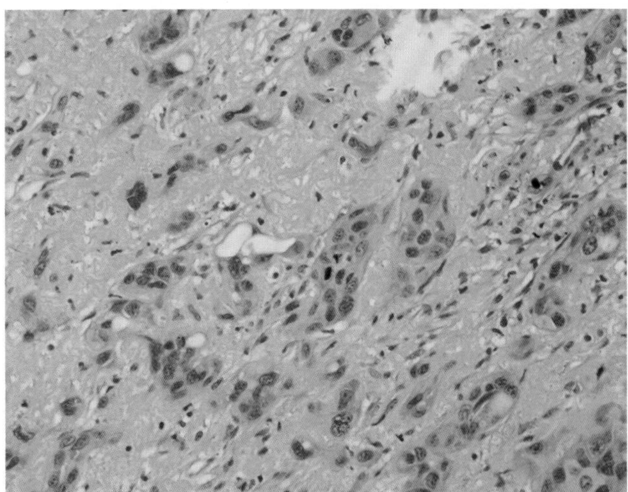

Figure 19.12 High-grade EHE shows nests and cords of epithelioid cells with brisk mitotic activity, pleomorphism, and apoptotic bodies admixed with a gray-blue myxoid stroma.

Part 4

Kaposi Sarcoma

Kaposi sarcoma (KS) is a vascular tumor commonly associated with acquired immunodeficiency syndrome (AIDS), immunosuppression following solid organ transplantation, and long-term immunosuppression for various conditions. KS may arise anywhere in the body, including the lungs. Grossly, lung lesions consist of hemorrhagic nodules that may coalesce. Differential diagnoses include angiosarcoma, arteriovenous malformation, inflammatory granulation tissue, and bacillary angiomatosis.

CYTOLOGIC FEATURES

- Bland to mildly atypical oval to spindle-shaped cells with variable hyaline globules in a background of abundant RBCs.

HISTOLOGIC FEATURES

- Diffuse infiltrative lesion along lymphatic pathways, interlobular septa, and pleura.
- Bland monomorphic spindle cells resembling fibroblasts separated by slit-like vascular spaces with RBCs.
- Admixed plasma cells and lymphocytes are common.
- PAS (periodic acid–Schiff)-positive, diastase-resistant intracellular and extracellular hyaline globules are common.

ANCILLARY TESTING

- Tumor cells are positive for vascular markers: ERG, CD34, and CD31.
- HHV-8 is positive in virtually all KS.

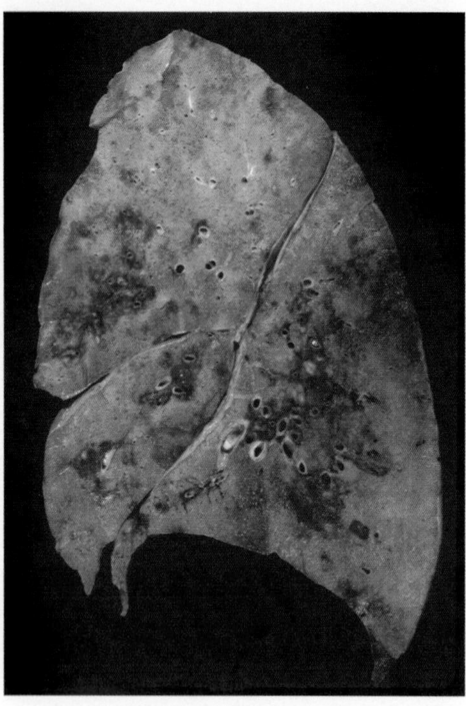

Figure 19.13 A gross image of the lung with KS shows multiple, diffuse, poorly demarcated, and coalescent hemorrhagic areas.

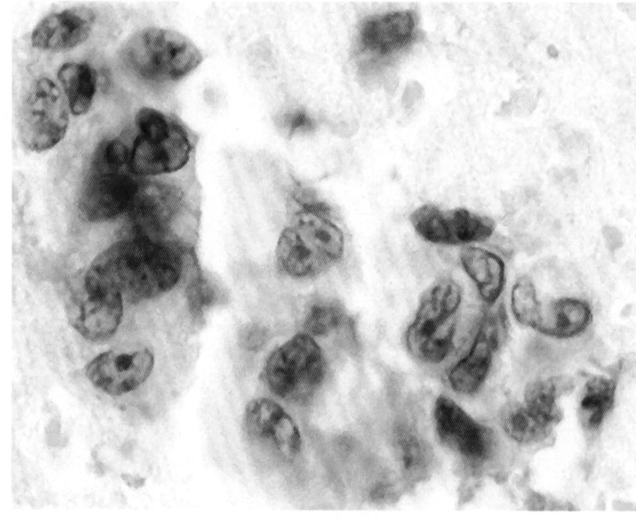

Figure 19.14 A cytology smear demonstrating mildly atypical oval to spindle-shaped cells with a background of RBCs.

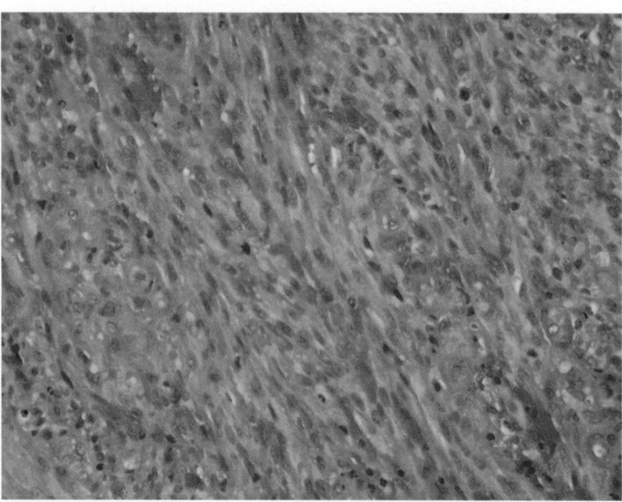

Figure 19.15 An example of KS consisting of plump spindle cells, with oval nuclei and occasional mitotic figures and apoptosis, and interposing slit-like vascular spaces.

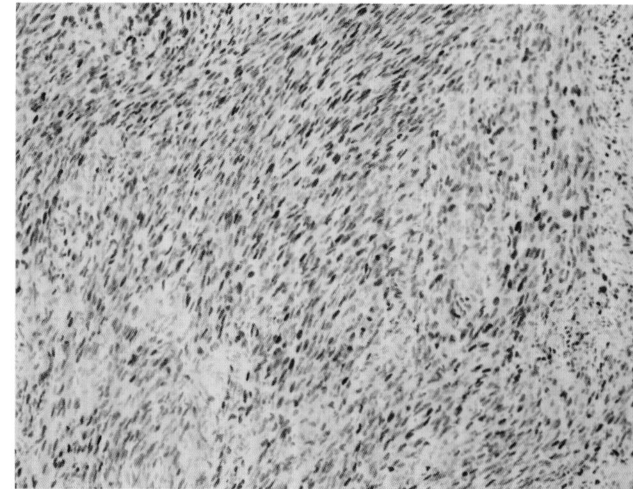

Figure 19.16 IHC for HHV-8 showing strong, diffuse positivity in the nuclei of the spindle-cell population.

Part 5

Synovial Sarcoma

Synovial sarcomas are sarcomas of uncertain origin, giving rise to mesenchymal and epithelial tumor cells, typically around large joints of the upper and lower extremities of patients aged 10 to 50 years. The lung is the most common organ-based site for primary synovial sarcoma, typically manifesting in the fifth decade of life, although most synovial sarcomas in the lung represent metastases. Grossly, synovial sarcomas are usually peripheral or pleural-based and are often nodular, circumscribed, tan-white, solid masses with focal necrosis, hemorrhage, and cystic change. By imaging, pulmonary synovial sarcomas typically show sharp borders without cavitation, calcification, or lymphadenopathy. They may be monophasic (spindled) or biphasic (spindled and epithelioid) and harbor a defining chromosomal translocation: t(X;18)(p11.2;q11.2). Primary pulmonary synovial sarcomas carry worse prognoses than soft tissue–derived synovial sarcomas.

CYTOLOGIC FEATURES

- Monomorphous spindled cells with round, vesicular nuclei, with occasional acinar structures with epithelial cells in biphasic synovial sarcomas.

HISTOLOGIC FEATURES

- Most often monophasic (spindled) when primary in the lung.
- The spindle-cell component consists of closely packed, small, monomorphic cells with indistinct cell borders and hyperchromatic nuclei often arranged in a "herringbone" pattern.
- The epithelial component, if present, consists of large, pale cells with round, vesicular nuclei and distinct cell borders arranged in solid nests, glands, or tubules and may be prominent (mimicking adenocarcinoma).
- Stroma may contain hemangiopericytoma-like vessels and variably thick collagen bundles. Necrosis is typically seen. Calcifications and mast cells are less common in primary pulmonary synovial sarcoma than in soft tissue synovial sarcoma.
- May be poorly differentiated with high mitotic index, round cell morphology, nuclear irregularity, and significant necrosis, resembling other small round blue cell sarcomas.

ANCILLARY TESTING

- Monophasic synovial sarcoma is usually focally positive for EMA and often focally positive for keratin; it typically shows strong diffuse nuclear TLE1 staining and multifocal CD99 reactivity. When present, the epithelial component reliably stains for EMA and keratin (AE1/AE3 and CK7).
- Cytogenetic evidence of t(X;18)(p11.2;q11.2) translocation or molecular detection of *SS18-SSX1* or *SS18-SSX2* fusion gene product is diagnostic.

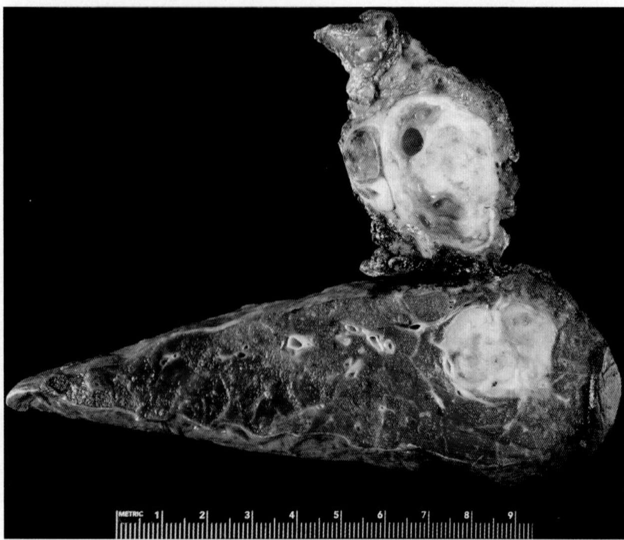

Figure 19.17 A gross image of a metastatic synovial sarcoma to the lung showing a lobulated, well-circumscribed, yellow-tan, solid, and cystic lesion.

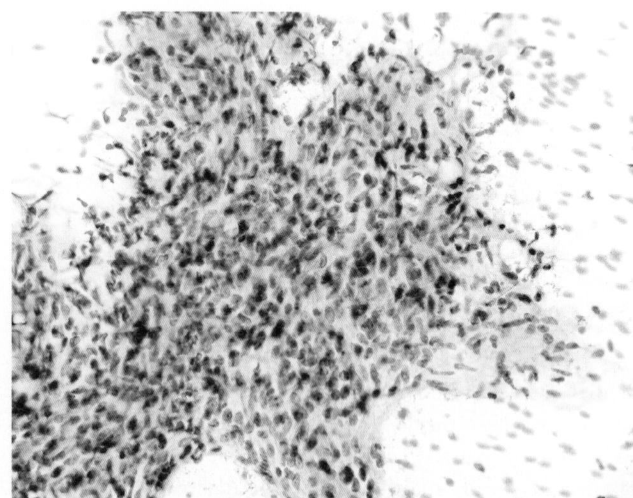

Figure 19.18 Cytology smear demonstrates dense clusters of spindled cells forming disorganized groups; epithelial cells may be identified in biphasic synovial sarcoma (not seen here).

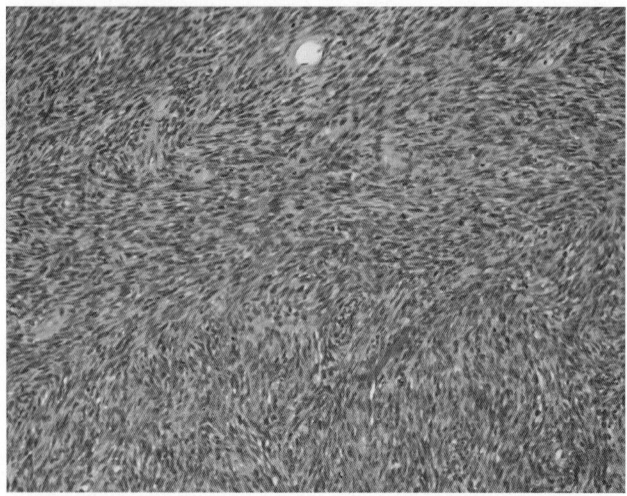

Figure 19.19 An example of monophasic synovial sarcoma showing a monomorphous population of plump spindle cells arranged in vague fascicles.

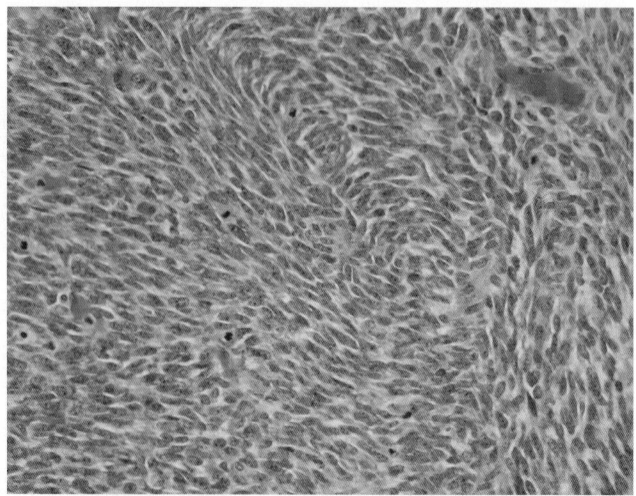

Figure 19.20 Numerous mitoses in the absence of significant nuclear pleomorphism.

Part 6

Malignant Solitary Fibrous Tumor

Solitary fibrous tumors (SFTs) are typically visceral pleural-based, spindle-cell neoplasms that occur in adults and are often detected incidentally on imaging studies. Intrapulmonary SFT is rare, representing <10% of all SFTs of the thorax. Although a great majority consists of benign tumors, a small subset of SFTs (~10%) exhibit local recurrence or distant metastasis and death years after surgical resection. Compared with their low-risk counterparts, malignant SFTs tend to be larger (about 13 cm on average) and may show infiltrative margins with necrosis.

CYTOLOGIC FEATURES

- Spindled to plump epithelioid cells with nuclear hyperchromasia forming variably cellular, cohesive groups without specific architectural patterns.

HISTOLOGIC FEATURES

- General features of SFT:
  - Fibroblastic neoplasm with spindled to ovoid cells with indistinct borders, pale cytoplasm, and oval nuclei with vesicular chromatin.
  - Cells are arranged haphazardly with variable cellularity ("patternless pattern").
  - Stroma contains distinctive thin-walled, branching ("staghorn") vessels, variable collagen deposition, occasional myxoid changes, and mast cells.
- Malignant behavior of SFT is correlated with parietal pleura origin, sessile growth, large size, high mitotic rate (≥4/10 high power fields), hypercellularity, and necrosis; cytologic atypia is usually limited.

ANCILLARY TESTING

- IHC for STAT6 protein shows diffuse and strong positivity (nuclear) with high specificity; CD34 is typically positive.
- Molecular testing for *NAB2-STAT6* gene fusion is characteristic and is secondary to an intrachromosomal inversion: inv(12)(q13q13); STAT6 IHC serves as a reliable surrogate for this molecular change.

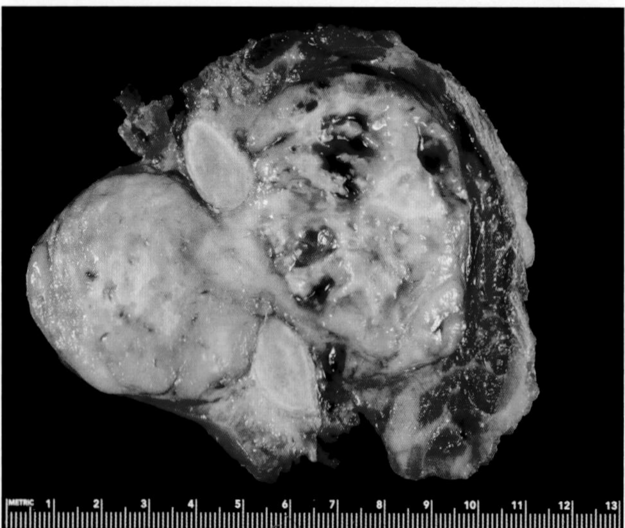

Figure 19.21 A gross image of a malignant SFT demonstrating a tan-white lobulated mass with extrathoracic extension, hemorrhage, cystic degeneration, and necrosis.

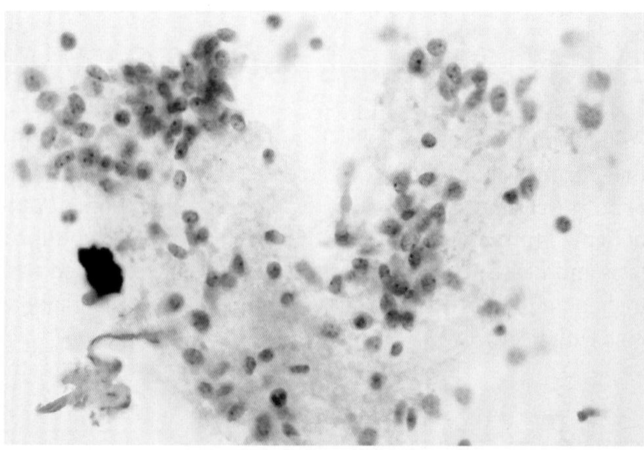

Figure 19.22 Variably cellular smear consisting of plump monomorphic spindle cells with finely dispersed chromatin and small, prominent nucleoli. Distinguishing malignant from benign is not possible on cytology.

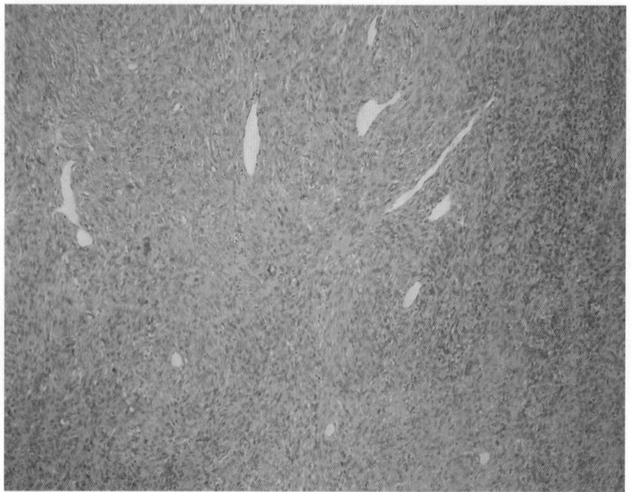

Figure 19.23 An example of malignant SFT characterized by sheets of spindled and epithelioid cells without distinct architectural pattern, scant fibrous stroma, and hemangiopericytoma-like vessels.

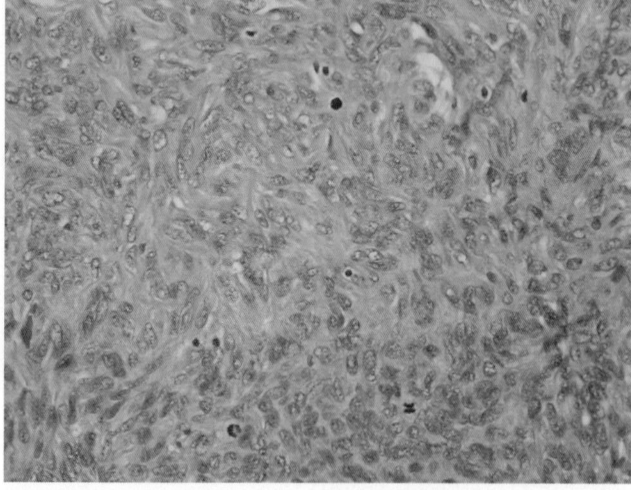

Figure 19.24 Plump spindled and epithelioid tumor cells with collagenous stroma and frequent mitoses.

Part 7

Intimal Sarcoma

Intimal sarcoma is an aggressive, rare primary sarcoma arising from multipotent mesenchyme associated with the intima of the pulmonary artery and pulmonary outflow tract in adults. Grossly, these tumors form fleshy, occasionally polypoid, masses that distend (and may obliterate) the pulmonary vasculature. Extravascular extension into adjacent structures and metastatic spread may occur, and the prognosis is poor.

CYTOLOGIC FEATURES

- Variable features, often revealing high-grade, pleomorphic cells with necrotic background.

HISTOLOGIC FEATURES

- Extremely variable with the largest group consisting of undifferentiated pleomorphic sarcomas, followed by low-grade spindle-cell sarcomas with a myxoid background.
- Heterologous elements, typically in the form of osteosarcoma or chondrosarcoma and less commonly in the form of angiosarcoma, rhabdomyosarcoma, and leiomyosarcoma.
- A primary diagnostic consideration is to rule out metastatic spread of a primary sarcoma of bone/soft tissue.

ANCILLARY TESTING

- IHC staining patterns will reflect the type of sarcomatous differentiation present, and undifferentiated tumors express vimentin and actin (focal).
- MDM2 overexpression is frequently seen by IHC, and cytogenetically, gain/amplification of 12q13-14 is also often present.

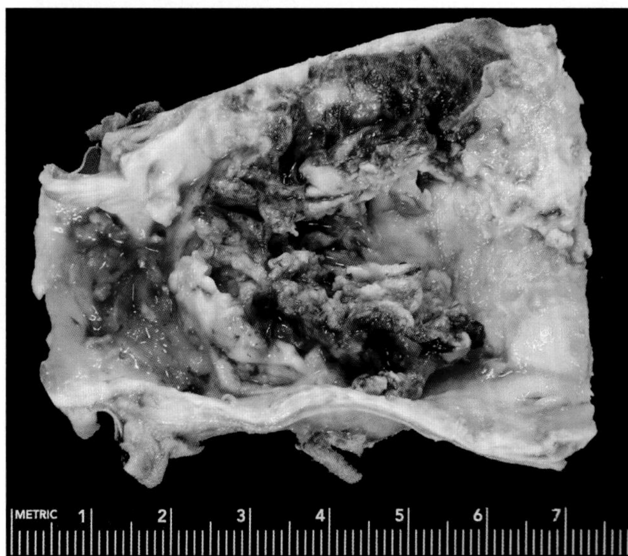

Figure 19.25 A gross image of intimal sarcoma demonstrating a fleshy mass with papillary endovascular growth with hemorrhage and necrosis (after fixation).

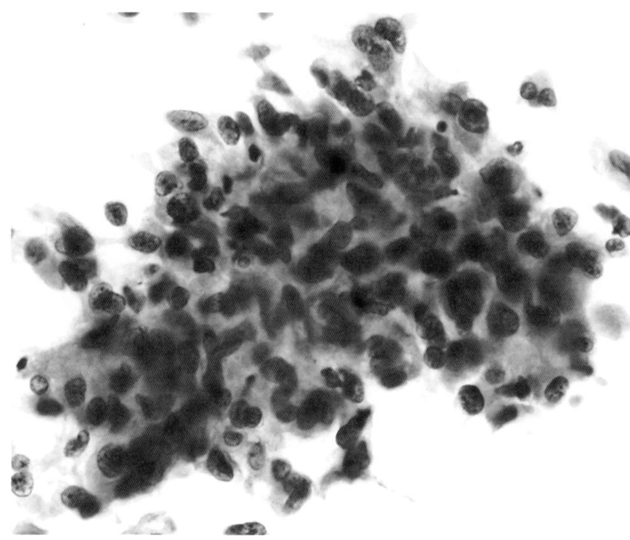

Figure 19.26 Cytology smear with cohesive groups of highly atypical spindle cells without specific line of differentiation.

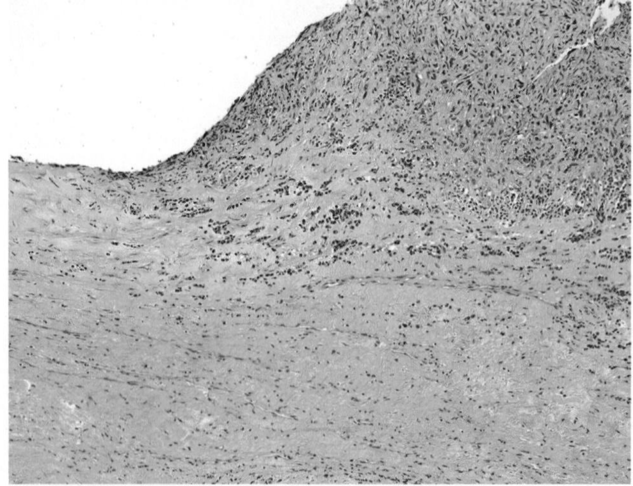

Figure 19.27 Proliferation of spindled and epithelioid cells is present in close association with the vascular intima. A transition between the underlying pulmonary artery *(on the left)* and sarcoma *(on the right)* is shown.

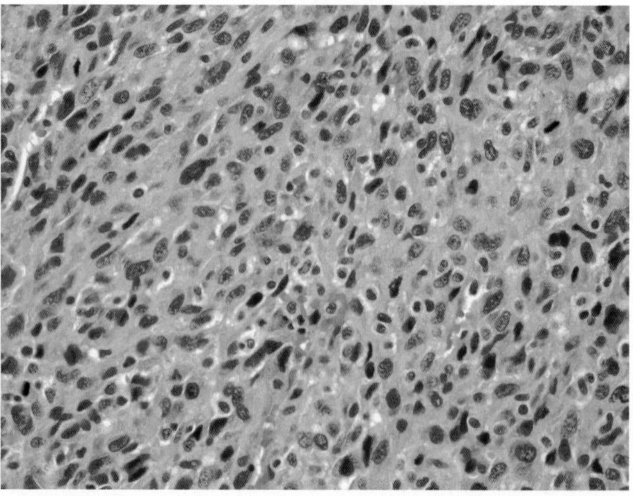

Figure 19.28 An undifferentiated component of intimal sarcoma characterized by spindled and epithelioid cells in sheets with frequent mitoses and pleomorphism.

Part 8

SMARCA4-Deficient Thoracic Sarcoma

SMARCA4-deficient thoracic sarcoma is a rare, aggressive round blue cell neoplasm, most commonly arising in the mediastinum and pleura in adult (30- to 40-year-old) male smokers and carries a poor prognosis (median survival of 7 months). Mediastinal lymphadenopathy may be prominent, mimicking lymphoma. Grossly, tumors tend to be large (>10 cm) and show extensive infiltration of adjacent structures, including the chest wall.

CYTOLOGIC FEATURES

- Nonspecific, showing discohesive epithelioid cells with high nuclear to cytoplasmic ratio with prominent nucleoli. Numerous mitoses may be seen.
- Background necrosis may be present.

HISTOLOGIC FEATURES

- Diffuse sheet-like growth of round, monomorphic, mildly discohesive epithelioid cells with scant to moderately abundant cytoplasm and prominent nucleoli with round to angulated nuclear membranes.
- Geographic necrosis and areas of hemorrhage may be seen.

ANCILLARY TESTING

- IHC typically shows loss of SMARCA4 expression, whereas SOX2, SALL4, and CD34 staining is often present. Keratin staining may be positive.
- Characterized by mutations leading to loss of function of SMARCA4, which may also be seen in small cell carcinoma (hypercalcemic type) of the ovary, malignant rhabdoid tumors, and a subset of lung and gastrointestinal carcinomas.

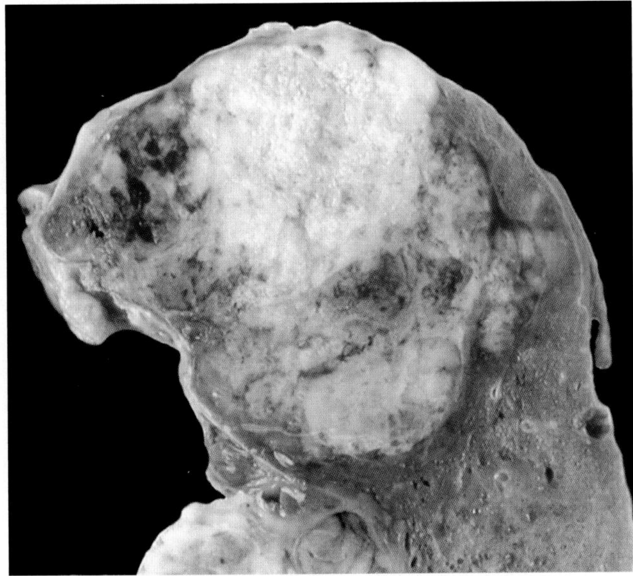

Figure 19.29 A gross image of SMARCA4-deficient thoracic sarcoma demonstrating a large, lobulated, well-circumscribed tan-white to gray mass with hemorrhage and necrosis. (Courtesy of Dr. Akihiko Yoshida.)

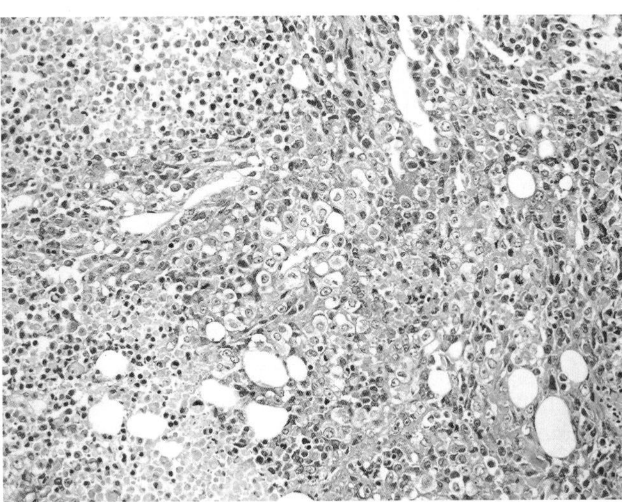

Figure 19.30 A microscopic image showing sheets of round and angulated monomorphous cells with geographic necrosis. (Courtesy of Dr. Akihiko Yoshida.)

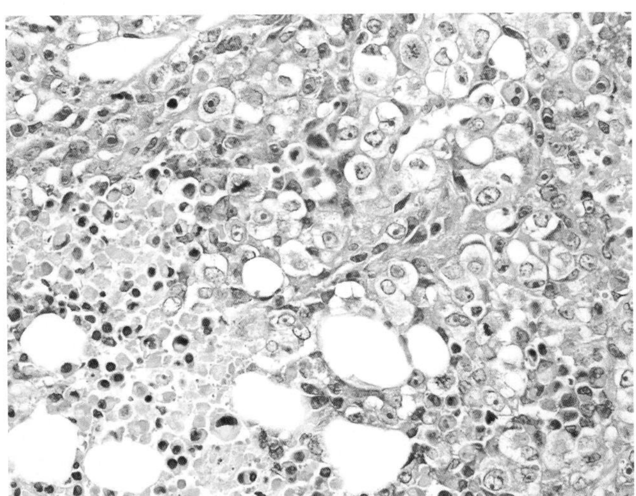

Figure 19.31 Tumor cells exhibit centrally located nuclei with prominent nucleoli, frequent mitoses, and necrosis. (Courtesy of Dr. Akihiko Yoshida.)

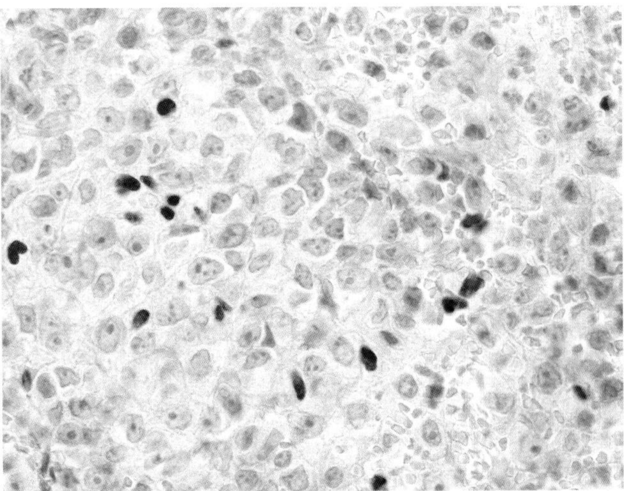

Figure 19.32 IHC for SMARCA4 (BRG1) shows loss of nuclear staining in tumor cells; interspersed inflammatory cells have retained staining. (Courtesy of Dr. Akihiko Yoshida.)

Part 9

Primary Pulmonary Myxoid Sarcoma with *EWSR1-CREB1* Translocation

Primary pulmonary myxoid sarcoma (PPMS) (with *EWSR1-CREB1* translocation) is an extremely rare and evolving entity, with intermediate biologic behavior, occurring in adults with an average age of 45 years. Clinically, PPMS often presents as a mediastinal mass on CT scan or chest radiograph and is frequently closely related to a bronchus, with predominant endobronchial growth that may lead to obstructive changes. Grossly, PPMS is generally small (<4 cm), well circumscribed, nodular, glistening, and yellow-white. Prognosis is favorable when PPMS is localized to the lung and excised completely but becomes poor if metastatic spread occurs. The *EWSR1-CREB1* translocation found in PPMS is characteristic but is also seen in other entities.

CYTOLOGIC FEATURES

- Cytologic features are not well described and likely reflect histologic findings of spindled to epithelioid cells with moderately abundant cytoplasm within a myxoid stroma.

HISTOLOGIC FEATURES

- At low-power magnification, PPMS is lobulated/nodular, with loosely cellular/myxoid areas separated by more dense fibrovascular bands.
- Often intimately associated with a bronchus.
- Tumor cells are spindled to epithelioid with moderately abundant eosinophilic cytoplasm arranged in loose reticular, nested, and corded groups embedded in a loose, myxoid matrix. An extraskeletal myxoid chondrosarcoma or myoepithelial tumor should be considered in the differential diagnosis.
- Generally, atypia is mild or absent, mitoses are <5 per 2 mm^2, and necrosis is focal.

ANCILLARY TESTING

- Immunohistochemical staining typically shows labeling for vimentin and occasionally for EMA. Other markers (keratin, S100, CD34, desmin, SMA, and neuroendocrine markers) are negative.
- *EWSR1-CREB1* rearrangement is characteristically seen by fluorescence in situ hybridization or polymerase chain reaction.
- Other entities harbor the *EWSR1-CREB1* rearrangement, including angiomatoid fibrous histiocytoma, clear cell sarcoma (of soft tissue), clear cell sarcoma–like tumor of the gastrointestinal tract, and hyalinizing clear cell carcinoma of the salivary gland; overlapping features between angiomatoid fibrous histiocytoma and PPMS have been described.

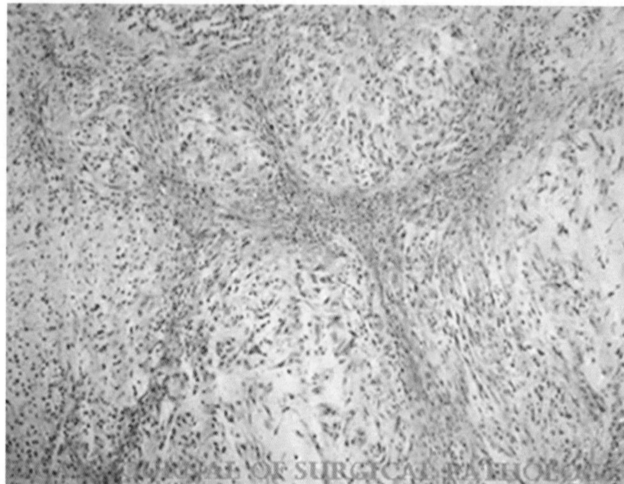

Figure 19.33 A low-power image demonstrating a nodular growth of tumor cells in cord-like arrangements with prominent myxoid stroma. (From Thway K, Nicholson AG, Lawson K, et al. Primary pulmonary myxoid sarcoma with EWSR1-CREB1 fusion: a new tumor entity. *Am J Surg Pathol.* 2011;35(11):1722–1132. doi:10.1097/PAS.0b013e318227e4d2.)

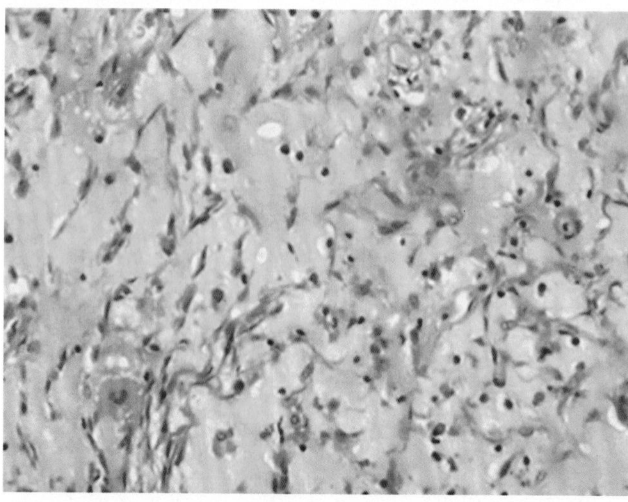

Figure 19.34 Tumor cells are spindle-shaped and stellate, with bland, ovoid, or elongated nuclei and small amounts of fibrillary cytoplasm. The stroma is myxoid rather than myxocollagenous. (From Thway K, Nicholson AG, Lawson K, et al. Primary pulmonary myxoid sarcoma with EWSR1-CREB1 fusion: a new tumor entity. *Am J Surg Pathol.* 2011;35(11):1722–1132. doi:10.1097/PAS.0b013e318227e4d2.)

Secondary Pulmonary Sarcomas

20

▸ Krzysztof Glomski
▸ Matthew W. Rosenbaum
▸ Ivan Chebib
▸ Mari Mino-Kenudson

Part 1

Leiomyosarcoma

Leiomyosarcoma is a malignant neoplasm with purely smooth muscle differentiation that occurs in older adults, most typically arising in the retroperitoneum and large vessels. In immunocompromised patients (patients with HIV/AIDS and transplant recipients), multicentric leiomyosarcomas involving parenchymal organs also occur and are associated with Epstein–Barr virus infection. Most leiomyosarcomas in the lung are metastatic, but rare primary tumors occur. Grossly, they are gray-white, fleshy, whorled, and often lobulated, with hemorrhage, necrosis, and cyst formation occasionally seen in large tumors.

CYTOLOGIC FEATURES

- Highly cellular fascicular arrangement of oval to spindle-shaped cells with mitotic activity.

HISTOLOGIC FEATURES

- Well-differentiated leiomyosarcomas show sharply demarcated intersecting fascicles of spindle cells with eosinophilic cytoplasm, elongated nuclei with rounded ends, and occasional hyalinized or myxoid stroma, necrosis, and hemorrhage.
- Poorly differentiated leiomyosarcomas show marked pleomorphism with abnormal mitotic figures.

ANCILLARY TESTING

- Immunohistochemistry (IHC) is typically positive for desmin, smooth muscle actin (SMA), and h-caldesmon in most cases.
- Poorly differentiated tumors may lose SMA and desmin immunoreactivity.
- No specific genetic molecular aberration. Loss of function mutations in *P53* and *RB1* may be seen.

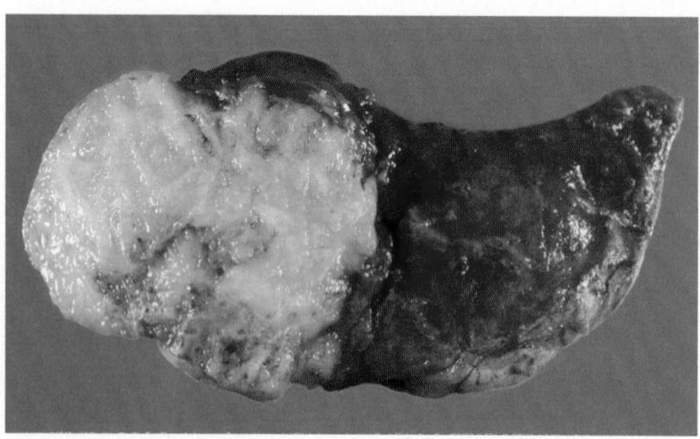

Figure 20.1 A gross image showing a fleshy, tan-white, well-circumscribed mass with focal hemorrhage.

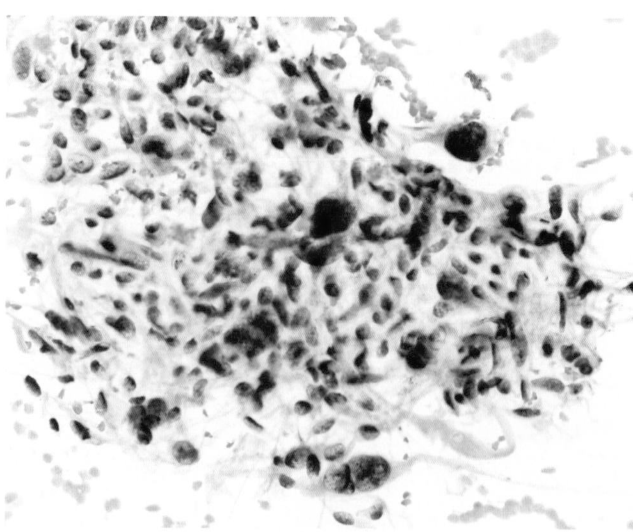

Figure 20.2 Cytology smear demonstrating pleomorphic and spindled cells with variable nuclear features (blunted elongate oval shapes being the most characteristic) and with elongated cytoplasmic processes.

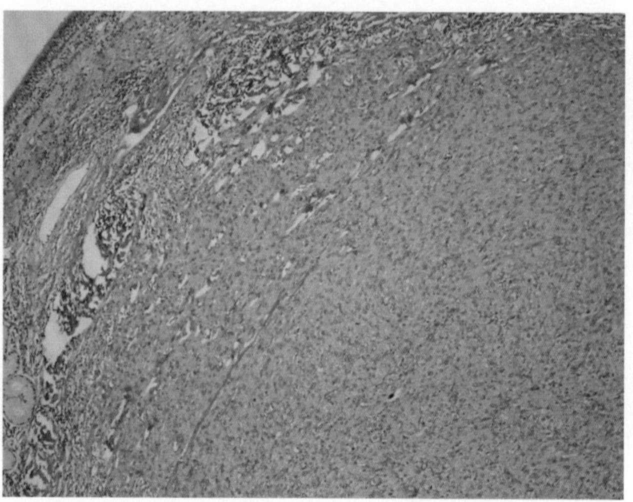

Figure 20.3 A well-demarcated mass underneath the respiratory mucosa composed of fascicles of spindle cells with eosinophilic cytoplasm.

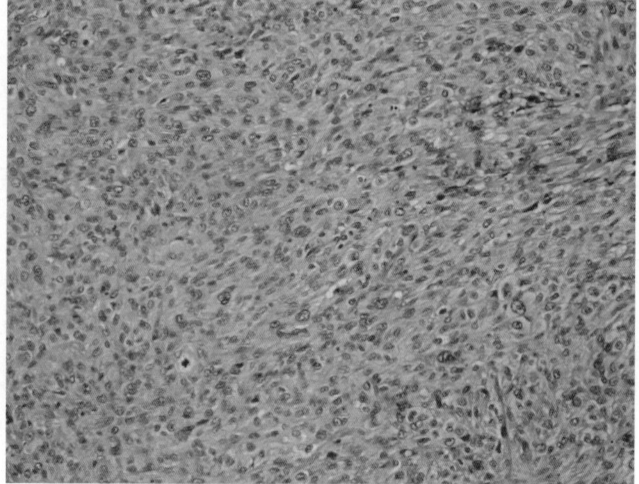

Figure 20.4 Fascicles of spindle cells with rounded, oval nuclei and moderately abundant, eosinophilic cytoplasm. Occasional mitotic figures and apoptotic debris are present.

Part 2

Angiosarcoma

Angiosarcomas of the lung usually represent metastases from other sites. They occur across a wide age distribution with peak incidence in older adults and have a slight male propensity. When they involve the lung, angiosarcomas are associated with hemoptysis and grossly appear as ill-defined, multinodular, hemorrhagic lesions with cystic degeneration and necrosis.

CYTOLOGIC FEATURES

- Atypical, pleomorphic cells that commonly disperse into single cells with epithelioid, spindled, or plasmacytoid morphology and vasoformative features (cytoplasmic lumina/vacuoles and endothelial wrapping).

HISTOLOGIC FEATURES

- Multiple histologic patterns within the same tumor may be seen.
- Well to moderately differentiated angiosarcomas show irregular anastomosing vascular spaces lined by dysplastic endothelial cells with hyperchromatic nuclei and abundant mitoses.
- Poorly differentiated angiosarcomas may show high-grade, pleomorphic spindle cells with rudimentary lumen formation and brisk mitotic activity.
- "Epithelioid" angiosarcoma describes tumors that contain solid areas of pleomorphic epithelioid cells with prominent, eosinophilic cytoplasm, large vesicular nuclei, and prominent nucleoli that may be misclassified as carcinoma (they may be keratin-positive).

ANCILLARY TESTING

- Ultrastructurally, angiosarcomas may show tight junctions, pinocytic vesicles, and Weibel–Palade bodies.
- Immunoreactive for CD34, CD31, ERG, and FLI1.
- Specific molecular aberrations are not well defined. MYC overexpression may be seen and often associated with radiation-induced angiosarcoma.

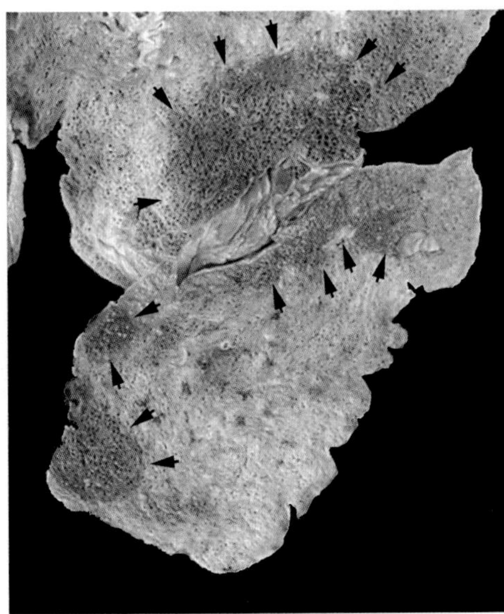

Figure 20.5 A gross image of angiosarcoma (after fixation) showing multiple hemorrhagic areas *(arrows)*. (Courtesy of Dr. Akihiko Yoshida.)

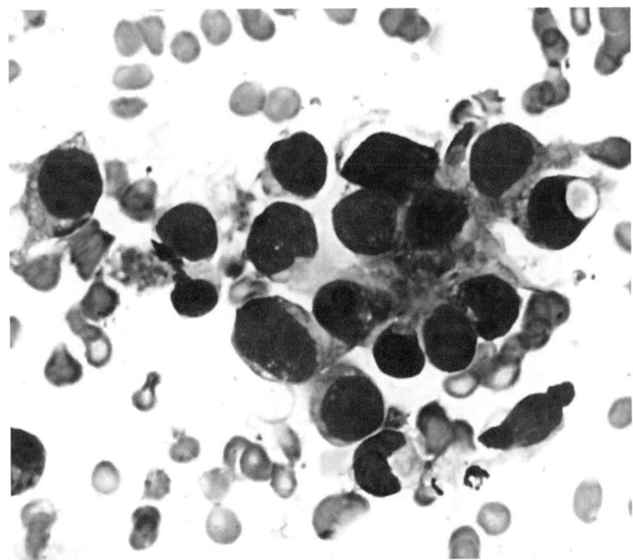

Figure 20.6 Bloody smear with epithelioid cells and rare intracytoplasmic inclusions (neolumens, which may contain red blood cells) may be identified.

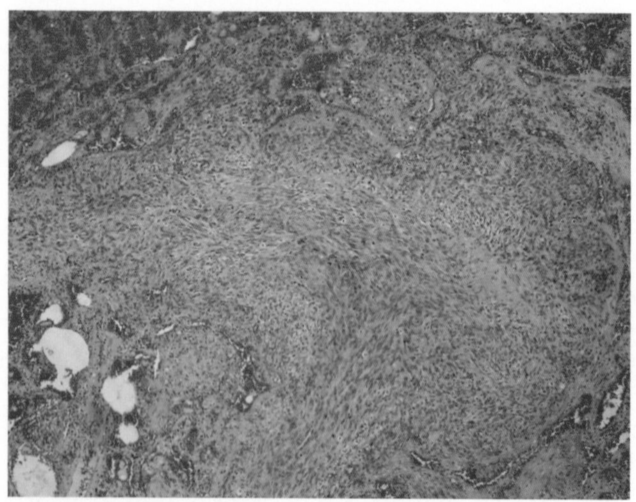

Figure 20.7 A low-power view demonstrating highly cellular spindle-cell proliferation with the background of blood-filled alveolar spaces.

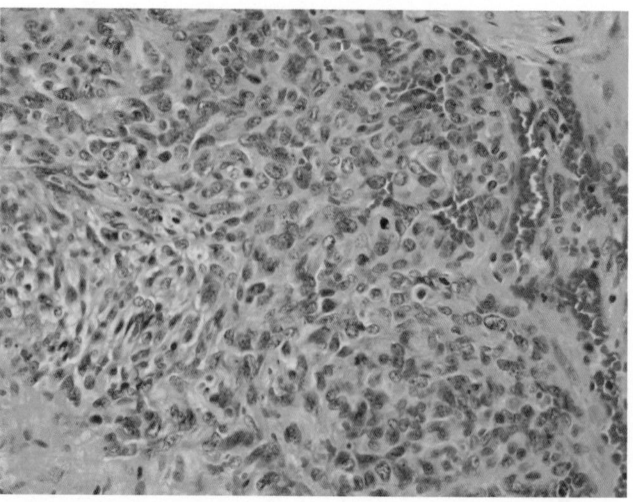

Figure 20.8 Spindled and atypical epithelioid cells line blood-filled lumina. Occasional tumor cells contain red blood cells in the cytoplasm. Mitotic figures and apoptotic bodies are conspicuous.

Part 3

Osteosarcoma

Conventional osteosarcoma is the most common primary sarcoma of the skeleton, most often arising in the metaphyses of long bones of the extremities in peripubescent children and older adults. It may also rarely arise in soft tissues of the trunk and thigh in older adults. Although primary pulmonary osteosarcoma is extremely rare, the lung is the most common site of metastatic osteosarcoma. Grossly, these lesions are gray-white with variable mineralization, hemorrhage, necrosis, and cystic changes. If found near the pulmonary artery, an osteosarcomatous component of pulmonary artery intimal sarcoma must be differentiated from metastasis.

CYTOLOGIC FEATURES

- Nonspecific, but will often contain high-grade pleomorphic cells with spindled to epithelioid morphology, multinucleated cells, fragments of bone/osteoid, cartilage, and necrosis.

HISTOLOGIC FEATURES

- Bone-forming sarcoma composed of neoplastic cells with highly variable morphology, including spindled, epithelioid, plasmacytoid, small and round, clear, or multinucleated.
- Lung metastases are commonly high-grade pleomorphic, with high mitotic index, with occasional chondroid component.

ANCILLARY TESTING

- IHC for SATB2 is typically positive. Variable immunopositivity for S100, SMA, CD99, EMA, and keratin.
- No recurrent molecular aberrations define conventional osteosarcoma, but *MYC* amplification and inactivation of P53 and RB1 are common.

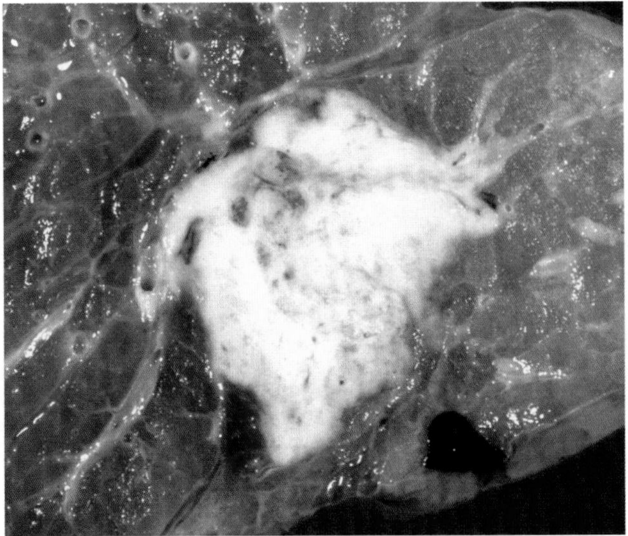

Figure 20.9 A gross image of osteosarcoma metastatic to the lung shows a white-tan, infiltrative mass with areas of hemorrhage.

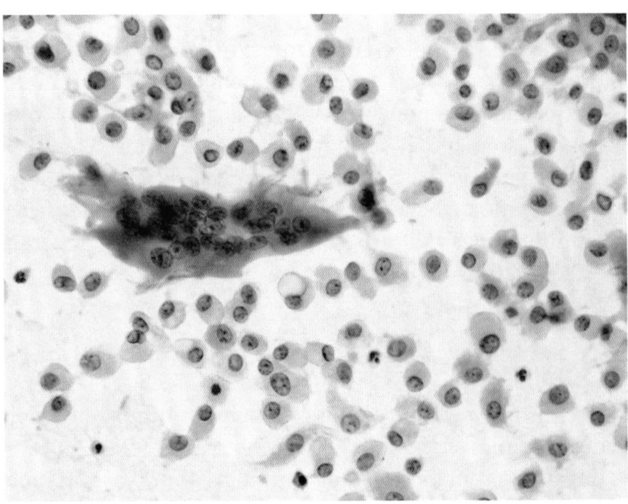

Figure 20.10 Cytology smear demonstrates abundant plasmacytoid cells and scattered osteoclasts; osteoid may be scant or only appreciated on cell block.

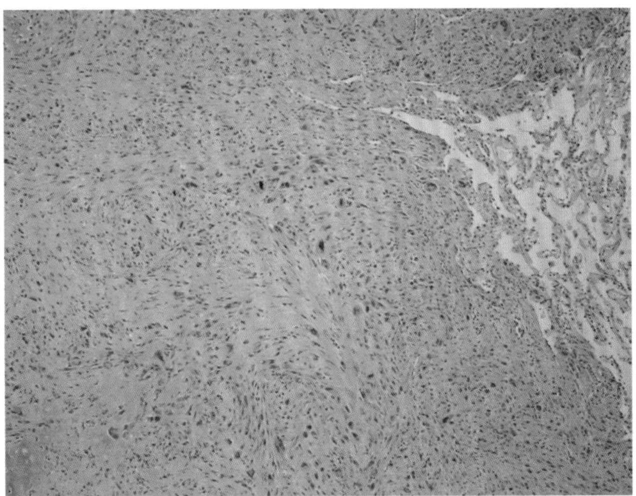

Figure 20.11 Spindled proliferation of pleomorphic cells; areas of bone formation are seen *(left of image)*.

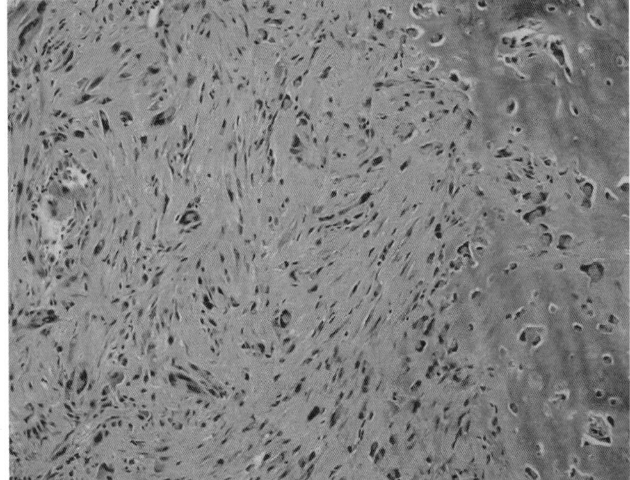

Figure 20.12 Pleomorphic spindled and epithelioid cells with eccentric, angulated, and hyperchromatic nuclei that form woven bone.

Part 4

Chondrosarcoma

Chondrosarcomas are malignant cartilage-producing tumors that most commonly arise in the pelvis, proximal femur, and proximal humerus of middle-aged and older adults with a slight male prominence. Low-grade lesions can occasionally give rise to high-grade dedifferentiated chondrosarcoma. In the lung, chondrosarcomas most commonly represent metastases. Grossly, they are lobulated, gray-white, glistening, gelatinous masses with occasional hemorrhage and necrosis.

CYTOLOGIC FEATURES

- Malignant chondrocytes with abundant vacuolated cytoplasm, large irregular nuclei, small to prominent nucleoli, and background chondromyxoid matrix material.

HISTOLOGIC FEATURES

- Lobules of gray-blue chondromyxoid matrix with embedded atypical chondrocytes (round to stellate cells with eosinophilic cytoplasm, multinucleation, condensed chromatin, and prominent nucleoli) arranged in variably loose clusters, rows, and nests.
- Lobules are typically separated by fibrous bands.
- Higher-grade lesions are more cellular, with greater pleomorphism and more mitotic figures.
- Dedifferentiated chondrosarcomas are typically undifferentiated spindled to pleomorphic sarcomas that arise abruptly from low-grade chondrosarcomas and may show osteosarcomatous differentiation.

ANCILLARY TESTING

- The distinct morphology of cartilaginous tumors often obviates the need for immunohistochemical staining.
- IHC using mutation-specific antibody (IDH1 R132H) may show reactivity and may be useful in identifying dedifferentiated components as arising from chondrosarcoma.
- Many chondrosarcomas harbor mutations in isocitrate dehydrogenase (*IDH-1* or *IDH-2*); higher-grade tumors also harbor activating mutations in *Rb1, p53*, or one of several receptor tyrosine kinases.

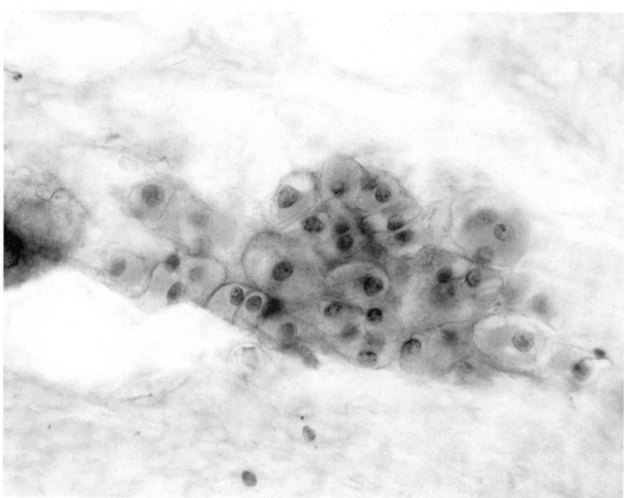

Figure 20.13 Cytology smear demonstrating low-grade-appearing chondrocytes with chondroid to chondromyxoid matrix.

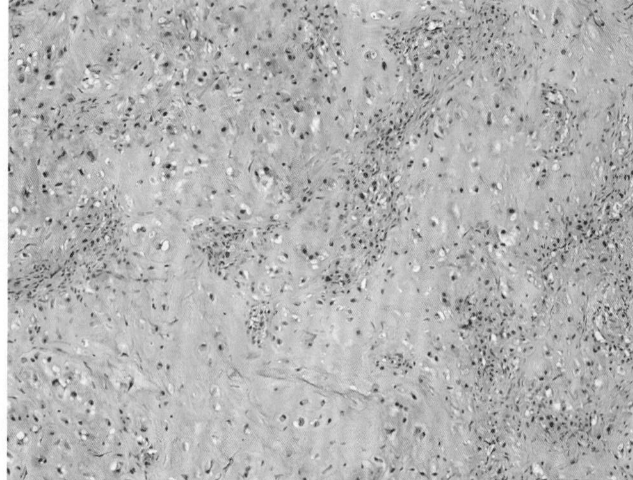

Figure 20.14 A low-power view of a high-grade chondrosarcoma showing a variably cellular neoplasm with gray-blue chondroid stroma.

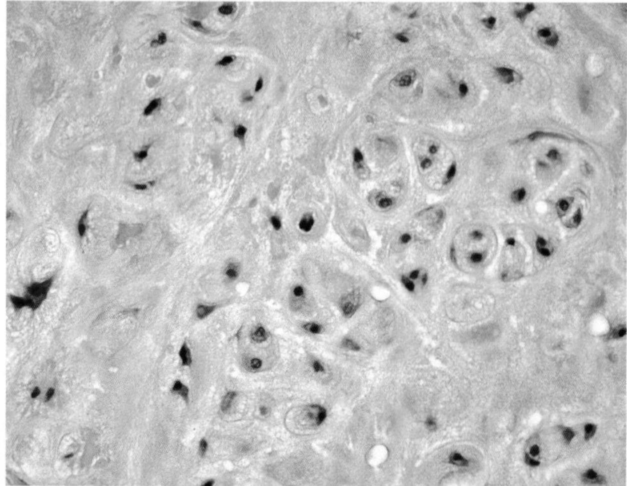

Figure 20.15 Low-grade chondrosarcoma contains a low density of epithelioid cells with amphiphilic cytoplasm, small round to oval nuclei, dense chromatin without conspicuous nucleoli, and rare binucleation.

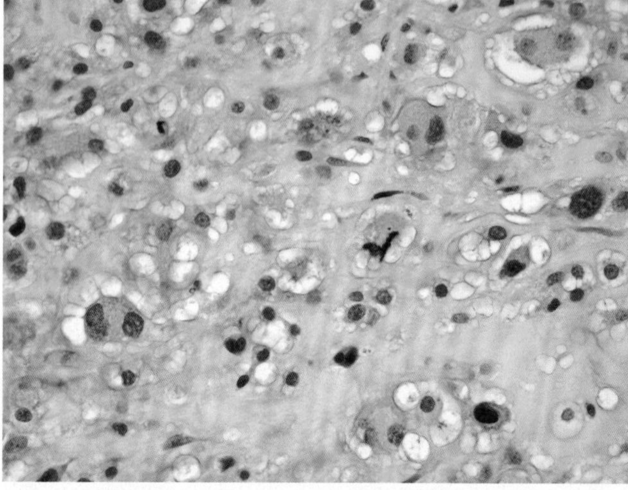

Figure 20.16 High-grade chondrosarcoma contains a moderate to high density of pleomorphic cells with amphiphilic cytoplasm, nucleoli, binucleation, and mitoses.

Part 5

Liposarcoma

Liposarcomas are malignant adipocytic tumors that generally occur in deep soft tissue sites (thigh, retroperitoneum, omentum, breast, mediastinum, and axilla) of older adults. Liposarcomas of the lung generally represent metastatic tumors; however, primary pulmonary liposarcomas rarely occur. Metastatic liposarcomas are typically higher-grade tumors with varied histology, including myxoid liposarcomas, dedifferentiated liposarcomas, and pleomorphic liposarcomas. Grossly, metastatic dedifferentiated liposarcomas of the lung are typically gray-white, nodular, fleshy to soft masses with areas of cystic change, hemorrhage, or necrosis.

CYTOLOGIC FEATURES

- Myxoid liposarcoma may show a delicate capillary network, foamy extracellular matrix, and lipoblasts.
- Dedifferentiated liposarcoma may consist only of malignant undifferentiated spindle cells with nuclear pleomorphism, hyperchromasia, and mitotic figures.

HISTOLOGIC FEATURES

- Myxoid liposarcomas contain small uniform cells with cytoplasmic vacuoles (signet ring lipoblasts) and small uniform nonlipogenic cells with scant cytoplasm within a myxoid stroma containing delicate arborizing vessels.
- Dedifferentiated liposarcoma is composed of a nonlipogenic high-grade sarcoma. Definitive diagnosis requires the identification of well-differentiated liposarcoma component.
- Pleomorphic liposarcoma contains pleomorphic to spindle cells with clusters of pleomorphic lipoblasts, which contain multiple cytoplasmic vacuoles. These tumors lack a well-differentiated liposarcomatous component.

ANCILLARY TESTING

- Myxoid liposarcomas contain characteristic *FUS-DDIT3* or *EWSR1-DDIT3* rearrangement. IHC is not necessary for diagnosis.
- Dedifferentiated liposarcomas will typically show staining with MDM2 and CDK4 by IHC and will harbor *MDM2* amplification by fluorescent in situ hybridization (FISH) and typically ring and giant marker chromosomes by karyotyping.
- Pleomorphic liposarcoma will typically show complex karyotypes, with no MDM2 or CDK4 staining or recurrent genetic alterations.

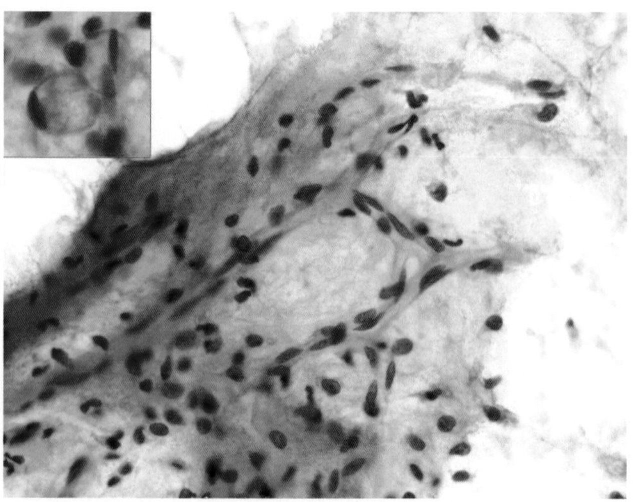

Figure 20.17 Cytology smear demonstrating delicate branching "chicken wire" vasculature, myxoid matrix, and scattered signet ring lipoblasts *(inset)*.

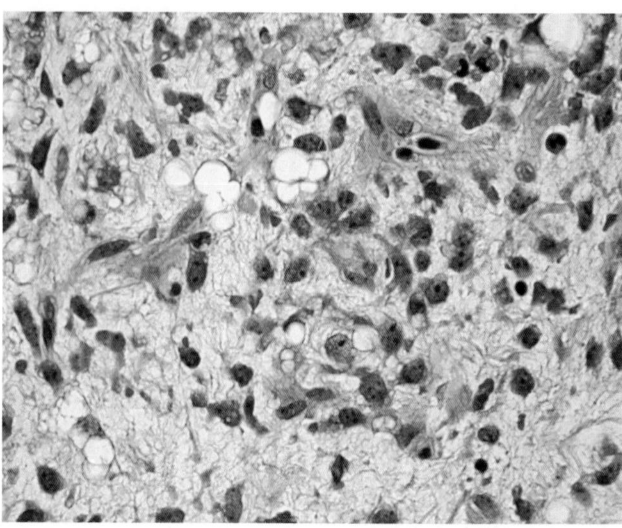

Figure 20.18 An example of myxoid liposarcoma with lipoblasts within a myxoid background.

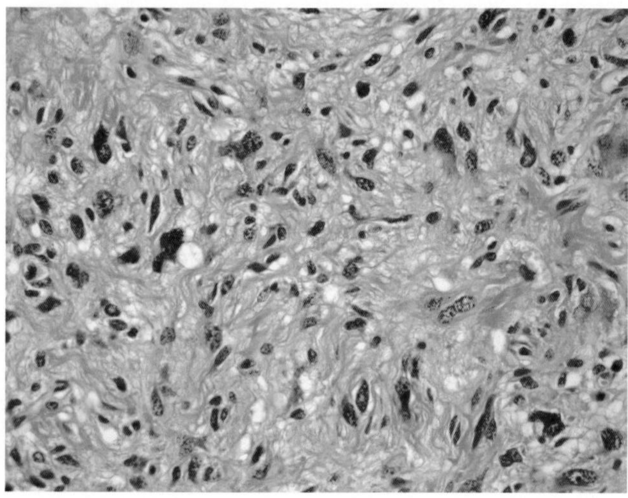

Figure 20.19 An example of dedifferentiated liposarcoma showing large, pleomorphic cells, with hyperchromatic nuclei.

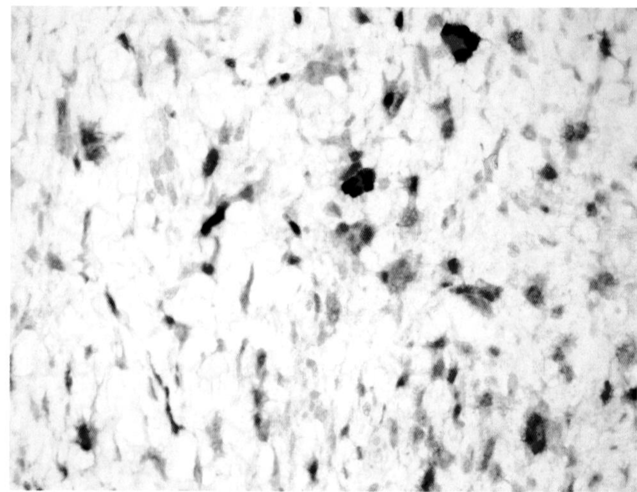

Figure 20.20 Immunohistochemistry for MDM2 shows nuclear staining within tumor cells.

Part 6

Malignant Peripheral Nerve Sheath Tumor

Malignant peripheral nerve sheath tumors (MPNSTs) most commonly arise from neurofibromas in patients with neurofibromatosis type 1 (NF1) and, less commonly, following radiation exposure or de novo from a preexisting nerve sheath tumor (usually neurofibroma). They most commonly arise in the extremities, trunk, and head/neck in young (particularly in NF1) and middle-aged adults. MPNSTs in the lung are predominantly metastatic and are grossly nodular with white-tan, fleshy cut surfaces with areas of hemorrhage and necrosis.

CYTOLOGIC FEATURES

- Often, clustered fascicles of spindle cells admixed with dissociated spindle cells with rounded nuclei, prominent nucleoli, variable pleomorphism, and frequent mitoses with a myxoid or fibrillary background.

HISTOLOGIC FEATURES

- Diverse appearance, but typically fascicular with densely cellular and hypodense regions with branching vasculature and geographic necrosis with viable cells often aggregating around blood vessels.
- Cells are typically tapered/spindled with wavy/comma-shaped nuclei and pale cytoplasm but may show marked pleomorphism.
- Heterologous elements are uncommon but may include skeletal muscle (malignant triton tumor), bone, and cartilage.
- Epithelioid MPNST is a rare variant containing plump, epithelioid cells, with abundant cytoplasm, lobulated growth, and myxoid matrix often arising in association with preexisting schwannomas in superficial sites.

ANCILLARY TESTING

- Focally positive for S100 in ~50% of MPNSTs, but higher-grade lesions may lose S100 expression completely. IHC may show loss of histone H3 lysine 27 trimethylation.
- Molecular alterations in *NF1* and *CDKN2A* have been reported.
- Epithelioid MPNST is diffusely S100-positive and often shows SMARCB1 (INI) loss by IHC in two-thirds of cases.

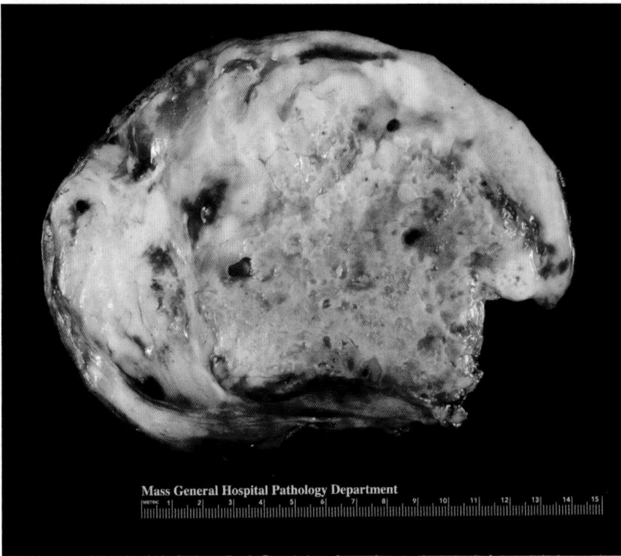

Figure 20.21 A gross image of malignant peripheral nerve sheath tumor shows a large, lobulated, tan-white, fleshy mass with areas of necrosis and hemorrhage invading into the chest wall. (Courtesy of Massachusetts General Hospital Pathology Department.)

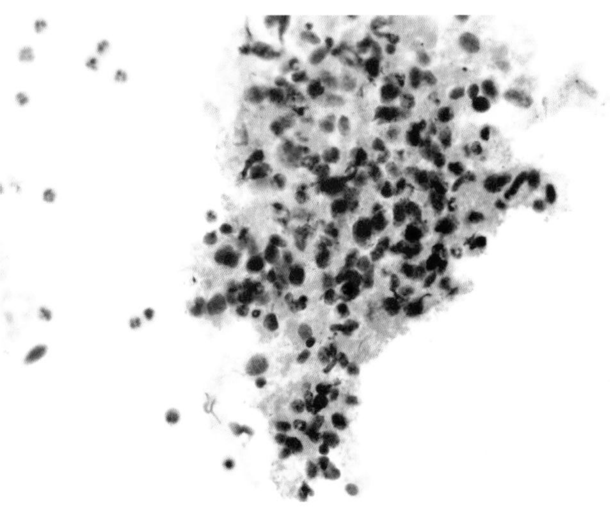

Figure 20.22 Cytology smear demonstrating high-grade spindle cells with hyperchromasia, pleomorphism, mitotic activity, and necrosis.

Figure 20.23 Moderately cellular spindle-cell proliferation arranged in whorled fascicles interposed with hypocellular collagen bands.

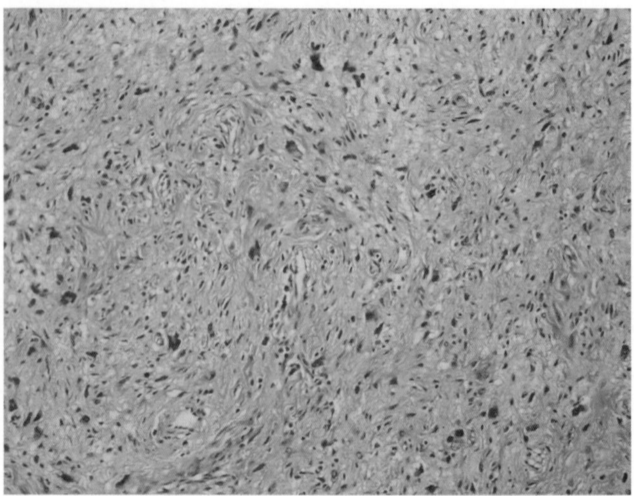

Figure 20.24 A high-power view reveals spindle cells with wavy, tapered nuclei, and occasional nuclear enlargement, pleomorphism, and hyperchromasia. Mitoses and necrosis (not shown) may be prominent.

Part 7

Rhabdomyosarcoma

Rhabdomyosarcoma (RMS) is a group of tumors that show skeletal muscle differentiation, with distinct clinicopathologic subtypes, including embryonal, alveolar, pleomorphic, and spindle cell/sclerosing. In the lung, RMS is usually metastatic. RMS is the most common soft tissue sarcomas of young children, often arising in the head and neck or urogenital systems (embryonal and spindle-cell RMS) and extremities (alveolar). Pleomorphic RMS typically arises in the extremities of adults. Grossly, lung metastases of RMS are nodular and expansile with fleshy-white cut surfaces with variable hemorrhage and/or necrosis.

CYTOLOGIC FEATURES

- Primitive-appearing small to medium round blue cells with hyperchromatic nuclei, scant or inconspicuous cytoplasm, occasional rhabdomyoblasts, rare multinucleation, and variable degrees of myogenic differentiation ("tadpole," "strap," or "spider" cell morphology).

HISTOLOGIC FEATURES

- Embryonal RMS contains variably cellular accumulations of primitive small round blue cells in differing stages of myogenesis and occasional rhabdomyoblasts. The stroma is often loose and myxoid, with occasional fibrosis. The "botryoid" variant of embryonal RMS has tumor cells in close abutment with epithelial surfaces, which grow as polypoid or pedunculated nodules.
- Alveolar RMS is a high-grade sarcoma containing densely cellular nests of primitive small round blue cells separated by fibrous septa, with discohesive cells toward the center of the nests, resulting in an alveolar pattern.

- Pleomorphic RMS contains sheets of undifferentiated large, atypical, and often multinucleated cells and scattered pleomorphic tumor cells showing skeletal muscle differentiation.
- Spindle-cell RMS shows a storiform growth pattern with spindled neoplastic cells with rare rhabdomyoblasts.

ANCILLARY TESTING

- RMS, in general, is typically positive for desmin, actin, MyoD, and myogenin by IHC.
- Alveolar RMS has a characteristic fusion of *PAX3* or *PAX7* with *FOXO1*, t(2;13) or t(1;13), respectively.
- Embryonal RMS has complex genetic alterations, often with loss of heterozygosity of ch11q15.5, but *PAX-FOXO1* fusion is absent.
- Pleomorphic and spindle cell subtypes show complex genetic alterations.

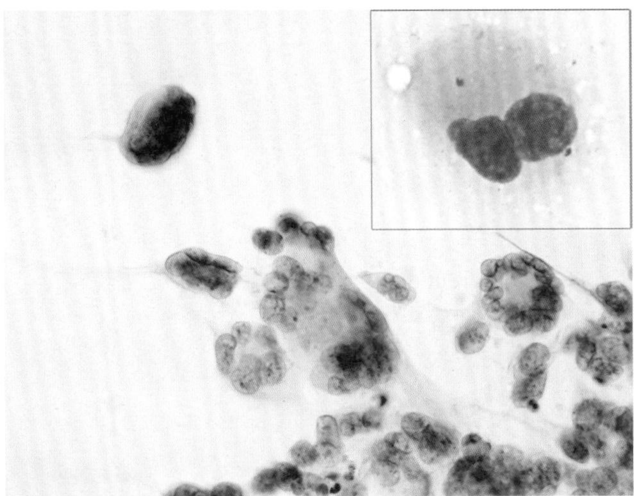

Figure 20.25 Cytology of alveolar rhabdomyosarcoma shows abundant tumor giant cells with peripheral wreath-like arrangement and highly atypical rhabdoid cells with prominent nucleoli; intracytoplasmic inclusions may also be seen.

Figure 20.26 A low-power image of metastatic pleomorphic rhabdomyosarcoma with highly cellular sheets of spindle cells.

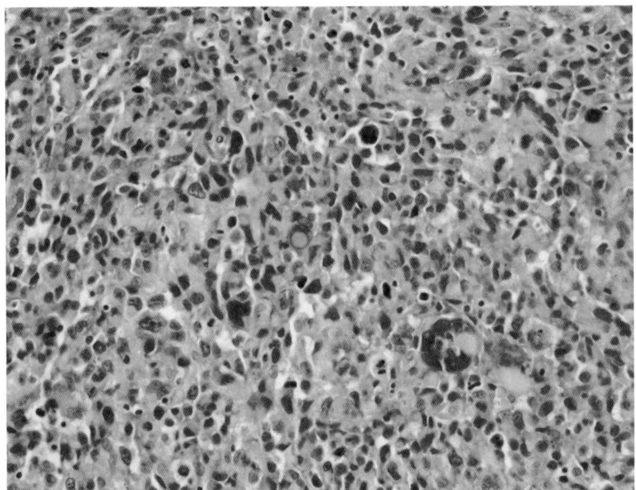

Figure 20.27 A high-power view of pleomorphic rhabdomyosarcoma demonstrating sheets of pleomorphic cells, some with rhabdoid features consisting of eccentric, hyperchromatic nuclei and prominent, glassy, eosinophilic cytoplasm.

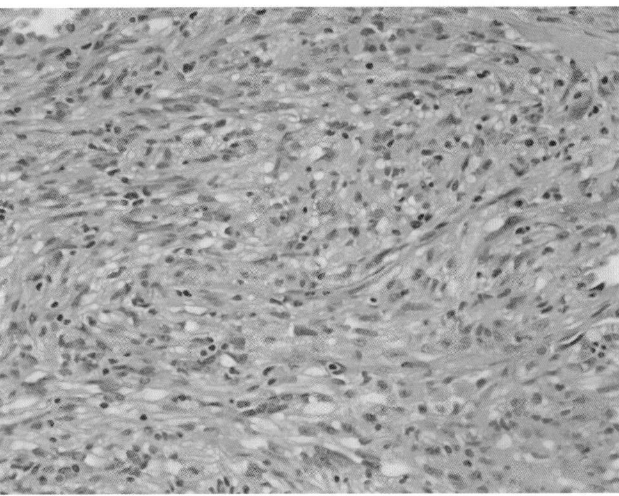

Figure 20.28 High-power image of pleomorphic rhabdomyosarcoma with plump spindle cells with elongated, angulated nuclei and prominent eosinophilic cytoplasm.

Part 8

Undifferentiated Soft Tissue Sarcoma

Undifferentiated sarcomas display no identifiable line of differentiation based on morphologic and ancillary studies (diagnosis of exclusion) and are generally metastatic when present in the lung. They account for approximately 20% of all sarcomas and typically arise in older adults, with no sex predilection. Grossly, their appearance may vary, but undifferentiated sarcomas often manifest as a white-tan nodular mass with necrosis.

CYTOLOGIC FEATURES

- Mixture of malignant spindle cells, and occasional giant cells, with areas of myxoid stroma and necrotic background.

HISTOLOGIC FEATURES

- High-grade sarcoma with variable growth patterns, brisk mitoses, occasional multinucleated tumor cells, necrosis, and hemorrhage.
- Morphologic subclassification includes undifferentiated spindle-cell sarcoma, undifferentiated pleomorphic sarcoma, undifferentiated round cell sarcoma, undifferentiated epithelioid sarcoma, and undifferentiated sarcoma, not otherwise specified, designated by the predominant morphologic appearance of sarcoma cells.

ANCILLARY TESTING

- No reproducible IHC pattern. Nonspecific or focal staining with keratin, actin, desmin, CD34, EMA, and CD99 may be seen.
- Recurrent genetic abnormalities are not seen.

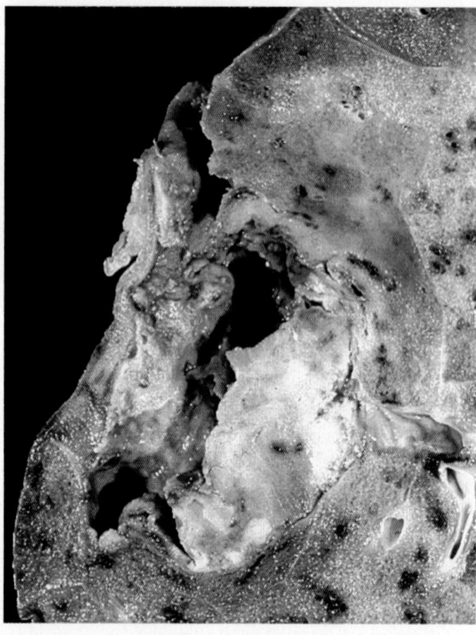

Figure 20.29 A gross image of undifferentiated pleomorphic sarcoma showing a tan-white mass with central necrosis.

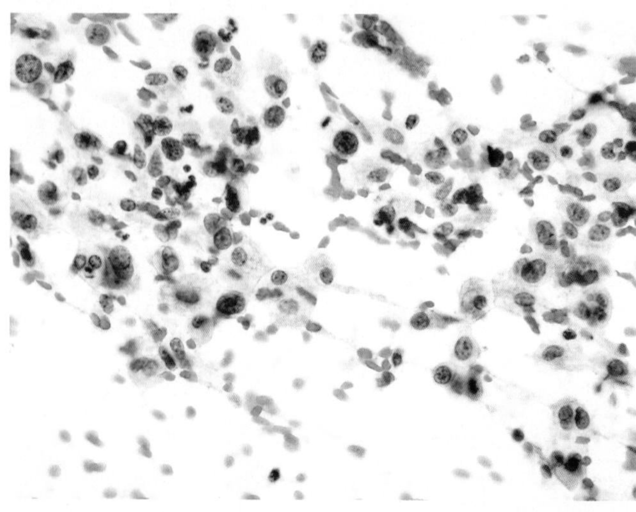

Figure 20.30 Cytology smear demonstrating pleomorphic, highly atypical epithelioid and spindle cells lacking other specific lines of differentiation.

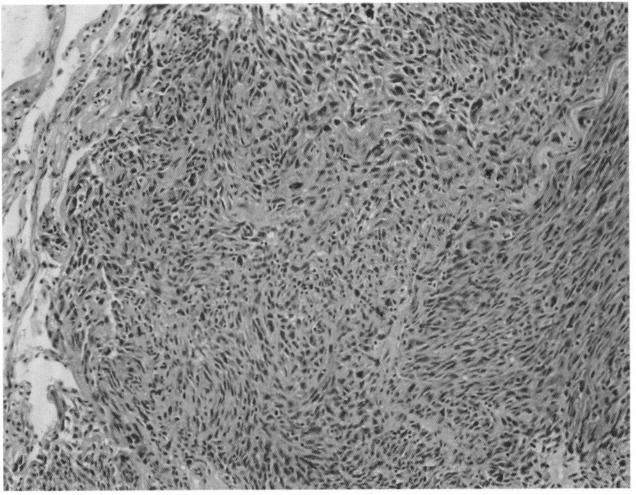

Figure 20.31 A low-power image characterized by a highly cellular, fascicular, spindle-cell neoplasm replacing the lung parenchyma.

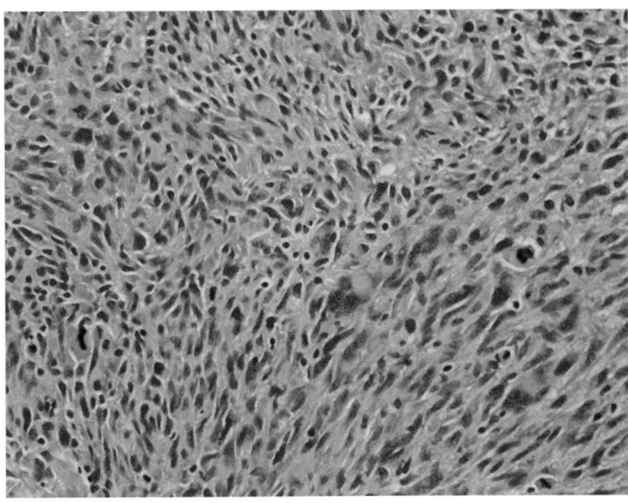

Figure 20.32 The tumor consists of atypical, pleomorphic spindle cells with numerous mitotic figures and apoptotic bodies.

Part 9

Ewing Sarcoma

Ewing sarcoma is a primitive, small round blue cell tumor that shows variable neuroectodermal differentiation and predominantly arises in metaphyseal/diaphyseal regions of long bones, pelvis, and ribs of children and young adults aged 10 to 30 years. Occasionally, they arise in extraskeletal locations; when found in the lung, it is most commonly due to metastatic spread. Grossly, these tumors are often tan-gray with prominent necrosis and hemorrhage.

CYTOLOGIC FEATURES

- Primitive-appearing small to medium round blue cells with granular to fine chromatin and scant or inconspicuous cytoplasm.

HISTOLOGIC FEATURES

- Most commonly sheet-like arrangement of small- to medium-sized round cells with fine chromatin, scant cytoplasm, and occasional neuroectodermal differentiation, including pseudorosettes.
- When neuroectodermal differentiation is prominent, Ewing sarcoma is sometimes termed primitive neuroectodermal tumor.
- Although histologically nonspecific, Ewing sarcoma is defined by recurrent genetic translocations (see below).

ANCILLARY TESTING

- IHC classically shows diffuse *membranous* staining for CD99 and nuclear FLI1 and may reveal focal neuroendocrine differentiation (synaptophysin, chromogranin, CD56 positivity).

- 85% of Ewing sarcomas carry an *EWSR1-FLI1* translocation, although many other translocations of *EWSR1* (and less commonly *FUS*) with ETS family of transcription factors (*ERG, ETV1, ETV4, FEV*) also occur.
- The diagnosis is confirmed by FISH or molecular testing detecting an *EWSR1* rearrangement.
- A small subset of small round blue cell tumors resembling Ewing sarcoma, which do not possess an *EWSR1* translocation, are termed *Ewing-like sarcomas* and have been found to have alternate translocations, including *CIC-DUX4* and *BCOR-CCNB3*.

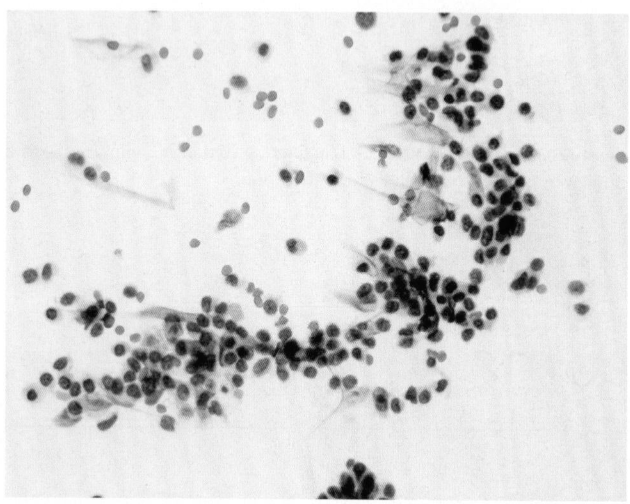

Figure 20.33 Cytology smear showing poorly cohesive monomorphic small round blue cells with scant cytoplasm.

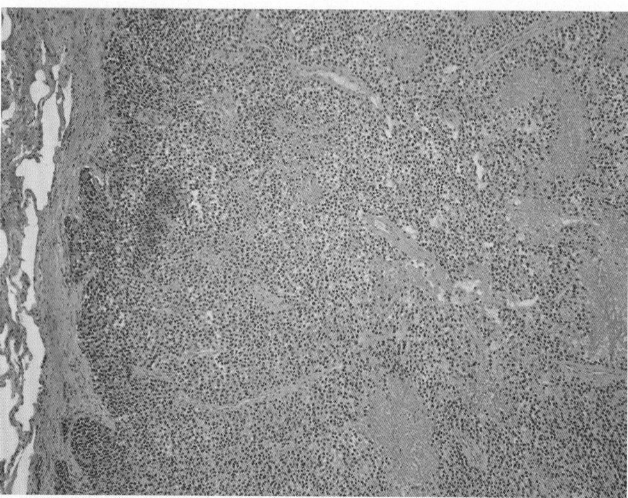

Figure 20.34 A low-power image demonstrating sheets of round, loosely cohesive cells with areas of necrosis and intervening fibrovascular septae.

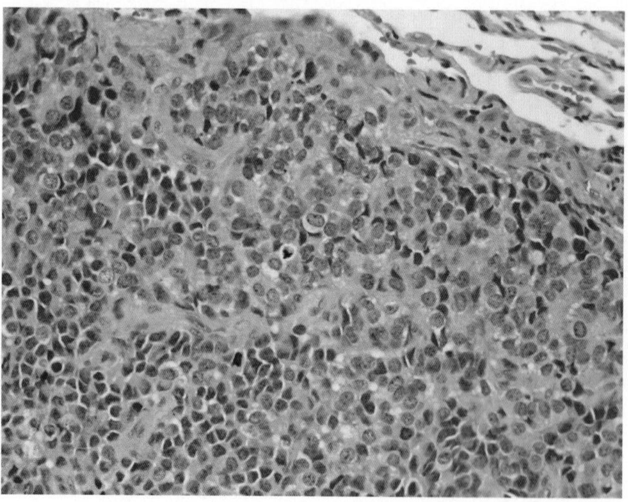

Figure 20.35 The tumor consists of homogenous cells with round to angulated nuclear contours, scant cytoplasm, and scattered mitoses.

21 Other Pulmonary Sarcomas

▸ Krzysztof Glomski
▸ Matthew W. Rosenbaum
▸ Ivan Chebib
▸ Mari Mino-Kenudson

Part 1

Alveolar Soft Part Sarcoma

Alveolar soft part sarcoma (ASPS) is a rare neoplasm typically arising in the deep soft tissues of the thigh or buttocks in adults and in the head/neck region (tongue or orbit) of infants and children. Other primary sites, including the lung, are possible, although metastatic disease is more common and often the presenting manifestation of the disease. Grossly, these tumors are poorly circumscribed, yellow-gray, and soft, with hemorrhage and necrosis.

CYTOLOGIC FEATURES

- Cells arranged in small clusters/acini or singly, with abundant clear to finely vacuolated cytoplasm (often disrupted), with central nuclei and prominent nucleoli.

HISTOLOGIC FEATURES

- Organoid/nesting architecture, with delicate fibrovascular stroma separating similarly sized nests.
- Tumor cells are uniform and epithelioid, with prominent cell borders, abundant, granular to clear cytoplasm, central uniform nuclei, with prominent nucleoli. Mitoses are uncommon, but vascular invasion may be seen.
- Occasional rhomboid intracytoplasmic crystalline inclusions are apparent within tumor cells.

ANCILLARY TESTING

- Electron microscopy occasionally shows membrane-bound lattice-like rhomboid crystals
- Periodic acid–Schiff highlights intracytoplasmic crystalline inclusions, which are typically focal.
- Immunohistochemistry (IHC) shows strong nuclear TFE3 staining and variable desmin staining. ASPS is negative for keratin, epithelial membrane antigen (EMA), chromogranin, synaptophysin, S100, and HMB45.
- Characteristic der(17)t(X;17)(p11.2;q25) translocation resulting in *TFE3-ASPSCR1* fusion may be detected by fluorescent in situ hybridization (FISH), reverse transcription polymerase chain reaction (RT-PCR), or related methods.

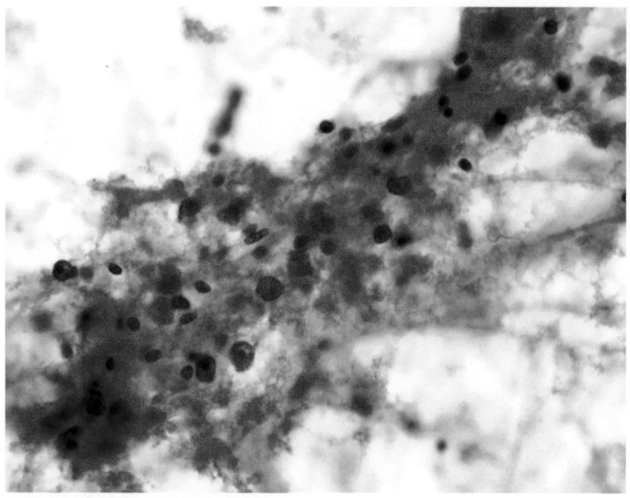
Figure 21.1 Cytology smear showing epithelioid tumor cells with prominent nucleoli and abundant granular cytoplasm.

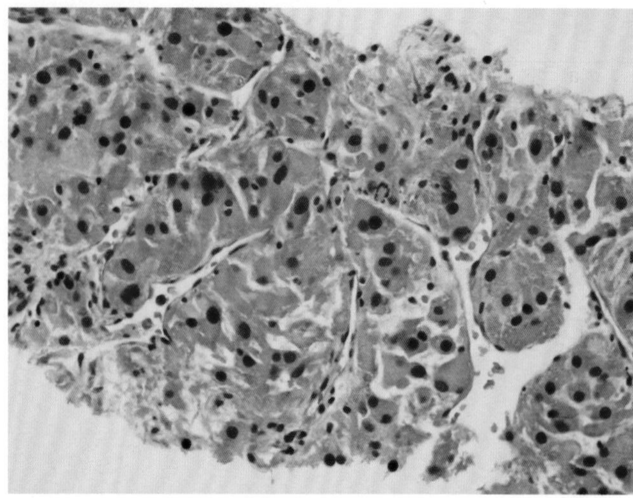
Figure 21.2 Nests of large cells with round, hyperchromatic, monomorphous nuclei and abundant, granular, eosinophilic cytoplasm.

Part 2

Clear Cell Sarcoma

Clear cell sarcoma of soft tissue (formerly known as melanoma of soft parts) is a rare, aggressive, malignant neoplasm usually arising in deep soft tissues around tendons/aponeurotic structures of the extremities (typically ankle/foot) in young adults. It less commonly arises from head/neck, trunk, or visceral structures, and when in the lung, it typically represents metastatic disease. Grossly, clear cell sarcomas are lobulated, gray-white, with variable hemorrhage and necrosis, and rare pigmentation.

CYTOLOGIC FEATURES

- Highly cellular neoplasm with variably cohesive cells; eosinophilic, eccentric cytoplasm; round nuclei; and prominent nucleoli.
- Pleomorphism, macronucleoli, and mitotic activity are usually less prominent than in metastatic melanoma.

HISTOLOGIC FEATURES

- Highly nested tumor separated by collagenous stroma.
- Neoplastic cells are relatively uniform and spindled to epithelioid, with pale eosinophilic or amphophilic cytoplasm, vesicular nuclei, and prominent nucleoli, although they can be as pleomorphic and mitotically active as metastatic melanoma.
- Wreath-like neoplastic cells are often scattered throughout the tumor.
- Melanin pigment is rarely seen on hematoxylin and eosin stain.

ANCILLARY TESTING

- Melanoma markers (such as S100, HMB45, MiTF, and Melan-A) are typically strongly expressed by IHC.
- Fontana-Masson stain reveals melanin in about half of cases.
- Characteristic fusion of *EWSR1-ATF1* seen in more than 90% of cases; less commonly *EWSR1-CREB1*.

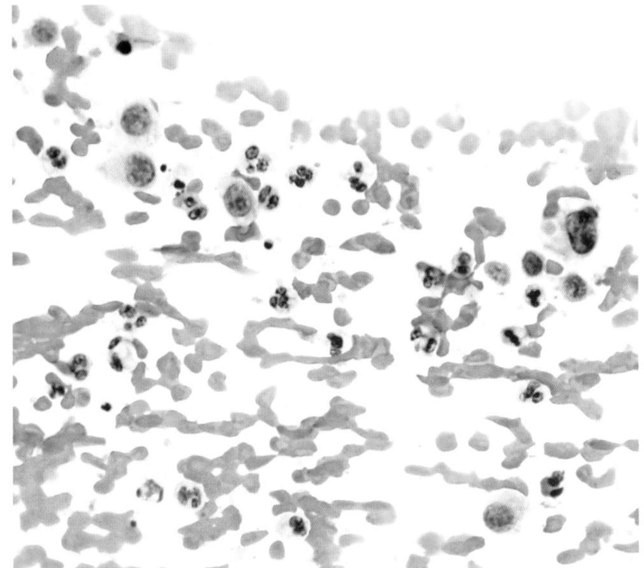

Figure 21.3 Cytology smear characterized by large epithelioid cells with round nuclei, prominent nucleoli, and abundant cytoplasm.

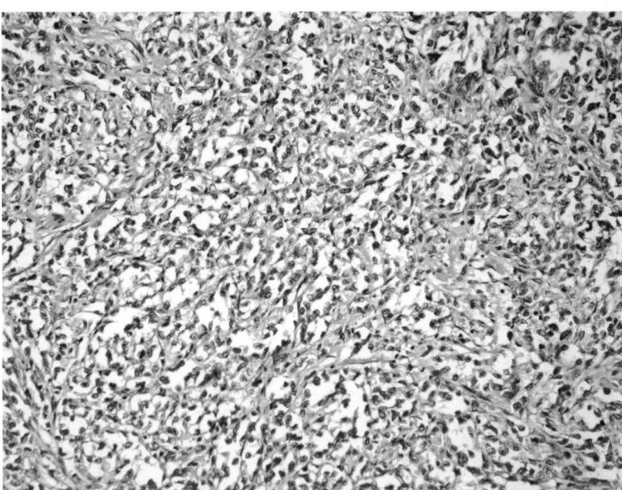

Figure 21.4 Sheets of spindled and epithelioid cells with abundant, cleared cytoplasm.

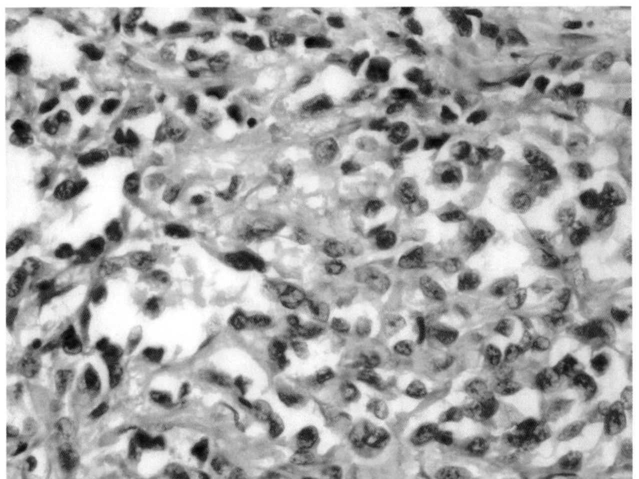

Figure 21.5 Round to spindle-shaped cells with large, pleomorphic nuclei with conspicuous nucleoli and vacuolated cytoplasm.

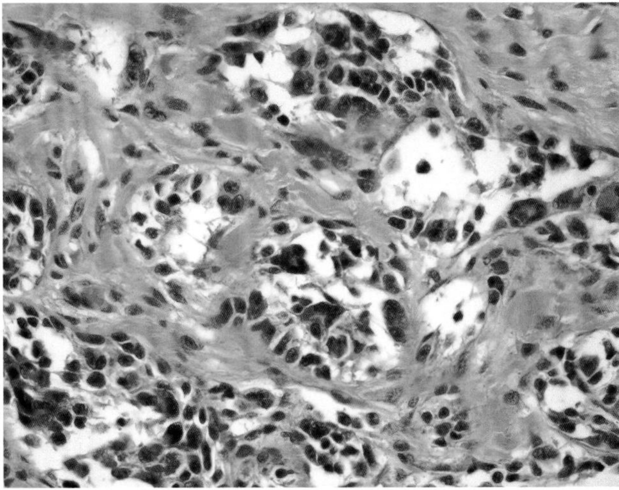

Figure 21.6 Occasionally nested/alveolar arrangement of pleomorphic cells with giant cells may be seen.

Part 3

Desmoplastic Small Round Cell Tumor

Desmoplastic small round cell tumor is an aggressive malignant neoplasm that most commonly presents as a multinodular mass studding the abdominal cavity (serosa, retroperitoneum, omentum, mesentery, pelvis) of young adults (with a peak in the 20s), with a strong male predilection. It rarely occurs outside the abdominal cavity and, when present in the lungs, typically represents metastatic disease. Metastatic nodules are typically gray-white, with hemorrhage and necrosis.

CYTOLOGIC FEATURES

- Primitive-appearing small to medium round blue cells with finely granular chromatin, indented nuclei, inconspicuous nucleoli, and scant cytoplasm. Nuclear molding and nucleic acid "streaking" may be seen.

HISTOLOGIC FEATURES

- Sharply delineated, highly cellular nests within a prominent collagenous or desmoplastic stroma are seen. Rosette formation may occur.
- The cells are usually uniform, small, and round, with hyperchromatic nuclei, scant cytoplasm, and inconspicuous borders.
- Mitoses are generally prominent, and necrosis is common.

ANCILLARY TESTING

- Desmin often shows dot-like cytoplasmic reactivity. Keratin, vimentin, and EMA are variably positive.
- WT1 IHC directed at C-terminal exons of the WT1 protein may be positive. However, most laboratories use clones directed toward the N-terminus of WT1, and so WT1 is often negative.
- Recurrent, characteristic *EWSR1-WT1* fusion is present and can be detected by PCR.

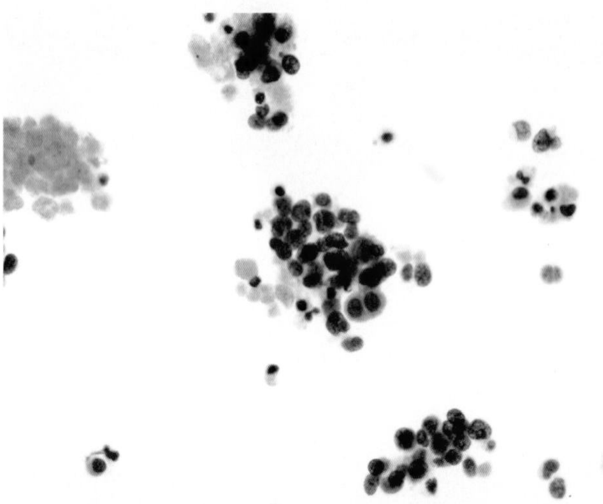

Figure 21.7 Cytology smear showing clusters of small round tumor cells with scant cytoplasm and necrosis. Fibrous (desmoplastic) stroma may be identified in a minority of cases.

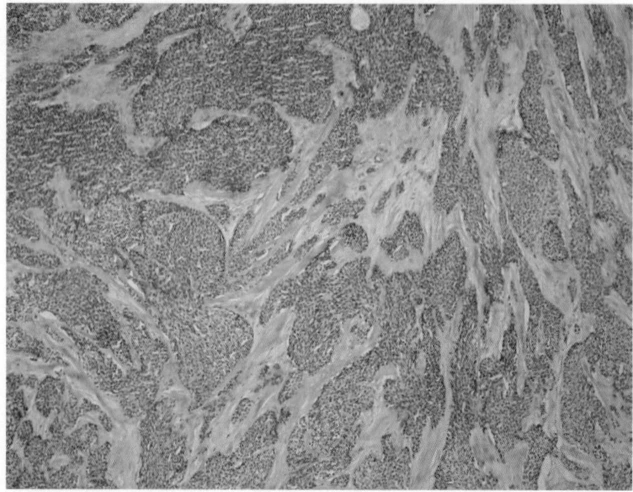

Figure 21.8 A low-power image demonstrating highly cellular sheets of cells separated by thick fibrous bands.

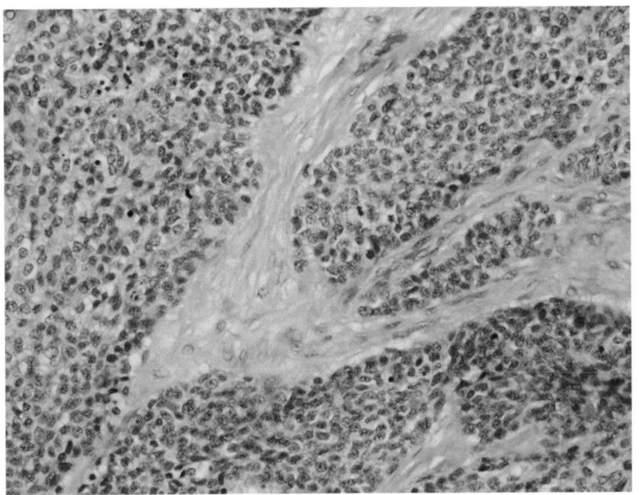

Figure 21.9 Small, round, blue monomorphous cells separated by hypocellular fibrous bands. Abundant mitoses and apoptotic bodies are present.

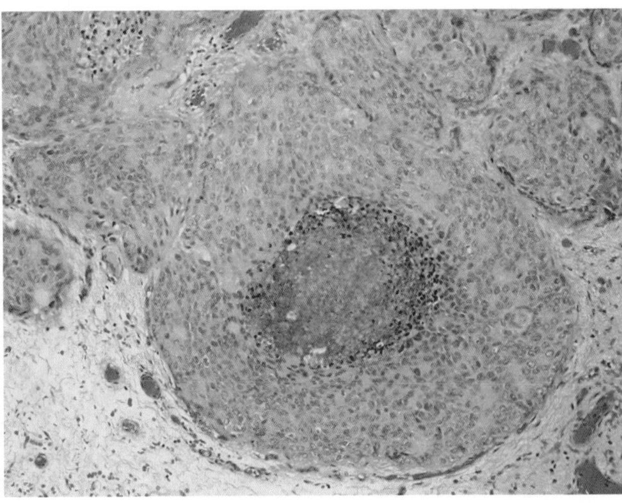

Figure 21.10 Central necrosis within large cellular nests and rosette formation may be seen.

Part 4

Extrarenal Rhabdoid Tumor

Extrarenal rhabdoid tumor is a malignant soft tissue tumor that arises in deep, central locations (neck, paraspinal, and perineum) in infants and young children. These tumors may arise in the extremities and are sometimes seen in visceral organs (most commonly liver) and, when in the lung, typically represent metastatic spread. These tumors are extremely aggressive with poor prognosis. Grossly, they are tan-gray, soft, with hemorrhage and necrosis.

CYTOLOGIC FEATURES

- Extrarenal rhabdoid tumors typically contain dispersed, epithelioid cells with eccentric, round nuclei with prominent nucleoli, and abundant cytoplasm with perinuclear cytoplasmic density (rhabdoid morphology).

HISTOLOGIC FEATURES

- Extrarenal rhabdoid tumors will often grow in sheets and cords of discohesive "rhabdoid" cells with eccentric, vesicular nuclei, prominent nucleoli, and perinuclear eosinophilic hyaline inclusions/globules.
- This may include a prominent "small, round, blue cell" component.
- Mitoses are typically prominent.

ANCILLARY TESTING

- By IHC, most extrarenal rhabdoid tumors shows loss of INI1 (SMARCB1) nuclear expression, and some tumors may be positive for EMA and keratin.
- Molecular analysis shows homozygous inactivation of the *SMARCB1* gene (also see in malignant rhabdoid tumors of the kidney, epithelioid malignant peripheral nerve sheath tumors, and atypical teratoid/rhabdoid tumors in the central nervous system).

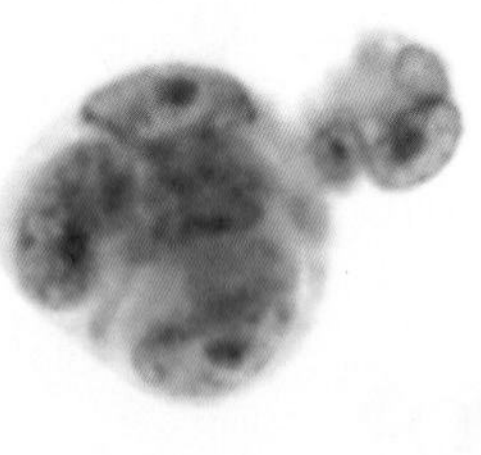

Figure 21.11 Cytology smear showing large cells with abundant cytoplasm, large nuclei with prominent nucleoli. Intracytoplasmic inclusions may also be identified (not seen here).

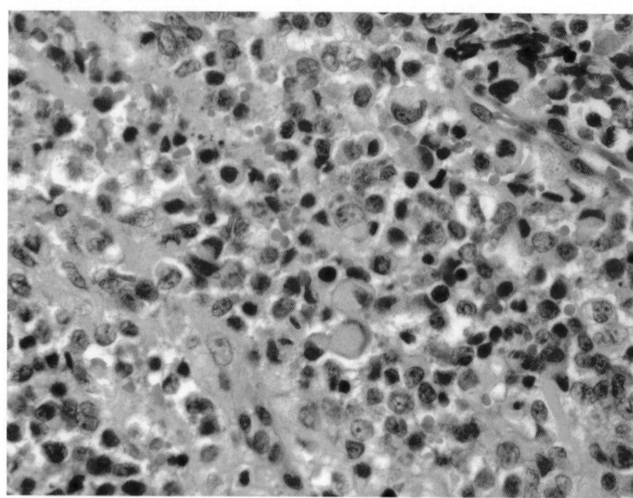

Figure 21.12 Pleomorphic cells with numerous rhabdoid forms with eccentric nuclei and prominent, central, glassy, eosinophilic cytoplasm. Numerous mitoses and apoptotic bodies are present.

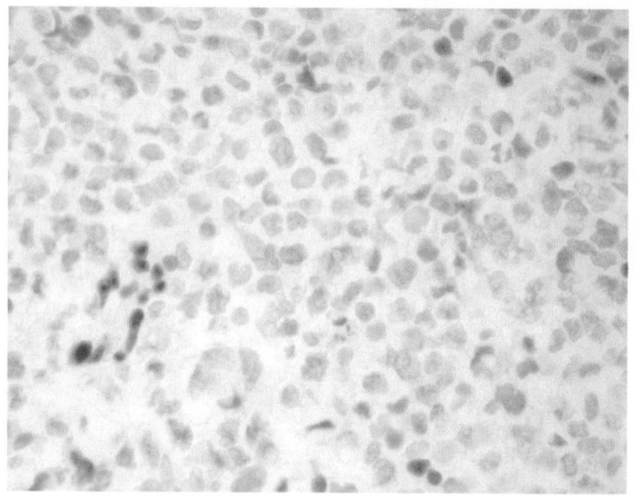

Figure 21.13 Immunohistochemistry for INI-1 shows loss in tumor cells, with retention in surrounding endothelial and stroma cells.

Part 5

Chordoma

Chordomas are malignant tumors of notochordal origin that most commonly affect the axial skeleton (sacrum, clivus, and vertebrae) of older adults, with slight male predilection but may occur at any age. Chordomas in the lung most commonly represent metastatic disease. Grossly, chordomas are lobulated, with blue-gray gelatinous cut surfaces.

CYTOLOGIC FEATURES

- Characteristic "physaliphorous" cells are large and round with vesicular chromatin and abundant "bubbly" cytoplasm.
- Smaller, round epithelial cells are also present with round nuclei and eosinophilic cytoplasm.
- Chondromyxoid background.

HISTOLOGIC FEATURES

- Typically lobulated with abundant chondromyxoid stroma separated by fibrous stroma.
- Embedded within the stroma are ribbons and cords of large, physaliphorous (bubbly) cells with variable nuclear atypia as well as smaller, epithelioid cells with round nuclei.
- Chondroid differentiation may be prominent (chondroid chordomas).
- High-grade undifferentiated sarcoma juxtaposed to a conventional chordoma component defines dedifferentiated chordoma.

ANCILLARY TESTING

- IHC is positive for brachyury (nuclear notochord-specific marker), EMA, keratin, and S100.
- Molecular alterations vary (no characteristic changes) and include monosomy for chromosome 1, gain of chromosome 7, loss of *CDKN2A* and *CDKNB*, and copy number gains of the brachyury locus.

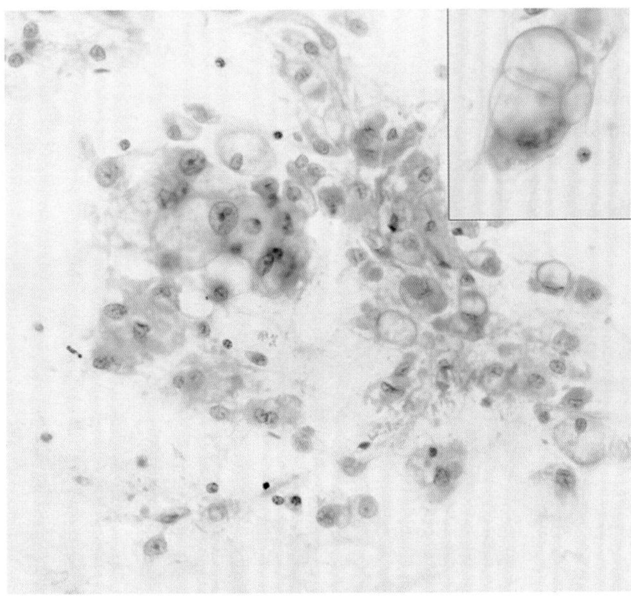

Figure 21.14 Cytology smear showing epithelioid to histiocytoid cells with abundant cytoplasm and prominent vacuoles, with some cells containing multiple vacuoles (physaliferous cells in inset).

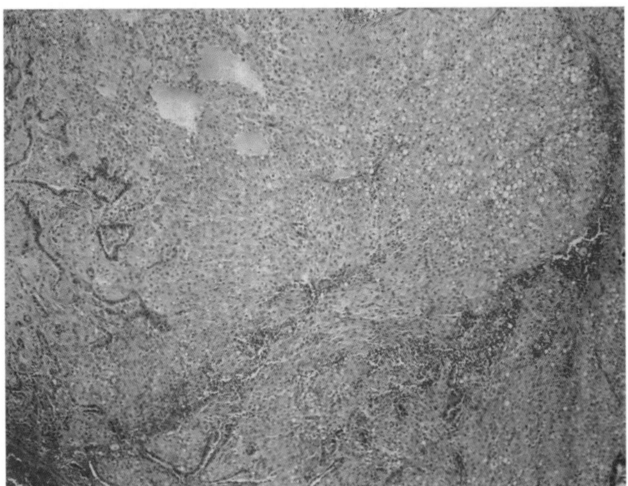

Figure 21.15 Moderately cellular sheets and cords of cells within a chondromyxoid stroma.

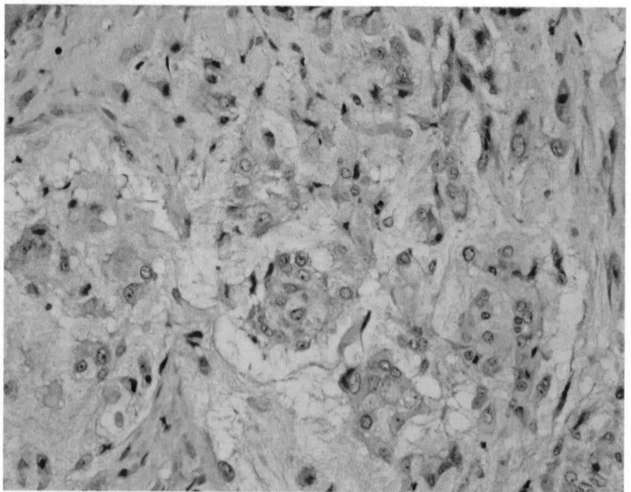

Figure 21.16 Epithelioid tumor cells with round vesicular nuclei and conspicuous nucleoli, moderately abundant eosinophilic cytoplasm with variable vacuolization embedded in a loose, chondromyxoid stroma.

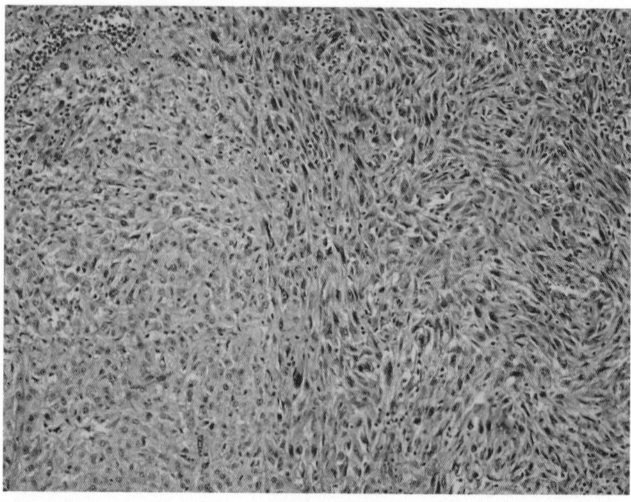

Figure 21.17 An example of dedifferentiated chordoma demonstrating highly cellular proliferation of spindled, pleomorphic tumor cells.

Part **6**

Extraskeletal Myxoid Chondrosarcoma

Extraskeletal myxoid chondrosarcoma (EMC) is a rare malignancy, most commonly arising in the deep soft tissues of the extremities in middle-aged adults with a skewed incidence toward males (2:1). When in the lungs, it is most commonly due to metastatic spread. Grossly, EMC is typically lobulated, with gray-white glistening, gelatinous cut surfaces separated by white-tan septae.

CYTOLOGIC FEATURES

- Round, uniform cells with moderate granular cytoplasm arranged in small clusters or chords with abundant myxoid background.

HISTOLOGIC FEATURES

- Multinodular tumor with abundant gray-blue, hypovascular stroma separated by fibrous septae.
- Embedded within the stroma are small, slightly elongated uniform cells with moderately abundant cytoplasm, which aggregate in loose clusters, cords, or nests.
- Chondroid differentiation is *not* seen.

ANCILLARY TESTING

- No specific IHC pattern defines EMC. May show focal S100 positivity and neuroendocrine marker positivity.
- Characteristic translocations generating NR4A3 fusion proteins, including *EWSR1-NR4A3* (most common), *TAF15-NR4A3*, and *TCF12-NR4A3*, are seen in most cases and may be detected by FISH or PCR.

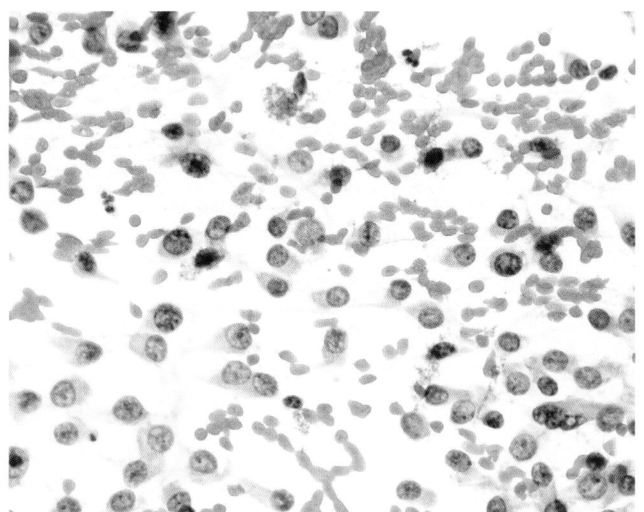

Figure 21.18 Cytology smear showing abundant plasmacytoid to epithelioid cells with large, round nuclei; chondromyxoid matrix may also be seen.

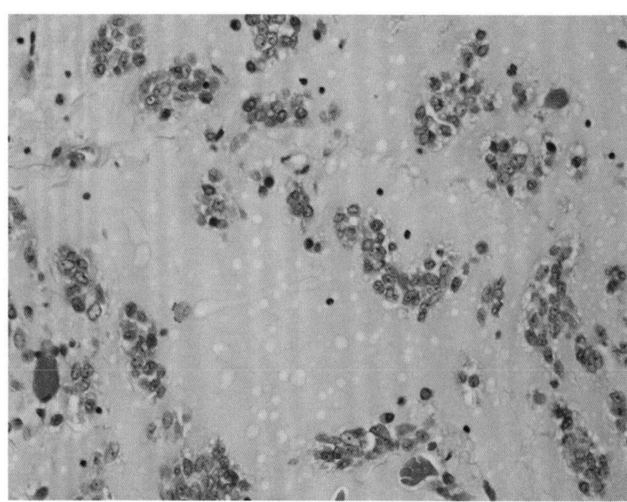

Figure 21.19 Clusters of epithelioid tumor cells with round nuclei, conspicuous nucleoli, and scant cytoplasm arranged in small, loose clusters within a prominent, loose chondromyxoid stroma.

Pulmonary B-Cell Lymphomas

22

Sergio Pina-Oviedo

INTRODUCTION

Primary pulmonary lymphomas are rare. They represent <1% of all primary lung tumors and 3% to 5% of extranodal lymphomas. Primary pulmonary lymphoma is defined as lymphoma confined to the lung with or without hilar lymph node involvement at the time of diagnosis or up to 3 months thereafter. The median age of presentation is 60 years. Patients may be asymptomatic or present with respiratory symptoms. On imaging, primary pulmonary lymphomas cannot be distinguished from infection, lung cancer, or metastatic disease, and therefore, their diagnosis must be established by histologic examination.

Extranodal marginal zone lymphoma (MZL) of the mucosa-associated lymphoid tissue (MALT lymphoma) is the most common type of primary pulmonary lymphoma (~80% of cases), followed by primary pulmonary diffuse large B-cell lymphoma (DLBCL) (~15%). Lymphomatoid granulomatosis (LyG), primary pulmonary plasmacytoma, primary pulmonary classical Hodgkin lymphoma (CHL), and other B-cell lymphomas add up to the remainder cases (~5%).

Secondary lung involvement by systemic B-cell lymphomas is by far more frequent than primary disease. Histologically, all these disorders are similar to their counterparts in lymph nodes or other extranodal sites. Primary and secondary B-cell lymphomas of the lung are morphologically identical and can only be distinguished as such by the clinical presentation.

Because some pulmonary B-cell lymphomas are composed of a polymorphous infiltrate (MALT lymphoma and low-grade LyG), the main differential diagnosis of these lesions includes reactive inflammatory conditions. Moreover, these lymphomas may be associated with organizing pneumonia that can further complicate the histologic interpretation. On the other hand, the differential diagnosis of monotonous large-cell pulmonary lymphomas (DLBCL and high-grade LyG) includes poorly differentiated lung carcinoma, metastasis, or other large-cell lymphomas.

Many cases of pulmonary lymphomas can be diagnosed using immunohistochemistry (IHC) and/or in situ hybridization (ISH) on paraffin sections. This material may also be used for the detection of B- or T-cell gene rearrangements (clonal vs non-clonal) by polymerase chain reaction (PCR). When fresh material is available, flow cytometry may confirm the clonality of B cells by the detection of monotypic light chain expression or the expression of aberrant markers in T cells. In certain instances, cytogenetic studies and fluorescence in situ hybridization (FISH) may be required to detect specific translocations associated with certain lymphomas.

Part 1

Primary and Secondary Lung Involvement

Subpart 1.1

Extranodal Marginal Zone Lymphoma (MZL) of the Mucosa-Associated Lymphoid Tissue (MALT Lymphoma)

Sergio Pina-Oviedo

Primary pulmonary MALT lymphoma is thought to arise from the existent bronchial-associated lymphoid tissue. It is the most common lymphoma affecting the lungs (~80% of cases) and comprises ~8% of all extranodal MALT lymphomas. The median age at presentation is 68 years, and it is slightly more common in women. Thirty percent of cases develop in association with an autoimmune disorder. A third of patients are asymptomatic at presentation, and it is discovered incidentally. On imaging, primary pulmonary MALT lymphoma usually presents as a solitary lung mass with ill-defined borders and air bronchograms, and less common it presents as multifocal disease. Pleural thickening may be seen in peripheral lesions. Hilar adenopathy is seen in ~30% of cases. Grossly, it consists of an ill-defined fleshy mass with preservation of the lung architecture. Visceral pleural involvement is seen as a thick white plaque. The 5-year survival rate is 90%. A lesion may be treated surgically if it is peripheral or by observation or single-agent chemotherapy if it is unresectable. Relapses may occur in the lungs, the stomach, salivary glands, and/or lymph nodes. Progression to DLBCL is seen in 10% of cases. Unlike gastric MALT lymphoma, no particular microorganism has been associated to the development of pulmonary MALT lymphoma. Secondary pulmonary MALT lymphoma may develop as a recurrence in patients with a previous MALT lymphoma elsewhere.

Differential diagnosis includes benign and borderline lymphoid proliferations, such as nodular lymphoid hyperplasia and lymphocytic interstitial pneumonia, and other small B-cell lymphomas such as chronic lymphocytic leukemia/small lymphocytic lymphoma (CLL/SLL), follicular lymphoma, mantle cell lymphoma, and lymphoplasmacytic lymphoma. Pulmonary MALT lymphoma with extensive plasmacytic differentiation may be difficult to distinguish from pulmonary plasmacytoma.

HISTOLOGIC FEATURES

- Dense lymphoid infiltrate with a lymphangitic distribution along septa and bronchovascular bundles.
- Large coalescent lesions form a solid mass that may show stromal sclerosis and effacement of lung parenchyma.
- Pleural involvement or erosion of bronchial cartilage may be seen; presence of these features favors lymphoma over a reactive process.
- Histologic triad: (1) reactive lymphoid follicles with expanded marginal zones with/without follicular “colonization”; (2) polymorphous infiltrate with centrocyte-like and monocytoid-like cells; and (3) lymphoepithelial lesions.

- Polymorphous infiltrate: small lymphocytes, centrocyte-like cells, monocytoid-like cells, plasmacytoid lymphocytes, plasma cells, and few scattered large cells with vesicular chromatin and distinct nucleoli.
- Follicular "colonization": infiltration of MZL cells into reactive germinal centers with effacement of the follicular architecture.
- Lymphoepithelial lesions: infiltration of ≥5 lymphoma cells into the respiratory epithelium. Very characteristic but not pathognomonic of MALT lymphoma, as they can be seen in reactive conditions.
- Dutcher bodies (nuclear pseudoinclusions) may be present in plasma cells or plasmacytoid lymphocytes; more common in malignant lymphomas than in reactive processes.
- Increase in large cells raises the possibility of transformation to DLBCL.
- Amyloid deposition, epithelioid granulomas, multinucleated giant cells, and large lamellar bodies (laminated eosinophilic whorls of surfactant protein) may be present.
- Pleural involvement with a plaque-like or polypoid lymphoid infiltrate.
- IHC: positive for B-cell markers CD19, CD20, CD22, CD79a, and PAX5; negative for CD5, CD10, CD23, cyclin D1, and bcl-6. Aberrant coexpression of CD43 on B cells is seen in a large percentage of cases but is not required for diagnosis.
- Extranodal and nodal MALT lymphomas may be positive for IRTA-1 (Immunoglobulin superfamily Receptor Translocation-Associated 1). This molecule is mainly found in the membrane and cytoplasm of lymphoma cells in lymphoepithelial lesions and those underlying the epithelium.
- Plasma cells are most often reactive, with polyclonal labeling for kappa and lambda light chains (IHC or ISH), whereas cases with extensive plasmacytic differentiation usually show light chain restriction.
- Monocytoid-like cells are bcl-2+, whereas reactive monocytoid lymphocytes are bcl-2–.
- CD21, CD23, and CD35 highlight disrupted follicular dendritic cell meshworks.
- Lymphoepithelial lesions highlighted with cytokeratin or CD20.
- Ki-67 is low in the neoplastic component and high in the reactive lymphoid follicles.
- In some cases, particularly small biopsies, the diagnosis may hinge on demonstration of clonality by either flow cytometry or analysis of immunoglobulin heavy chain genes by PCR.
- About 50% of cases harbor the translocation t(11;18)(q21;q21) between the *MALT1* gene (18q21) and *API2* gene (11q21). Other genetic alterations include trisomy 3 and 18, and t(1;14)(*IGH-BCL10*) in a subset of cases.
- These translocations can be detected by FISH on paraffin-embedded tissues or cytologic imprints or by reverse transcription PCR in fresh or frozen material.

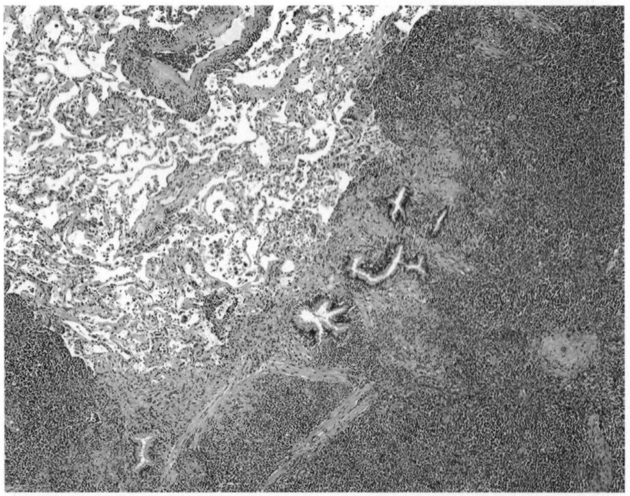

Figure 22.1 MALT lymphoma and adjacent uninvolved lung parenchyma. The lymphangitic distribution of the tumor is appreciated at the *periphery* of the lesion (**top, left**).

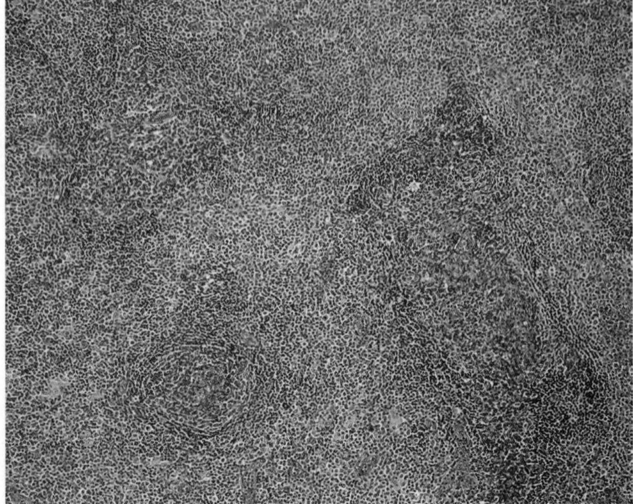

Figure 22.2 Sheets of lymphoma cells expand the interfollicular areas *(paler areas)* and invade or "colonize" residual lymphoid follicles and germinal centers.

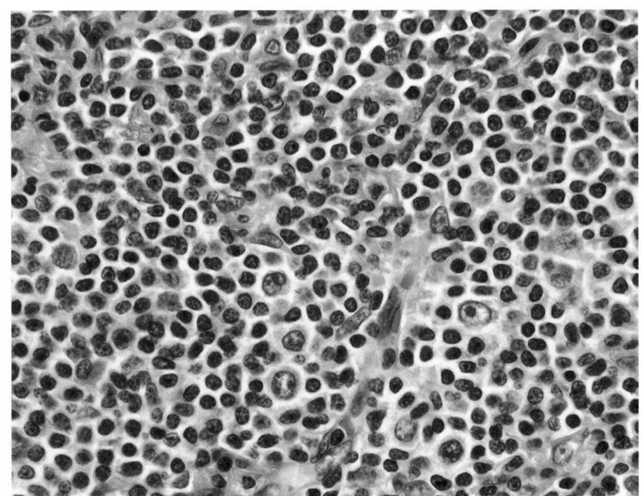

Figure 22.3 MALT lymphoma is characterized by a polymorphous infiltrate composed of small lymphocytes, centrocyte-like cells, monocytoid-like cells, plasma cells, and few scattered large cells with vesicular chromatin and distinct nucleolus.

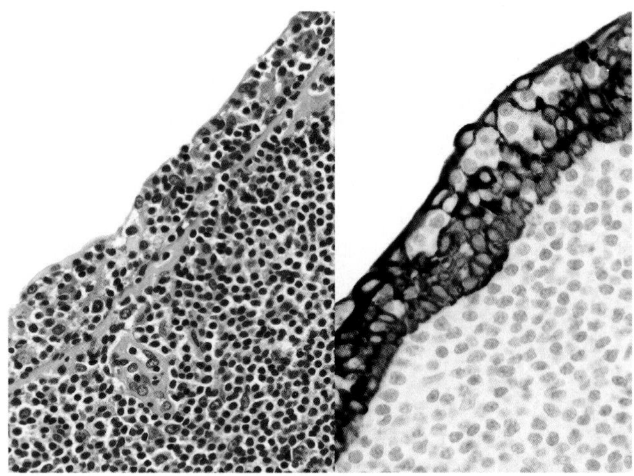

Figure 22.4 Lymphoepithelial lesions. The bronchiolar epithelium is almost completely effaced by lymphoma (**left**). Cytokeratin highlights the epithelium and the intraepithelial keratin-negative neoplastic lymphocytes (**right**).

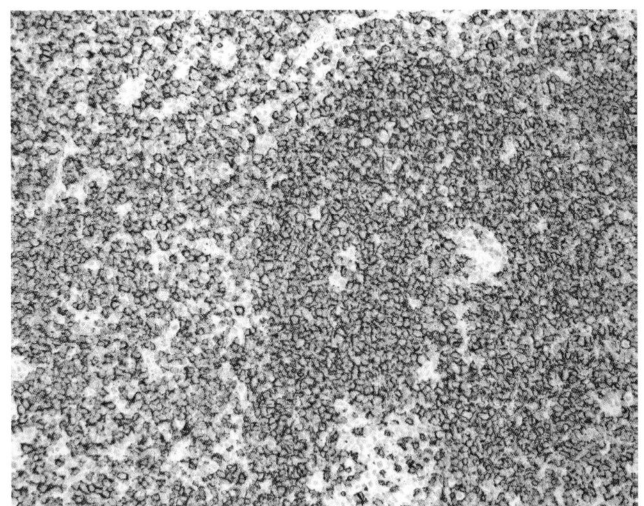

Figure 22.5 Immunostain for CD20 is positive in the neoplastic lymphocytes.

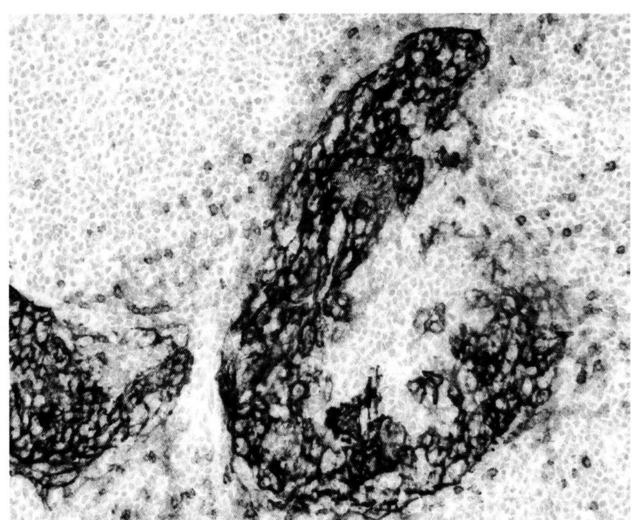

Figure 22.6 Follicular "colonization" is better appreciated by CD23, which highlights the disrupted follicular dendritic cell meshwork of residual follicles. MALT lymphoma cells are negative for CD23.

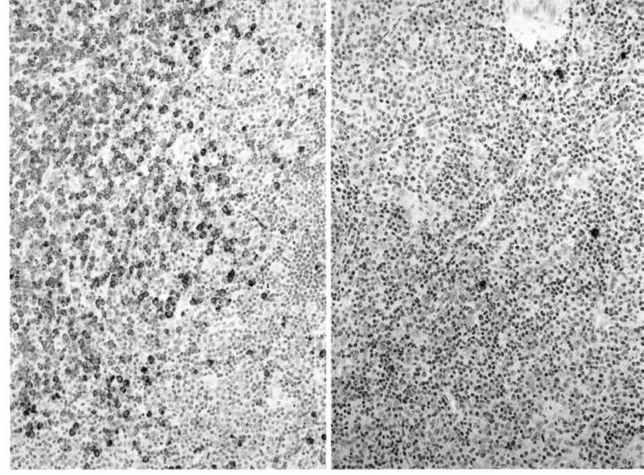

Figure 22.7 MALT lymphoma with focal increase of plasma cells showing monotypic labeling for kappa light chain by IHC (**left**). Lambda light chain is negative in the same region (**right**).

Subpart 1.2

Diffuse Large B-Cell Lymphoma (DLBCL)

▶ Sergio Pina-Oviedo

Primary pulmonary DLBCL is the second most common type of primary pulmonary lymphoma (~15% of cases). Most cases arise from a preexisting primary pulmonary MALT lymphoma, and few arise de novo. The mean age at presentation is 60 years, but some cases may develop in younger individuals. Patients usually present with dyspnea, chest pain and/or hemoptysis, and B symptoms. On imaging, primary pulmonary DLBCL is observed as a peripheral mass with well-defined borders and central necrosis or as an infiltrative lesion with extension into the mediastinum or the chest wall. Hilar adenopathy is more frequent than in MALT lymphoma (~50% of cases). Grossly, tumors are well circumscribed and fleshy and tend to be hemorrhagic and have central necrosis. Prognosis is poor with a median survival of 3 to 5 years despite chemotherapy. Differential diagnosis includes poorly differentiated carcinoma, small-cell carcinoma, metastatic carcinoma, melanoma, other large-cell lymphomas (anaplastic large-cell lymphoma [ALCL], peripheral T-cell lymphoma, CHL, high-grade LyG) or mediastinal large-cell lymphomas extending into the lung (primary mediastinal large B-cell lymphoma (LBCL), CHL).

HISTOLOGIC FEATURES

- Confluent sheets of discohesive large lymphoid cells that have a nucleus larger or about the size of a macrophage nucleus, with frequent mitoses and apoptosis.
- Destruction of the lung parenchyma, bronchial walls, angioinvasion with necrosis, with or without extension to the pleura.
- Edges of the lesion often show infiltration in a lymphangitic distribution.
- Variable cytomorphology. Centroblastic: nucleus with fine chromatin, ≥1 small basophilic nucleoli adjacent to the nuclear membrane. Immunoblastic: vesicular chromatin with a central prominent nucleolus and moderate amount of cytoplasm (>90% of cells to call immunoblastic variant). Anaplastic: mimics carcinoma, metastases, or ALCL.
- "Tumoral pneumonia": lymphoma cells admixed with fibrin filling alveolar spaces, mimicking a pneumonic process.
- In core needle biopsies, DLBCL may show artifactual spindle morphology.
- IHC: positive for CD19, CD20, CD22, CD79a, PAX5, and CD45 (leukocyte common antigen); negative for T-cell markers, cyclin D1, keratin, and melanoma markers.
- Necrotic DLBCL: CD20 is the best marker to highlight "ghost" tumor cells.
- Immunoblastic and anaplastic LBCLs are more frequently positive for CD30.
- IHC can be used as surrogate of the gene expression profiling data, which has certain implications in prognosis. Germinal center B cell–like (GCB) phenotype: CD10+, bcl-6+, MUM1–. Activated B cell–like (ABC) phenotype or non-GCB: CD10–, bcl-6+/–, MUM-1+. Primary extranodal DLBLCs usually have an ABC phenotype.
- High Ki-67 (>40%): if Ki-67 is >90%, it is suggestive of a "high-grade BCL" or a "double-hit lymphoma." Important to request FISH for *c-MYC*, *BCL2*, and *BCL6* gene rearrangements.
- Flow cytometry may yield a false-negative result because of necrosis and/or cell fragility.

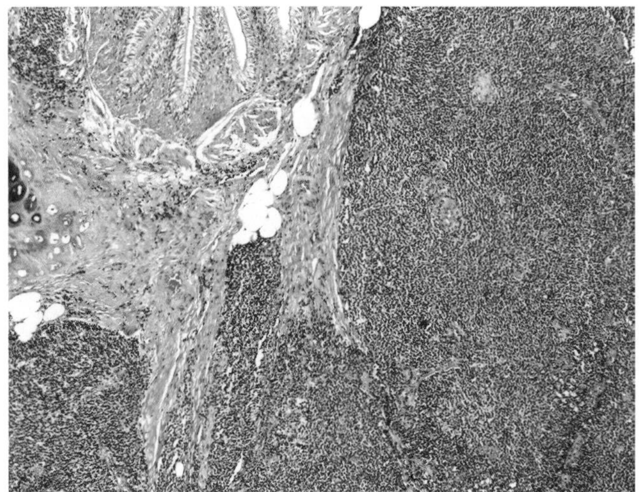

Figure 22.8 DLBCL with effacement of the lung architecture and extension into a bronchial wall.

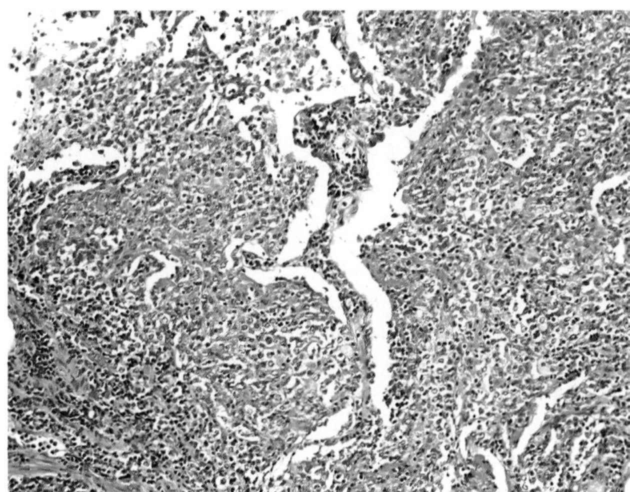

Figure 22.9 Tumoral pneumonia. The alveolar spaces are filled with large lymphoma cells admixed with fibrin resembling a pneumonic process.

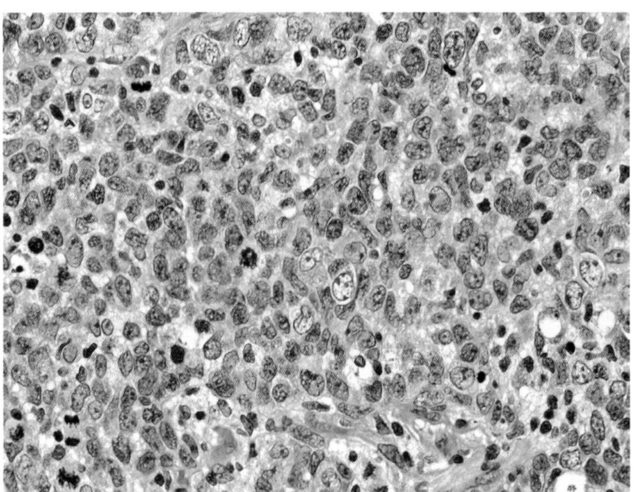

Figure 22.10 DLBCL with centroblastic features. The lymphoma cells have fine chromatin and >1 small basophilic nucleoli adjacent to the nuclear membrane. There are abundant mitoses and apoptotic cells.

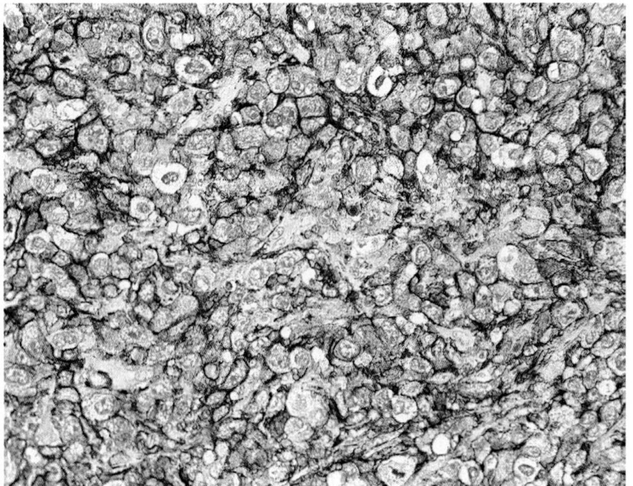

Figure 22.11 The large lymphoma cells are positive for CD20.

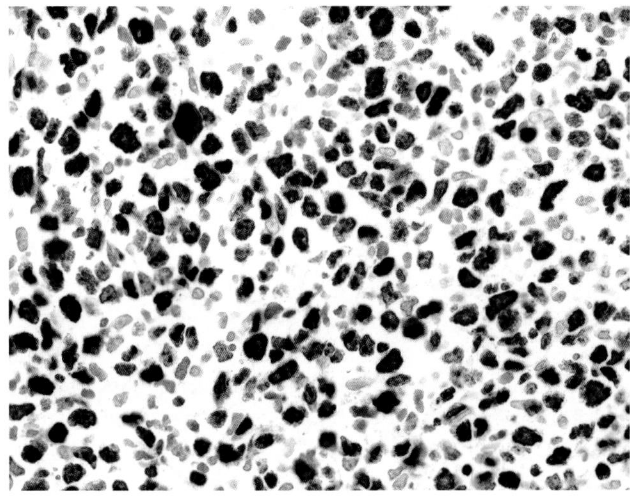

Figure 22.12 High proliferation index by Ki-67 immunostain.

Subpart 1.3

Lymphomatoid Granulomatosis (LyG)

▸ Sergio Pina-Oviedo

LyG is a T cell–rich LBCL in which the malignant B cells are EBV+. The term *granulomatosis* is a misnomer because granulomas are not a feature of the disease. It usually presents in middle-age individuals—more commonly men—who are immunosuppressed (human immunodeficiency virus, postchemotherapy), or children or young individuals with a congenital immunodeficiency. Rarely, LyG develops in an immunocompetent host. The lungs are the most common organ involved followed by the skin, brain, and kidneys. Clinical symptoms include intermittent and recurrent fevers, cough, dyspnea, and/or hemoptysis. On imaging, LyG appears as multiple bilateral lung nodules of variable size with bronchovascular distribution. The nodules may disappear and reappear ("migratory" nodules) or may become confluent to form a large necrotic mass. Rarely, LyG presents as a solitary mass or with hilar adenopathy. On gross examination, the nodules are well delimited with variable degree of necrosis and hemorrhage and a rim of viable white-yellow tissue. The disease is aggressive in most patients, although occasional cases may be more indolent. Patients with confined lung disease usually have a longer survival than those with systemic or brain involvement.

LyG is classified in three grades (see *Histologic Features*). Low-grade lesions have better prognosis than high-grade lesions. Differential diagnosis of low-grade lesions includes inflammatory conditions (Wegener granulomatosis and bronchocentric granulomatosis) or polymorphous lymphomas (CHL, T cell/histiocyte-rich LBCL, and peripheral T-cell lymphoma). Differential diagnosis of high-grade lesions includes large-cell lymphoma, carcinoma, melanoma, or metastasis. Necrotic lesions should be distinguished from necrotizing infections, necrotizing sarcoid, or a pulmonary infarct. The diagnosis of LyG should not be made in patients treated with methotrexate or after allogeneic transplant, conditions in which an EBV+ lymphoproliferative disorder is likely related to the drug or the post-transplant state, respectively.

HISTOLOGIC FEATURES

- Diagnosis of LyG must be established in the appropriate clinical setting: no history of transplant or therapy with immunomodulatory agents.
- Well-circumscribed nodules composed of a polymorphous lymphoid infiltrate with predilection for blood vessels (angiocentric) and variable degree of necrosis. The surrounding lung parenchyma is usually unremarkable.
- Tracheobronchial lesions cause mucosal ulceration.
- Necrosis is of coagulative type (eosinophilic), devoid of neutrophils or karyorrhectic debris.
- Granulomas and eosinophils are uncommon. The presence of granulomas or eosinophils favors an alternate diagnosis.
- Classic lesion: polymorphous infiltrate of small lymphocytes, macrophages, and plasma cells with occasional scattered large atypical lymphoid cells with immunoblastic or Hodgkin/Reed–Sternberg-like morphology.
- IHC: most small lymphocytes are CD3+ T cells (CD4 > CD8).
- Large cells are of B-cell lineage, positive for CD20, CD79a, and PAX5, variably positive for CD30, and negative for CD15. The large cells are also positive for EBV (EBER+ and LMP-1+).
- Grading of LyG is based on the number of EBER+ large cells and degree of necrosis. Grade 1: <5 EBV+ cells per 10 high-power fields (hpf) and minimal to no necrosis. Grade 2: 5 to 20 EBV+ cells per 10 hpf and more abundant necrosis. Grade 3: numerous EBV+ cells and extensive necrosis, indistinguishable from EBV+ LBCL.

- Alternative grading counting the number of CD20+ large cells, instead of EBER, has been suggested.
- Diagnostic areas, including large cells, may be focal, and thorough sampling is warranted.
- High-grade LyG may contain areas of low-grade LyG at the periphery of a nodule. Therefore, a biopsy with low-grade LyG may not reflect the highest possible grade in a nodule.
- B-cell clonality is commonly detected in high-grade lesions. In contrast, low-grade lesions have a high rate of false-negative results due to the paucity of tumor cells.

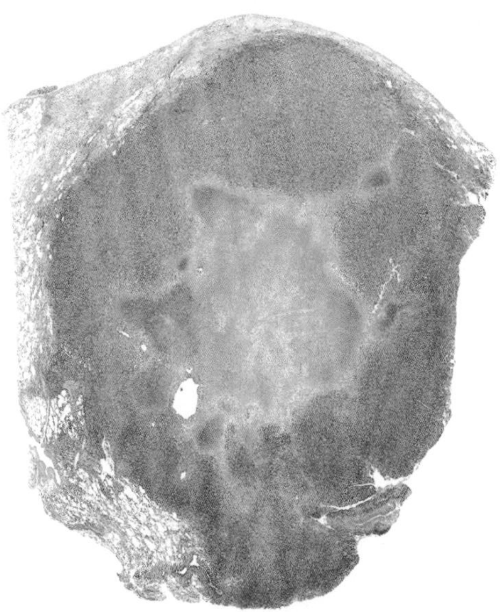

Figure 22.13 Wedge resection of a peripheral lung nodule diagnosed as high-grade LyG. The nodule is well delimited and has central necrosis. Residual bronchovascular bundles are seen at the lower aspect of the nodule.

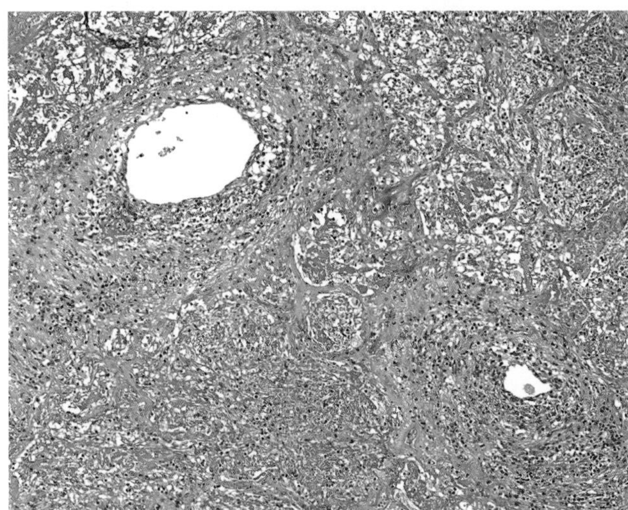

Figure 22.14 Coagulative-type (eosinophilic) necrosis of the lung and necrotizing vasculitis. The necrotic areas contain sparse karyorrhectic debris and no neutrophils. The degree of vasculitis and necrosis is variable in LyG.

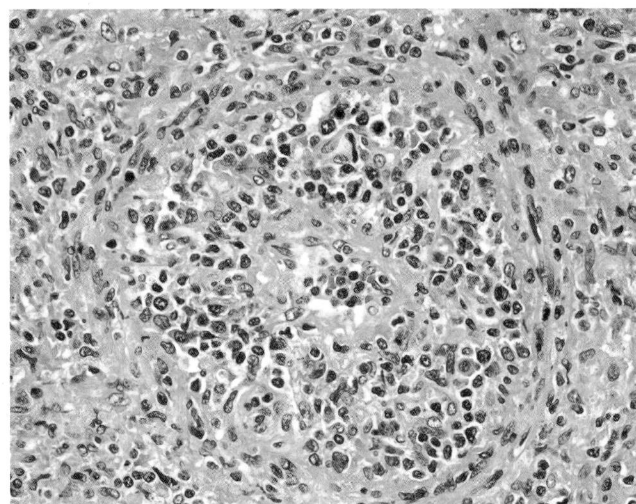

Figure 22.15 Vasculitis in high-grade LyG. The angiocentric infiltrate is mostly composed of large atypical lymphoid cells, similar to a large-cell lymphoma with angiocentricity.

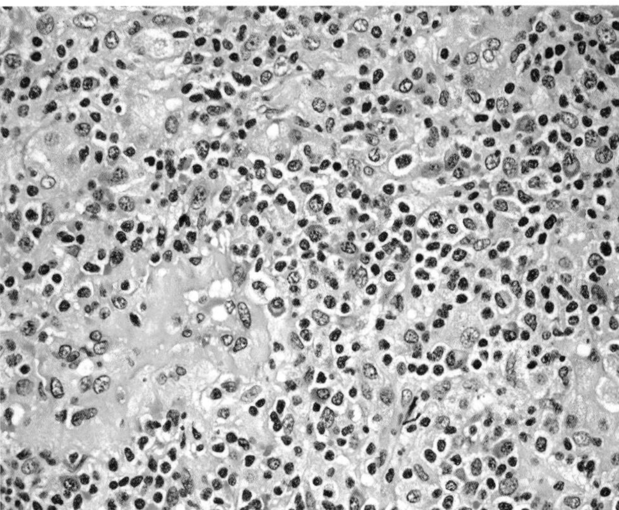

Figure 22.16 Low-grade LyG. Polymorphous lymphoid infiltrate composed of small lymphocytes, macrophages, and plasma cells with occasional scattered large atypical lymphoid cells.

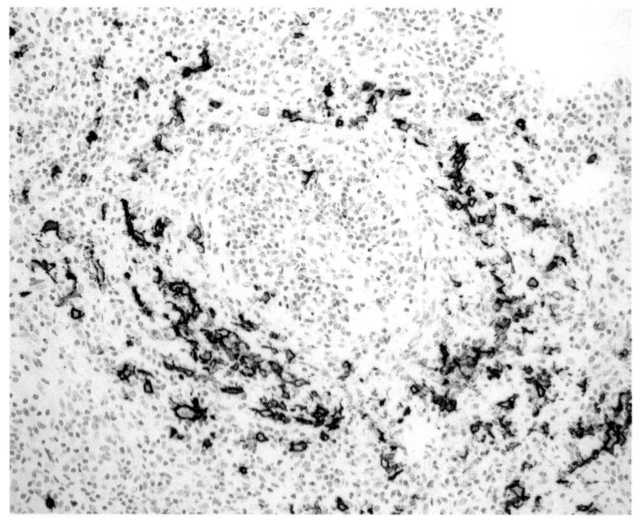

Figure 22.17 The large atypical lymphoid cells in LyG are positive for CD20, confirming their B-cell lineage.

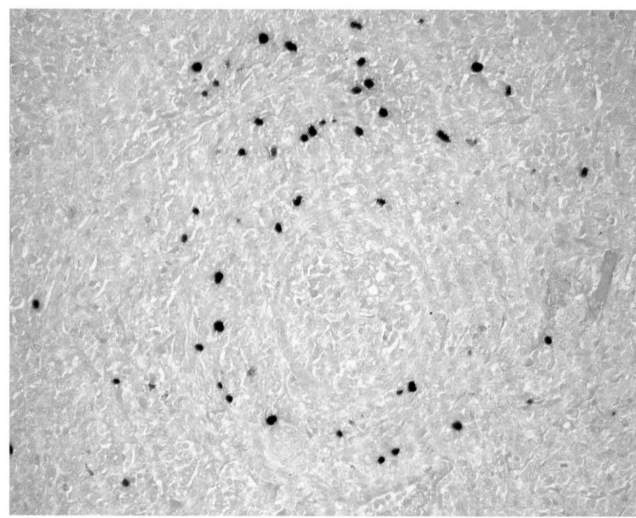

Figure 22.18 The large atypical lymphoid cells in LyG are characteristically positive for EBV (EBER in situ hybridization). LyG lesions are classified as low grade or high grade based on the amount of EBER-positive large cells.

Part 2

Systemic B-Cell Lymphomas with Secondary Lung Involvement

Sergio Pina-Oviedo

Primary lung involvement by CLL/SLL, follicular lymphoma, mantle cell lymphoma, and lymphoplasmacytic lymphoma is extremely rare. Secondary lung and pleural involvement by their systemic counterparts is much more common. On imaging, systemic small B-cell lymphomas usually present as bilateral reticulonodular infiltrates and/or pleural lesions. The presence of a lung mass in a patient with history of low-grade B-cell lymphoma suggests large-cell transformation. Alternatively, a new lung mass or an infiltrate in a patient known to have a low-grade B-cell lymphoma may show a different pathologic process (carcinoma, pneumonia, and granulomatous inflammation) with or without associated lymphoma.

Neoplastic small B-cell infiltrates may be distinguished in most cases by IHC of flow cytometry. An IHC panel for differentiating small B-cell lymphomas includes CD20, CD3, CD5, CD10, CD23, CD43, bcl-2, bcl-6, cyclin D1, SOX11, LEF1, and LMO2. Some of these may or may not be used depending on the morphologic differential diagnosis.

Pulmonary Burkitt lymphoma and intravascular LBCL are also discussed in this section.

Subpart 2.1

Small B-Cell Lymphomas

Sergio Pina-Oviedo

CHRONIC LYMPHOCYTIC LEUKEMIA/SMALL LYMPHOCYTIC LYMPHOMA (CLL/SLL)

- Small lymphocytes with clumped chromatin and scant cytoplasm with a lymphangitic distribution. Large nodules of CLL/SLL may contain proliferation centers. Rarely, CLL/SLL may involve the lung in a bronchiolocentric pattern.
- IHC: positive for CD20 (weak), CD5, CD23, CD43, bcl-2, and LEF1 (Lymphoid Enhancer binding Factor 1).
- Negative for CD10, bcl-6 and cyclin D1.
- Main differential diagnosis: mantle cell lymphoma.

FOLLICULAR LYMPHOMA

- Back-to-back neoplastic lymphoid follicles with a lymphangitic distribution. The follicles are composed of small to intermediate size cells with cleaved nucleus (centrocytes) admixed with large cells with vesicular chromatin and distinct nucleolus (centroblasts). The follicles are not polarized and do not contain tingible-body macrophages in contrast to reactive follicles.
- Diffuse pattern of follicular lymphoma is more difficult to differentiate from other small B-cell lymphomas.
- IHC: positive for CD20, CD10, bcl-2, bcl-6, and LMO2 (LIM domain Only 2), variable CD23.
- bcl-2 is positive in the follicles in contrast to reactive follicles, which are negative. (Note that most other subtypes of low-grade B-cell lymphoma are also bcl-2+.)
- Negative for CD5, CD43, and cyclin D1.
- Main differential diagnosis: florid follicular hyperplasia, follicular bronchiolitis, MALT lymphoma with extensive follicular "colonization."
- FISH: translocation t(14;18)(*BCL2-IGH*) may be used to support the diagnosis.

MANTLE CELL LYMPHOMA

- Monotonous small to intermediate size lymphocytes with indented nucleus, similar to centrocytes. Larger nodules of lymphoma may show vague nodular arrangement, hyalinized blood vessels, and epithelioid ("pink") macrophages.
- IHC: positive for CD20, CD5, CD43, cyclin D1, and SOX11.
- Negative for CD10, CD23, bcl-6, LEF1, and LMO2.
- Main differential diagnosis: CLL/SLL and follicular lymphoma.
- Prognosis is significantly worse than that for other small B-cell lymphomas.
- FISH: translocation t(11;14)(*CCND1-IGH*) may be used to support the diagnosis.

Subpart 2.2
Other B-Cell Lymphomas

Sergio Pina-Oviedo

BURKITT LYMPHOMA

- Exceedingly rare as primary lung disease. May present as an endobronchial mass.
- Sheets of cells of intermediate size with oval to round nucleus, fine chromatin, inconspicuous nucleoli, and scant basophilic cytoplasm; usually no nuclear molding. Abundant mitoses and apoptosis, and evenly dispersed tingible-body macrophages, given the tumor a "starry-sky" appearance.
- IHC: positive for CD20, CD10, CD19, CD45, and bcl-6. Ki-67 is typically >95%; negative for CD3, CD5, CD34, bcl-2, and TdT.
- Main differential diagnosis: small-cell carcinoma, lymphoblastic lymphoma, high-grade DLBCL, other small blue round cell tumors.
- FISH: most common translocation t(8;14)(*MYC-IGH*) in ~80% of cases, less frequent t(2;8) and t(8;22).

INTRAVASCULAR LARGE B-CELL LYMPHOMA

- Rare variant of LBCL with aggressive behavior that usually occurs in adults.
- Radiologically this variant may present as bilateral ground glass opacities, but imaging may be normal.
- Patients often present with systemic disease involving brain, skin, lung, and other organs, with occasional initial pulmonary presentation. Unfortunately, a significant number of patients remain undiagnosed until postmortem examination.
- The infiltrate is subtle and can be missed at low magnification.
- Large lymphoma cells with round nucleus, fine chromatin, and distinct nucleolus fill small vessels and capillaries and expand the alveolar septae mimicking interstitial pneumonia.
- Blood vessels filled with lymphoma cells may or may not contain fibrin thrombi.
- IHC: positive for CD20 and other B-cell markers, usually of ABC phenotype.
- Lymphoma cells lack homing receptor molecules needed to exit blood vessels and enter tissues.
- Main differential diagnosis: interstitial pneumonia, carcinomas or metastasis with lymphangitic spread, intravascular leukemic infiltrates.

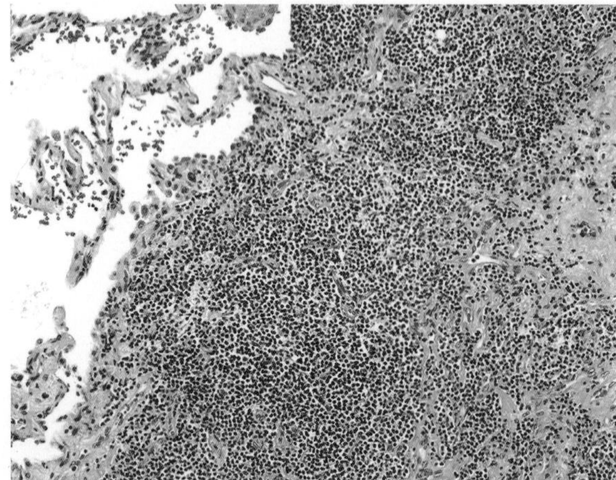

Figure 22.19 CLL/SLL involving the lung. The lung resection was done for a pulmonary adenocarcinoma (not shown). The surrounding parenchyma was involved by lymphoma. The patient had a history of CLL/SLL.

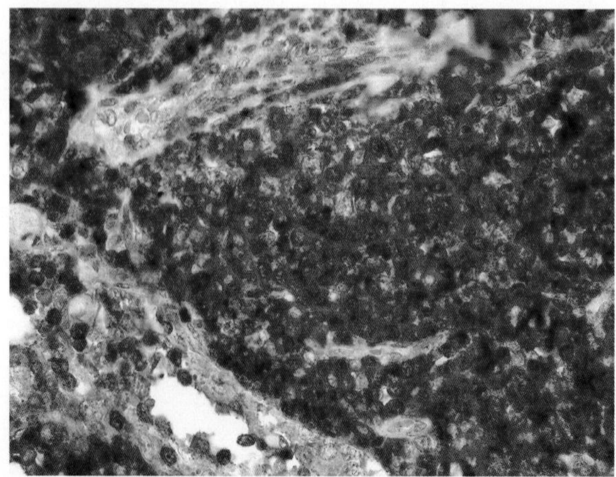

Figure 22.20 Double IHC for PAX5 *(brown nuclear labeling)* and CD5 *(red cytoplasmic labeling)* in CLL/SLL. The lymphoma cells show coexpression of PAX5 and CD5.

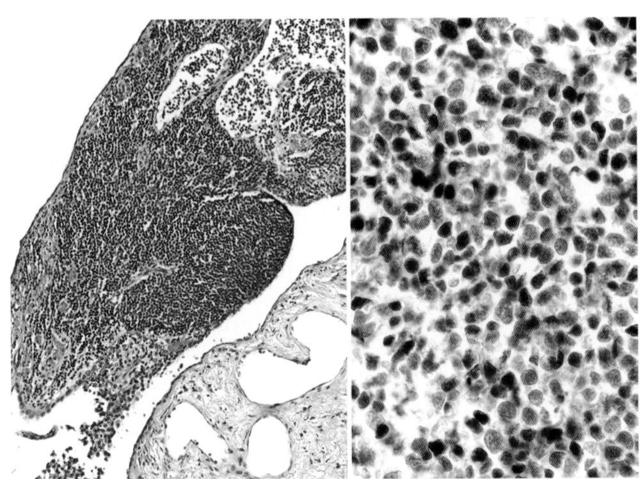

Figure 22.21 Mantle cell lymphoma involving the pleura. The resection was done for a pulmonary adenocarcinoma (not shown). The lymphoma cells have a variable positivity for cyclin D1 (**right**). The patient had a history of mantle cell lymphoma.

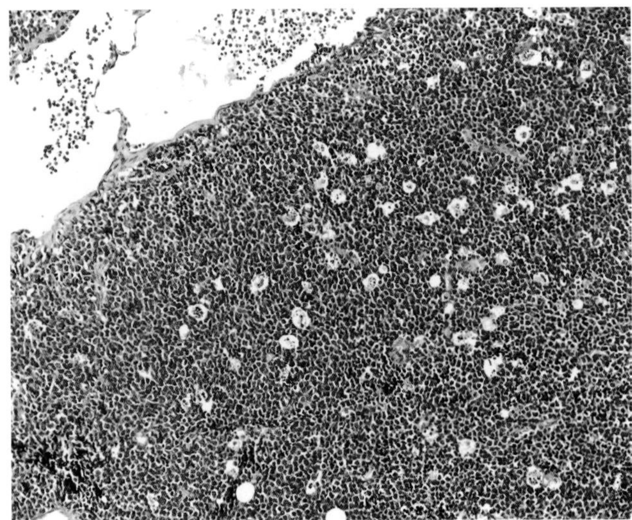

Figure 22.22 Burkitt lymphoma involving lung. The tumor effaces the lung parenchyma and has a "starry-sky" pattern. This patient had a history of Burkitt lymphoma elsewhere.

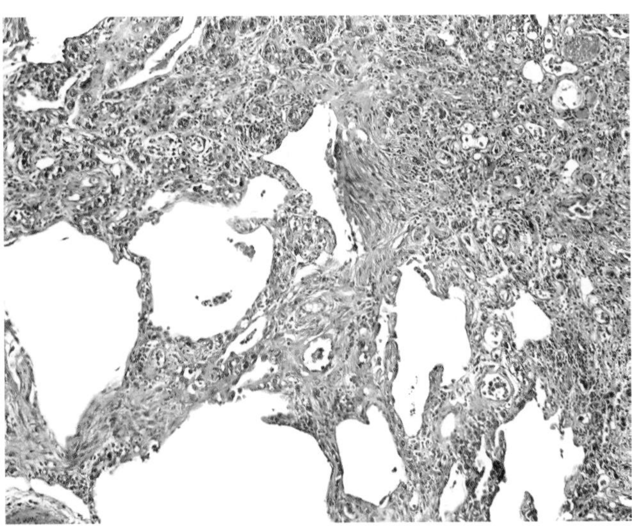

Figure 22.23 At low and intermediate magnification, intravascular LBCL may appear deceptively benign or mimic the pattern of interstitial pneumonia. The alveolar septae are expanded and more cellular than normal septae.

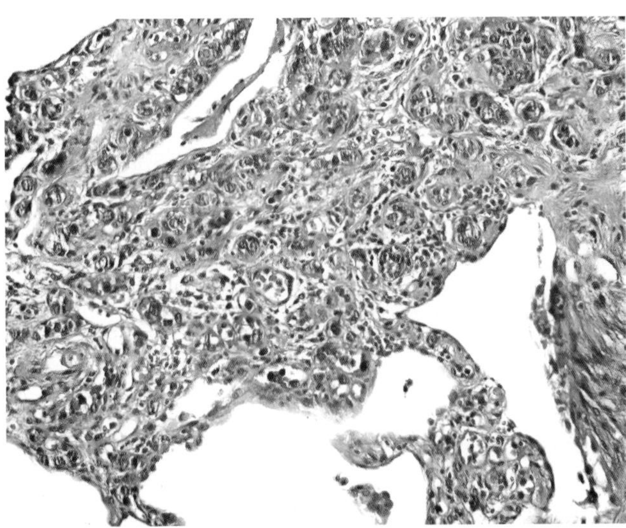

Figure 22.24 Intravascular LBCL. At higher magnification, the capillaries are expanded and filled with large lymphoma cells.

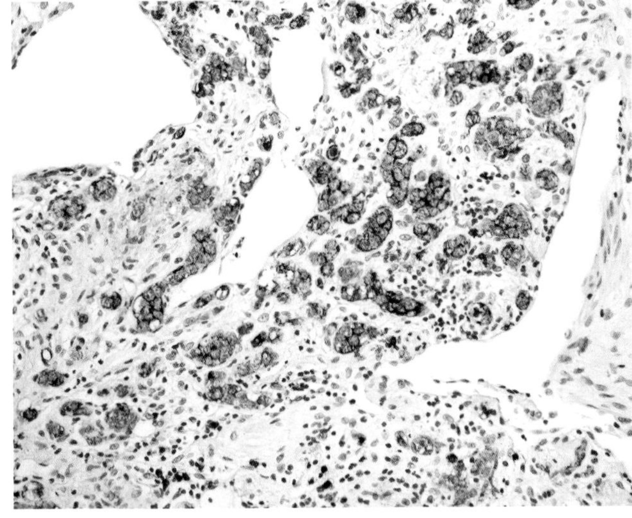

Figure 22.25 Intravascular LBCL. CD20 highlights the lymphoma cells within capillary lumina.

Pulmonary Classical Hodgkin Lymphoma

23

▶ Sergio Pina-Oviedo

PRIMARY AND SECONDARY LUNG INVOLVEMENT: CLASSICAL HODGKIN LYMPHOMA (NODULAR SCLEROSIS AND MIXED CELLULARITY)

Primary pulmonary classical Hodgkin lymphoma (CHL) is rare. Exclusion of mediastinal involvement is mandatory to establish the diagnosis of primary disease. Patients often present with cough, dyspnea, and B symptoms. The age of presentation is older than that of nodal or mediastinal disease (~40 years), and it is more common in women. On imaging, primary pulmonary CHL usually presents as bilateral masses but may also manifest as a solitary nodule with or without cavitation or as a localized infiltrate. Secondary pulmonary involvement by CHL is far more common than primary disease. CHL may (1) involve the visceral pleura and lung by direct extension from the mediastinum, particularly in bulky disease; (2) recur in the lung just outside the field of radiation therapy of a mediastinal primary CHL or (3) involve the lung in the form of metastatic disease (stage IV). The prognosis depends on the age of the patient and the extent of lung involvement. Differential diagnosis includes inflammatory and infectious processes, large-cell lymphoma, lymphomatoid granulomatosis, poorly differentiated carcinoma, metastasis, primary mediastinal large B-cell lymphoma (LBCL) extending into the lung, and a mediastinal germ cell tumor extending into the lung. Recurrent or posttherapy CHL may resemble sarcomatoid carcinoma or sarcoma.

HISTOLOGIC FEATURES

- CHL has a lymphangitic pattern of spread into airways, pulmonary vessels, and pleura.
- Necrosis, granulomatous inflammation, and neutrophilic microabscesses are common.
- Most common subtypes of CHL involving the lung are nodular sclerosis and mixed cellularity, but traditionally extranodal primary disease is not subdivided.
- Polymorphous infiltrate composed of small lymphocytes, plasma cells, eosinophils, neutrophils, and macrophages with a variable number of large (20 to 60 μm) pleomorphic Hodgkin/Reed–Sternberg (HRS) cells.
- Reed–Sternberg cells have a bilobated or multilobated nucleus with prominent eosinophilic nucleoli surrounded by a clear halo. Hodgkin cells are monolobated. Both cells may contain abundant eosinophilic or vacuolated cytoplasm or may show marked cytoplasmic retraction artifact ("lacunar" cells). The nucleus of HRS cells may be pyknotic or show smudged chromatin without a nucleolus and glassy eosinophilic cytoplasm ("mummified" cells).
- HRS cells may be found in large clusters or sheets or can be sparse and difficult to find.
- CHL can have an exuberant granulomatous component that may obscure HRS cells and mimic sarcoid, infection, or a burnout germ cell tumor with granulomatous reaction.
- HRS-like cells may be seen in non-Hodgkin lymphomas and even carcinomas (e.g., giant cell and anaplastic). The presence of an appropriate inflammatory background is essential for the diagnosis of CHL.
- Nodular sclerosis CHL shows dense collagen bands that are polarizable.

- Immunohistochemistry (IHC): HRS cells are positive for CD30 (>95%) and CD15 (~70%), with a membranous and Golgi pattern of labeling. CD15 may only be cytoplasmic and granular.
- HRS cells are weakly positive for PAX5 compared with B cells and can be positive for CD20 in ~30% of cases. MUM1/IRF4 is positive in >90% of cases.
- HRS cells are negative for CD3, CD45, CD79a, and the B cell–associated transcription factors OCT2 and BOB.1. HRS cells rarely express T-cell markers or cytotoxic molecules.
- Mixed cellularity CHL is commonly positive for Epstein–Barr virus (EBV) (EBER+, LMP1+), whereas nodular sclerosis CHL is usually negative for EBV.
- Recurrent pulmonary CHL may show increased number and pleomorphism of the HRS cells, with reduction in the accompanying inflammatory background cells, resembling LBCL, anaplastic large-cell lymphoma, anaplastic carcinoma, or sarcoma.

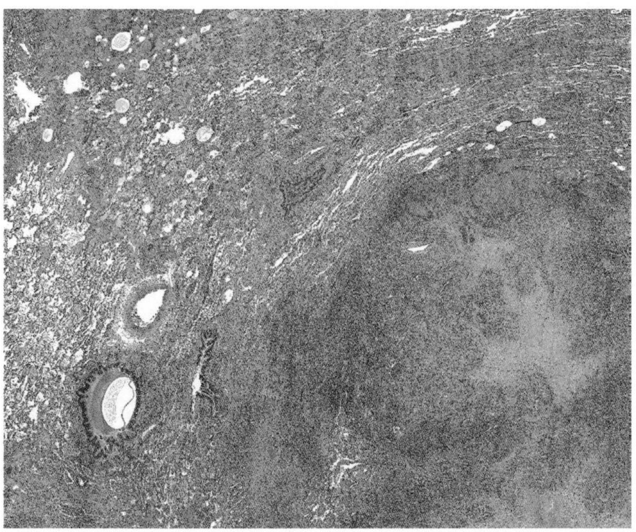

Figure 23.1 Primary pulmonary classical Hodgkin lymphoma. The mass has a bronchovascular distribution and compresses the surrounding lung parenchyma. The lesion contains central necrosis and resembles lymphomatoid granulomatosis at low magnification.

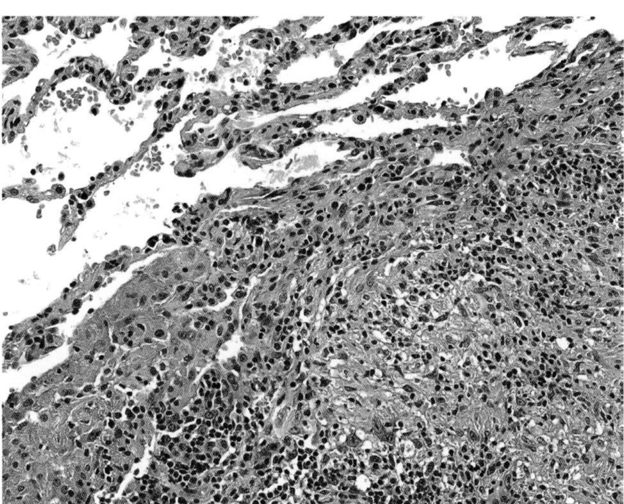

Figure 23.2 Primary pulmonary classical Hodgkin lymphoma. The edge of a lesion containing a polymorphous infiltrate of small lymphocytes, macrophages, eosinophils, and scattered Hodgkin/Reed–Sternberg cells *(bottom center)*.

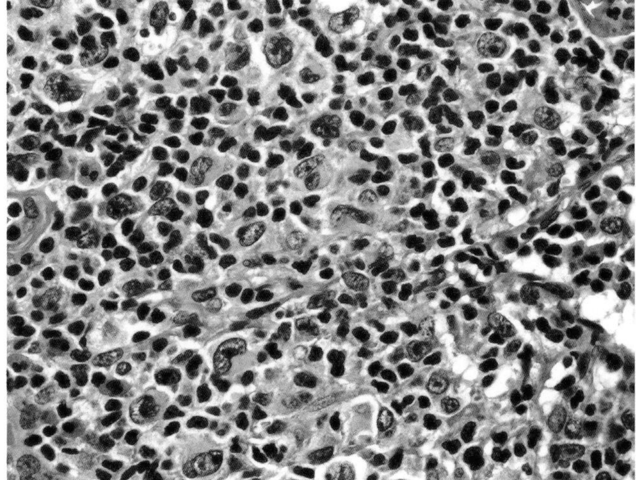

Figure 23.3 Primary pulmonary classical Hodgkin lymphoma. Higher magnification of the mass from Figure 23.1. The lesion contains small lymphocytes, macrophages, eosinophils, and scattered Hodgkin/Reed–Sternberg cells.

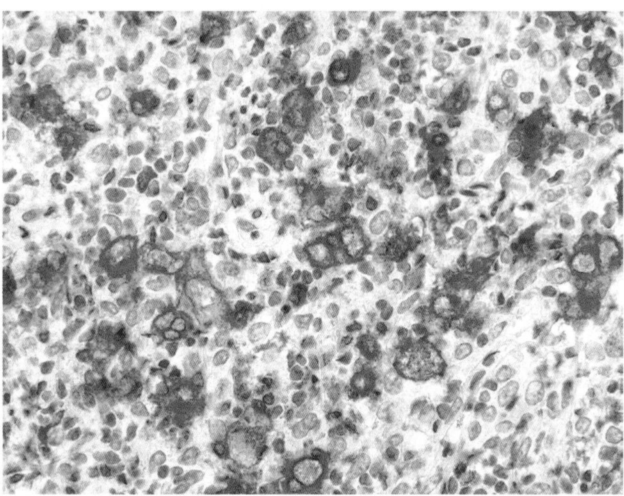

Figure 23.4 Double IHC for CD30/PAX5. Hodgkin/Reed–Sternberg cells are positive for CD30 *(red cytoplasmic labeling)* and weakly positive for PAX5 *(light-brown nuclear labeling)*.

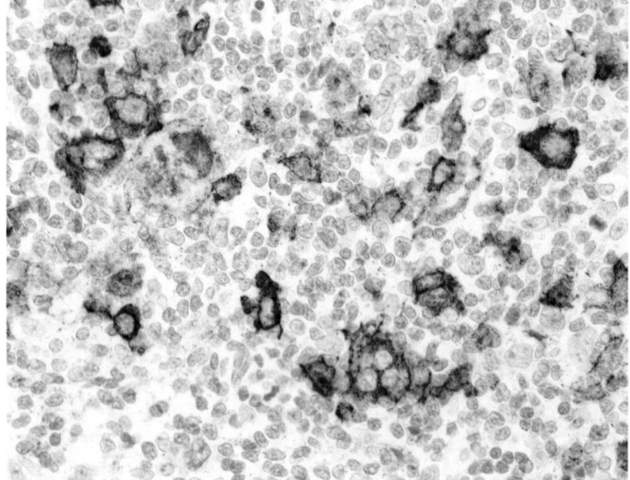

Figure 23.5 Hodgkin/Reed–Sternberg cells are positive for CD15 in about 70% of cases.

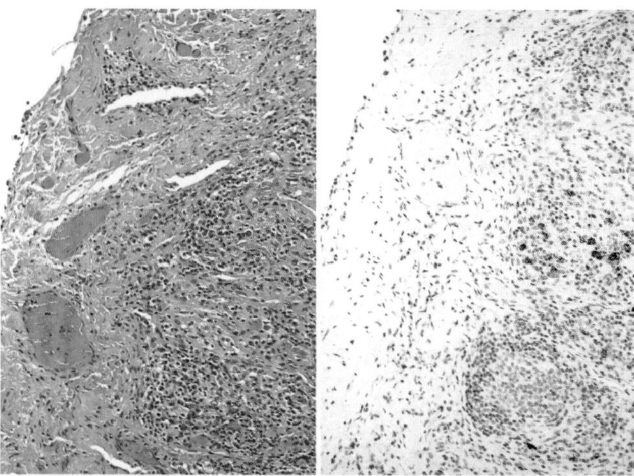

Figure 23.6 Secondary pulmonary classical Hodgkin lymphoma involving the pleura. The primary tumor was located in the mediastinum and infiltrated the visceral and parietal pleura and the lung. The Hodgkin/Reed–Sternberg cells are not obvious on hematoxylin and eosin stain (**left**). The CD30 immunostain highlights Hodgkin/Reed–Sternberg cells within the infiltrate (**right**).

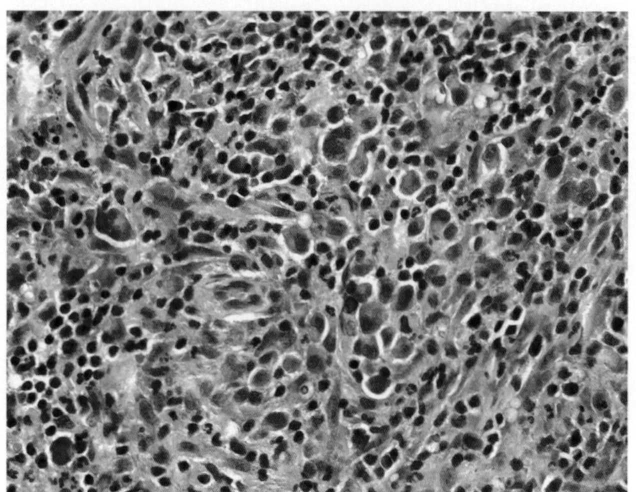

Figure 23.7 Recurrent classical Hodgkin lymphoma. There are several Hodgkin/Reed–Sternberg cells, some with spindle morphology and a less prominent inflammatory background.

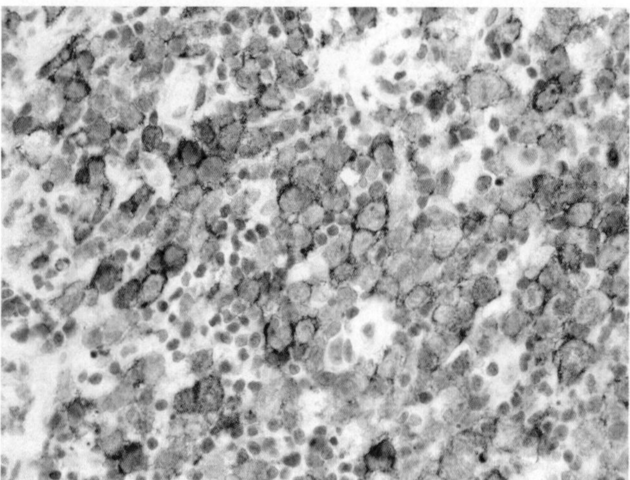

Figure 23.8 CD30 immunostain in a case of recurrent classical Hodgkin lymphoma highlights sheets of Hodgkin/Reed–Sternberg cells.

Pulmonary T-Cell Lymphomas

24

Sergio Pina-Oviedo

INTRODUCTION

T-cell lymphomas involve the lungs rarely. Primary lung involvement is limited to sporadic reports (usually anaplastic large-cell lymphoma [ALCL] and peripheral T-cell lymphoma, not otherwise specified [NOS]), whereas systemic involvement is sometimes seen in the late stages of disease. Thus, clinical history is crucial. Mycosis fungoides is a cutaneous T-cell lymphoma that, in the late stages, commonly involves the lungs ("visceral" mycosis fungoides). On imaging, these lesions can present as a mass, a nodule, or as a diffuse infiltrate. Most cases have an intermediate to poor prognosis. Differential diagnosis of "visceral" mycosis fungoides includes reactive or infectious processes or a low-grade B-cell lymphoma. Differential diagnosis of large T-cell lymphomas involving the lung (ALCL, some peripheral T-cell lymphomas, large-cell transformation in mycosis fungoides) includes lung carcinoma, metastasis, melanoma, diffuse large B-cell lymphoma (DLBCL), or classical Hodgkin lymphoma (CHL).

Part 1

Peripheral T-cell Lymphoma, NOS

Sergio Pina-Oviedo

HISTOLOGIC FINDINGS

- Variable morphology: some cases are composed of only monomorphic small cells or monomorphic large cells, whereas others are composed of a polymorphous infiltrate of small, intermediate, and large atypical cells, including Hodgkin/Reed–Sternberg–like cells.
- Lymphoma cells often have convoluted nuclei with thick nuclear membranes, condensed chromatin, with or without clear cytoplasm. Usually accompanied by granulomatous inflammation and variable number of eosinophils.
- Angiocentricity and necrosis may be present.
- Immunohistochemistry (IHC): positive for T-cell markers, namely CD2, CD3, CD5, CD7, CD43, or CD45RO, with loss or quantitative alterations in the expression of some of these markers; positive for CD4 or CD8, double positive (CD4+/CD8+), or double negative (CD4–/CD8–). CD30 may be positive in T-cell lymphomas with large cells.
- EBER is positive in extranodal NK/T-cell lymphoma (not discussed here).
- Negative for B-cell markers.
- Flow cytometry is more sensitive than IHC for identifying aberrations in T-cell markers.
- Main differential diagnosis: inflammatory or infectious processes, vasculitis, DLBCL, CHL, and lymphomatoid granulomatosis.
- Molecular analysis of *TCR* gene rearrangements may be used to confirm clonality. However, a negative result does not exclude the diagnosis.

Part 2

Systemic T-cell Lymphomas with Secondary Lung Involvement

Subpart 2.1

Pulmonary (Visceral) Involvement by Mycosis Fungoides/Sézary Syndrome

▸ Sergio Pina-Oviedo

HISTOLOGIC FINDINGS

- By definition, a history of mycosis fungoides or Sézary syndrome is required.
- Infiltrate in a lymphangitic distribution, along bronchovascular bundles and septa.
- Lymphoma cells are usually small to intermediate in size with hyperchromatic and convoluted "cerebriform" nuclei. In the stage of large-cell transformation, the cells are larger, with convoluted nuclei, vesicular chromatin, and prominent nucleoli.
- Association with granulomatous inflammation may be found.
- IHC: positive for T-cell markers, namely CD2, CD3, CD5, CD7, CD43, or CD45RO, with loss or quantitative alterations in the expression of some markers (usually CD7).
- Nearly all cases positive for CD4, with few cases positive for CD8. Remaining cases may be double positive (CD4+/CD8+) and rarely double negative (CD4–/CD8–).
- CD30 is usually positive in cases of large-cell transformation, but may be negative.
- Flow cytometry is more sensitive than IHC for identifying aberrations in T-cell markers.
- Main differential diagnosis: inflammatory or infectious processes; DLBCL, ALCL, carcinoma, or metastasis in cases of large-cell transformation.
- Molecular analysis of *TCR* gene rearrangements may be used to confirm clonality. However, a negative result does not exclude the diagnosis.

Subpart 2.2

Pulmonary Anaplastic Large-Cell Lymphoma (ALCL)

▸ Sergio Pina-Oviedo

HISTOLOGIC FINDINGS

- Most common primary pulmonary T-cell lymphoma. Mostly reported in adults, but some cases have been reported in children.
- Pulmonary ALCL may present as a solitary mass, multiple lesions, or an endobronchial mass.
- Sheets of large cells with marked pleomorphism, "hallmark" cells (horseshoe-shaped nucleus), and multinucleated cells; abundant mitoses; and may have a "starry-sky" pattern.

- Several morphologic variants: lymphohistiocytic, neutrophil-rich, small cell, sarcomatoid, etc.
- IHC: positive for CD30 and variable T-cell markers, namely CD2, CD4, CD5, less frequently positive for CD3 and CD8; may show a "null" phenotype with lack of T-cell markers.
- ALK+ (Anaplastic lymphoma kinase) and ALK negative cases.
- Positive for clusterin and EMA and negative for CD15, CD45 (LCA), B-cell markers, melanoma, keratins, and EBER.
- Main differential diagnosis: DLBCL, CHL, anaplastic carcinoma, melanoma, or metastasis.
- ALK+ cases correlate with the presence of a fusion protein resulted from a translocation between the *ALK* gene (2p23) and several gene partners, most commonly *NPM* (5q35). The subcellular localization of the protein depends on the function of the gene partner involved.
- Majority show TCR gene rearrangements, but "null" phenotype cases may lack rearrangement.
- ALK negative cases can show rearrangement of the *DUSP22* or *TP63* genes, which are associated with prognosis. Fluorescence in situ hybridization for these rearrangements is not widely available yet.

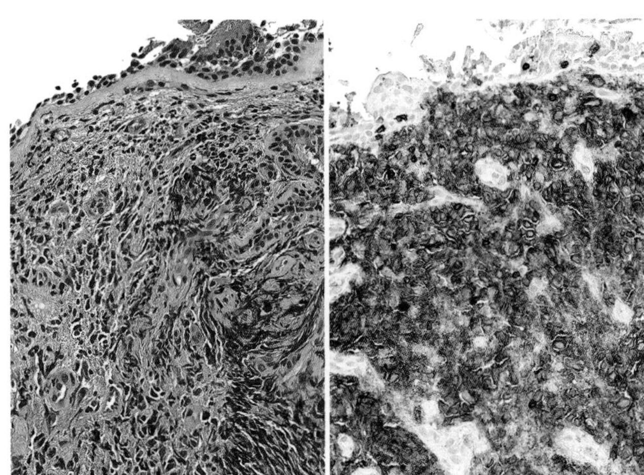

Figure 24.1 Peripheral T-cell lymphoma, NOS, involving the bronchus. The lymphoma cells have artifactual distortion, but in better preserved areas they appear monotonous and hyperchromatic (**left**). The infiltrate is diffusely positive for CD3 (**right**) and was negative for CD7 (not shown). The patient had a history of peripheral T-cell lymphoma.

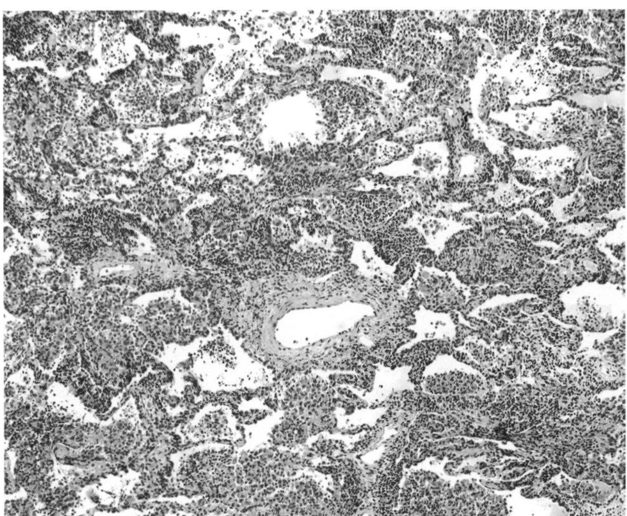

Figure 24.2 Mycosis fungoides involving the lung ("visceral" mycosis fungoides). The lung contains an extensive lymphoid infiltrate with perivascular and septal distribution. Most cells have small to intermediate size. The patient had a long-standing history of mycosis fungoides.

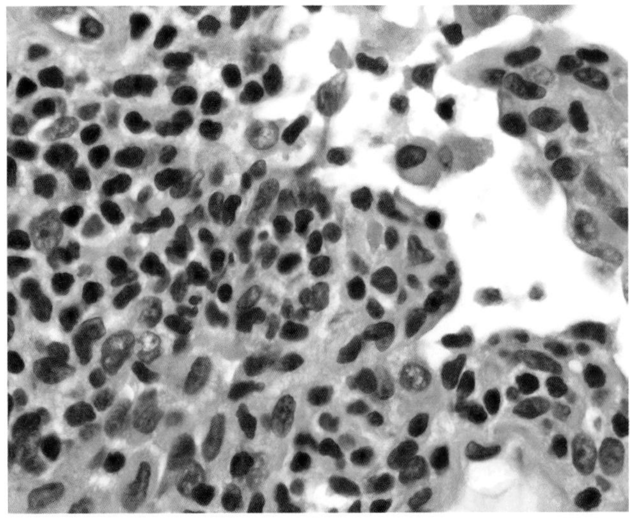

Figure 24.3 The cells in mycosis fungoides are small to intermediate in size and have hyperchromatic and cerebriform nuclei. The lymphoma cells fill the alveolar septa and infiltrate the alveolar epithelium in a similar fashion to lymphoepithelial lesions of MALT lymphoma.

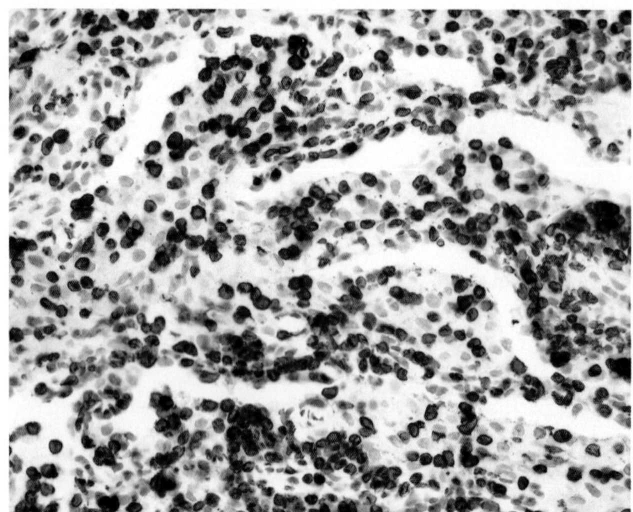

Figure 24.4 Mycosis fungoides involving the lung. Lymphoma cells are positive for CD3.

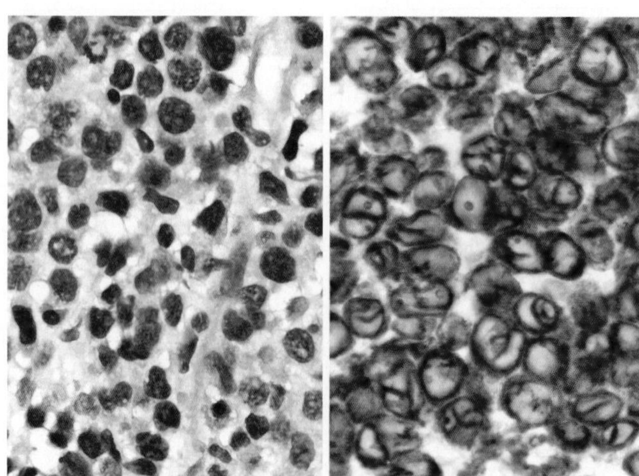

Figure 24.5 Large-cell transformation of mycosis fungoides. The cells are large with markedly convoluted nuclei. Mitotic figures are also seen (**left**). CD3 highlights the marked degree of nuclear irregularity of the neoplastic T cells (**right**).

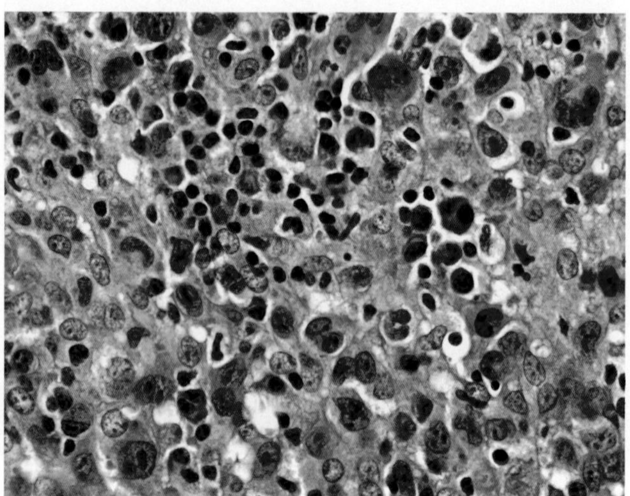

Figure 24.6 Anaplastic large-cell lymphoma. The tumor contains large cells with marked pleomorphism, cells with horseshoe-shaped nucleus ("hallmark" cells), and scattered multinucleated cells.

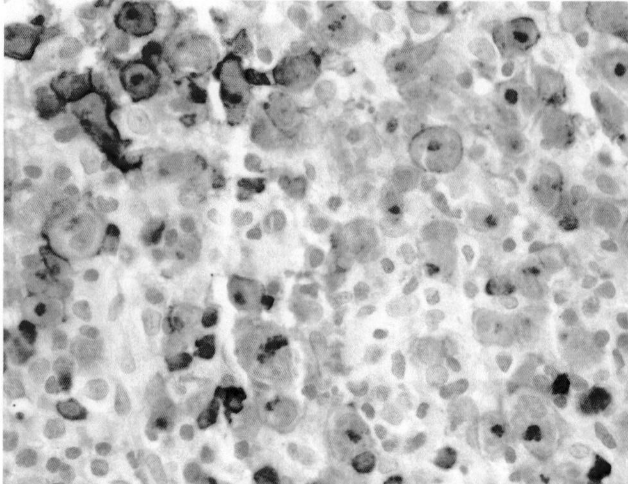

Figure 24.7 Anaplastic large-cell lymphoma cells are positive for CD30. The tumor cells are decorated in the cell membrane and the Golgi region.

Pulmonary Plasma Cell Neoplasms and Related Conditions

25

Part 1

Primary Pulmonary Plasma Cell Neoplasms

▸ Sergio Pina-Oviedo

PULMONARY PLASMACYTOMA

Primary pulmonary plasmacytoma is rare. It affects adults in the fifth to seventh decades of life and presents with cough, dyspnea, or hemoptysis. Elevated serum M-peak is detected in ~50% of cases. On imaging, it presents as a solitary mass with well-defined borders in a central or a peripheral location. The 5-year overall survival is 40%. Surgical resection may be accomplished in proximally located plasmacytomas, whereas chemoradiation is used for unresectable disease. Differential diagnosis includes reactive plasmacytosis or diseases with significant increase in plasma cells (inflammatory pseudotumor, IgG4-related disease, chronic inflammation with reactive plasmacytosis) and lymphomas with plasmacytic differentiation (mucosa-associated lymphoid tissue [MALT] lymphoma, lymphoplasmacytic lymphoma, and rarely other small B-cell lymphomas).

Part 2

Systemic Plasma Cell Neoplasm with Secondary Lung Involvement

▸ Sergio Pina-Oviedo

Secondary lung involvement by systemic plasma cell myeloma is uncommon and may occur in the late stages of the disease.

HISTOLOGIC FEATURES

- Nodules of plasma cells in a lymphangitic pattern or sheets of plasma cells forming a mass, usually with effacement of the lung architecture.

- Plasma cells may appear small and mature with eccentric round nucleus with cartwheel chromatin, no nucleolus, and basophilic cytoplasm with a clear Golgi zone (Marschalkó type), or may show atypical features, such as nuclear enlargement, anisonucleosis, binucleation or multinucleation, and/or prominent nucleoli.
- Russell bodies (cytoplasmic eosinophilic globules), Mott cells (plasma cells laden with Russell bodies), or Dutcher bodies (intranuclear pseudoinclusions) are variably observed.
- Stromal amyloid deposition or "amyloid-like" deposits may be present in some cases.
- No lymphoid follicles, monocytoid-like cells, lymphoepithelial lesions, or desmoplastic stroma should be present.
- A lymphoplasmacytic neoplasm with >20% of a non-plasma cell component is unlikely to be a plasmacytoma.
- Immunohistochemistry (IHC): neoplastic plasma cells are positive for CD38, CD138, CD79a, MUM1, with kappa or lambda light chain restriction. Light chain status can also be evaluated by in situ hybridization (ISH).
- Neoplastic plasma cells usually show aberrant expression of CD56 and CD117.
- Negative for CD19, CD20, PAX5, and variable CD45 (leukocyte common antigen). Some cases may show weak CD20 and PAX5 (MALT and lymphoplasmacytic lymphomas are strongly positive for these markers).
- Flow cytometry may be used to determine aberrant markers on plasma cells and light chain clonality. Plasma cells are sticky and fragile and may be lost during processing a sample for flow cytometry, thus yielding few events to analyze by this method (false-negative result).
- By flow cytometry, aberrant plasma cells are usually negative for CD27 and CD81.

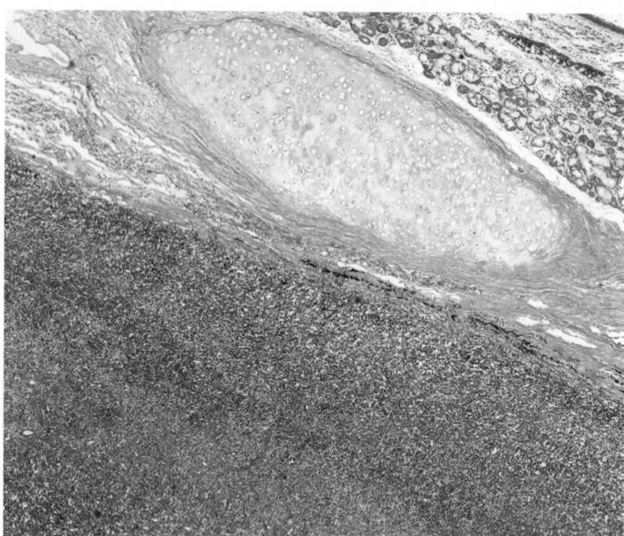

Figure 25.1 Primary pulmonary plasmacytoma. The tumor shows a sharp border and abuts the bronchial wall.

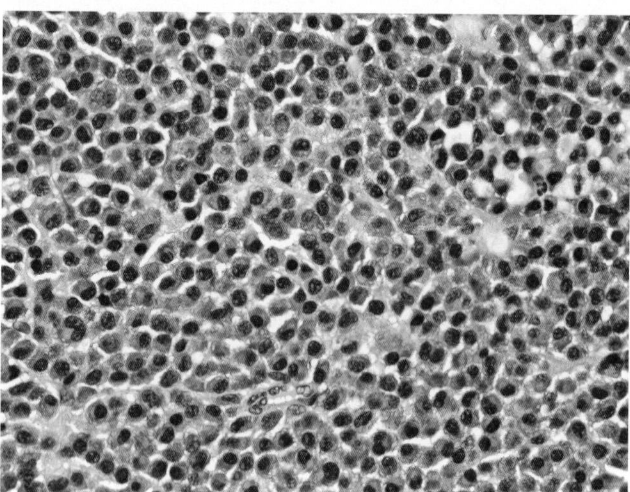

Figure 25.2 Primary pulmonary plasmacytoma. Most plasma cells have mature morphology. Occasional binucleated forms and cells with open chromatin and small nucleolus are seen.

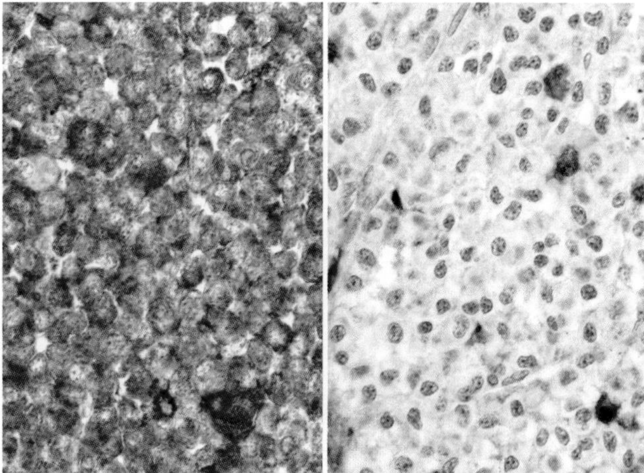

Figure 25.3 The plasma cells are positive for kappa light chain (**left**) and negative for lambda light chain by IHC (**right**). Rare lambda-positive cells represent residual non-neoplastic plasma cells.

Other Systemic Hematolymphoid Neoplasms with Secondary Lung Involvement

26

Sergio Pina-Oviedo

Part 1

Acute Leukemia or Myeloproliferative Neoplasms

Although neoplastic pulmonary infiltrates occur in patients with acute leukemias and myeloproliferative neoplasms, most patients do not have pulmonary symptoms except in cases when extremely high peripheral white cell counts are present. The infiltrates usually manifest as bilateral ground glass opacities, as reticulonodular infiltrates, and rarely as a mass. Acute myeloid leukemia forming a mass is also referred to as myeloid sarcoma. Pulmonary involvement in myeloproliferative neoplasms may also be accompanied by extramedullary hematopoiesis. Most pulmonary manifestations of acute leukemia are secondary to chemotherapy and radiation therapy, including opportunistic infections. Differential diagnosis of acute leukemia involving the lung includes inflammatory infiltrates, diffuse large B-cell lymphoma, Burkitt lymphoma, or any other small blue round cell tumor. Differential diagnosis of myeloproliferative neoplasms includes extramedullary hematopoiesis and extramedullary hematopoietic tumor.

Subpart 1.1

Acute Leukemia

Sergio Pina-Oviedo

HISTOLOGIC FEATURES

- Pulmonary leukemic infiltrates are not uncommonly found in patients with leukemia in postmortem examination.
- Infiltrates of blasts of intermediate to large size, high nuclear to cytoplasmic ratio, vesicular chromatin, prominent nucleolus, and granular cytoplasm.

- Infiltrates may be intravascular or have lymphangitic and perivascular distribution. Larger collections of blasts may form nodules or extensive infiltrates filling the alveolar spaces.
- Lesions may be extensively necrotic, especially after therapy.
- Look for opportunistic organisms (viral cytopathic changes, fungi, bacteria).
- Acute leukemias can be myeloid or lymphoid. If possible, it is extremely useful to know the original phenotype of the acute leukemia to evaluate a tissue infiltrate with a more specific set of markers. Rarely leukemias may switch phenotype, especially after therapy.
- Immunohistochemistry (IHC): myeloblasts are usually positive for myeloperoxidase, CD11c, CD33, CD34, CD117, CD123, and lysozyme. Lymphoblasts are usually positive for CD10, CD34, TdT, and CD3 or CD19 (if T- or B-cell derived, respectively). Additional specific markers may be present or absent depending on the type of the original leukemia (monocytic, megakaryocytic, erythroid, lymphoid, etc.).
- If a fresh sample is available, flow cytometry is preferred over IHC to confirm the immunophenotype.

Subpart 1.2

Myeloproliferative Neoplasms

Sergio Pina-Oviedo

HISTOLOGIC FEATURES

- Infiltrates composed of variable amounts of immature granulocytes, sometimes with eosinophils, mast cells, and with or without other hematopoietic elements.
- Infiltrates may be intravascular or have lymphangitic and perivascular distribution. Larger lesions may fill the alveolar spaces.
- Infiltrates may be associated with a myxoid or a desmoplastic stroma.
- Myeloproliferative neoplasms can rarely transform to acute leukemia (blast crisis) in tissues.
- IHC: usually not required for diagnosis; sometimes required for confirmation of cell types: myeloperoxidase, CD4, CD14, CD42, CD61, glycophorin, CD117, or tryptase. If suspicion for blast crisis, see above points for acute leukemia.

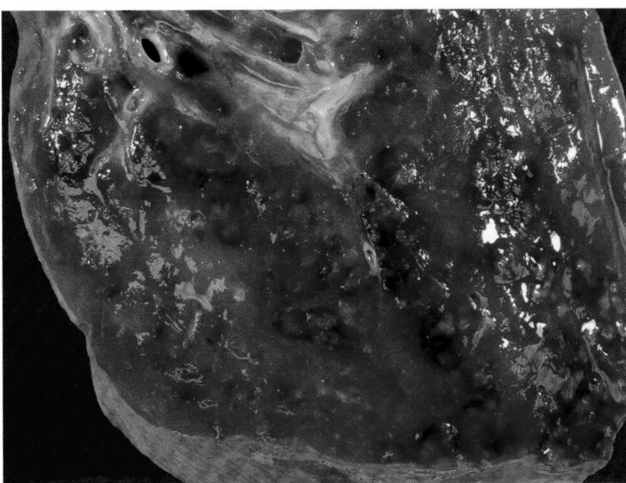

Figure 26.1 Autopsy lung specimen from a patient with acute promyelocytic leukemia. The patient had marked leukocytosis at the time of death. The lung parenchyma is hemorrhagic and congested with numerous tiny nodules in a miliary distribution.

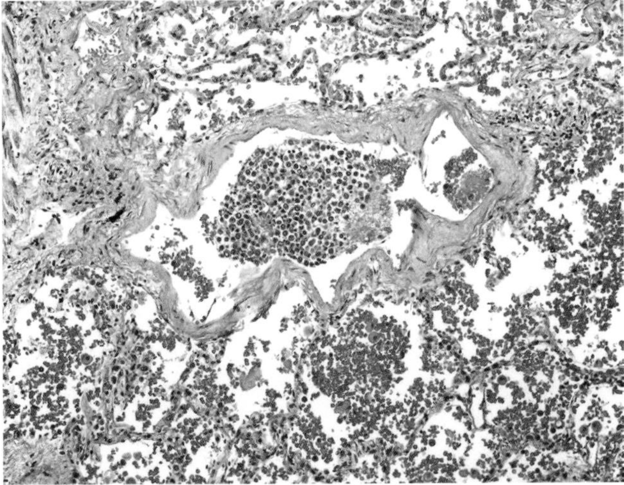

Figure 26.2 Tissue section of the lung from Figure 26.1. The lung parenchyma has diffuse hemorrhage. A blood vessel has a cluster of leukemic cells in the lumen.

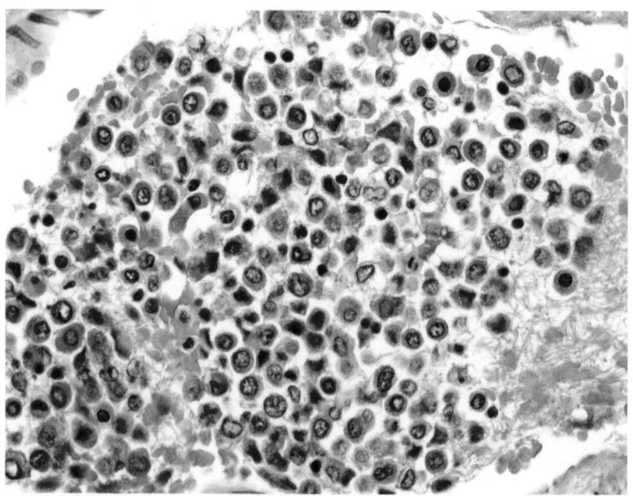

Figure 26.3 High magnification from Figure 26.2. The leukemic cells have round to reniform nucleus with fine chromatin, occasional nucleolus, and moderate amount of eosinophilic and granular cytoplasm. These cells correspond to promyelocytes.

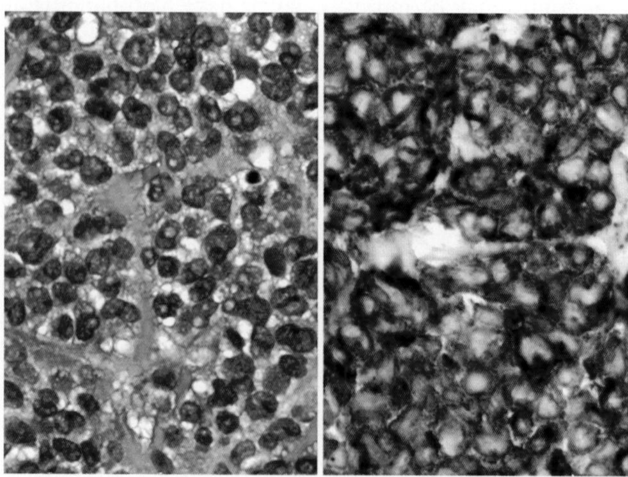

Figure 26.4 Myeloid sarcoma. The leukemic cells have cleaved nucleus with fine chromatin and amphophilic cytoplasm (**left**). The tumor cells are positive for myeloperoxidase (**right**).

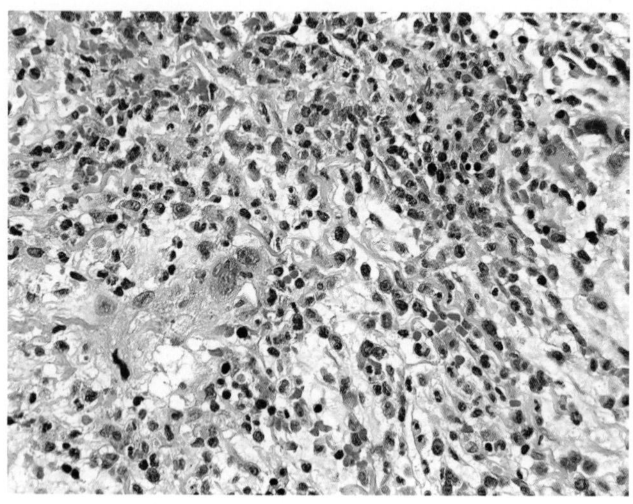

Figure 26.5 Myeloproliferative neoplasm with extramedullary hematopoiesis. The patient presented with hyperleukocytosis and large coalescent lung infiltrates. The lung biopsy shows replacement of the parenchyma by hematopoietic elements and dysplastic megakaryocytes in a myxoid background. The patient was later shown to have chronic myeloid leukemia.

27 Other Neoplasms of the Lung

Ross A. Miller

The neoplasms presented in this section include an assortment of unusual benign and malignant primary lung tumors not covered in other sections of this book. For the *malignant* tumors presented in this section (melanoma, malignant thymoma, and malignant germ cell tumors), it is emphasized that an extrapulmonary primary site must be excluded before diagnosing a primary lung malignancy with one of these histotypes as lung involvement is almost invariably a direct extension or metastasis. Although primary lung malignancies with these histotypes have been described in the medical literature, they are extraordinarily rare.

Part 1

Malignant Melanoma

Ross A. Miller

There are rare reports of primary malignant melanoma of the lung; diagnosis is dependent on excluding metastatic melanoma from other sites (cutaneous, ocular, other mucosal origins, etc.). As such, definitive diagnosis requires a thorough investigation of the past medical history (a current or previous diagnosis of melanoma excludes a diagnosis of primary malignant melanoma of the lung) and an extensive clinical examination looking for occult melanoma. Because metastatic pulmonary involvement is a relatively common occurrence in those with melanoma, some have suggested that primary malignant melanoma of the lung can only be retrospectively diagnosed following postmortem examination to exclude a primary site from elsewhere.

Most primary lung cases described are endobronchial in location; there are occasional reports of tracheal origin tumors. If a peripheral lung melanoma is encountered (even if solitary), it is almost invariably a metastasis. The described primary endobronchial melanomas are typically solitary and polypoid; some of the described tracheal lesions have been flat. Pigmentation is variable and the reported age range is between 29 and 80 years. Reported gender distributions are variable among the very limited series reports, and owing to the rarity of the tumor, meaningful conclusions cannot be made regarding gender predilection. The histologic and cytologic findings mirror melanoma presenting in other locations (see typical cytologic and histologic features below); the cells are typically positive for the following markers by immunohistochemistry: S100, SOX10, Melan-A, Mart-1, and HMB-45. Of note, melanomas composed of spindle cells (spindle-cell melanoma) are often only positive for S100 and SOX10 (Melan-A, Mart-1, and HMB-45 are usually negative in spindled variants). The differential diagnosis includes poorly differentiated neoplasms (both primary and metastatic), neuroendocrine tumors (generally positive for synaptophysin and chromogranin; CD56 staining is not specific for neuroendocrine tumors in this setting), and PEComas (perivascular epithelioid tumors are typically positive for HMB-45, Melan-A, Mart-1, and SMA [smooth muscle actin]).

CYTOLOGIC FEATURES

- Typically, cells are dyshesive.
- Often nonspecific features, can mimic a wide range of malignancies.
  - Cells can be spindled, epithelioid, or quite small.
- When present, the following nuclear characteristics can be helpful.
  - Eccentrically placed (also termed *plasmacytoid*) nuclei.
  - Binucleation.
  - Intranuclear inclusions.
  - Prominent nucleoli.
- Scattered mitotic figures and/or necrosis may be seen.
- Melanin pigment may be seen (not a diagnostic requirement and often absent).

HISTOLOGIC FEATURES

- Primary lung melanoma described to be centrally located, typically having an endobronchial component.
- Dyshesive cells; melanin pigment may or may not be seen.
- Scattered mitotic figures; necrosis may be seen.
- Tumor cells can have a variety of morphologic patterns (see cytologic features aforementioned).
- Immunohistochemistry profile:
  - Positive stains: S100, SOX10, Mart-1, Melan-A, and HMB-45.

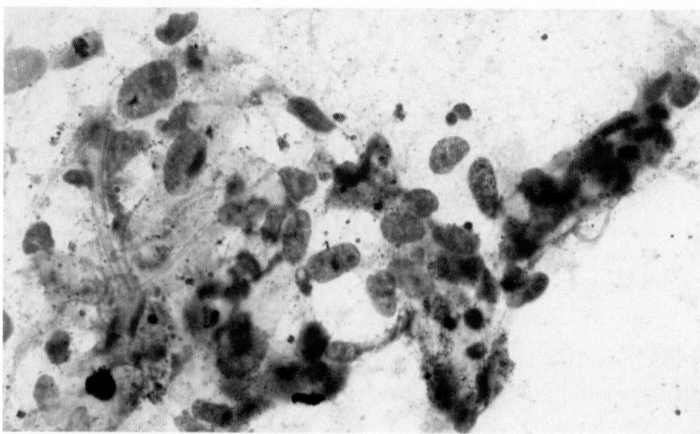

Figure 27.1 Cytology preparation, Papanicolaou stain: dyshesive spindled to epithelioid cells with large nuclei. Occasional conspicuous nucleoli can be seen along with background melanin pigment.

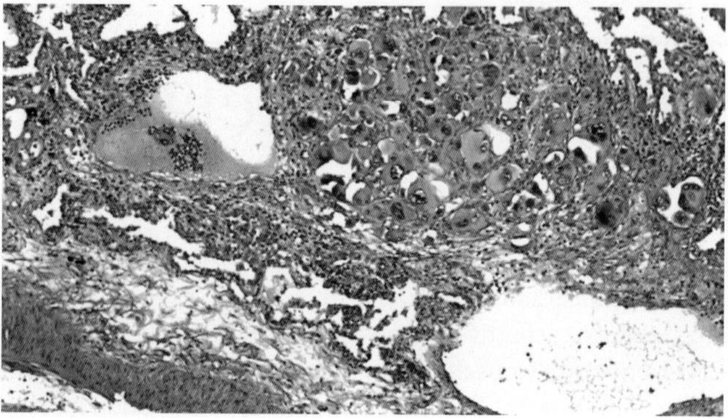

Figure 27.2 Melanoma seen adjacent to bronchial wall composed of large epithelioid cells with prominent nuclei and conspicuous nucleoli. Pronounced cellular atypia is seen.

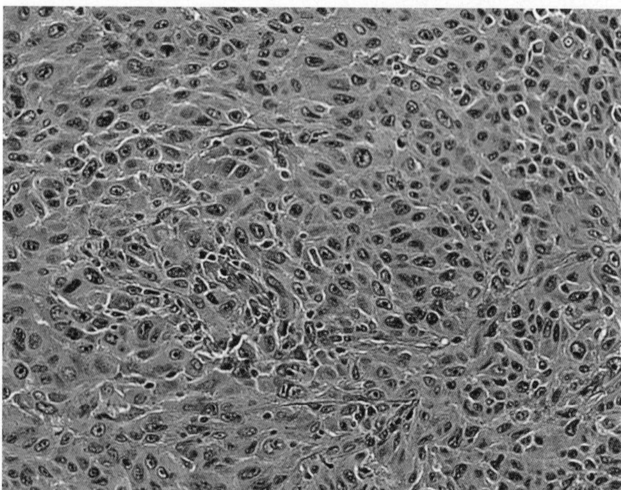

Figure 27.3 Large cells with eccentrically placed nuclei and prominent nucleoli.

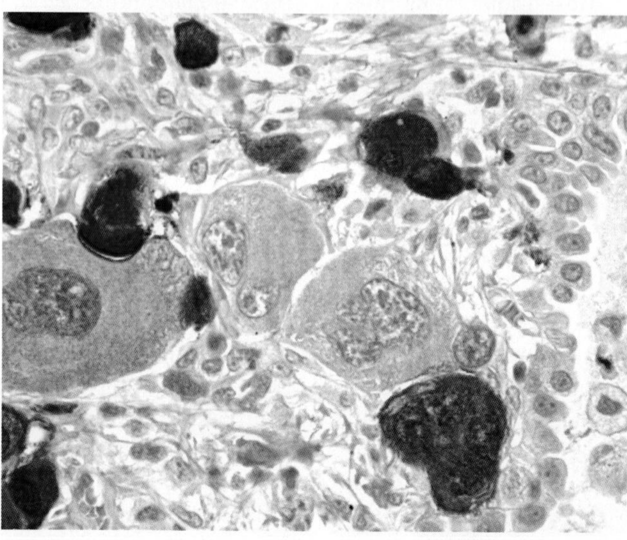

Figure 27.4 An immunohistochemical stain for S-100 highlights the malignant melanoma cells.

Part 2

Pleuropulmonary Thymoma

Ross A. Miller and Cesar Moran*

Pleuropulmonary thymomas are intrapulmonary or pleural-based thymomas likely developing from thymic epithelial rests. The majority of described cases have been solitary; however, multifocal lesions involving the same lung have been described. The lesions are often well circumscribed; however, they can be infiltrative like those in the mediastinum. Some have focal intralesional cystic change or areas of calcification. A minority of cases are associated with paraneoplastic syndromes related to thymoma (myasthenia gravis, red cell aplasia, Good syndrome [combined B-cell and T-cell immunodeficiency occurring with thymoma]). Treatment is generally complete surgical excision and prognosis is typically quite favorable. Perhaps the most relevant pathologic factor is the presence of capsular invasion. The various types have a similar behavior with the exception of type B3, which tends to be more aggressive.

The differential diagnosis is dependent on the type of thymoma seen (see histologic features below). Lymphoma may be a consideration, particularly in thymomas with numerous lymphocytes (most notably, type B1). A keratin stain (CK5/6) or p63 can be helpful as lymphoma should not show keratin- and/or p63-positive epithelioid cells. Solitary fibrous tumor may be a consideration in thymomas composed of spindle cells (type A or AB). The spindle cells in solitary fibrous tumor typically are positive for CD34 and STAT6 and are negative for keratin. Rosette-like structures can occasionally be seen in thymoma, which may lead one to consider a neuroendocrine tumor. The rosette structures seen in thymomas will be positive for keratin and negative for neuroendocrine markers (synaptophysin and chromogranin).

CYTOLOGIC FEATURES

- Epithelioid cells, spindle cells, or both (depending on the type of thymoma); background lymphocytes in variable proportions.

HISTOLOGIC FEATURES

- Similar characteristics to thymomas in the anterior mediastinum; findings depend on the type of thymoma. The spindle and/or epithelioid cells are typically positive for keratin stains (CK5/6) and p63.
  - World Health Organization (WHO) classification:
    - Type A: oval-spindle cells, no mitotic activity.
    - Type AB: oval-spindle cells (like type A) with admixed lymphocytes.
    - Type B1: round-epithelioid cells with abundant cytoplasm admixed with numerous T lymphocytes.
    - Type B2: approximately equal numbers of round-epithelioid cells and lymphocytes.
    - Type B3: sheets of large epithelioid cells; scant lymphocytes.

*The author would like to acknowledge the work of Dr. Moran, who contributed to the previous edition.

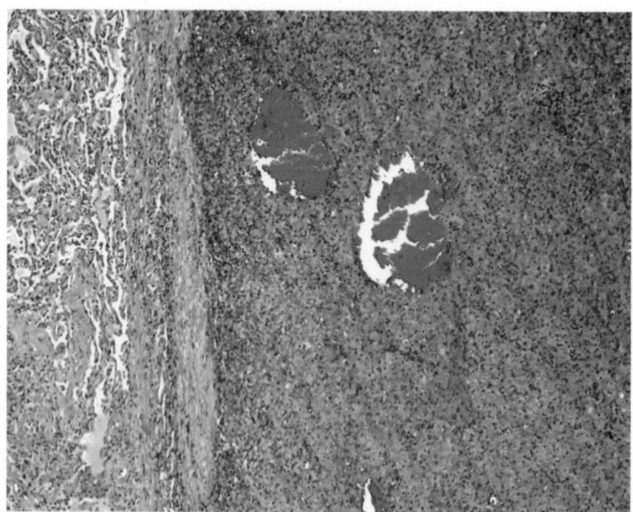

Figure 27.5 A well-demarcated cellular proliferation is seen within the lung tissue.

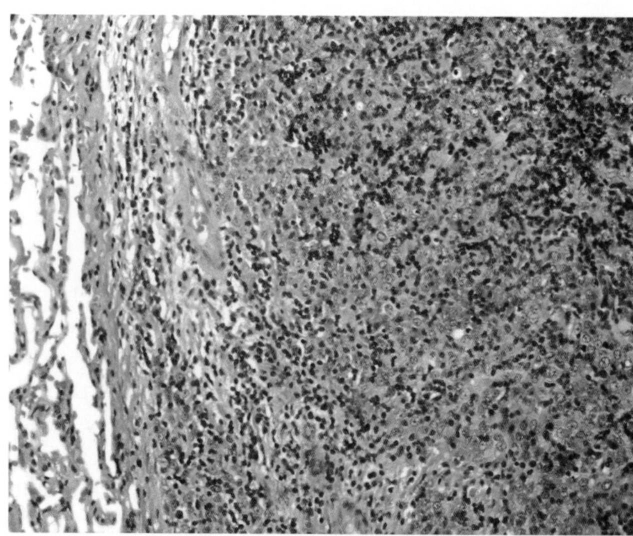

Figure 27.6 The tumor is made up of a biphasic cellular proliferation composed of epithelial cells and lymphocytes.

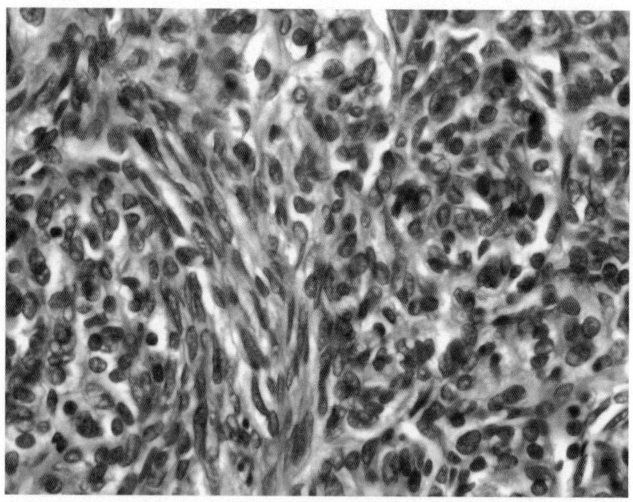

Figure 27.7 An intrapulmonary thymoma showing spindled cells with interspersed lymphocytes.

Part 3

Malignant Germ Cell Tumors

Ross A. Miller and Paloma del C. Monroig-Bosque

Primary germ cell tumors of the lung are extraordinarily rare; diagnoses of a primary tumor is dependent on excluding metastasis. The majority of primary germ cell tumors reported in the lung have been teratomas, which are derived from at least two of three embryonic germinal lines. The presumed etiology is ectopic tissues likely arising from the third pharyngeal pouch; the lesions typically occur in the upper lobe, particularly on the left side. The majority of described cases have occurred between the second and fourth decades of life, and there seems to be slight male predominance. Most described tumors have been mature teratomas and are therefore benign. Immature teratomas have also been described (albeit extraordinarily rare) and are associated with a very poor prognosis. There are very few accounts of primary malignant germ cell tumors other than immature teratomas reported in the literature. The cytologic and histologic features depend on which germinal elements are present. As this section is being devoted to malignant neoplasms, the following listed features will focus on malignant germ cell tumors.

CYTOLOGIC FEATURES

Immature Teratoma

- Primitive round to spindle-shaped cells with minimal cytoplasm.
- Hyperchromatic nuclei.
- Mitoses and apoptotic figures are common.

Seminoma

- Dual cell population of dyshesive large cells with prominent nucleoli and reactive lymphocytes.
- Background described as "tigroid," which is due to the glycogen material in cells, best seen on Diff-Quik–stained preparations.

Embryonal Carcinoma

- Poorly differentiated large malignant cells; necrotic background.

Yolk Sac Tumor (Endodermal Sinus Tumor)

- Relatively uniform cells with vacuolated cytoplasm and irregular nuclei; hyaline globules or Schiller–Duval bodies may be seen.

Choriocarcinoma

- Syncytiotrophoblasts and cytotrophoblasts.

HISTOLOGIC FEATURES

Immature Teratoma

- Immature elements recapitulate embryonic elements; most commonly seen are immature neuroepithelial elements.

Seminoma

- Sheets or nest of neoplastic cells with clear to slightly pink cytoplasm; background lymphocytes.
- Immunohistochemistry: positive for SALL4, PLAP, OCT3/4, and CD117.

Embryonal Carcinoma

- Highly malignant cells in a glandular to sheet-like growth pattern.
- Immunohistochemistry: positive for SALL4, CD30, PLAP, and OCT3/4.

Yolk Sac Tumor (Endodermal Sinus Tumor)

- The tumor can have a variety of growth patterns; reticular and/or microcystic patterns are most common.
- Eosinophilic globules and Schiller–Duval bodies.
- Immunohistochemistry: positive for SALL4, AFP, glypican-3, and PLAP (variable).

Choriocarcinoma

- Lots of hemorrhage, syncytiotrophoblasts and cytotrophoblasts.
- Immunohistochemistry: syncytiotrophoblasts are positive for SALL4, hCG, HPL, inhibin, glypican-3, and cytokeratin; cytotrophoblasts are positive for SALL4, GDF3, GATA3, and p63.

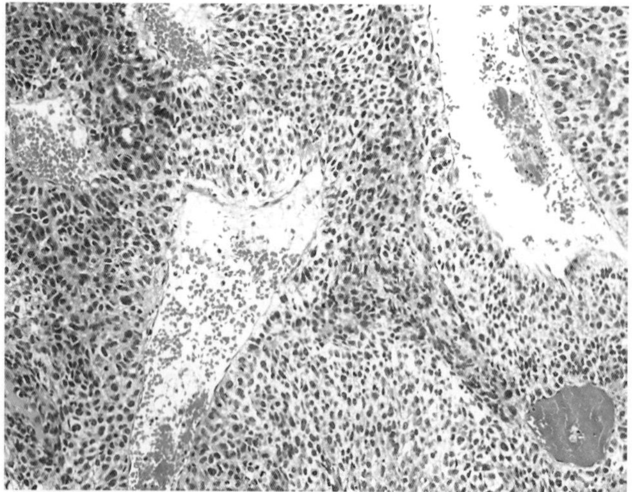

Figure 27.8 Immature neuroepithelium is the most common element seen in an immature teratoma. It is characterized by true rosettes, pseudorosettes, primitive tubules, or mitotically active glia.

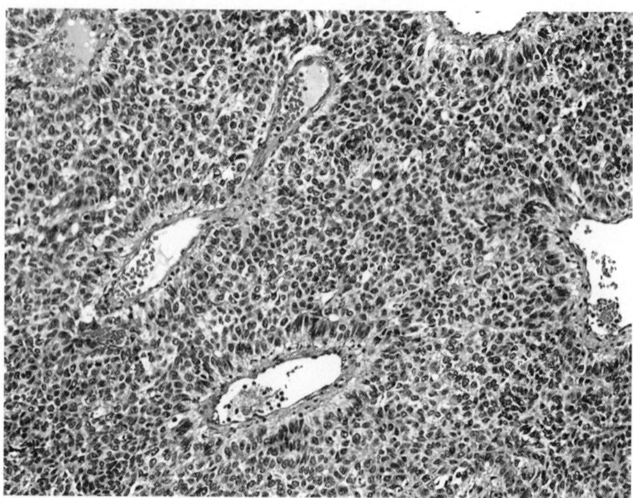

Figure 27.9 Another image of immature neuroepithelium.

Part 4

Lymphangioleiomyomatosis

Ross A. Miller and Paloma del C. Monroig-Bosque

Neoplasms thought to be derived from perivascular epithelioid cells (often referred to as *PEComas*) can be seen throughout the body. These tumors are typically composed of spindled and/or epithelioid cells and coexpress smooth muscle markers (SMA and calponin) and melanocytic-related markers (Melan-A and HMB-45). This family of tumors includes angiomyolipomas, clear cell "sugar" tumors, lymphangioleiomyomatosis (LAMM), and PEComas of various other sites (falciform ligament/ligamentum teres, skin, uterus, soft tissues, and viscera). These neoplasms have an association with tuberous sclerosis, and most are benign. The two main PEComas involving the lung include clear cell "sugar" tumor and LAMM. A discussion on clear cell "sugar" tumor is seen in Chapter 43.

LAMM is essentially only seen in women of reproductive range. It is a very rare condition, and around 15% of cases are associated with tuberous sclerosis. The classic imaging findings include a reticular interstitial pattern in the lung parenchyma along with chylous pleural effusion and pneumothorax. Honeycomb changes can be seen in advanced disease. Histologically, nodules and plaque-like lesions are seen surrounding cystically dilated airways. These nodules and lesions are composed of spindled cells with fibrillary to vacuolated eosinophilic cytoplasm. Sometimes, admixed epithelioid cells are seen intermixed with the spindled cells.

CYTOLOGIC FEATURES

- Cells typically spindled with fibrillary to finely vacuolated cytoplasm.
- Some of the nuclei have irregular nuclear contours.
- Occasionally, admixed epithelioid cells are seen with clear to vacuolated cytoplasm.

HISTOLOGIC FEATURES

- Nodules or plaque-like lesions composed of cells with features as outlined above (see cytologic features above) which surround or are adjacent to dilated airspaces.
- Cells express smooth muscle markers (SMA and calponin) and melanocytic-associated markers (Melan-A and HMB-45).

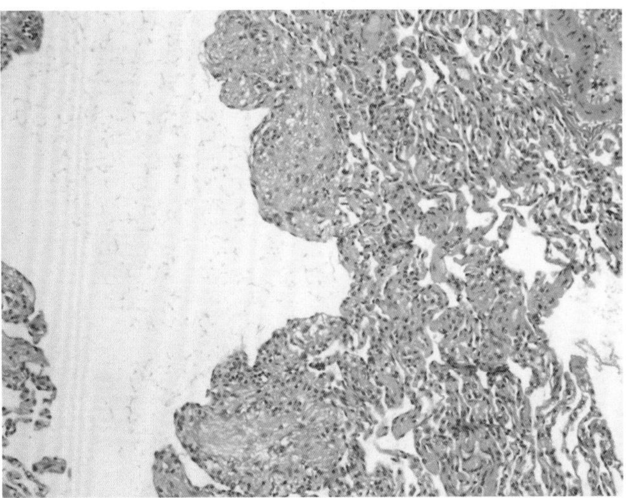

Figure 27.10 LAMM is a rare progressive and systemic disease that can result in cystic lung destruction. It is characterized by the classic presence of smooth muscle proliferation that can obliterate the normal alveolar lining or vascular walls.

Part 5

Ciliated Muconodular Papillary Tumor of the Lung

Ross A. Miller, Yi-Chen Yeh, and Yen-Wen Lu

Ciliated muconodular papillary tumor of the lung is a rare entity that is not defined in the 2015 WHO classification of thoracic tumors. There are just over 30 reported cases in the medical literature to date; of these reported cases, most patients are in their sixth to eighth decades of life. However, the lesion has been reported in a patient of age as young as 19 years. The tumor is most often incidentally discovered during imaging studies and is typically located in the peripheral lung fields. A gelatinous or mucinous cut surface is often grossly described; microscopic findings include papillary structures containing ciliated columnar and goblet cells. Often, free-floating neoplastic cells are seen in the mucin. Given the findings, the lesion can be easily misclassified as an adenocarcinoma, particularly mucinous adenocarcinoma. The ciliated columnar cells can be a clue; in addition, ciliated muconodular papillary tumors of the lung have a continuous layer of basal cells. Variable staining can be seen with CK7 and TTF-1 by immunohistochemistry. CK5/6 or p40 will highlight the continuous basal cell layer. The lesions have a seemingly indolent clinical course as no metastases or recurrences have been reported. Various mutations have been described including alterations in BRAF, EGFR, and ALK. No specific molecular alteration has been found to date.

CYTOLOGIC FINDINGS

- Ciliated columnar and goblet cells.
- Abundant mucin.
- Presence of basal cells.

HISTOLOGIC FINDINGS

- Papillary structures lined by ciliated columnar cells and goblet cells.
- Continuous basal cell layer.
- Detached, free-floating cells in mucin pools.

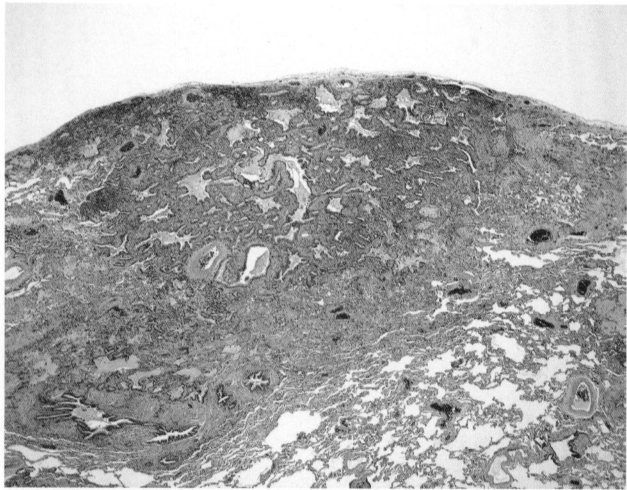

Figure 27.11 A fairly well-demarcated lesion is seen with papillary-like structures lined by ciliated columnar cells and goblet cells.

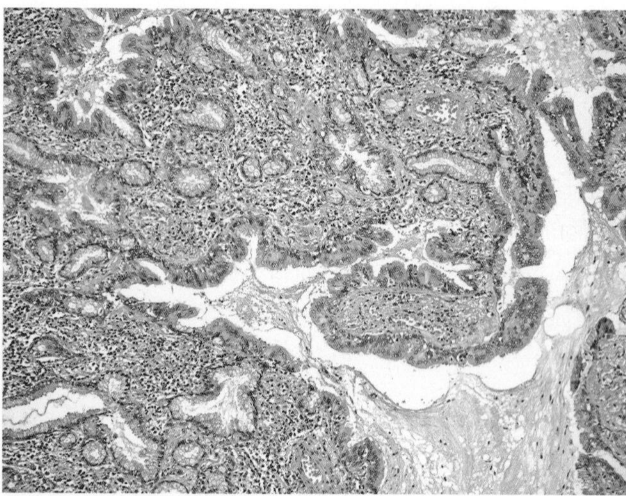

Figure 27.12 Papillary-like structure lined by ciliated columnar cells and goblet cells. Abundant mucin material is seen and a continuous layer of basal cells can be seen.

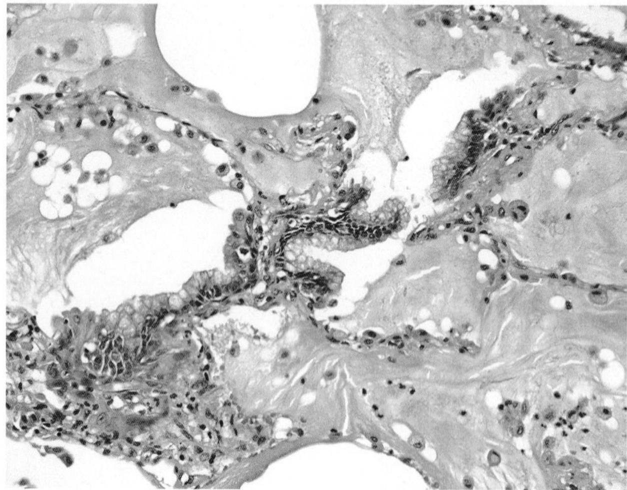

Figure 27.13 Abundant mucin along with ciliated columnar cells and goblet cells.

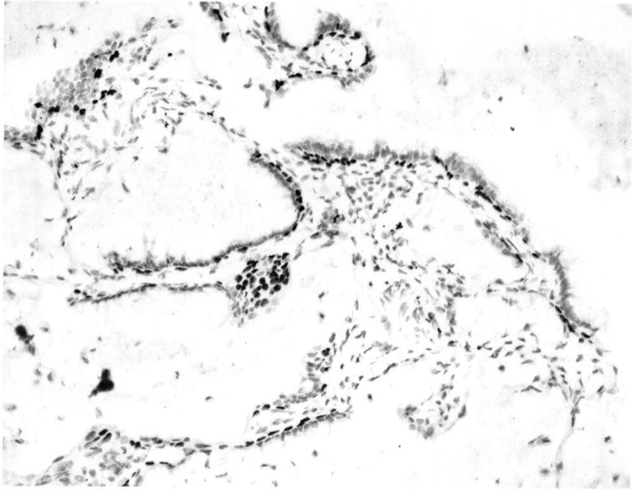

Figure 27.14 An immunohistochemical stain for p40 highlights the continuous basal cell layer.

Metaplastic, Dysplastic, and Premalignant Lesions

28

Part 1

Atypical Adenomatous Hyperplasia

Sanja Dacic

Atypical adenomatous hyperplasia (AAH) is a small, usually ≤0.5 cm, localized proliferation of mildly to moderately atypical type II pneumocytes and/or Clara cells lining alveolar walls. AAH is considered to be a precursor to a subset of nonmucinous adenocarcinomas. It is typically an incidental microscopic finding. If it is grossly visible than appears as a poorly defined yellow-tan nodule. AAH often arises in centriacinar region close to respiratory bronchioles. Clara cells are recognized as columnar, with cytoplasmic snouts and pale eosinophilic cytoplasm. Type II pneumocytes are cuboidal or dome-shaped with fine cytoplasmic vacuoles or clear to foamy cytoplasm. Intranuclear eosinophilic inclusions may be present. In contrast to adenocarcinoma in situ (AIS), there are gaps along the surface of the basement membrane between the cells. The differential diagnosis includes reactive pneumocyte hyperplasia and nonmucinous AIS. Reactive pneumocyte hyperplasia usually occurs in the background of inflammatory process in the lung, such as pneumonia or chronic interstitial fibrosis. The distinction from AIS is more difficult in some cases, but AIS is usually larger than 0.5 cm, more cellular, and composed of crowed and uniform cells. *KRAS* and *EGFR* mutations have been reported in AAH.

HISTOLOGIC FEATURES

- Small localized frequently centriacinar lesion usually ≤0.5 cm.
- AAH is composed of Clara cells and/or type II pneumocytes.
- Clara cells are columnar, with cytoplasmic snouts and pale eosinophilic cytoplasm.
- Type II pneumocytes are cuboidal or dome-shaped with fine cytoplasmic vacuoles or clear to foamy cytoplasm.
- Intranuclear eosinophilic inclusions may be present.
- Gaps between the cells and along the surface of the basement membrane.

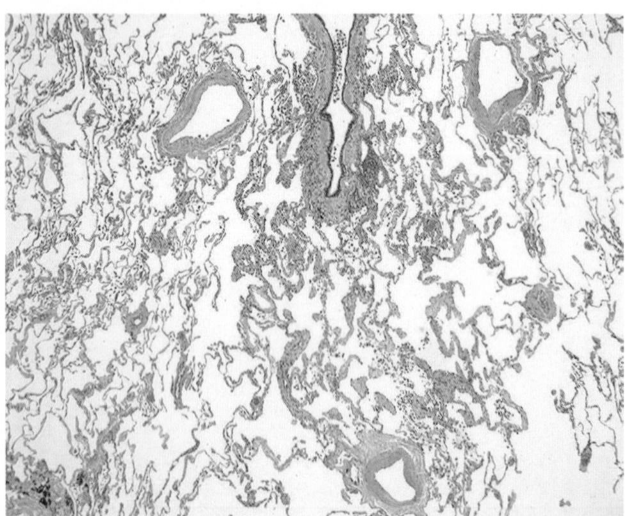

Figure 28.1 Localized centriacinar proliferation of type II pneumocytes along thickened alveolar septa.

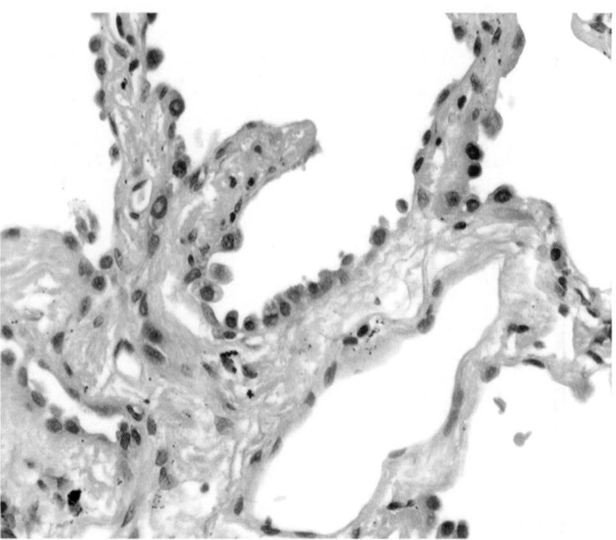

Figure 28.2 Mildly atypical pneumocytes with gaps between the cells and occasional intranuclear inclusions.

Part 2

Adenocarcinoma In Situ

Sanja Dacic

AIS (formerly *bronchioloalveolar carcinoma*) is defined by 2015 World Health Organization (WHO) as a localized small (≤3.0 cm) adenocarcinoma with growth restricted to neoplastic cells along preexisting alveolar structures (lepidic growth), lacking stromal, vascular, or pleural invasion. Invasive patterns, such as acinar, papillary, micropapillary, and solid, should be absent. AIS is further subdivided into nonmucinous and mucinous variants. Nonmucinous variant is more frequent than mucinous. Similar to AAH, nonmucinous variant may show type II pneumocyte or Clara cell differentiation. This distinction is of no clinical significance. Patients with AIS have 100% disease-free and recurrence-free survival if lesion is completely resected.

Grossly, AIS appears as a tan or pale, circumscribed, and poorly defined nodule, usually in the subpleural location. A definitive diagnosis of AIS can be established on the resection specimens only and may be suggested on the biopsy or cytology specimen when they should be reported as a lepidic adenocarcinoma.

The main differential diagnosis includes minimally invasive adenocarcinoma (MIA), which requires identification of invasion. Mucinous AIS always require clinical correlation with imaging studies to exclude a metastatic mucinous adenocarcinoma, particularly from pancreas.

HISTOLOGIC FEATURES

- Nonmucinous AIS grows in a pure lepidic pattern without evidence of invasion and shows either type II pneumocyte and/or Clara cell differentiation.
- Mucinous AIS consists of tall columnar cells with basal nuclei and abundant cytoplasmic mucin; sometimes resemble goblet cells.
- Nuclear atypia in nonmucinous AIS is minimal to mild, whereas it is virtually absent in mucinous AIS.
- Alveolar septal sclerosis is common, particularly in nonmucinous AIS.

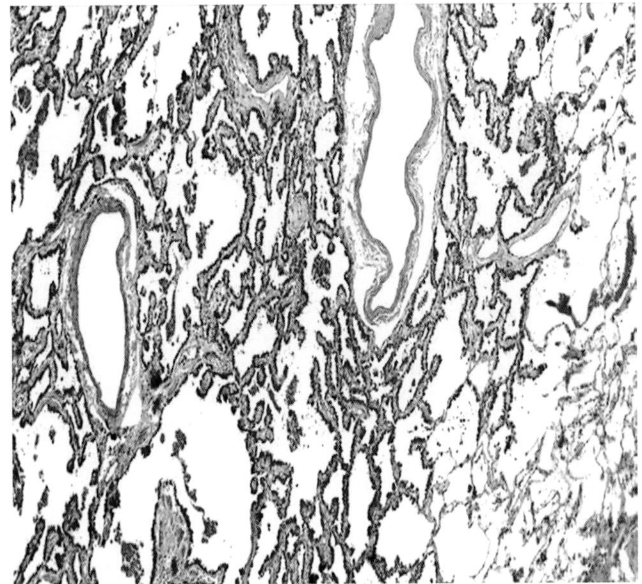

Figure 28.3 Nonmucinous AIS showing a pure lepidic growth pattern without evidence of invasion.

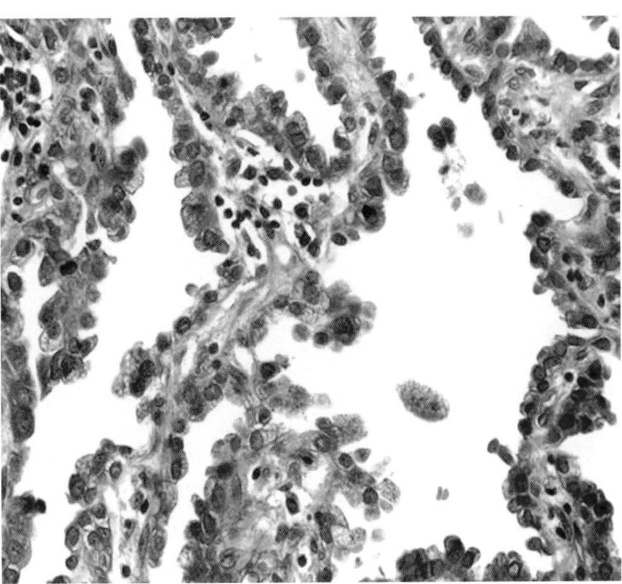

Figure 28.4 Mildly atypical crowded pneumocytes along thickened alveolar septa.

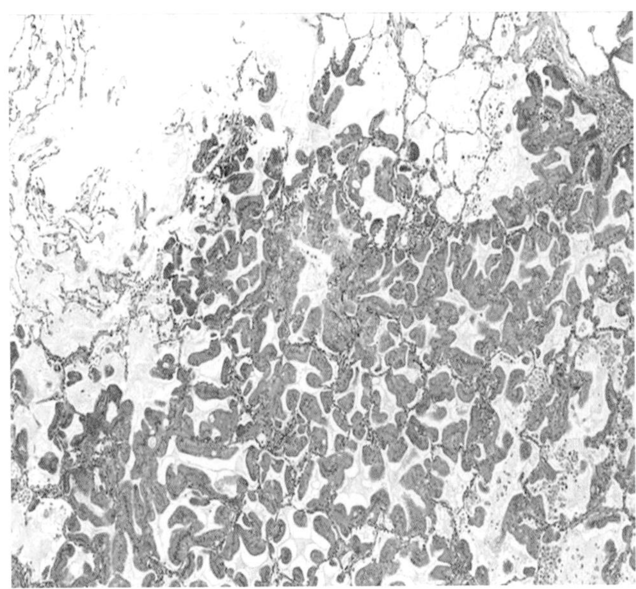

Figure 28.5 Mucinous AIS with tall columnar cell growing along alveolar septa without evidence of invasion and associated with extracellular and intracellular mucin.

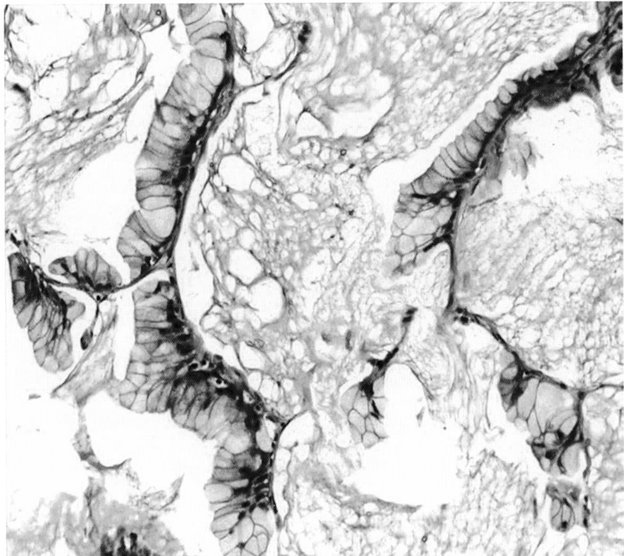

Figure 28.6 Mucinous AIS showing columnar cells with abundant cytoplasmic mucin and small basally oriented nuclei resembling goblet cells.

Part 3

Minimally Invasive Adenocarcinoma

▶ Sanja Dacic

MIA is defined by 2015 WHO as a small (≤3.0 cm) solitary adenocarcinoma with a predominantly lepidic growth pattern and ≤5 mm invasion. MIA is usually nonmucinous but rarely may be mucinous or mixed. Similar to AIS, the diagnosis of MIA can be established on the resection specimens only. Nonmucinous MIA and mucinous MIA are cytologically and architecturally similar to AIS, but with the presence of invasion. The size of invasion should be measured in the largest dimension. The invasive component to be measured is defined by histologic types other than lepidic (acinar, papillary, micropapillary, and solid) or tumor cells infiltrating the stroma. MIA is excluded if angiolymphatic, pleural, or air-space invasion is identified; tumor shows necrosis or spread through airspaces. MIA must be distinguished from invasive adenocarcinoma. Patients with entirely surgically resected MIA should have 100% disease-free and recurrence-free survival.

HISTOLOGIC FEATURES

- Nonmucinous MIA grows in a pure lepidic pattern with ≤5 mm invasion and shows either type II pneumocyte and/or Clara cell differentiation.
- Mucinous AIS shows ≤5 mm invasion of tall columnar cells with basal nuclei and abundant cytoplasmic mucin, often resembling goblet cells.
- The invasion component is defined by histologic subtypes other than lepidic.

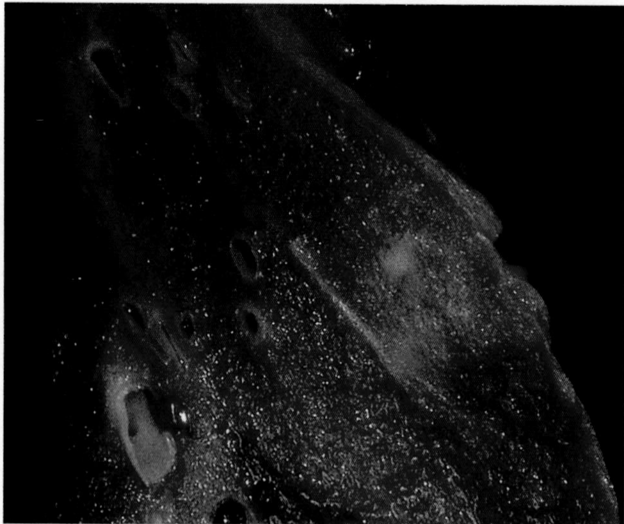

Figure 28.7 Gross appearance of MIA as a poorly circumscribed, pale–tan peripheral nodule with slightly more prominent central area.

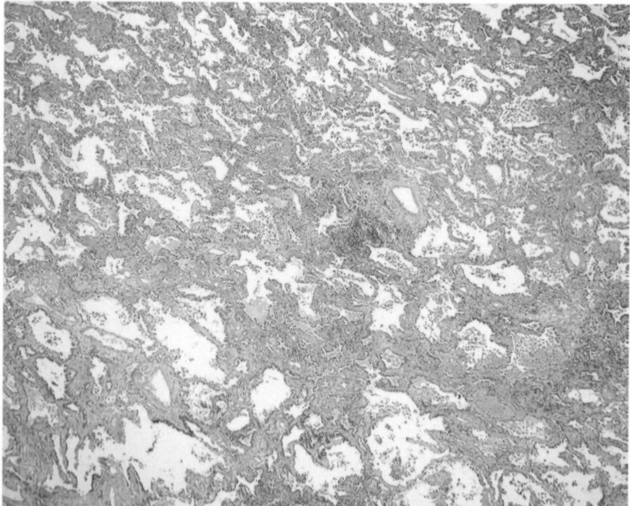

Figure 28.8 Low-power magnification of mostly lepidic adenocarcinoma with multiple areas of crowded gland-like structures associated with more prominent stroma and lymphocytic reaction.

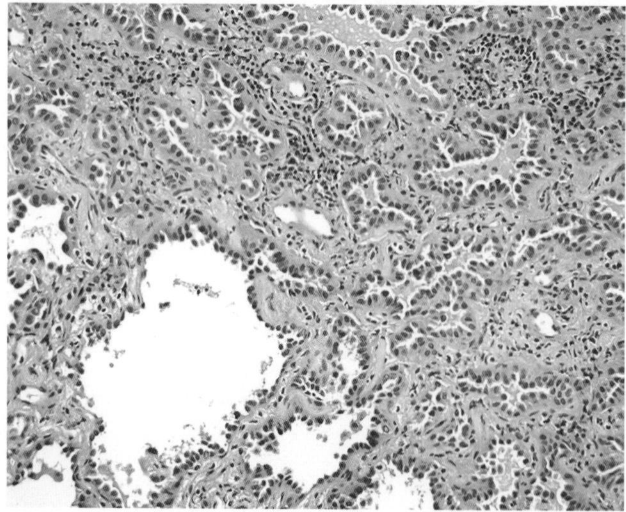

Figure 28.9 High-power magnification of the same case demonstrating invasion measuring less than 5 mm.

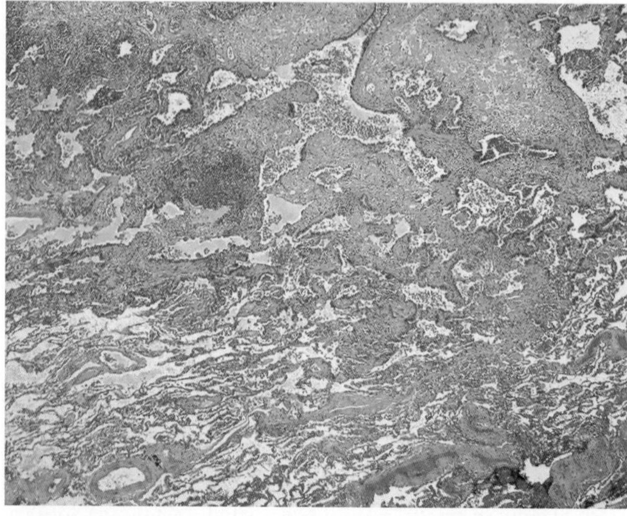

Figure 28.10 Another example of MIA demonstrating lepidic-predominant pattern with stromal invasion at the periphery of the preexisting scar.

Part 4

Squamous Metaplasia, Squamous Dysplasia, and Squamous Carcinoma In Situ

Ross A. Miller

Squamous metaplasia, dysplasia, and carcinoma in situ are a spectrum of changes that can be seen in the bronchial epithelium thought to precede invasive squamous-cell carcinoma. The progression from metaplasia–dysplasia–carcinoma in situ–invasive squamous-cell carcinoma is considered a stepwise process as increasing molecular alterations accumulate. Metaplasia is reversible and is a physiologic response to injury. Dysplasia can persist in the airways for years; often, progression to a more severe lesion never occurs. Squamous carcinoma in situ is classified as Tis in the TNM classification system utilized by the Union for International Cancer Control (UICC) and the American Joint Committee on Cancer (AJCC) and is considered a *pre*invasive malignant process.

Subpart 4.1

Squamous Metaplasia

Ross A. Miller

The normal physiologic response of the bronchial epithelium after encountering an irritant is basal cell hyperplasia followed by squamous metaplasia. The metaplastic epithelium replaces the normal goblet and ciliated respiratory cell types seemingly as a protective response. Irritants to the bronchial mucosa can be carcinogens and/or noncarcinogens; as such, squamous metaplasia may be a resultant of a purely inflammatory process or it may be the first step in the development of a neoplasm (i.e., a preneoplastic finding). Squamous metaplasia (along with dysplasia) is often multifocal in cigarette smokers, a so-called field effect of the carcinogenic irritant resulting from inhaled smoke coming into contact with all areas of the tracheobronchial tree. Of note, squamous metaplasia can be seen in specimens from posttransplant patients and may represent inflammatory and/or reparative changes; it is often seen at the site of anastomosis and marked reactive changes can be encountered.

CYTOLOGIC FEATURES

- Squamous metaplastic cells characterized by dark nuclei, glassy cytoplasm, defined cytoplasmic borders, and possible keratinization.

HISTOLOGIC FEATURES

- Squamous cells lining the airway; organization maintained.
- Loss of goblet and ciliated respiratory cells.
- Metaplastic epithelium may occlude underlying bronchial mucous glands.

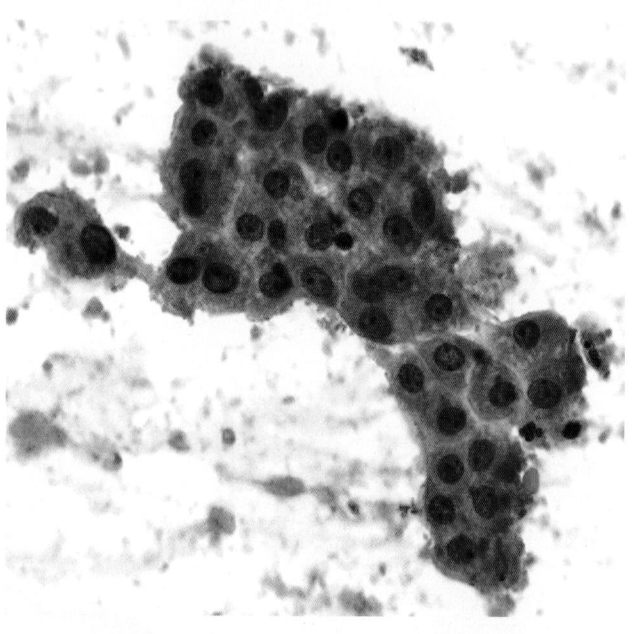

Figure 28.11 Lung cytology specimen showing squamous metaplasia. The cytoplasmic borders are well-defined and the nuclear and cytoplasm show squamous features opposed to ciliated respiratory features typically seen from specimens from this site.

Subpart 4.2

Squamous Dysplasia

Ross A. Miller

With continued irritant exposure, squamous metaplasia can progress to dysplasia. In smokers, dysplasia is often multifocal (similar to metaplastic changes seen in smokers) likely due to a field effect of inhalational exposure to carcinogens. Dysplastic change can persist for many years and may or may not progress to squamous carcinoma in situ. Dysplasia can be stratified into mild, moderate, and severe; this grading system is based on epithelial thickness, cell size, nuclear atypia, and cellular maturation/organization seen in the epithelium. Epithelial thickness, cell size, and nuclear atypia increase, and cell maturation is progressively lost with increasing degrees of dysplasia. The basal zone is typically expanded to varying degrees: the lower third with mild dysplasia, the lower two-thirds with moderate dysplasia, and the upper third with severe dysplasia.

CYTOLOGIC FEATURES

- Cells show progressively increasing anisocytosis and pleomorphism with increasing degrees of dysplasia.
- Dysplasia is not typically graded on cytology specimens; if dysplastic cells are seen on cytology specimens, the assigned diagnostic category is typically "atypical" or "suspicious." This being said, cytologic features are described with varying degrees of dysplasia. These are typically described in histologic (surgical biopsy) specimens.
  - Mild dysplasia: mild alteration of the nuclear to cytoplasmic ratio, rare mitotic figures, and absent or inconspicuous nucleoli.
  - Moderate dysplasia: moderate changes in the nuclear to cytoplasmic ratio, nuclear angulations and grooves, and occasional mitotic figures.
  - Severe dysplasia: variable nuclear to cytoplasmic ratios, coarse chromatin, conspicuous nucleoli, and more numerous mitotic figures.

HISTOLOGIC FEATURES

- Progressive maturation loss and expansion of the basal layer with increasing dysplasia.
- Mild dysplasia: basal layer expanded and crowded with vertically oriented nuclei in the lower third; superficial flattening of cells (maturation toward the epithelial surface). Only rare mitotic figures are seen, confined to the area of basal layer expansion.
- Moderate dysplasia: basal layer expanded and crowded with vertically oriented nuclei in the lower two-thirds of the epithelium; cells at the surface flatten out (some degree of maturation). Mitotic figures may be seen, confined to the lower third.
- Severe dysplasia: little maturation present; basal zone expanded into the upper third of the epithelium. Superficial cells still flatten out. Mitotic figures are often seen, confined to the lower two-thirds of the epithelium.

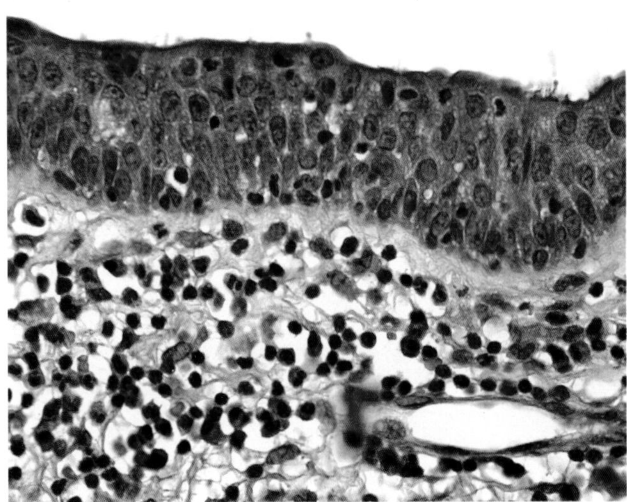

Figure 28.12 Severe squamous dysplasia: there is little maturation present and the basal zone is expanded into the upper third. Superficial cells flatten out *(top right of the image)*. The cells have large nuclei containing coarse chromatin; occasional nucleoli are seen.

Subpart 4.3

Squamous Carcinoma In Situ

Ross A. Miller

Carcinoma in situ is characterized by full-thickness epithelial atypia with an intact basement membrane (i.e., no invasion). Foci of squamous carcinoma in situ tend to arise at bifurcations in the bronchial tree and may extend proximally and/or distally. Grossly, the lesions can be flat and may resemble leukoplakia or erythroplakia. Some lesions may have a nodular to polypoid configuration. There is significant overlap with carcinoma in situ and high-grade dysplasia, which may lead to intraobserver variability on how to classify the lesion. The presence of an intact basement membrane separates squamous carcinoma in situ (no invasion) from invasive squamous-cell carcinoma. As such, examining multiple levels from a tissue section with carcinoma in situ can be helpful to rule out an invasive process. Carcinoma in situ can extend into bronchial glands, which may mimic invasion. When this occurs, an intact basement membrane layer should remain. A ragged, infiltrative appearance, presence of single cells, necrosis, and a defined endobronchial mass are all features favoring invasive carcinoma.

CYTOLOGIC FEATURES

- Highly variable nuclear to cytoplasmic ratios, coarse chromatin, conspicuous nucleoli, often numerous mitotic figures.

HISTOLOGIC FEATURES

- No maturation from the basal layer to the surface; mitotic figures can span the entire thickness of the epithelium; intact basement membrane.
- Mucosal thickening may occur; polypoid or nodular lesion may be present.
- Extension into bronchial glands can be seen.

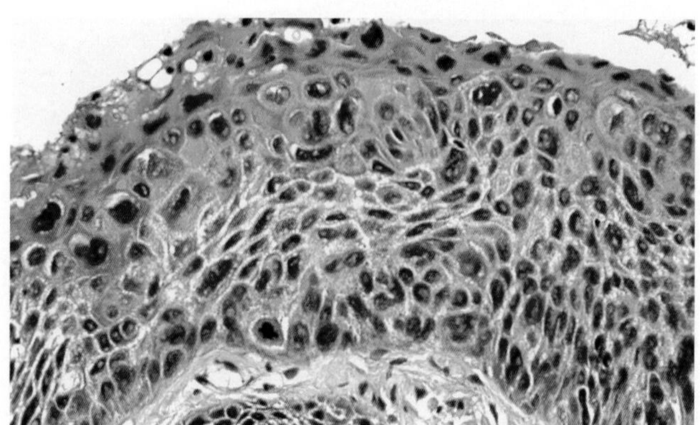

Figure 28.13 Carcinoma in situ: the mucosa has full-thickness atypia; the basement membrane remains intact (i.e., no invasion).

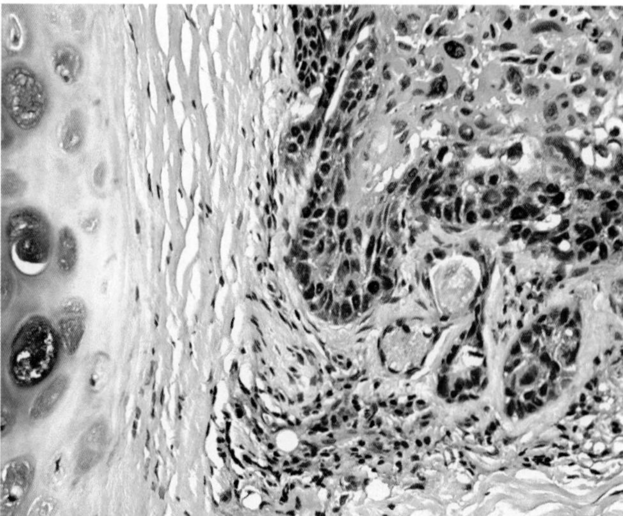

Figure 28.14 Extension into the bronchial glands can be seen. This findings should not be misinterpreted as invasion, note the relatively smooth and intact basement membrane.

Part 5

Squamous Papilloma and Papillomatosis

Ross A. Miller

Squamous papillomas can be exophytic or inverted and solitary or multiple. When lesions occur, they are most often multiple (papillomatosis) and can involve the tracheobronchial tree or even lung parenchyma. Papillomatosis is more commonly seen in the larynx and can be aggressive in children. The term *invasive papillomatosis* is sometimes used when papillomas extend into the lung parenchyma. This can result in significant morbidity when airway obstruction occurs.

The human papilloma virus (HPV) plays a pathogenic role in nearly all cases where multiple lesions are seen. HPV serotypes 6 and 11 are seen in simple papillomas. The same HPV high-risk serotypes associated with cervical cancer (serotypes 16, 18, 31, 33, and 35) tend to play a role when malignant transformation occurs in lesions of the respiratory tract. Solitary lesions are extraordinary rare and the HPV is thought to play a role in only a minority of such lesions. Most patients described with solitary lesions have been tobacco smokers.

Papillomas consist of delicate connective tissue fronds lined by squamous epithelium; acanthosis and parakeratosis are common findings. Some cases have HPV cytopathic effects including koilocytic atypia, binucleate cells, and wrinkled nuclei. When dysplasia is seen, it should be graded accordingly (see section on squamous dysplasia for grading, part 4, subpart 4.2). Papillomas can be inverted (inverted papillomas) and are characterized by invagination of squamous epithelium into the submucosal tissues. Typically, the invaginated squamous nests have orderly cell maturation and are surrounded by a basement membrane material.

CYTOLOGIC FEATURES

- Squamous cells; HPV cytopathic effects (koilocytic atypia) or even dysplasia may be seen (see section on squamous dysplasia, part 4, subpart 4.2).

HISTOLOGIC FEATURES

- Papillae composed of connective tissue fronds containing fibrovascular cores with overlying squamous epithelium.
- Varying degrees of acanthosis, parakeratosis, and associated inflammatory cells may be seen.
- Inverted papillomas have fronds of squamous epithelium invaginating into the submucosa; significant cellular atypia, single cells in stroma, necrosis, and mitotic figures should be absent.
- Condylomatous atypia (HPV cytopathic effects in cells) may be seen.
- Dysplasia (see section on dysplasia for findings and grading, part 4, subpart 4.2) may be seen.

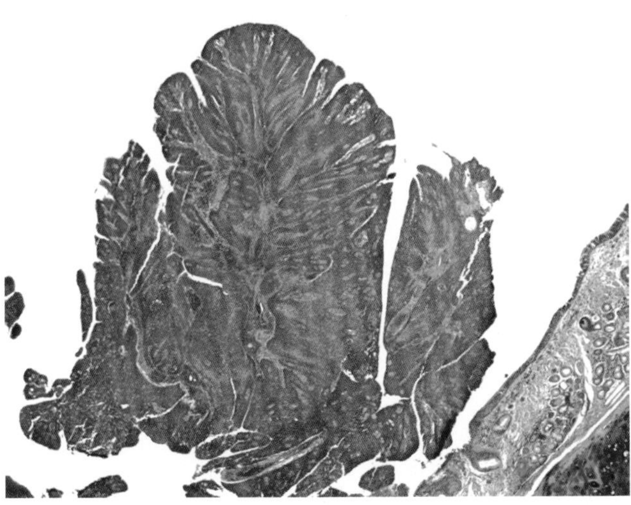

Figure 28.15 Squamous papilloma, papillary lesion composed of fibrovascular cores and squamous epithelium.

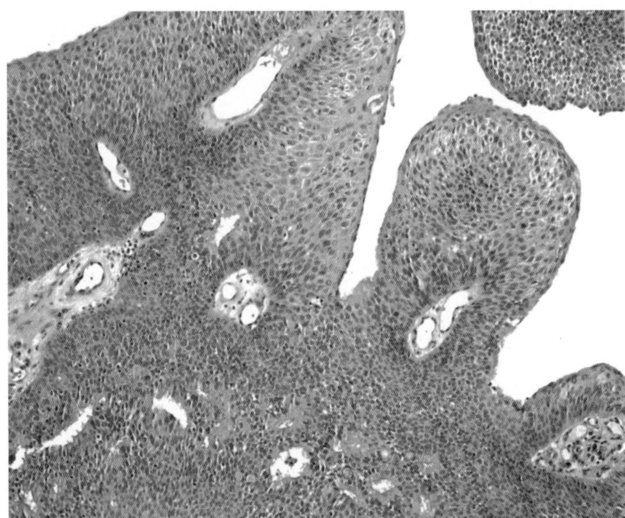

Figure 28.16 Higher power view of fibrovascular cores, varying degrees of acanthosis, parakeratosis, and associated inflammatory cells can be seen in squamous papillomas.

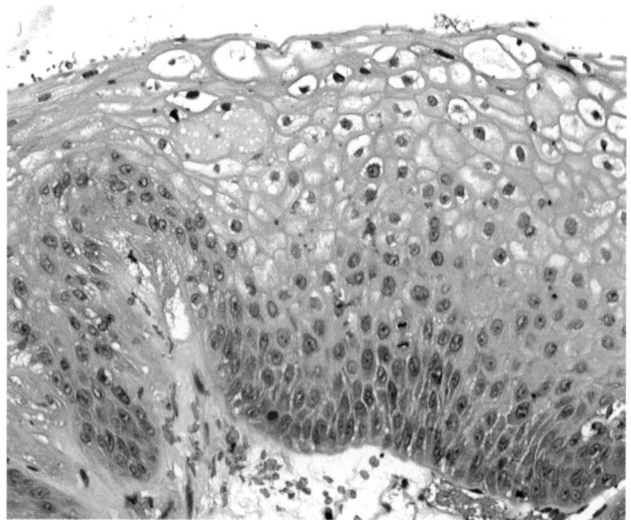

Figure 28.17 Squamous papilloma with HPV cytopathic effect (condylomatous atypia).

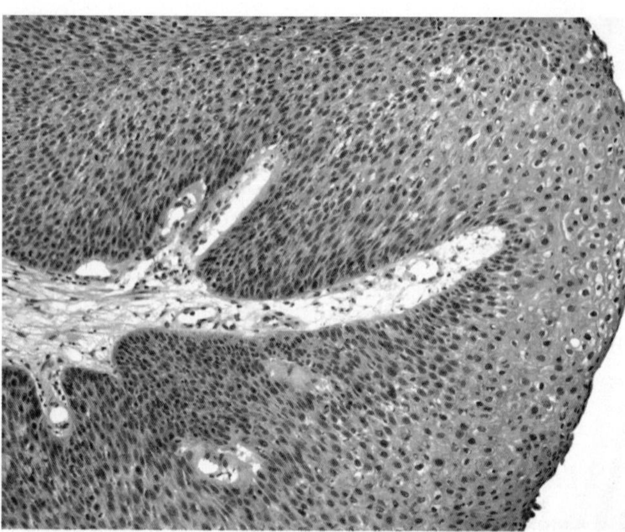

Figure 28.18 Squamous papilloma with moderate dysplasia. There is basal layer expansion and occasional mitotic figures in the lower third of the mucosa.

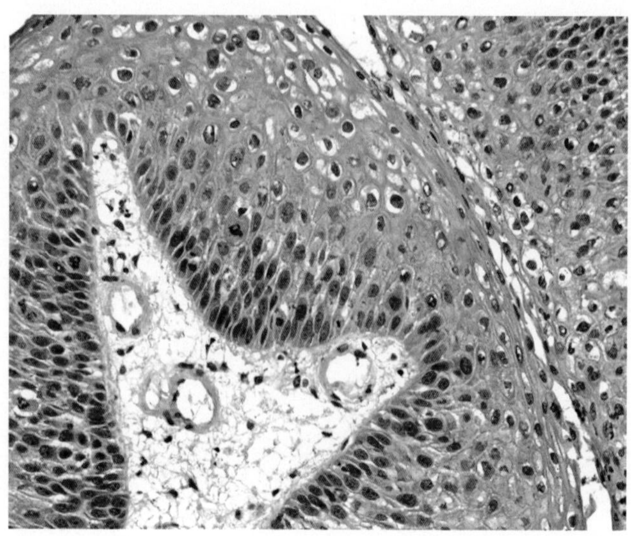

Figure 28.19 Higher power view; squamous papilloma with moderate dysplasia. There is basal layer expansion and occasional mitotic figures in the lower third of the mucosa.

Subpart 5.1

Glandular Papilloma and Mixed Squamous and Glandular Papilloma

Ross A. Miller

Glandular papillomas and mixed squamous and glandular papillomas are rare benign endobronchial lesions treated by complete surgical excision. Patients with either type of papilloma typically present with obstructive symptoms, cough, wheezing, or hemoptysis. Glandular papillomas are papillary lesion lined by ciliated or nonciliated columnar type cells often containing admixed goblet and cuboidal cells in varying proportions. A mixed squamous cell and glandular papilloma has both squamous and glandular lining components; the glandular component is supposed to make up at least one-third of the lining otherwise the lesion is better classified as a squamous papilloma. Mixed squamous and glandular papillomas typically have bland glandular cells. Varying degrees of atypia can be seen in the squamous component; HPV has not been identified in studied cases.

CYTOLOGIC FEATURES

- Cytology specimens may show glandular cells (in glandular papilloma) or an admixture of glandular and squamous cells (in mixed-type papilloma). The findings are not specific for the lesion.

HISTOLOGIC FEATURES

- Papillary structures with hyalinized or vascular cores.
- Lining cells: pseudostratified or stratified columnar cells with admixed cuboidal and/or goblet cells in varying proportions (glandular papilloma); in mixed squamous and glandular papillomas, interspersed squamous islands are seen.
- Necrosis, atypia, and mitotic figures are absent in glandular lining; the squamous lining in mixed papillomas can have varying degrees of atypia.

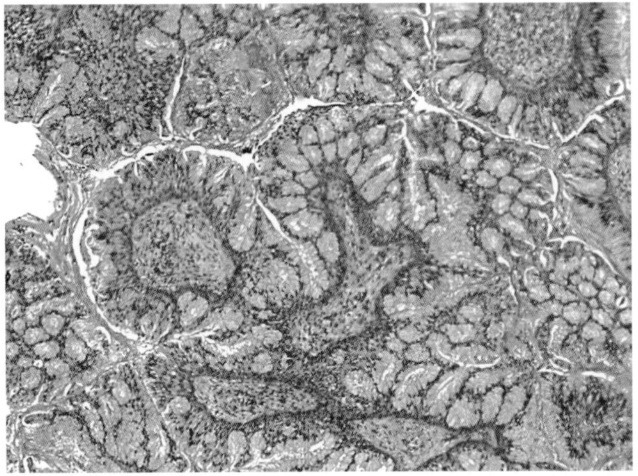

Figure 28.20 Glandular papilloma, note the papillary structures and glan dular lining. Numerous goblet cells are seen in this lesion.

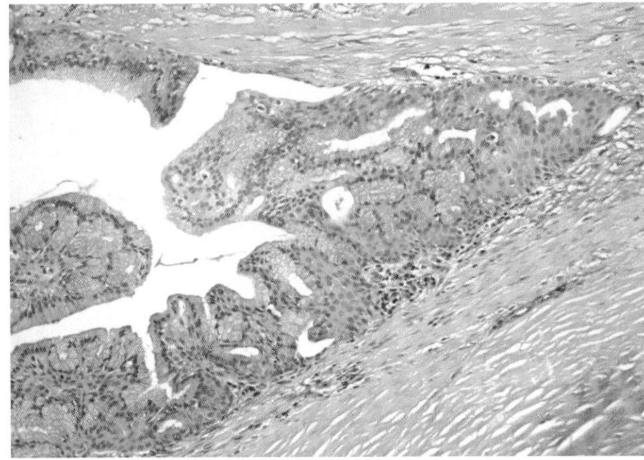

Figure 28.21 A mixed squamous and glandular papilloma. The lining is composed of both squamous and glandular cells. The glandular cells make up more than one-third of the lining cells.

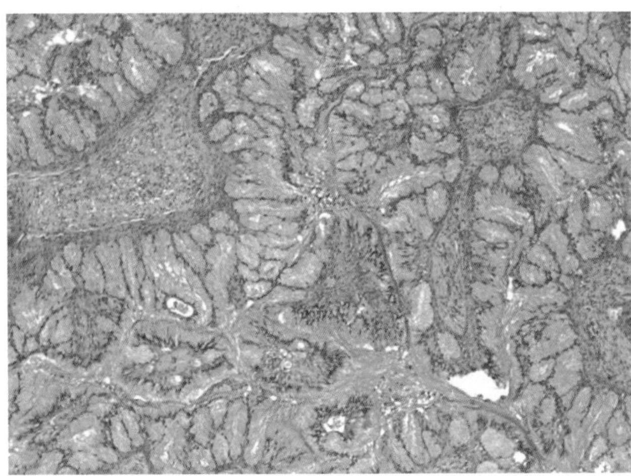

Figure 28.22 A higher power view of a mixed squamous and glandular papilloma. The lining is composed of both squamous and glandular cells. The glandular cells make up more than one-third of the lining cells.

Part 6

Diffuse Idiopathic Pulmonary Neuroendocrine-Cell Hyperplasia (DIPNECH)

Ross A. Miller and Paloma del C. Monroig-Bosque

Diffuse idiopathic pulmonary neuroendocrine-cell hyperplasia (DIPNECH) typically presents in the fifth or sixth decade of life and has a female predominance. DIPNECH is an idiopathic proliferation of pulmonary neuroendocrine cells seen throughout the lung parenchyma. Often, associated chronic inflammation and fibrosis of involved airways (particularly findings of constrictive bronchiolitis) is seen. The neuroendocrine proliferations can form tumorlets (aggregates of neuroendocrine cells less than 5 mm in diameter) or even carcinoids (greater than 5 mm by definition). The risk of developing carcinoids is seemingly small; when carcinoid tumors develop, they are almost always typical carcinoids. There are only rare reports of atypical carcinoid tumors developing in the setting of DIPNECH and no described cases of small-cell or large-cell neuroendocrine carcinomas.

The differential diagnosis includes neuroendocrine tumors (tumorlet and carcinoid), reactive hyperplasia in chronically injured lungs, and peritumoral neuroendocrine proliferations seen around carcinoid tumors. The presence of a diffuse neuroendocrine proliferation distinguishes it from an isolated tumorlet or carcinoid. Of course, tumorlets and carcinoids are a part of DIPNECH, and neuroendocrine markers (synaptophysin, chromogranin, and CD56) will often highlight neuroendocrine cells that may be overlooked on examination of routine stained sections. The presence of chronic lung injury and neuroendocrine hyperplasia favors a reactive proliferation secondary to chronic injury over DIPNECH and the neuroendocrine hyperplasia that can be seen around carcinoids is typically confined to tissue immediately adjacent to the carcinoid opposed to the diffuse process seen in DIPNECH.

DIPNECH is considered a "preinvasive" condition and therefore is not staged. If a carcinoid tumor does develop, the carcinoid tumor should be stage accordingly. Of note, some patients may go on to develop obliterative bronchiolitis which may require transplantation. At this time, it is not known if the resulting neuroendocrine hyperplasia is secondary to an unrecognized pulmonary process (as accompanying airway inflammation and fibrosis is often seen) or if the airway changes are secondary to the effects of the proliferating neuroendocrine cells. Currently, by definition, the process is considered idiopathic. Occasional described cases have been associated with multiple endocrine neoplasia type 1.

CYTOLOGIC FEATURES

- Neuroendocrine cells can be round to spindle-shaped with round to oval nuclei and characteristic salt-and-pepper chromatin.

HISTOLOGIC FEATURES

- Diffuse neuroendocrine proliferations occurring along airways; lesions may traverse across the basal lamina and form tumorlets (less than 5 mm by definition).
- Some patients may develop carcinoids (greater than 5 mm by definition).

- Associated findings include chronic inflammation and fibrosis of the airways, which may take the form of constrictive bronchiolitis.
- Some patients may develop obliterative bronchiolitis.
- Immunohistochemical profile:
  - Neuroendocrine cells are positive for: synaptophysin, chromogranin, and CD56.

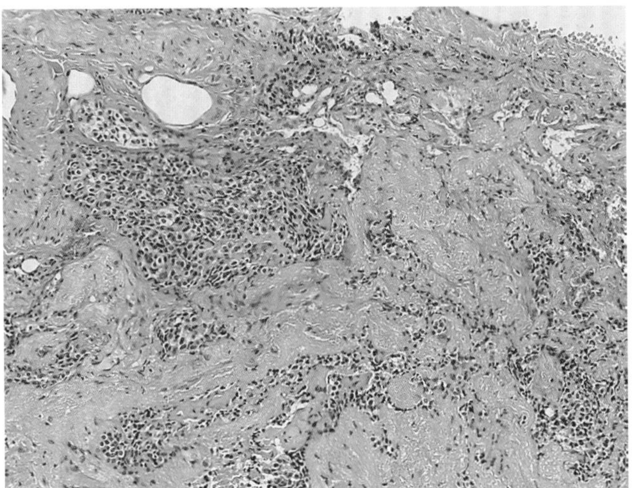

Figure 28.23 Pulmonary neuroendocrine cells in DIPNECH are arranged in small groups or in a monolayer arrangement. The cells may be confined to the mucosa, protrude into the lumen of the airway, or invade across the basal lamina forming tumorlets.

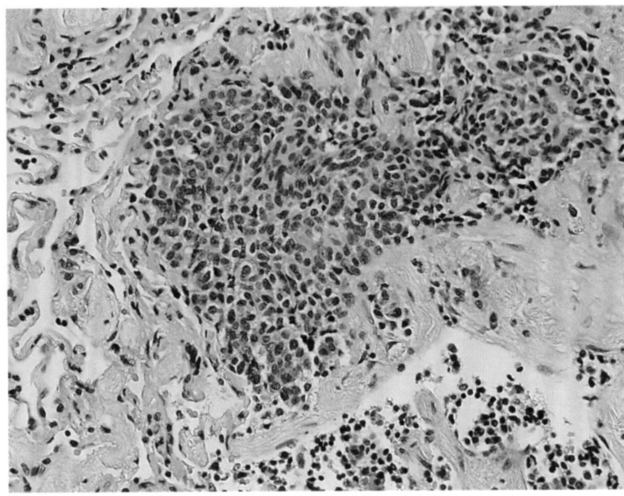

Figure 28.24 Pulmonary neuroendocrine cells arranged in a small group forming a tumorlet.

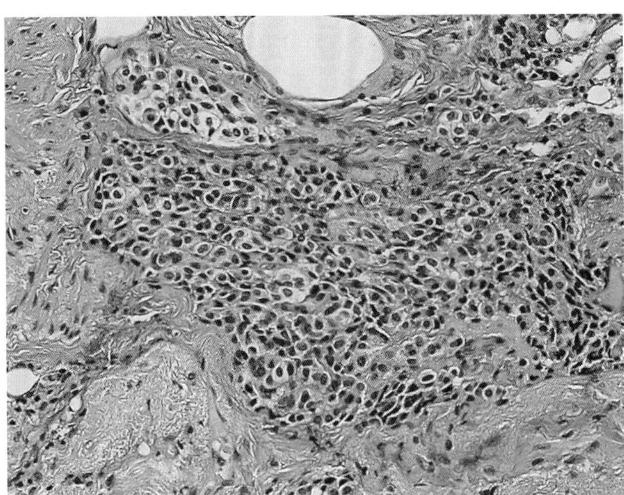

Figure 28.25 Another image of a tumorlet in a patient with DIPNECH.

29 Neoplasms of the Pleura

Part 1

Diffuse Malignant Mesothelioma

Sanja Dacic

Diffuse malignant mesothelioma (DMM) of the pleura is a malignant tumor originating from mesothelial cells. It most frequently occurs in adult males of the age ≥60 years. The most common cause of mesothelioma is asbestos exposure, followed by therapeutic radiation for other neoplasms (e.g., mediastinal lymphoma and breast cancer) and the mineral fiber erionite in Turkey. Some mesotheliomas do not have an identifiable cause. Typical imaging studies in patients with mesothelioma show a diffuse circumferential rind of nodular pleura often associated with ipsilateral lung volume loss and a pleural effusion. Less often, they may present as a pleural effusion without obvious pleural mass. The presence of calcified pleural hyaline plaques is suggestive of asbestos exposure. The 2015 WHO classification of tumors of the lung and pleura recognizes three major histologic subtypes of a DMM, including epithelioid, sarcomatoid, and biphasic. The diagnosis of DMM can be challenging particularly on the limited specimens, such as effusion specimens and small tissue biopsies. The first requirement for the diagnosis is that the process is recognized as mesothelial, which requires recognition of morphology and use of the appropriate immunohistochemistry depending on morphology (e.g., epithelioid mesothelioma vs adenocarcinoma and sarcomatoid mesothelioma vs sarcoma). The presence of tissue invasion into either chest wall or lung parenchyma is considered the most reliable morphologic feature to distinguish benign from malignant mesothelial proliferations. Advances in molecular profiling of DMM resulted in the identification of diagnostic markers of malignant mesothelial proliferations, such as *p16* deletion and BAP1 mutations/protein loss.

CYTOLOGIC FEATURES

- DMM cells in the effusions are always of epithelioid morphology, as sarcomatoid DMMs do not shed cells into the pleural fluid.
- The typical morphologic features of DMMs include "more and bigger cells in more and bigger clusters" with lobulated or flower-like contours, in addition to nuclear atypia and prominent nucleoli, without a foreign or second population.
- Epithelioid DMMs in fluids may form sheets, clusters, morules, or papillae.

- Epithelioid DMMs show a large spectrum of cytologic appearances ranging from bland to pleomorphic cells but frequently without atypia associated with adenocarcinoma.
- Psammoma bodies, glandular formations, and bizarre multinucleated cells may be present.
- Distinction between benign and malignant mesothelial proliferations can be difficult, as reactive mesothelial processes may show increased cellularity, nuclear pleomorphism, and mitoses.

HISTOLOGIC FEATURES

- Epithelioid DMMs show a wide range of histologic patterns, and several patterns are often present within the same tumor.
- Typical epithelioid DMM is composed of polygonal, oval, or cuboidal cells with bland vesicular chromatin and eosinophilic cytoplasm. Mitoses are infrequent. Stroma can be scant to prominent with variable cellularity.
- The most common histologic subtypes include solid, tubulopapillary, and trabecular.
- Less common histologic subtypes include micropapillary, adenomatoid (microcystic), clear cell, transitional, deciduoid, and small cell.
- The solid pattern consists of sheets and/or nests of polygonal to round tumor cells.
- The tubulopapillary subtype shows combinations of tubules and papillary structures lined by relatively bland, flat, cuboidal, or polygonal tumor cells.
- The trabecular subtype consists of uniform, small cells infiltrating the stroma in thin cords, sometimes with a single-file appearance. Psammoma bodies may be present.
- The micropapillary pattern shows papillary structures with tufts lacking central fibrovascular cores.
- The adenomatoid pattern shows microcystic structures, with lace-like or signet ring appearance.
- Pleomorphic DMM is composed of anaplastic or prominent giant and multinucleated cells that are arranged in a pleomorphic pattern.
- Sarcomatoid DMM is composed of spindle cells that are arranged in fascicles or that show a haphazard pattern. Nuclear atypia, mitoses, and necrosis are more common than those in epithelioid DMM.
- Desmoplastic DMM is composed of dense, hyalinized stroma with atypical spindle cells arranged in the so-called patternless pattern. Bland necrosis and cellular stromal nodules are additional helpful criteria that favor malignancy.
- Biphasic mesothelioma has a combination of both epithelioid and sarcomatoid subtypes, with each constituting at least 10% of the tumor.
- The diagnosis of DMM has to be confirmed by immunohistochemical studies. The most common mesothelial markers include calretinin, CK5/6, WT-1, and D2-40. Adenocarcinoma markers are MOC31, Ber-EP4, BG8, B72.3, and monoclonal CEA. Organ-specific markers such as TTF-1 and napsin A (lung) may be included and their choice depends on the differential diagnosis.

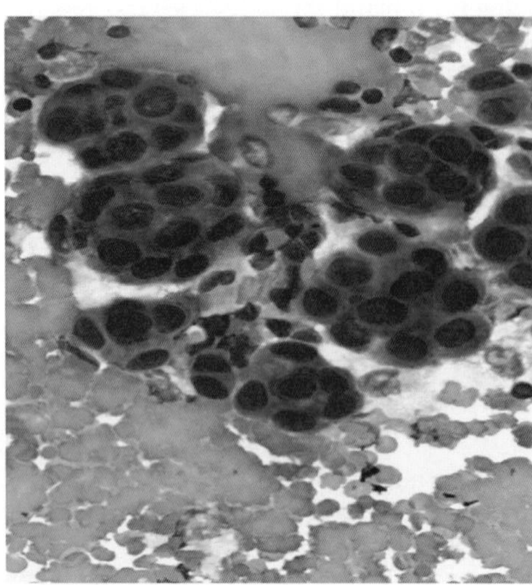

Figure 29.1 Pleural fluid specimen with three-dimensional morules of mesothelial cells.

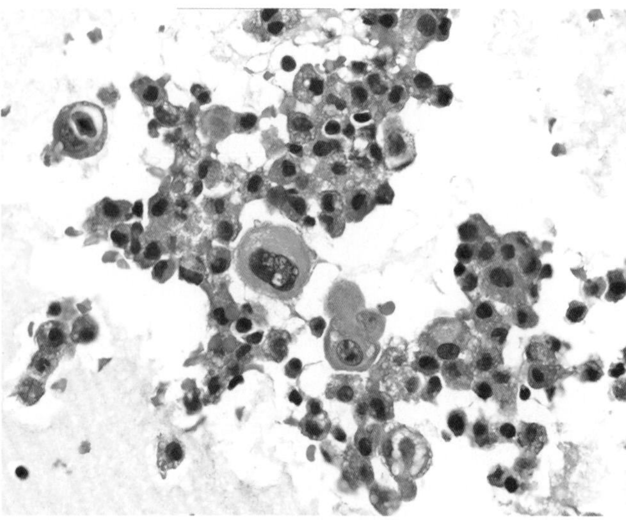

Figure 29.2 Cell block preparation of pleural fluid specimen with clusters of atypical cells, some of which have large bizarre nuclei.

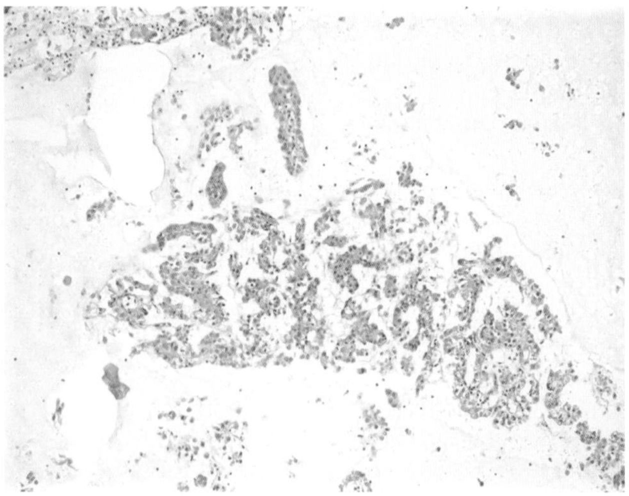

Figure 29.3 Cell block preparation of a hypercellular pleural fluid specimen with complex papillary structures lined by malignant mesothelial cells.

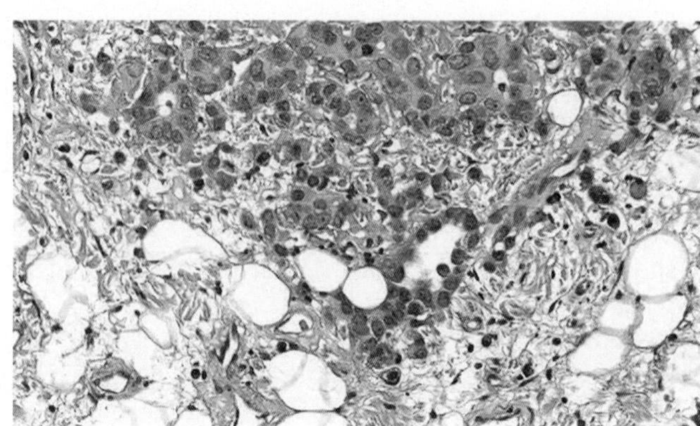

Figure 29.4 Chest wall biopsy showing invasion of mesothelial cells into chest wall adipose tissue, an unequivocal evidence of malignancy.

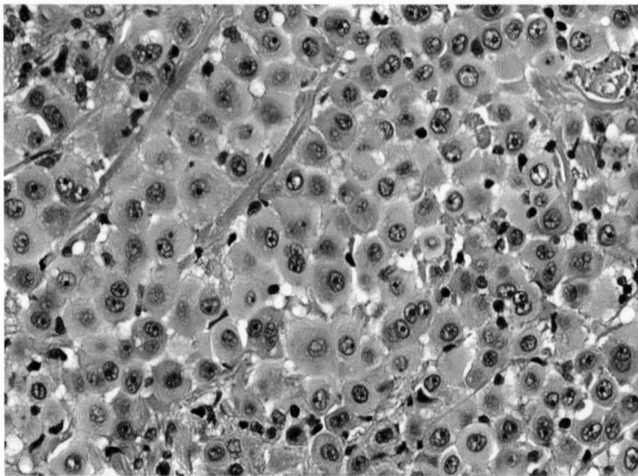

Figure 29.5 Solid pattern of epithelioid DMM consists of solid, monotonous relatively noncohesive sheets of polygonal cells.

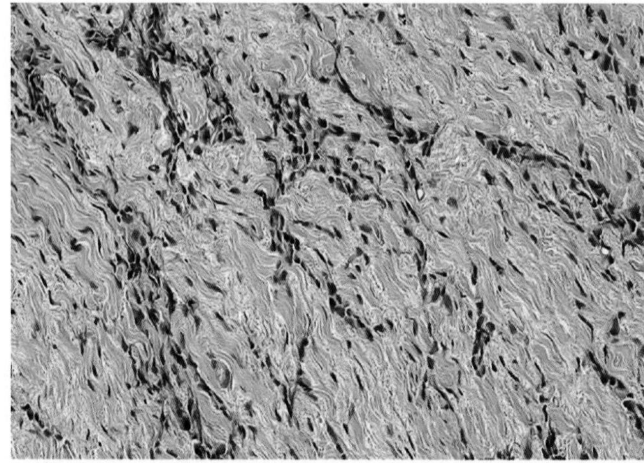

Figure 29.6 Trabecular pattern of epithelioid DMM consists of relatively small, uniform cells arranged in thin cords.

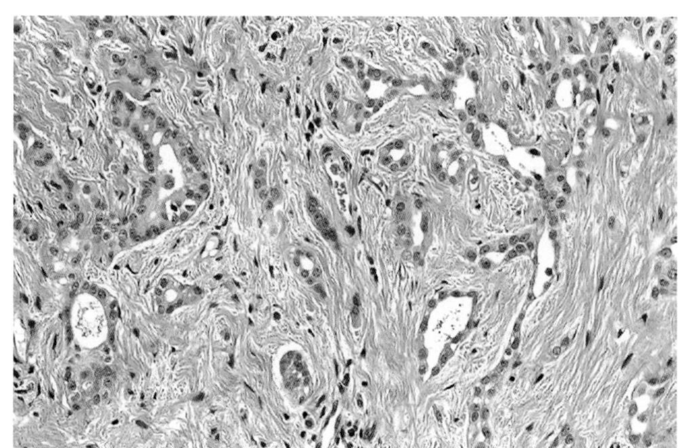

Figure 29.7 Tubular pattern of epithelioid DMM consists of tubules lined by relatively bland-appearing mesothelial cells.

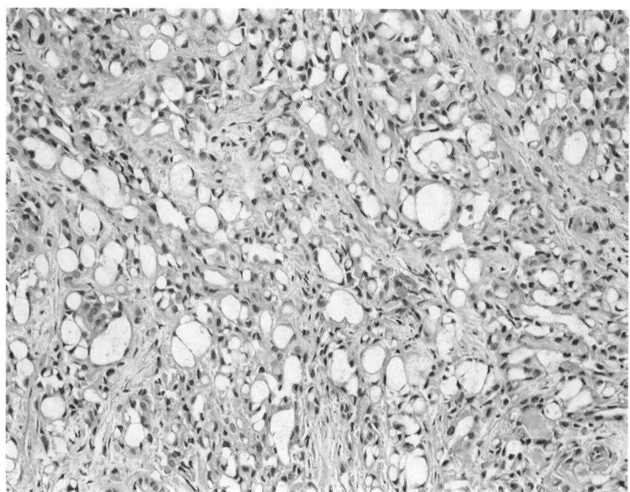

Figure 29.8 Microcystic (adenomatoid) pattern shows microcystic structures with signet ring appearance.

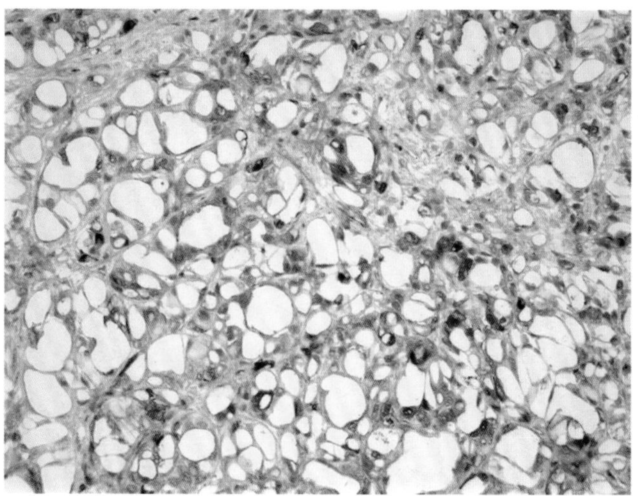

Figure 29.9 Calretinin stain confirms mesothelial origin of cells forming microcystic (adenomatoid) pattern.

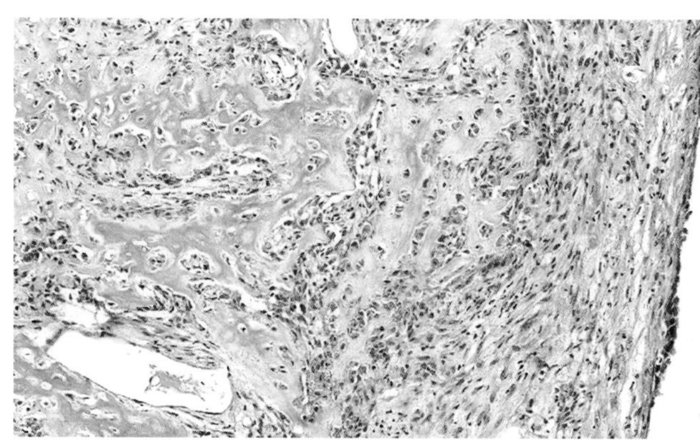

Figure 29.10 DMM with heterologous elements (osteoid).

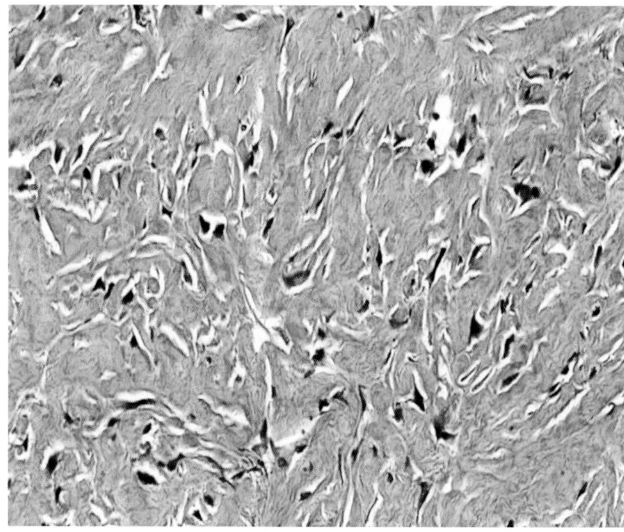

Figure 29.11 Desmoplastic DMM showing paucicellular atypical spindle-cell proliferation within hyalinized stroma.

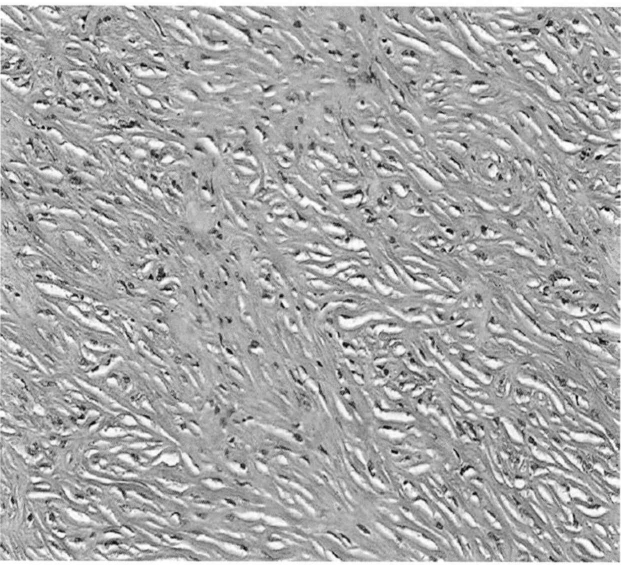

Figure 29.12 Hypercellular proliferation of spindle cells within hyalinized stroma of desmoplastic DMM.

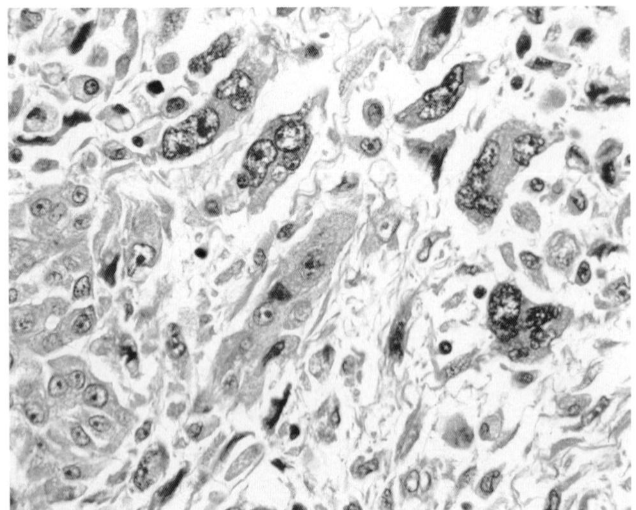

Figure 29.13 Pleomorphic DMM with giant and multinucleated cells.

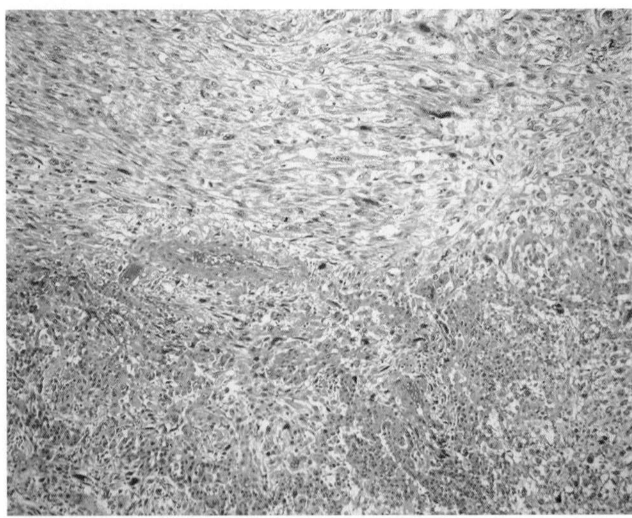

Figure 29.14 Biphasic DMM composed of an epithelioid component (mostly solid pattern) and a sarcomatoid component.

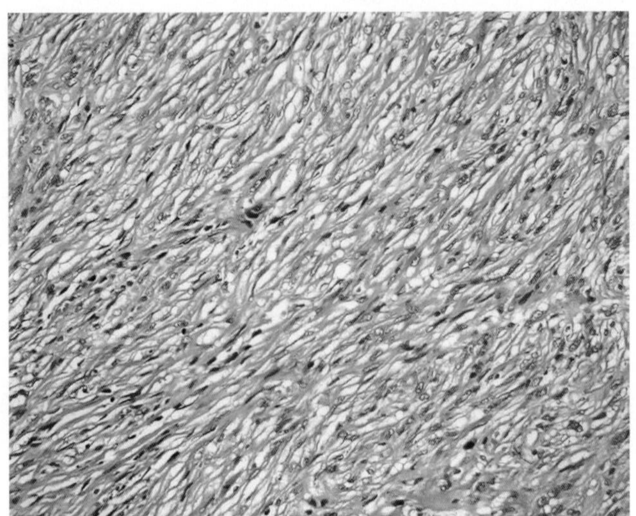

Figure 29.15 Sarcomatoid DMM showing high spindle cellularity and mitoses.

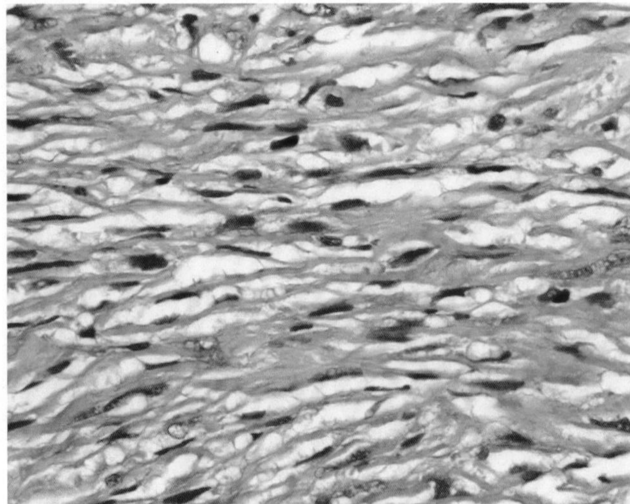

Figure 29.16 High-power magnification of sarcomatoid DMM composed of plump spindle cells with elongated atypical nuclei.

Part 2

Localized Malignant Mesothelioma

▶ Sanja Dacic

Localized malignant mesothelioma (LMM) is a rare tumor that grossly appears as a distinct localized nodular pleural-based mass that is either sessile or pedunculated and has morphologic, immunohistochemical, and ultrastructural features of DMM. It is often an incidental finding. Localized mesotheliomas have a better prognosis than DMM and may be cured by surgical resection.

HISTOLOGIC FEATURES

- Nodular, discrete, well-circumscribed, pedunculated, or sessile mass arising from visceral or parietal pleura.
- Morphologically, immunohistochemically, and ultrastructurally identical to DMM.
- The tumors may show epithelioid, sarcomatoid, and biphasic morphologies.
- The differential diagnosis depends on morphology and may include carcinoma, solitary fibrous tumor (SFT), and synovial and other sarcomas.

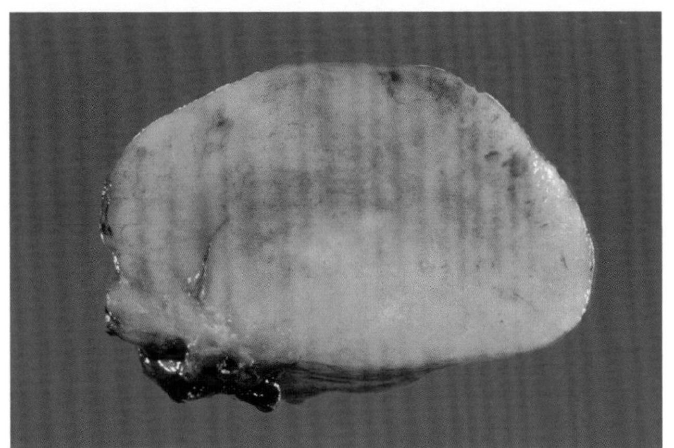

Figure 29.17 Gross appearance of LMM showing a solitary, well-circumscribed pleural-based mass.

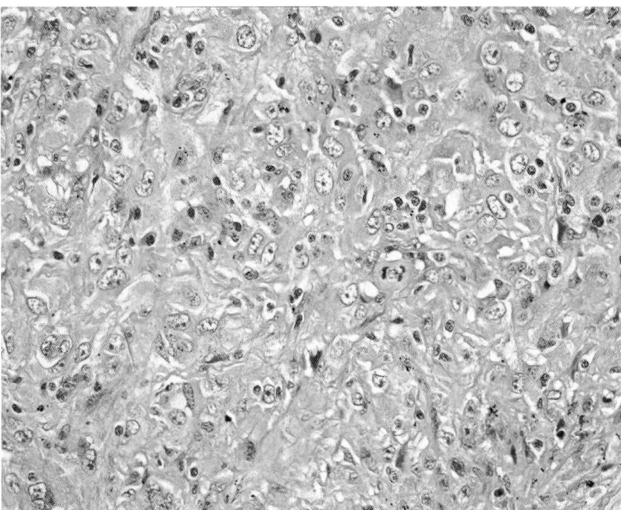

Figure 29.18 Epithelioid LMM morphologically indistinguishable from DMM. Clinical correlation with imaging studies is essential.

Part 3

Well-Differentiated Papillary Mesothelioma

Sanja Dacic

Well-differentiated papillary mesothelioma (WDPM) of the pleura is a rare tumor of mesothelial origin characterized by papillary architecture and bland cytology. It has a tendency toward superficial spread without invasion. WDPM is clinically, morphologically, and prognostically different from the papillary subtype of DMM. It occurs more frequently in the peritoneum than in the pleura. WDPMs of the pleura are considered clinically benign if completely surgically resected and are associated with a long survival. Rare cases of WDPM with invasive foci show superficial invasion and should be followed up more closely, as they may show less favorable outcome. It remains uncertain if WDPM may progress to DMM.

HISTOLOGIC FEATURES

- WDPM is characterized by a prominent papillary architecture composed of papillae with myxoid cores covered by a single layer of flat to cuboidal mesothelial cells without atypia or mitoses.
- Macrophages may be present in the cores of the papillae.

- Rare cases with superficial invasion should be called WDPM with foci of invasion.
- The immunohistochemical profile of WDPM is mesothelial.
- The most important differential diagnosis is a papillary subtype of epithelioid DMM. Helpful features favoring DMM include grossly apparent diffuse or multinodular disease and microscopic evidence of other growth patterns, such as solid or tubular and complex papillae lined by stratified cells.

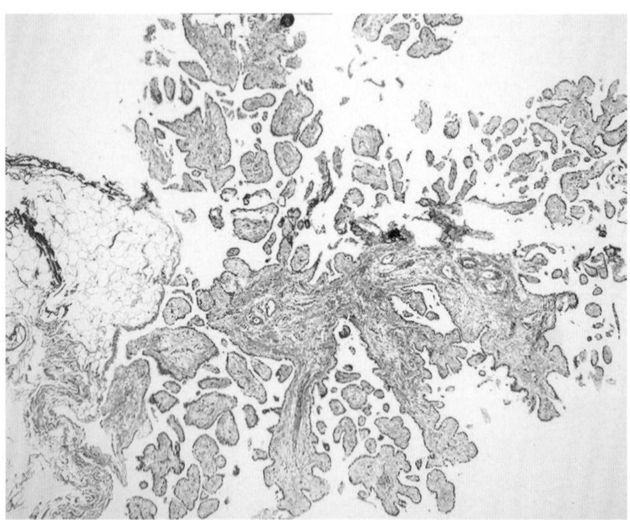

Figure 29.19 Pleural WDPM showing exophytic growth.

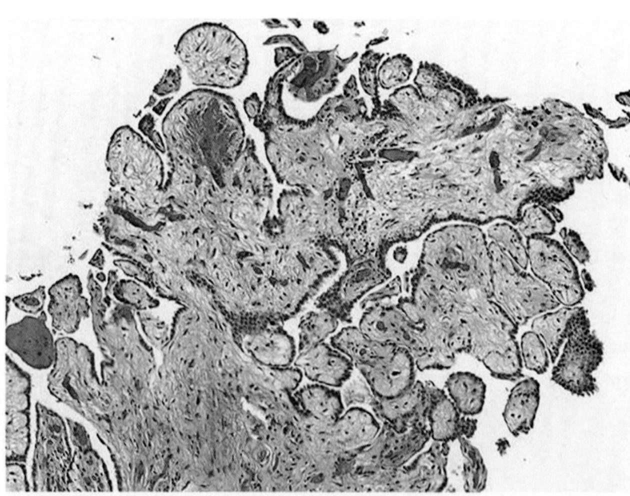

Figure 29.20 Pleural WDPM composed of multiple papillae with myxoid cores covered by a single layer of cuboidal mesothelial cells.

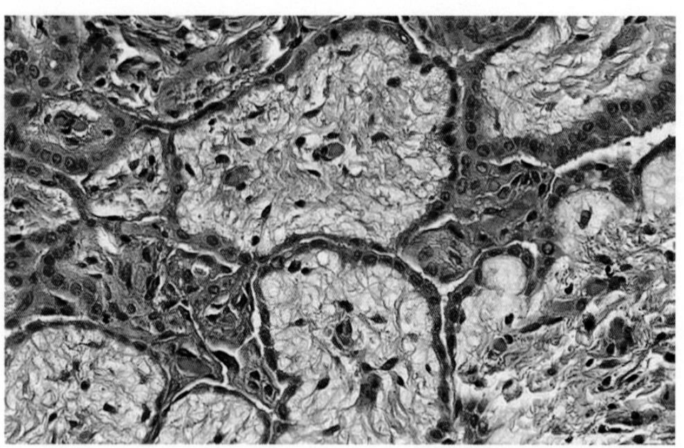

Figure 29.21 Higher power magnification showing a single layer of bland, cuboidal epithelioid cells with round to oval nuclei without atypia or mitoses.

Part 4

Synovial Sarcoma

▶ Sanja Dacic

Pleural synovial sarcoma is rare and often involves the lung. Most patients are adults with a median age of 40 years and presenting with chest pain. Before the case is considered to represent a primary neoplasm of the pleura, the possibility of metastasis should be excluded. Pleural synovial sarcomas are often localized large solid tumors but can also present with diffuse pleural thickening mimicking DMM grossly. Morphologic, immunoprofile, and ultrastructural features of pleural synovial sarcomas are the same as those described in synovial sarcomas in other locations. Most primary pleural synovial sarcomas are monophasic. Synovial sarcomas are typically immunopositive for at least one epithelial marker (EMA or cytokeratin) and often coexpress vimentin, CD99, and Bcl2. Calretinin and S100 may be focally positive. Smooth muscle actin, desmin, and CD34 are negative. The most important differential diagnosis is malignant mesothelioma, sarcomatoid carcinoma, and SFT. These entities can be easily distinguished by the combination of clinical presentation, morphology, immunohistochemistry, and cytogenetic findings. The diagnostic translocation t(X:18)(p11;q11) occurs in synovial sarcomas only. TLE1 immunostain can be used as a surrogate for cytogenetic studies. Pleural synovial sarcomas are aggressive and the median survival is about 2 years. In contrast to its counterparts in somatic soft tissues, no well-defined prognostic factors have been defined for pleural synovial sarcomas.

CYTOLOGIC FEATURES

- Monophasic synovial sarcomas show spindle cells with irregular nuclei and sparse cytoplasm.
- Biphasic synovial sarcomas contain an epithelial component, which is reminiscent of mesothelial cells, but they tend to be plumper.

HISTOLOGIC FEATURES

- Both monophasic and biphasic synovial sarcomas contain sheets or fascicles of uniform, elongated spindle cells with scant cytoplasm and indistinct cell borders.
- The epithelial component of biphasic synovial sarcoma contains glands or slit-like structures with single or multiple layers of cuboidal cells with round nuclei, occasional nucleoli, and a moderate amount of eosinophilic cytoplasm.
- Other features include hemangiopericytoma-like blood vessels, hyalinized or eosinophilic stroma, and necrosis.
- Calcifications and mast cells are less common than in soft tissue synovial sarcomas.

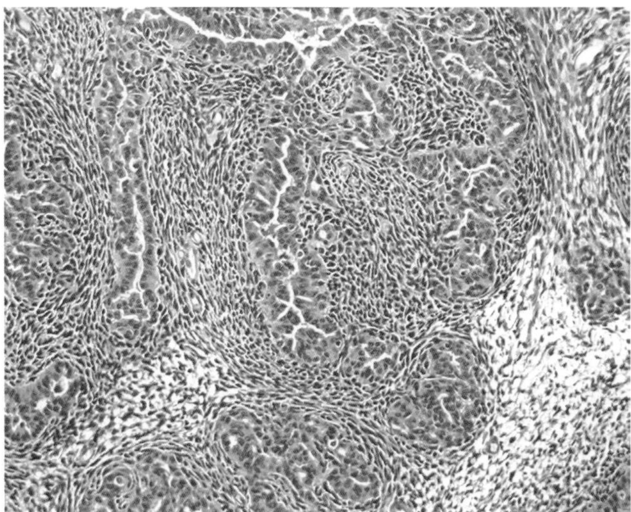

Figure 29.22 Biphasic synovial sarcoma with glandular structures surrounded by spindle and myxoid stroma.

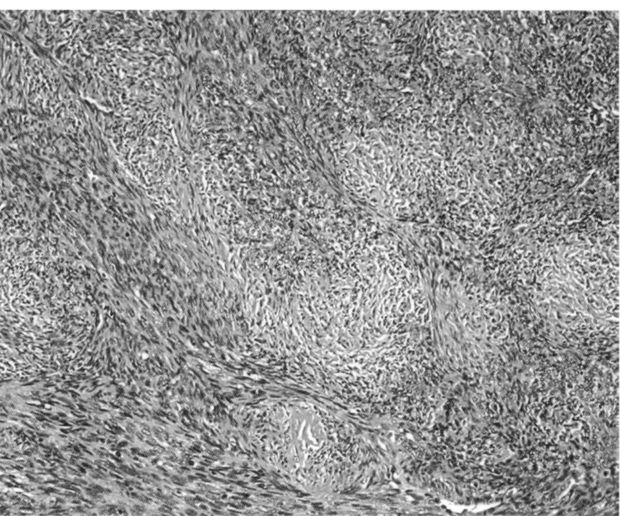

Figure 29.23 Monophasic synovial sarcoma with spindle cells.

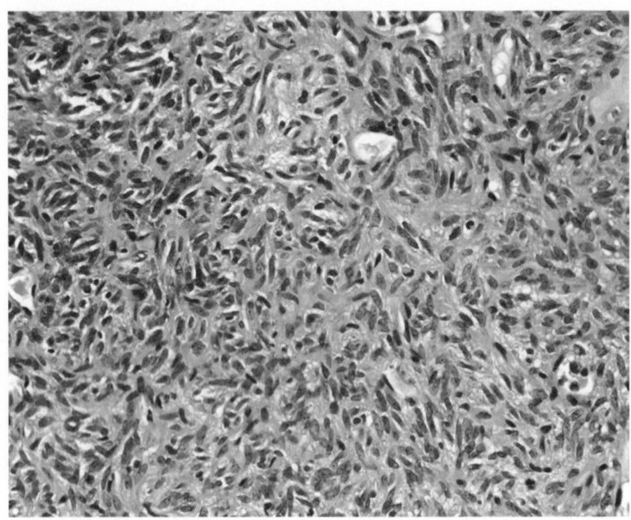

Figure 29.24 Higher power magnification of uniform, elongated spindle cells with scant cytoplasm and indistinct borders.

Part 5

Vascular Sarcomas

Sanja Dacic

Primary pleural vascular sarcomas are rare tumors that generally occur in adult men and with invariable aggressive behavior and poor outcome. The most common vascular tumors arising in pleura include epithelioid hemangioendothelioma and angiosarcoma. An association between primary pleural angiosarcoma and chronic tuberculous pyothorax or asbestos exposure in Japanese patients has been reported. No such association has been confirmed in patients from Western countries. Grossly, primary pleural vascular sarcomas often show diffuse involvement of the pleura and may mimic DMM. Most of the epithelioid hemangioendotheliomas have a specific diagnostic translocation (1;3)(p36;q2325), which results most frequently in *WWTR1-CAMTA1* gene fusion. Less often, *YAP1-TFE3* fusion occurs resulting in overexpression of TFE3 protein.

HISTOLOGIC FEATURES

Epithelioid Hemangioendothelioma

- Cords, strands, and nests of epithelioid endothelial cells with glassy eosinophilic cytoplasm within a myxohyaline stroma.
- Cytoplasmic vacuoles (lumina), some of which may contain red blood cells, are common.
- Mitoses are infrequent.
- CD31, ERG, and CD34 are positive; about a third of the cases are positive for keratin.
- TFE3 is positive in cases with *YAP1-TFE3* fusion.

Epithelioid Angiosarcoma

- Sheets of large cells with copious cytoplasm and irregular vesicular nuclei and prominent nucleoli.
- Intracytoplasmic vacuoles (lumina) may be focally present.

- May be morphologically indistinguishable from carcinomas and mesotheliomas, and detection of endothelial antigens is essential.
- Express endothelial antigens CD31, ERG, or CD34 and are often keratin-positive, at least focally.

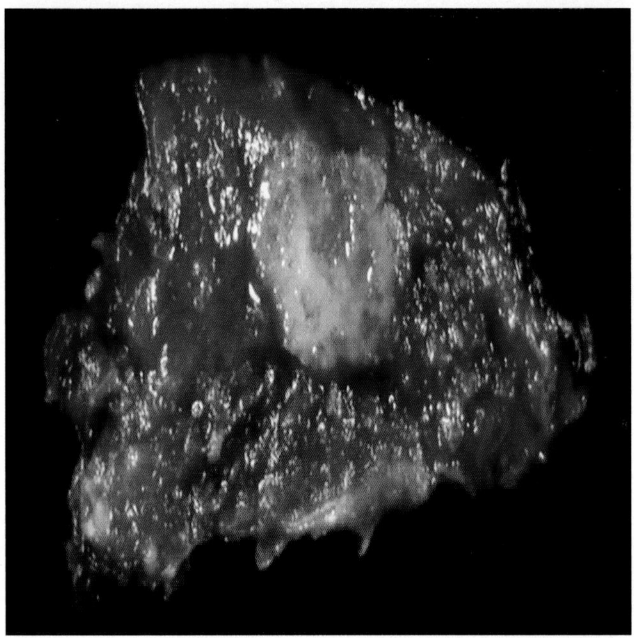

Figure 29.25 Epithelioid hemangioendothelioma showing pleural thickening and nodule.

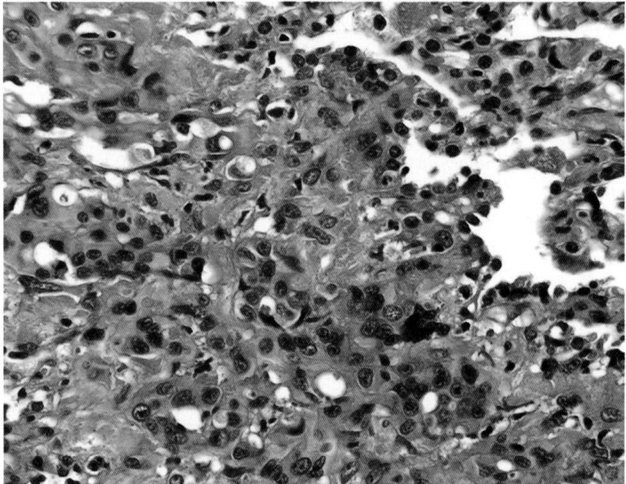

Figure 29.26 Epithelioid hemangioendothelioma with sheets of epithelioid endothelial cells with nuclear atypia and hyperchromasia, some with cytoplasmic vacuoles containing red blood cells.

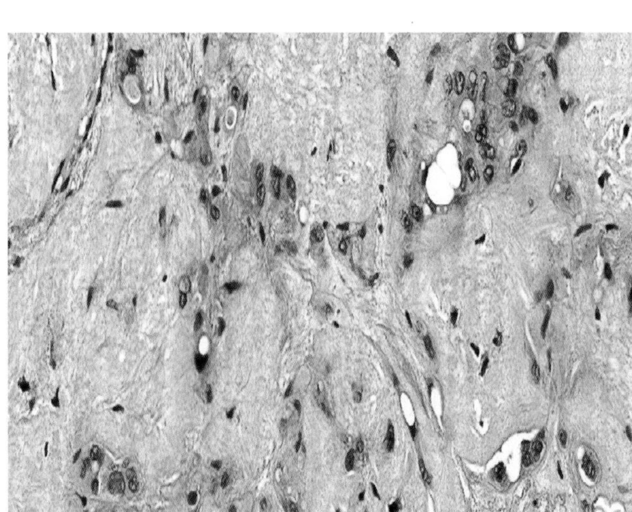

Figure 29.27 Epithelioid hemangioendothelioma with clusters of epithelioid cells, some with cytoplasmic vacuoles, infiltrating hyalinized stroma.

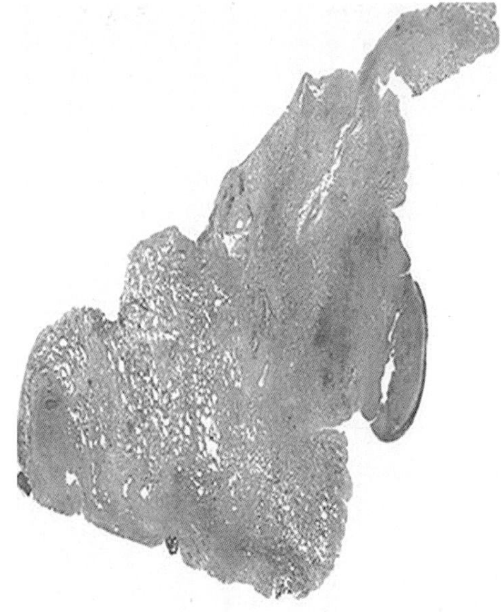

Figure 29.28 Low-power magnification of pleural epithelioid angiosarcoma showing a well-circumscribed pleural-based hemorrhagic mass.

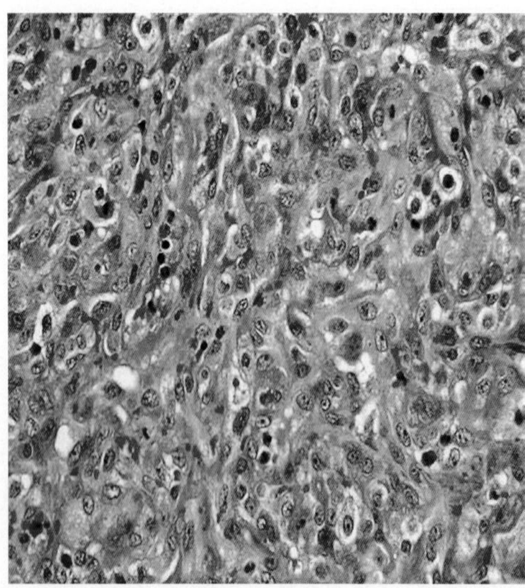

Figure 29.29 Epithelioid angiosarcoma composed of sheets of large cells with large vesicular nuclei and prominent nucleoli. Focal intracytoplasmic vacuoles (lumina) are present.

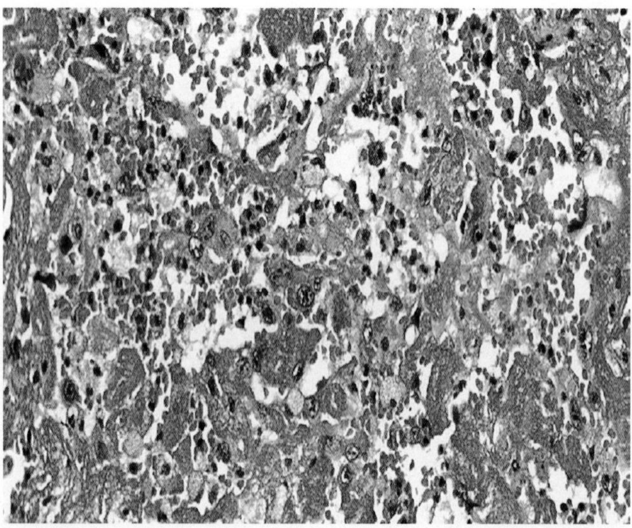

Figure 29.30 Epithelioid angiosarcoma with more prominent hemorrhage and scattered highly atypical epithelioid cells.

Part 6

Malignant SFT

Sanja Dacic

SFTs of the pleura are most often benign but up to 10% are malignant. Clinically, malignant SFTs present with chest pain, shortness of breath, and pleural effusion. Malignant SFTs are often large (>10 cm) solitary nodules, but may be multiple, attached to the parietal pleura or mediastinum. Histologically, malignant SFTs, in addition to typical morphology of benign SFTs, also show hypercellular areas, cytologic pleomorphism, necrosis, and more than four mitoses per 2 mm^2. Rare cases may show dedifferentiation. They often recur locally, may metastasize, and may result in the patient's death. Malignant SFTs are positive for bcl-2 and CD99 and may be negative for CD34. Much more specific STAT6 is positive. Overexpression of STAT6 is a result of gene fusion *NAB2-STAT6,* which results from the intrachromosomal inversion inv(12)(q13q13). This translocation is diagnostic of SFT. Some cases may also express smooth muscle actin, EMA, keratin, S100, or desmin. The differential diagnosis includes synovial sarcoma, sarcomatoid mesothelioma, and nerve sheath tumors. Immunohistochemistry and gene rearrangements are helpful in the distinction.

CYTOLOGIC FEATURES

- Cytologic features on fine needle aspiration of SFT with additional features of malignancy, such as necrosis, mitotic figures, and nuclear pleomorphism.

HISTOLOGIC FEATURES

- Cellular lesions composed of spindle cells with mitoses and often necrosis.
- Frequently, areas typical of benign SFT are present.

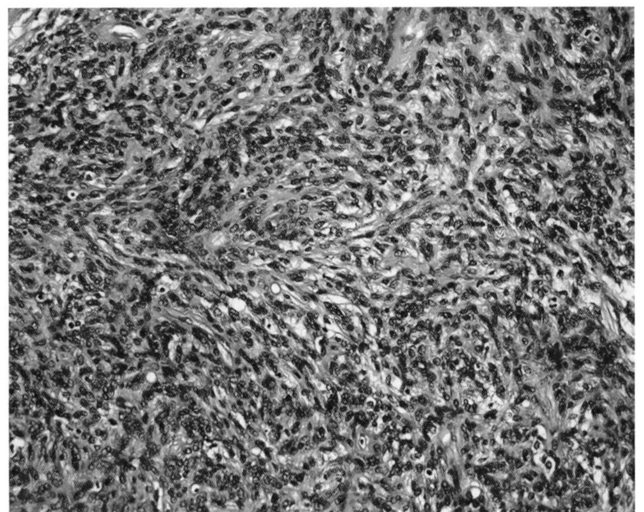

Figure 29.31 Malignant SFT with increased cellularity and mitoses.

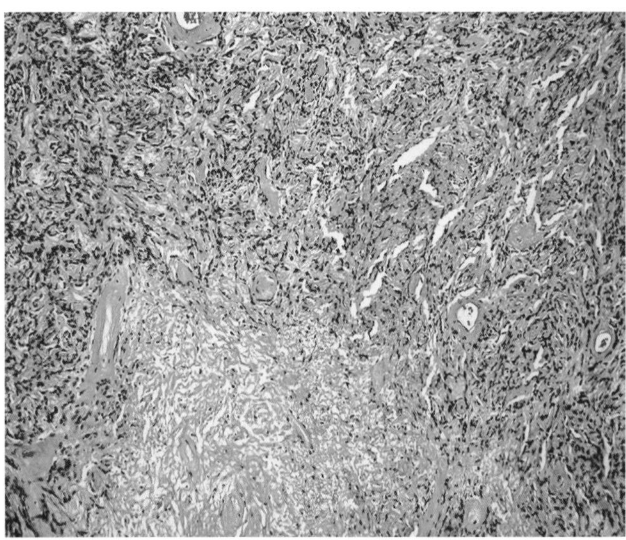

Figure 29.32 Malignant SFT with atypical spindle-cell proliferation and necrosis.

Part 7

Pseudomesotheliomatous Carcinoma

Sanja Dacic

The term *pseudomesotheliomatous carcinoma* is used to describe carcinomas that grow over the pleural surface and encase the lung in a manner mimicking DMM. They often mimick DMM clinically, radiographically, and morphologically. These tumors most frequently present as pleural effusion. The term may be used for any carcinoma that metastasizes to the pleura and grows in this fashion, but primarily it has been used to describe peripheral lung adenocarcinomas exhibiting growth along the pleural surface. The presumed primary site of these peripheral adenocarcinomas within the subpleural lung parenchyma may be difficult to identify. The prognosis for these carcinomas is poor, with high similarity to that of DMM.

HISTOLOGIC FEATURES

- Pleural infiltration by nests of cells that focally form glands or tubulopapillary structures.
- Psammoma bodies can be found, particularly in the papillary component.
- Isolated glands within a desmoplastic stroma are a common finding.
- Immunoprofile is that of a carcinoma including expression of polyclonal CEA and low-molecular-weight cytokeratins in most cases; immunopositivity for Ber-EP4, Leu-M1, and B72.3 can be seen in some cases.

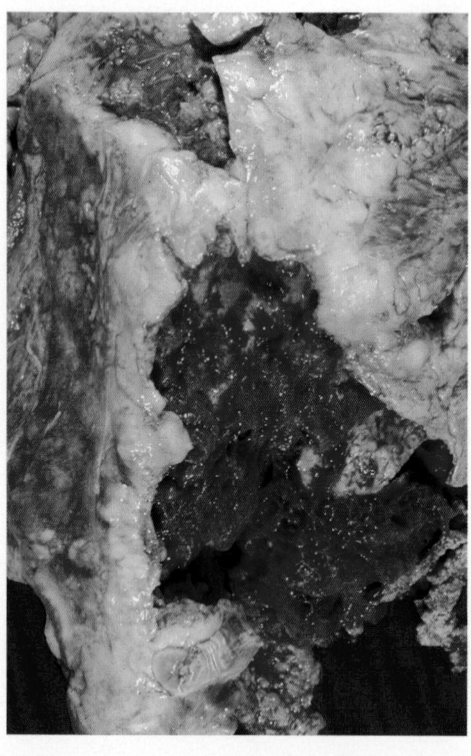

Figure 29.33 Gross appearance of pseudomesotheliomatous adenocarcinoma growing along pleural surface and without obvious subpleural lung mass.

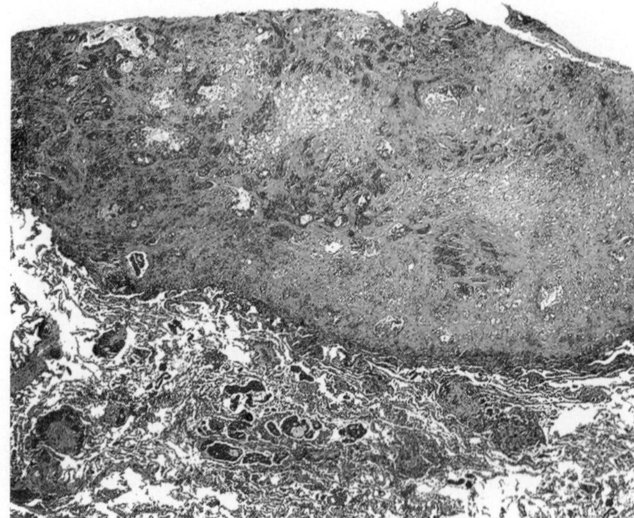

Figure 29.34 Low-power magnification of adenocarcinoma growing along pleural surface.

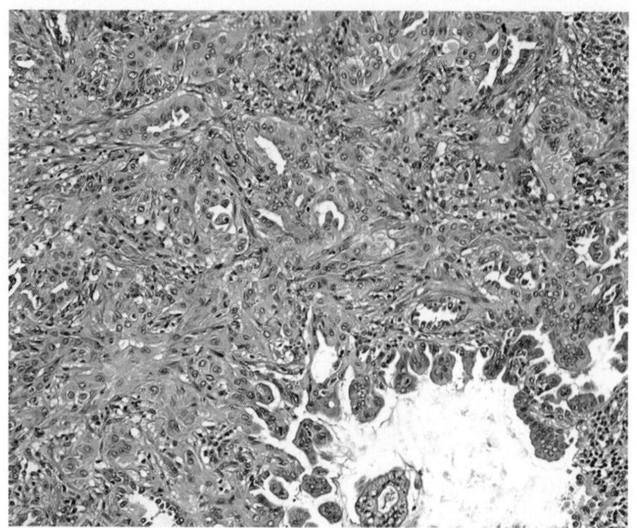

Figure 29.35 High-power magnification of the same adenocarcinoma exhibiting acinar growth pattern.

Part 8

Calcifying Fibrous Tumor

Sanja Dacic

Calcifying fibrous tumor is a rare, benign tumor occurring in visceral pleura. Most patients are women with a median age of 39 years. Multiple disseminated tumors are mostly reported in Asian patients. Patients may be asymptomatic or may present with chest pain. Imaging studies show either a single or multiple pleural-based nodular masses. Calcifying fibrous tumor is typically limited to the pleura and does not involve the underlying lung parenchyma. Grossly, the tumor is well circumscribed, unencapsulated, and solid, with gritty texture. Microscopically, the tumor is hypocellular, diffusely hyalinized with cytologically bland fibroblasts. Dystrophic or psammomatous calcification may be numerous. A lesion may be positive for CD34 but negative for beta-catenin and ALK1. SFT may be in the differential diagnosis, but it is more cellular. Local recurrence may occur in 10% to 15% of the cases, but there is no metastasis.

HISTOLOGIC FEATURES

- Single or multiple pleural-based nodular masses limited to visceral pleura and without extension into underlying lung parenchyma.
- Hyalinized and hypocellular stroma with scattered cytologically bland fibroblasts, scattered lymphoplasmacytic inflammation, and frequently numerous psammomatous calcifications.

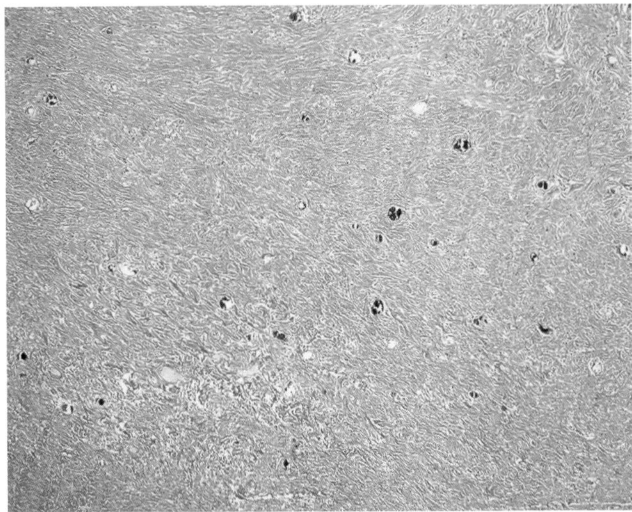

Figure 29.36 Low-power magnification of calcifying fibrous tumor showing a prominent collagenous stroma

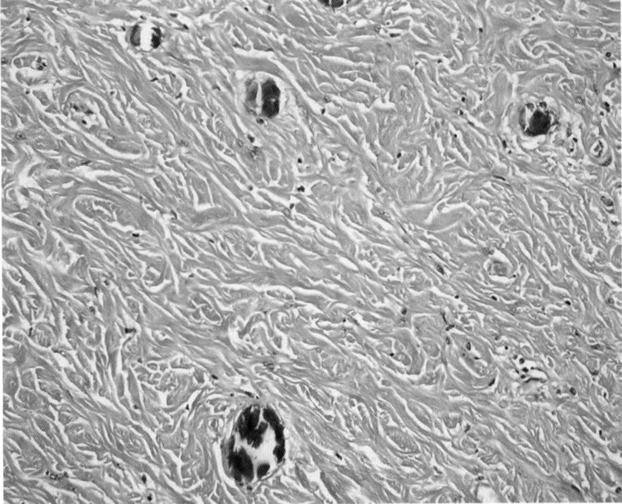

Figure 29.37 Cytologically bland fibroblasts and psammomatous calcifications.

Part 9

Desmoplastic Small Round Cell Tumor

Sanja Dacic

Desmoplastic small round cell tumor (DSRCT) of the pleura is exceedingly rare malignant mesenchymal neoplasm with round cell morphology, complex immunophenotype, and consistent *EWSR1-WT1* gene fusion. It usually presents with chest pain and pleural effusion in teenagers and young adult males. DSRCT forms multiple pleural-based nodules encasing the lung and usually spreads into the mediastinum. Bilateral pleural involvement and metastases into lung parenchyma may occur. The tumor is composed of small, round, uniform tumor cells organized in nests in a desmoplastic stroma. The tumor cells have hyperchromatic nuclei, scant cytoplasm, and indistinct cell borders; intracytoplasmic eosinophilic rhabdoid inclusions may be present. Mitoses and cell necrosis are common. Most DSRCTs are immunopositive cytokeratins, EMA, desmin (with a perinuclear dot-like pattern), WT-1, and NSE. Myogenin and MyoD are negative. All cases are characterized by diagnostic *EWSR-WT1* gene fusion.

HISTOLOGIC FEATURES

- The tumor is composed of irregularly shaped islands of tumor cells in a desmoplastic stroma.
- The small round cells with scant cytoplasm are admixed with occasional cells with rhabdoid inclusions.
- DSRCT usually shows immunohistochemical evidence of epithelial (cytokeratin-positive) and muscle (desmin-positive) differentiation.

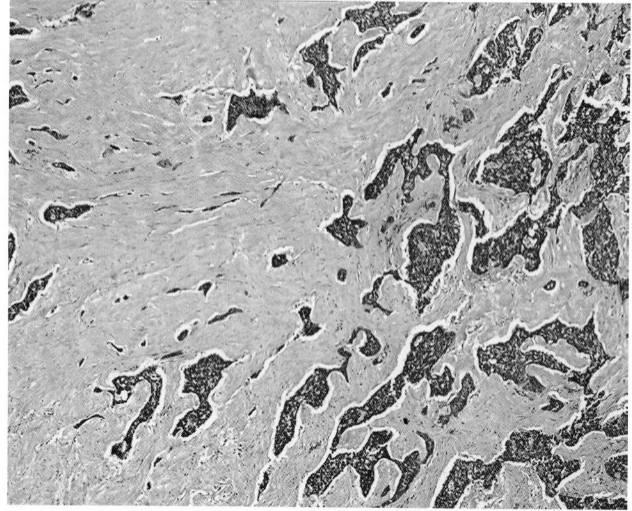

Figure 29.38 Nests of tumor cells in the desmoplastic stroma.

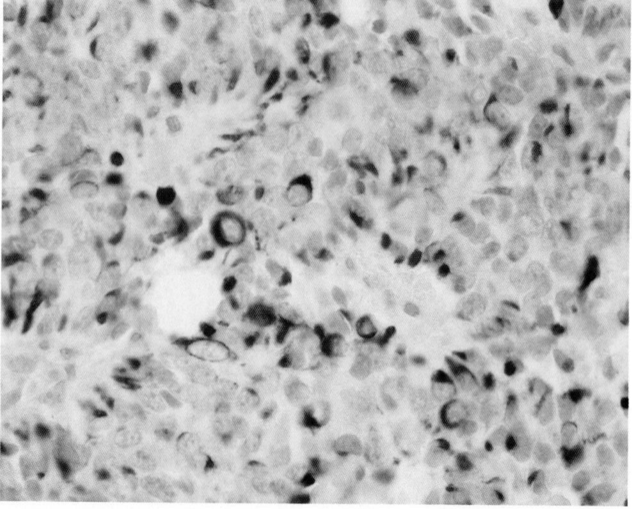

Figure 29.39 A typical dot-like expression of desmin.

Section 4

Benign Neoplasms

▸ Natasha Rekhtman

30

Pulmonary Hamartoma

Charles Leduc
Darren Buonocore
Natasha Rekhtman

Pulmonary hamartomas are benign tumors that are composed of at least two mesenchymal elements commonly associated with entrapped benign pulmonary epithelium. Molecular studies have confirmed recurrent cytogenetic aberrations involving *HMGA2* in the majority of cases, clearly suggesting a neoplastic rather than a truly hamartomatous etiology. They tend to occur in the periphery of the lung and are generally less than 4 to 5 cm. The classic radiologic description includes a well-circumscribed nodule (coin lesion) with compression of adjacent lung parenchyma. A Fat component and/or popcorn-like calcification(s) are present in a subset of cases and, if detected, are virtually pathognomonic. The tumor consists of lobules of mesenchymal tissue, which, as they expand, entrap benign parenchymal epithelium in cleft-like spaces. Mesenchymal elements most commonly encountered are hyaline cartilage, adipose tissue, fibroblastic connective tissue (often with a myxoid/chondromyxoid matrix), and occasionally smooth muscle. Cytologic atypia, mitotic activity, and necrosis are consistently absent. The pathologic diagnosis is based on histologic features, and immunohistochemistry is generally noncontributory. The differential diagnosis includes pulmonary chondroma and primary or metastatic low-grade chondrosarcoma or liposarcoma. With the exception of dedifferentiated liposarcoma, which can be recognized by clear cut cytologic atypia, these lesions are monophasic, whereas pulmonary hamartoma has, by definition, at least two distinct mesenchymal elements. Correlation with radiologic features can be helpful on small biopsy specimens.

CYTOLOGIC FEATURES

- Fine needle aspiration shows variable proportions of chondromyxoid matrix, mature cartilage, benign glandular epithelium, and adipocytes.

HISTOLOGIC FEATURES

- Well-circumscribed or lobulated borders with entrapped benign epithelial cells in the form of cleft-like spaces lined by benign pulmonary epithelium (can be ciliated or nonciliated).
- Presence of at least two mesenchymal components.

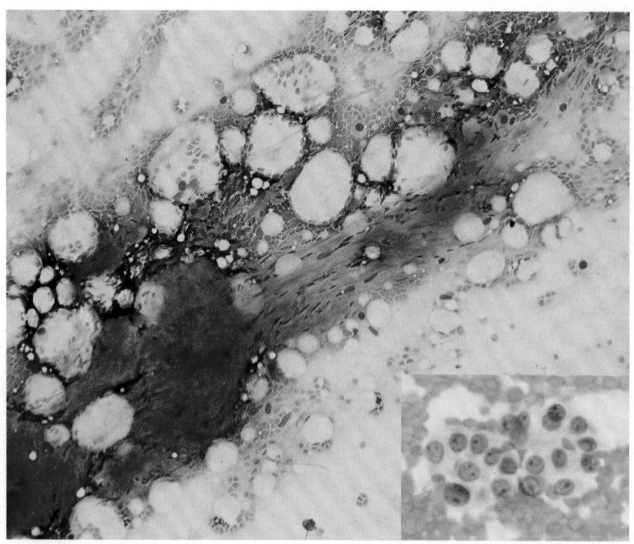

Figure 30.1 Diff-Quik smears show a metachromatic fibrillary matrix admixed with adipocytes. Other areas demonstrate bland glandular epithelium (*inset*, Papanicolaou-stained).

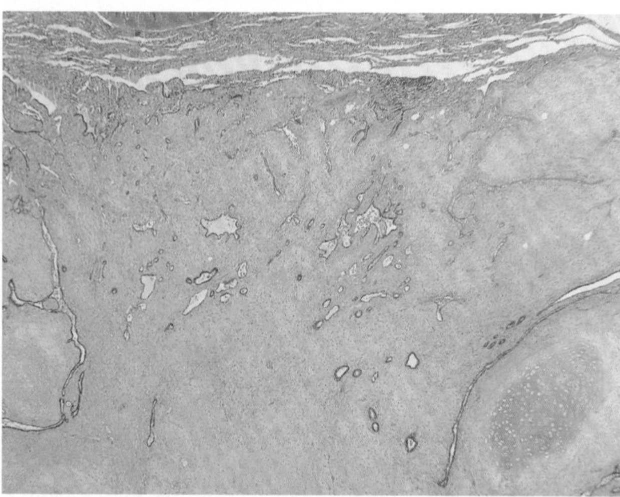

Figure 30.2 Well-delineated and slightly lobulated pushing tumor border with compression of adjacent lung parenchyma and multiple entrapped epithelial-lined spaces.

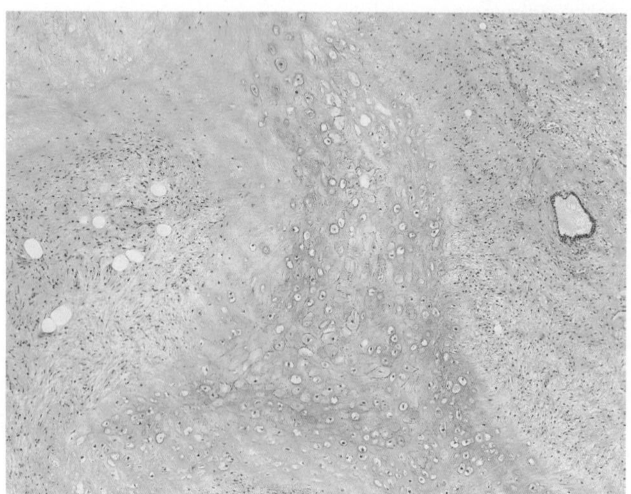

Figure 30.3 Lesional elements most commonly encountered in pulmonary hamartoma including mature adipocytes *(left)*, hyaline cartilage *(center)*, entrapped pulmonary epithelium *(right)*, and myxoid/chondromyxoid connective tissue with scattered bland fibroblasts.

31 Pulmonary Chondroma

Charles Leduc
Melanie C. Bois
Natasha Rekhtman

Pulmonary chondromas are rare benign tumors of mature and immature cartilaginous tissue. They can occur sporadically or in the context of Carney triad, in which case they tend to be multiple and peripherally located, generally in young women. They are well-circumscribed intraparenchymal lesions, composed of lobules of immature-appearing cartilaginous tissue, separated from adjacent lung by a thin fibrous pseudocapsule. Myxoid degeneration, infarct-type necrosis, and calcification (often in the form of osseous metaplasia) are frequently encountered. The pathologic diagnosis is based on histologic features, and immunohistochemistry is generally noncontributory. The differential diagnosis includes primarily pulmonary hamartoma and primary or metastatic chondrosarcoma. The former has entrapped epithelial-lined spaces, lacks a fibrous pseudocapsule, and by definition has more than one mesenchymal component. The latter can be distinguished by higher cellularity and the presence of cytologic atypia.

HISTOLOGIC FEATURES

- Lobules of mature-appearing cartilage separated from adjacent parenchyma by a thin fibrous pseudocapsule.
- Myxoid degeneration and ossification are frequently encountered.
- Absence of epithelial-lined clefts or nonchondromatous differentiated mesenchymal elements.

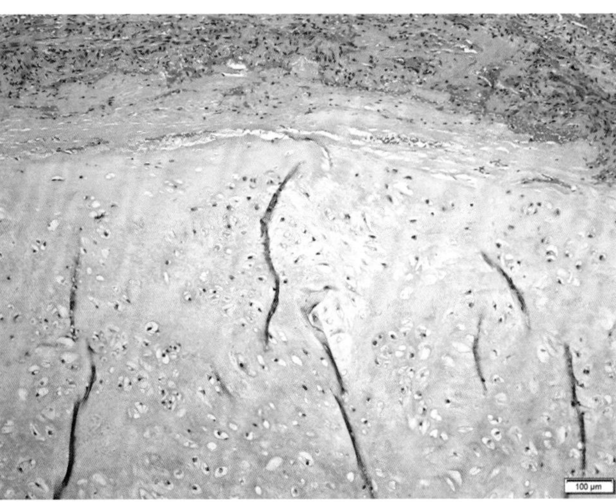

Figure 31.1 Homogeneous proliferation of purely chondroid tissue with well-circumscribed border defined by a thin fibrous pseudocapsule.

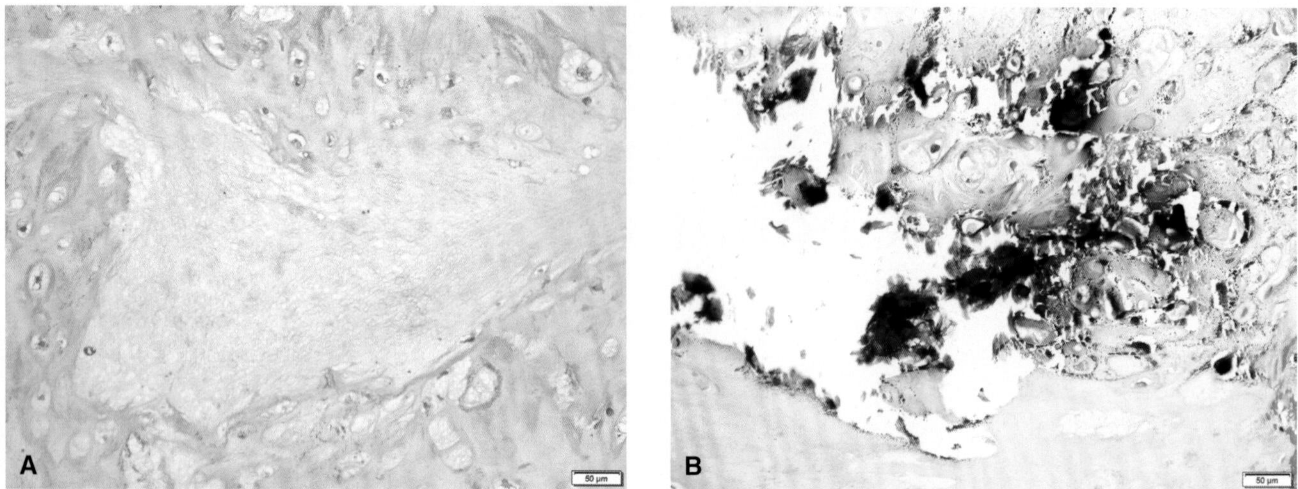

Figure 31.2 Foci of acellular myxoid degeneration (**A**) and calcification (**B**) are common.

32 Solitary Fibrous Tumor

▸ Charles Leduc
▸ Darren Buonocore
▸ Natasha Rekhtman

Solitary fibrous tumor (SFT) is a spindle-cell neoplasm, which generally originates in the pleura (rarely intraparenchymal). On low-power magnification, it appears as a rounded circumscribed tumor with patchy areas of hypocellular dense collagenized stroma, numerous thin-walled vessels that are often dilated and branched (so-called hemangiopericytoma-like), and often several areas of entrapped pulmonary epithelium in cleft-like spaces. The lesional cells are haphazardly arranged, with bland plump oval to spindle-shaped nuclei with inconspicuous nucleoli, open chromatin, and scant to inapparent clear cytoplasm. As the name implies, the tumor matrix consists of abundant dense ropy hyalinized collagen, which is interwoven between tumor cells. The tumors are characterized by the *NAB2-STAT6* gene fusion, which manifests with diffuse nuclear immunoreactivity to antibodies directed against the STAT6 protein. The tumor cells also tend to be positive for CD34 and BCL2, although these are nonspecific. Although the vast majority of SFTs are benign, malignant variants are well recognized and should be considered if the tumor harbors any of the following features: frank cytologic atypia, tumor necrosis, or greater than 4 mitoses per 10 high-power fields. The differential diagnosis includes synovial sarcoma, desmoid-type fibromatosis, spindle-cell carcinoid tumor, and primary or metastatic spindle-cell lesions of neural or smooth muscle origin. The recognition of relatively characteristic histologic features along with a concise immunohistochemical panel usually allow for relatively clear distinction between these entities.

CYTOLOGIC FEATURES

- Fine needle aspiration yields a bloody specimen with a variable amount of stromal fragments composed of irregular fascicles of bland spindle cells surrounding a meshwork of branching vessels.
- Spindle cells contain fusiform nuclei with evenly distributed, finely granular chromatin.
- Intermixed ropy collagen fibers.

HISTOLOGIC FEATURES

- Well-circumscribed borders with numerous branching thin-walled vessels.
- Alternating hypercellular/collagen-poor and hypocellular/collagen-rich areas.
- Haphazard arrangement of bland plump spindle cells with abundant thick hyalinized ropy collagen.

Figure 32.1 Cytology of complex branching vessels (*black arrows*—branch points, *white arrows*—vessels) traversing through spindle cells and intermixed ropy collagen (*inset*).

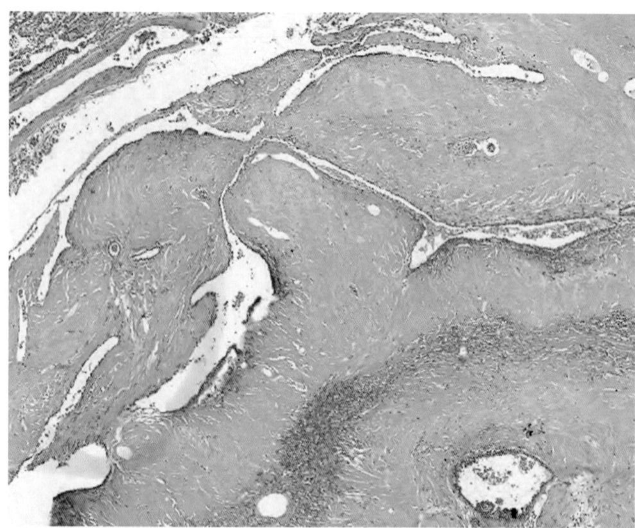

Figure 32.2 Sharp tumor–parenchymal interface with respiratory epithelium entrapped in cleft-like spaces, and alternating areas of hypocellular dense hyalinized stroma and hypercellular tumor cell aggregates.

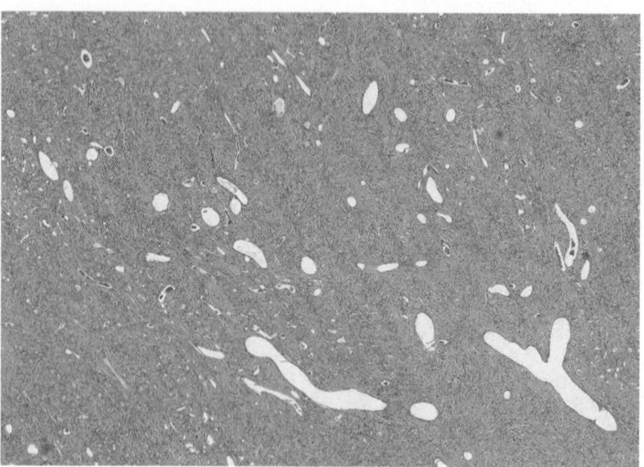

Figure 32.3 Numerous characteristic dilated thin-walled branching vessels.

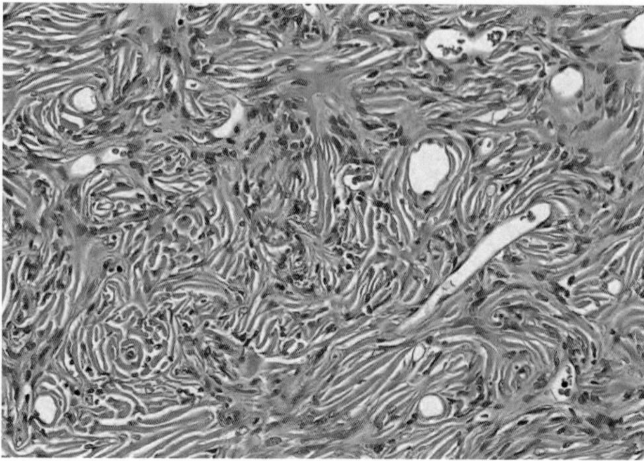

Figure 32.4 Haphazardly arranged cytologically bland plump oval to spindle-shaped tumor cells intimately associated with abundant ropy collagen.

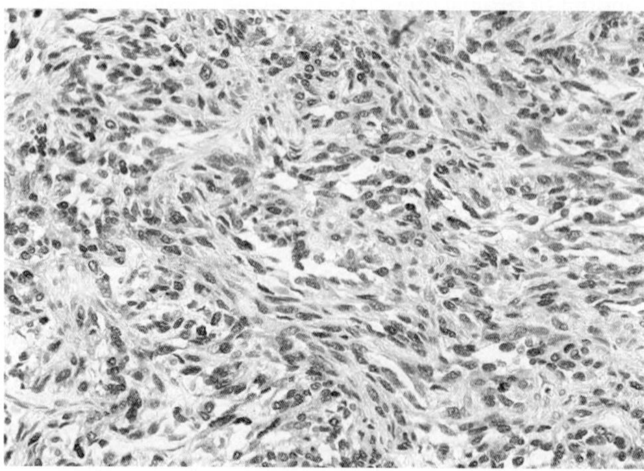

Figure 32.5 Diffuse nuclear reactivity for STAT6 antibodies is characteristic.

Desmoid-Type Fibromatosis

33

Charles Leduc
Natasha Rekhtman

Desmoid-type fibromatosis (desmoid tumor) of the thorax is a fibroblastic neoplasm that generally originates in the chest wall with secondary intrathoracic involvement, although rare cases of primary pleuropulmonary origin have been described. Although they are considered benign because of their inability to metastasize, they are locally aggressive tumors. On low-power magnification, they appear as a relatively uniform and hypocellular lesion with irregular and infiltrative borders. The tumor cells are medium-sized filiform to plump fibroblasts with characteristic pale nuclei, often in parallel orientation, embedded in a variably dense but usually loose fibrillar collagenous stroma with scattered arterioles. Most cases arise sporadically, with antecedent trauma/surgery and female sex (particularly pregnancy) as risk factors, whereas a minority of cases occur in the setting of Gardner syndrome. Mutations in the genes encoding proteins involved in the Wnt/β-catenin pathway have been identified in both sporadic (most commonly *CTNNB1*) and hereditary (most commonly *APC*) cases, which manifest as diffuse nuclear and cytoplasmic immunoreactivity to antibodies directed against β-catenin. Tumor cells are negative for S100, allowing for distinction from neural lesions, as well as for CD34 and STAT6, which are useful in distinguishing fibromatosis from solitary fibrous tumor (which can also occasionally be positive for β-catenin). The differential diagnosis also includes low-grade fibromyxoid sarcoma, which can be morphologically similar but generally has prominent myxoid areas and is negative for β-catenin.

HISTOLOGIC FEATURES

- Irregular infiltrative borders.
- Uniform appearance with low to at most moderate cellularity with abundant variably dense collagenous stroma with scattered venules and arterioles.
- Nuclear immunoreactivity to β-catenin.

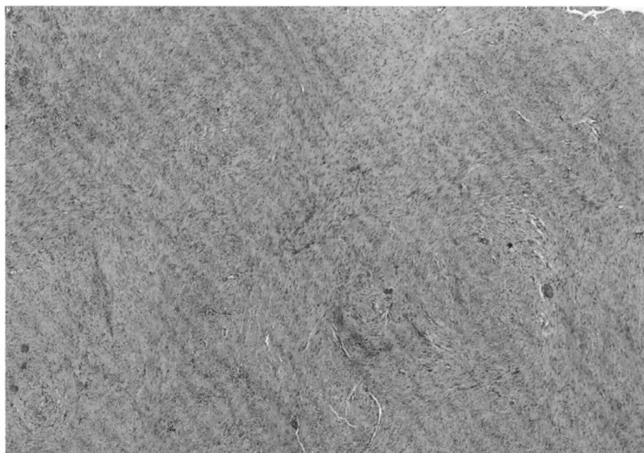

Figure 33.1 Relatively homogeneous appearing proliferation of spindle cells with pale nuclei within a collagenous matrix with scattered arterioles.

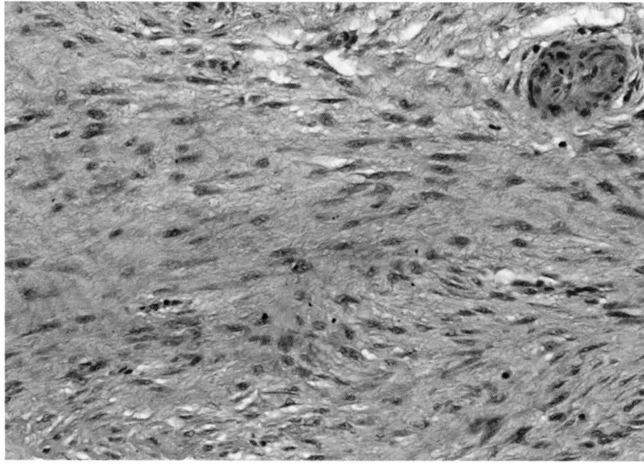

Figure 33.2 Variably sized irregular fibroblasts in vaguely parallel orientation associated with a fibrillary collagenous stroma.

34 Carcinoid Tumorlet

▶ Charles Leduc
▶ Natasha Rekhtman

Carcinoid tumorlets are benign neuroendocrine neoplasms, which are, by definition, less than 0.5 cm in greatest dimension. They are generally isolated lesions discovered incidentally in resection specimens, however, occasionally are multiple and can produce a diffuse micronodular pattern with radiologic mosaic attenuation, such as in the setting of diffuse idiopathic pulmonary neuroendocrine cell hyperplasia. Although both neuroendocrine cell hyperplasia and carcinoid tumorlets are believed to originate from naturally occurring bronchial neuroendocrine cells (Kulchitsky cells), the latter extend beyond the basement membrane of the bronchiolar epithelium, whereas the former do not. Other than overall size, they are morphologically identical to typical carcinoid tumors of the lung, and thus the same spectrum of histologic (trabecular, nested, pseudoglandular) and cytomorphologic (round, spindle, oncocytic) features can be observed. Similarly, carcinoid tumorlets are diffusely immunoreactive to antibodies directed against the neuroendocrine proteins, chromogranin and synaptophysin, while variably positive (often negative) for TTF-1. They are generally (but not universally) positive for broad-spectrum cytokeratins. Because of their small size and occasional peripheral location, they can be confused with meningothelioid nodules. Although both these lesions are CD56 positive, the latter tend not to arise centrilobularly, lack neuroendocrine architecture and cytology, and are negative for other neuroendocrine markers. When tumorlets are multiple, metastatic neuroendocrine tumor should be considered, and careful examination of tumor location (peribronchiolar vs intravascular) and clinicopathologic correlation is necessary.

HISTOLOGIC FEATURES

- Bronchiolar/peribronchiolar location and less than 0.5 cm in greatest dimension.
- Neuroendocrine architecture most commonly consisting of organoid nesting with adjacent fibrotic stromal response and delicate vasculature.
- Cytologically bland round, epithelioid, or spindle-shaped tumor cells with granular chromatin, inconspicuous nucleoli, and diffuse immunoreactivity to neuroendocrine markers.

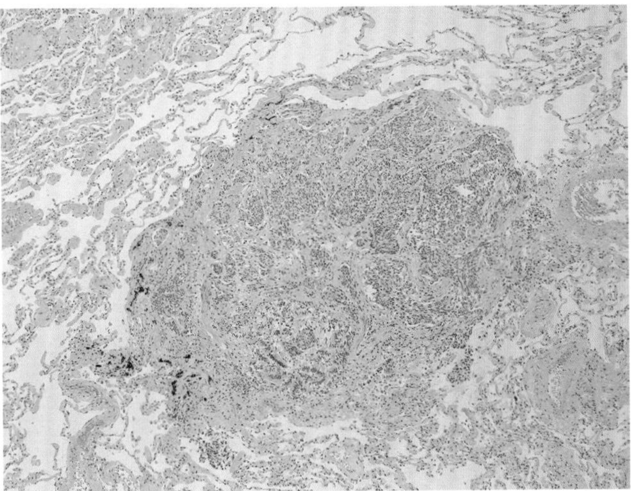

Figure 34.1 Small (<0.5 cm) nodular proliferation of nested round to spindle-shaped tumor cells with associated desmoplastic response, involving a bronchiole.

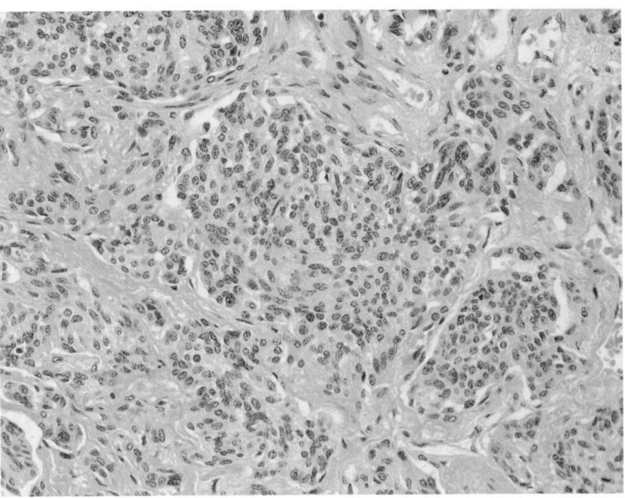

Figure 34.2 Tumor nests with rare rosette-like structures, predominantly spindled cell cytomorphology, and typical granular chromatin with inapparent nucleoli.

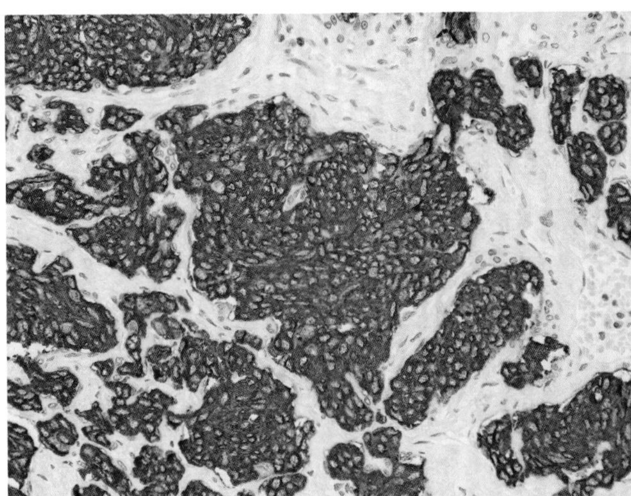

Figure 34.3 Diffuse strong cytoplasmic staining for chromogranin is characteristic.

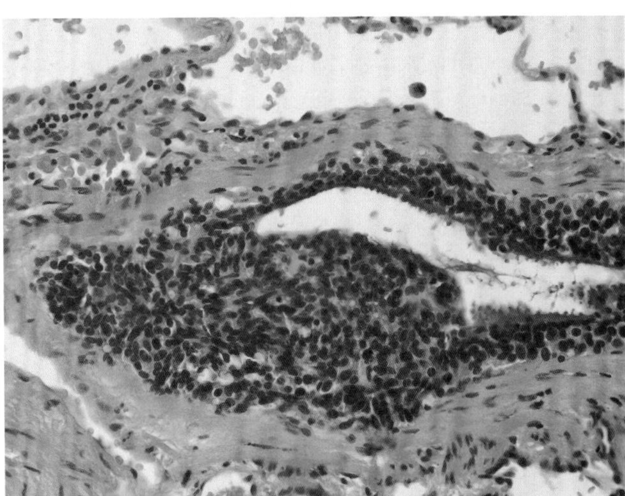

Figure 34.4 Focus of neuroendocrine cell hyperplasia undermining but restricted to the bronchiolar epithelium.

Pulmonary Meningothelial Nodule

35

Charles Leduc
Natasha Rekhtman

Pulmonary minute meningothelioid nodules are discrete interstitial proliferations of benign round to spindle-shaped cells of uncertain origin and function. As their name implies, they are small (generally <5 mm), but otherwise morphologically and immunohistochemically identical to intracranial and extracranial meningiomas. They are generally incidentally identified in resection specimens, often adjacent to interlobular septa and/or pulmonary venules, proliferating in small whorls within and expanding the interstitium, resulting in a vaguely stellate lesion. Cytologically the lesional cells are oval to spindle-shaped with dense eosinophilic cytoplasm, indistinct cell borders, finely granular chromatin, and indistinct nucleoli. Intranuclear inclusions are common. They are positive for the immunohistochemical markers EMA, progesterone receptor, and CD56. In contrast to meningiomas, minute meningothelioid nodules are considered reactive lesions, although there is some evidence to suggest that they may harbor neoplastic molecular driver aberrations in the setting of diffuse bilateral disease ("diffuse pulmonary meningotheliomatosis"). The differential diagnosis is relatively limited and includes carcinoid tumorlets, which are peribronchiolar and positive for chromogranin and synaptophysin, and small vascular proliferations such as plexiform lesions. Rarely, diffuse pulmonary meningotheliomatosis can simulate metastasis of well-differentiated carcinoma; however, immunohistochemical workup and close clinical and radiologic correlation can generally resolve this diagnostic dilemma.

HISTOLOGIC FEATURES

- Small (usually <5 mm) interstitial proliferations, generally perivenular or periseptally located.
- Bland spindled to epithelioid cells arranged in whorls.
- Immunoreactivity for EMA, PR, and CD56.

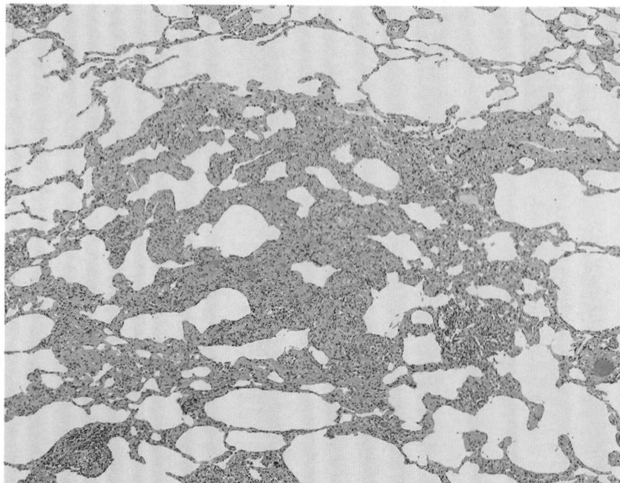

Figure 35.1 Proliferation of monomorphic cytologically bland ovoid cells, which expand the interstitium.

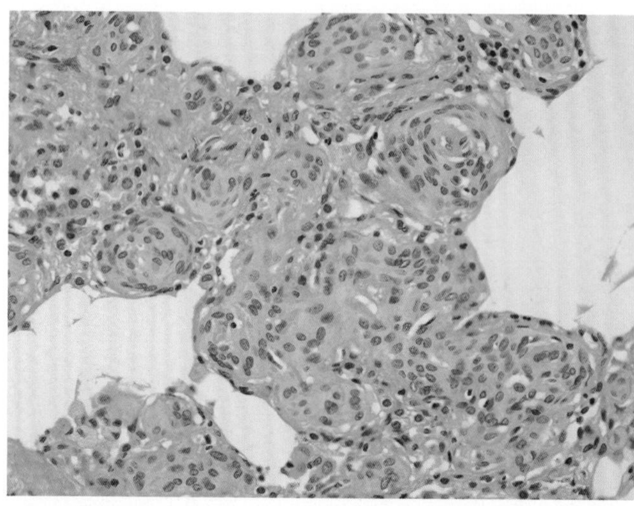

Figure 35.2 Meningothelioid cells are arranged in whorls with relatively indistinct cell borders.

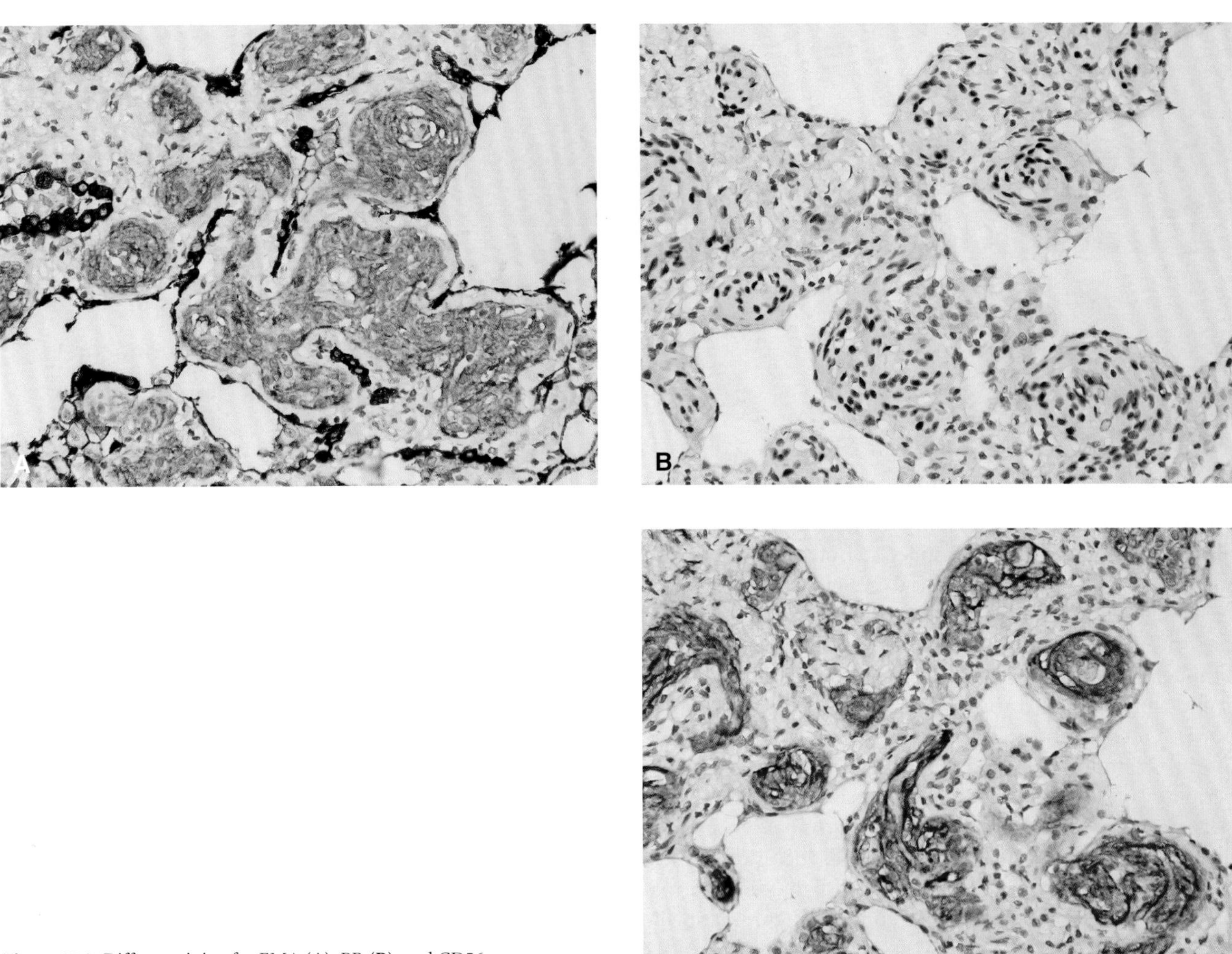

Figure 35.3 Diffuse staining for EMA (**A**), PR (**B**), and CD56 (**C**) is characteristic.

Sclerosing Pneumocytoma

36

- Charles Leduc
- Darren Buonocore
- Natasha Rekhtman

Sclerosing pneumocytoma (formerly sclerosing hemangioma) is a benign biphasic neoplasm consisting of a two distinct cell populations: surface cuboidal cells and stromal round cells. Immunohistochemical and molecular studies have shown that both cell types are clonal and believed to originate from a common primitive respiratory epithelial precursor. They occur more commonly in women and are generally peripheral and solitary, although multifocal cases have been reported. Tumor borders are well circumscribed and, as the name implies, variable amounts of dense tumoral fibrosis can be seen even at low power. Often several architectural patterns occur within the same lesion, including papilliform, sclerotic, solid, and hemorrhagic. The lesional cells are often best viewed at the periphery of the lesion, as stromal fibrosis frequently obscures them centrally. The stromal cells are round, with a moderate amount of pale eosinophilic cytoplasm, generally vesicular chromatin, and small visible nucleoli (occasional nuclear grooves can be seen). The surface cells are cuboidal, tend to appear slightly smaller than the round cells, with denser eosinophilic cytoplasm and more condensed chromatin. Both cell types are positive for TTF-1 and EMA, whereas only the surface cells are positive for cytokeratins and napsin A. Diagnosis on small biopsy specimens can be challenging and the differential diagnosis includes pulmonary adenocarcinoma, metastatic papillary thyroid or renal cell carcinoma, papillary adenoma, hemangioma, and Langerhans cell histiocytosis. The key to the correct diagnosis is the lack of significant cytologic atypia of the surface cells as well as recognition and immunohistochemical characterization of the stromal round cells.

CYTOLOGIC FEATURES

- Fine needle aspiration yields cellular smears with a biphasic population.
- Bland stromal cells with round to oval nuclei surrounding small blood vessel and sclerotic cores.
- Loosely cohesive epithelial cells present as single cells, small clusters, rosettes, and surrounding stromal fragments with round nuclei and occasional pseudoinclusions.
- Hemosiderin-laden macrophages and giant cells may be seen.

HISTOLOGIC FEATURES

- Well-circumscribed tumor–parenchymal interface with generally numerous architectural patterns within individual tumors, including papilliform, sclerotic, solid, and hemorrhagic.
- Two distinct cell populations consisting of surface cuboidal cells and stromal round cells, both of which are positive for TTF-1, whereas only the former are positive for cytokeratins.

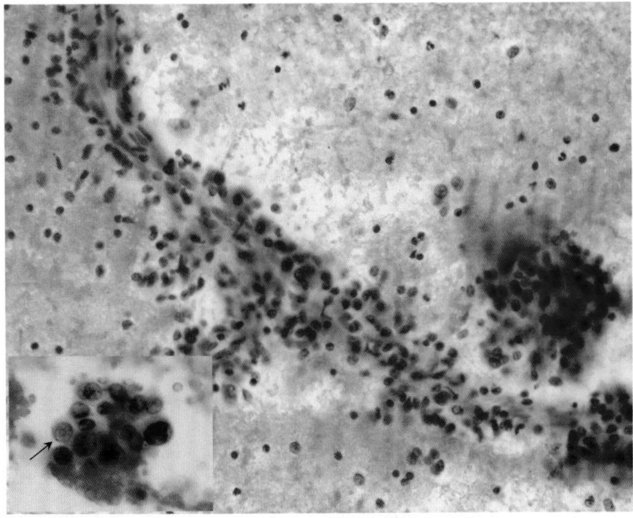

Figure 36.1 Bland stromal cells surrounding a small blood vessel. Epithelial cells are present singly and in rosettes *(inset)*, with occasional intranuclear pseudoinclusions *(arrow)*.

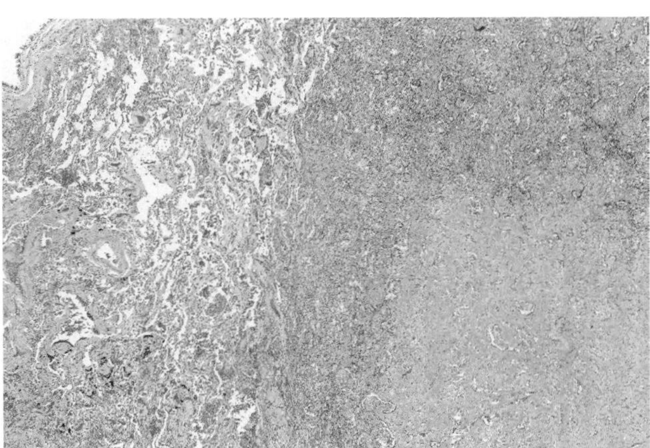

Figure 36.2 Relatively sharp tumor–parenchymal interface with condensed papilliform structures at the periphery and more dense sclerosis centrally.

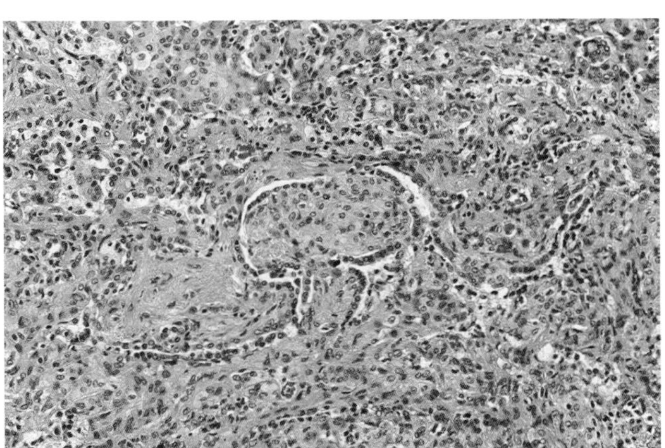

Figure 36.3 Papillary-like structures lined by cuboidal epithelial cells and round stromal cells centrally with variable fibrosis. A fair number of capillary-sized vessels are generally seen.

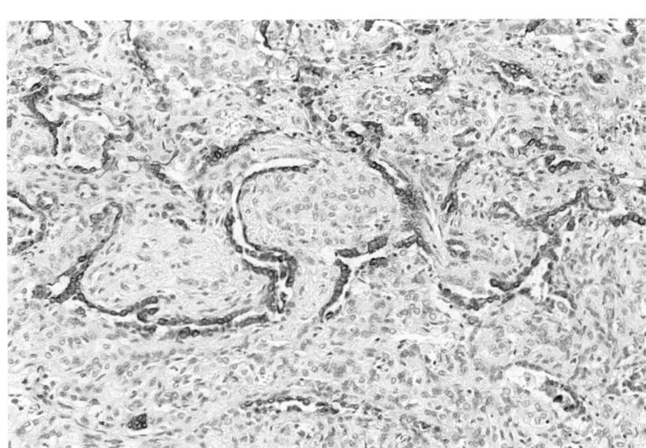

Figure 36.4 Broad-spectrum cytokeratin generally stains only the surface cells.

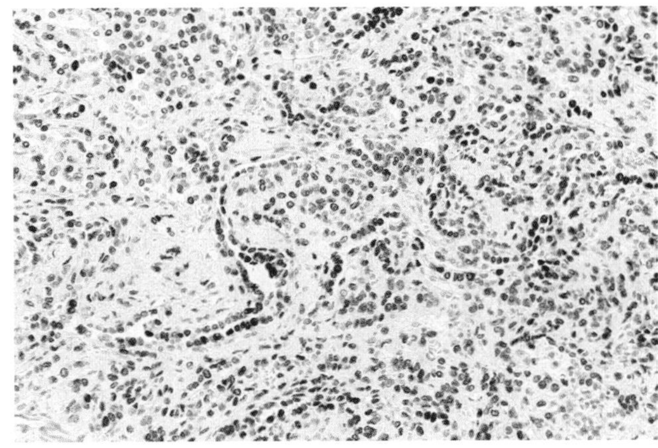

Figure 36.5 Both surface and stromal round cells are positive for TTF-1.

37 Alveolar Adenoma

Charles Leduc
Natasha Rekhtman

Alveolar adenoma is a rare benign biphasic tumor consisting of mesenchymal fibroblast-like interstitial cells and epithelial cells of pneumocytic lineage. It is believed to be a neoplasm; however, it remains unclear if only one or both of the components are neoplastic, and studies to date suggest that it is unlikely that the two cell populations originate from a common progenitor. They are benign, and generally peripherally located. On low-power magnification, the tumor is characterized by well-circumscribed borders, with multiple variably sized cystic spaces, which are lined by plump epithelial cells (often discontinuous) and are often filled with amphophilic granular debris and rare macrophages. The intratumoral and peritumoral interstitium contains plump ovoid to spindle-shaped fibroblast-like cells in a variably myxoid matrix with occasional mast cells and/or lymphocytes and plasma cells. Immunohistochemistry demonstrates pneumocytic differentiation in the epithelial cells (positive for CK7 and TTF-1), whereas the interstitial cells are cytokeratin-negative with an immunoprofile somewhat akin to fibroblasts (variable positivity for CD34 and SMA). The morphologic differential diagnosis includes lymphangioma, atypical adenomatous hyperplasia, sclerosing pneumocytoma, and pulmonary hamartoma. Recognition of the prominent cystic spaces, biphasic morphology without differentiated mesenchymal elements, and lack of cytologic atypia, generally allows for distinction from these entities.

HISTOLOGIC FEATURES

- Well-circumscribed tumor with multiple cystic spaces filled with granular debris and lined by plump pneumocytes.
- The tumor stroma is variably myxoid with ovoid to spindle-shaped fibroblast-like cells.

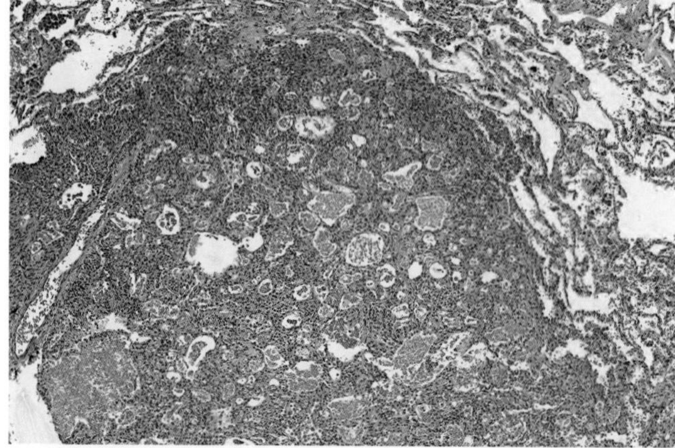

Figure 37.1 The tumor demonstrates multiple variably sized cystic spaces, prominent interstitium, and well-circumscribed tumor–parenchymal interface.

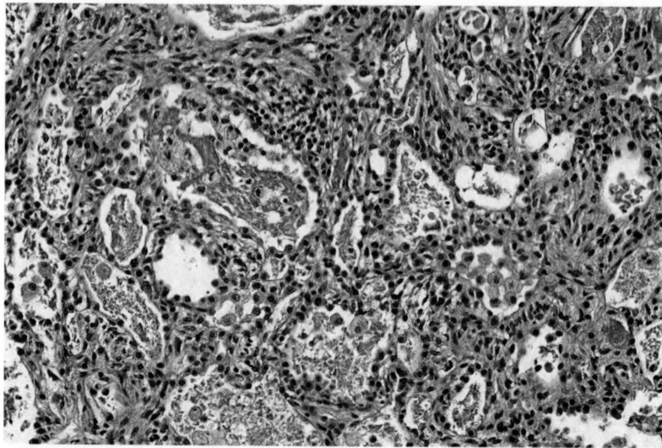

Figure 37.2 The cystic spaces are lined by plump pneumocytes and filled with granular debris and occasional foamy macrophages, whereas the interstitium contains ovoid to spindle-shaped cells with variable number of chronic inflammatory cells.

38 Papillary Adenoma

▶ Charles Leduc
▶ Bruno Murer*
▶ Natasha Rekhtman

Papillary adenoma is an exquisitely rare benign epithelial neoplasm consisting of a well-circumscribed proliferation of true papilla lined by cuboidal to columnar respiratory epithelial cells. They are generally peripherally located and solitary, and tend to occur more commonly in males. On low-power magnification, they appear as multiple simple and focally branching papillary structures that compress adjacent and intratumoral interstitium, occasionally giving rise to dilated-appearing alveolar airspaces filled with papillae. The core of the papillae typically consists of loose fibrovascular tissue. The lining of the papilla consists of a continuous single row of cuboidal to columnar epithelial cells with pneumocytic differentiation. The lining epithelial cells are positive for CK7 and TTF-1, whereas the stromal cells are negative for these markers. Although several studies have demonstrated lack of *EGFR* and *KRAS* mutations, the precise driver aberration underlying this neoplasm remains unknown. The main entities in the differential diagnosis are primary or metastatic papillary adenocarcinoma and sclerosing pneumocytoma. Papillary adenoma can be differentiated from the former by the complete lack of cytologic atypia or other malignant features (such as necrosis and elevated mitotic activity) and from the latter by the absence of TTF-1-positive stromal round cells.

HISTOLOGIC FEATURES

- Proliferation of simple to occasionally branching papillae with well-circumscribed pushing borders.
- Papillae consisting of fibrovascular cores with loose connective tissue, lined by a continuous single row of cuboidal to columnar cells with pneumocytic differentiation.

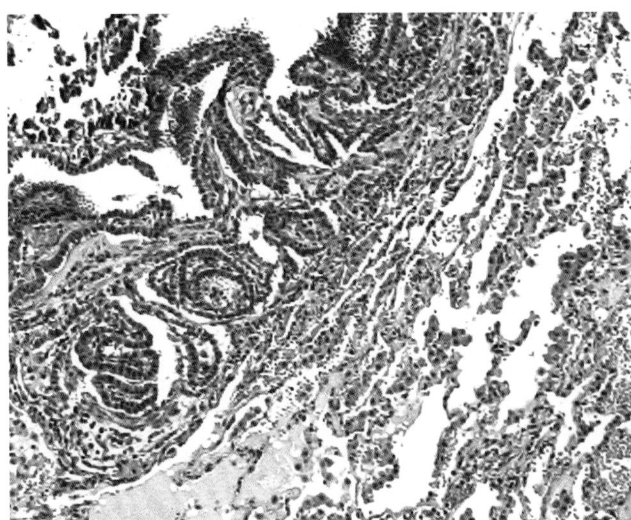

Figure 38.1 Pushing, noninfiltrative border, with well-developed true papillae.

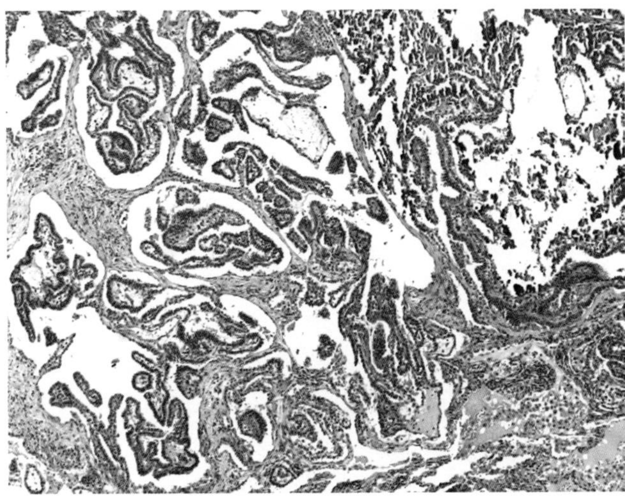

Figure 38.2 Numerous dilated alveolar airspaces filled with papillary fronds.

*The authors would like to acknowledge the work of Dr. Murer, who contributed to the previous edition.

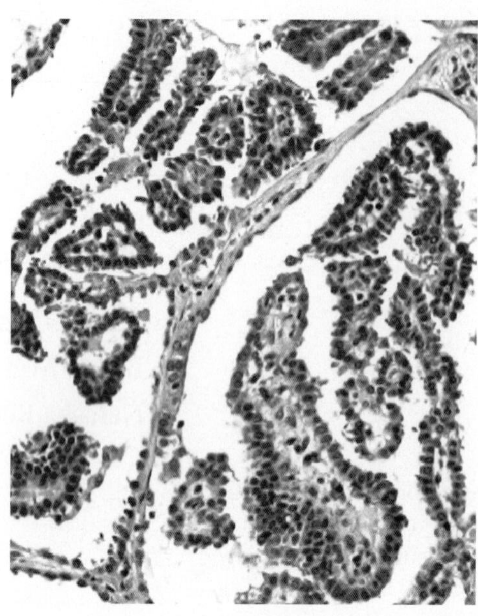

Figure 38.3 Papillae characterized by loose fibrovascular connective tissue lined by a single row of cytologically bland epithelial lining cells.

39 Mucous Gland Adenoma

▸ Charles Leduc
▸ Bruno Murer*
▸ Natasha Rekhtman

Mucous gland adenoma is a rare benign neoplasm of the mucin-producing cells of the bronchial submucosal seromucinous glands. As their origin implies, they tend to occur centrally, in a peribronchial or endobronchial location, and frequently manifest with clinical signs and symptoms of obstruction. The tumor typically has well-circumscribed pushing borders and consists of multiple glandular spaces lined by uniform nonciliated columnar cells with basally oriented nuclei and abundant clear intracytoplasmic mucin. Focal papillary architecture is occasionally present. The intervening stroma is generally compressed and contains scattered spindle cells and collagen. The mucous cells are positive for broad-spectrum cytokeratins whereas negative for TTF-1. The stromal cells demonstrate focal positivity for broad-spectrum cytokeratin and S100, suggesting a myoepithelial component. Molecular characterization of these neoplasms has been limited by their rarity, and driver aberrations have yet to be identified. The main entities in the differential diagnosis are primary invasive or metastatic mucinous adenocarcinoma, mucinous cystadenoma, low-grade mucoepidermoid carcinoma, and glandular papilloma. Differentiating between these entities on small biopsy samples may be challenging and close clinical and radiologic correlation is instrumental. Both mucinous cystadenoma and primary invasive mucinous adenocarcinoma typically occur in the periphery of the lung, with the former characterized by large dilated mucin-filled cysts and the latter generally harboring areas of lepidic growth. Low-grade mucoepidermoid carcinoma and glandular papilloma occur centrally, but both have multiple cell types, with the former harboring squamous and intermediate cells and the latter having a pseudostratified ciliated epithelium containing only occasional mucous cells.

HISTOLOGIC FEATURES

- Endobronchial or peribronchial location with well-circumscribed pushing border.
- Uniform population of columnar epithelial cells with abundant clear mucin and basally oriented nuclei, arranged in variably sized glandular structures with scant intervening stroma.

*The authors would like to acknowledge the work of Dr. Murer, who contributed to the previous edition.

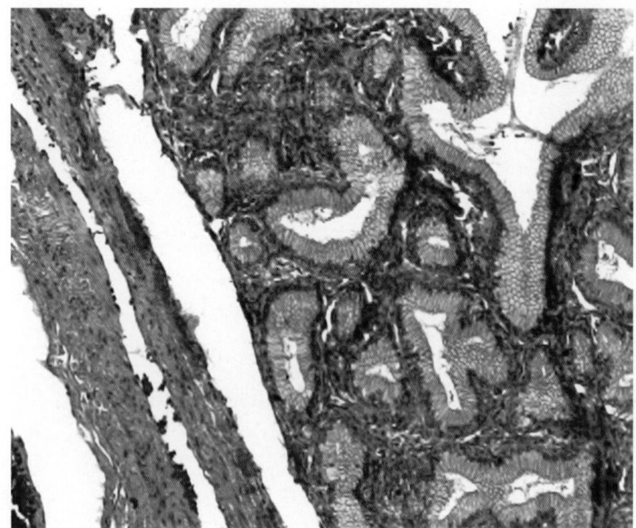

Figure 39.1 Well-circumscribed tumor border with numerous irregular but rounded glandular spaces and scant intervening stroma.

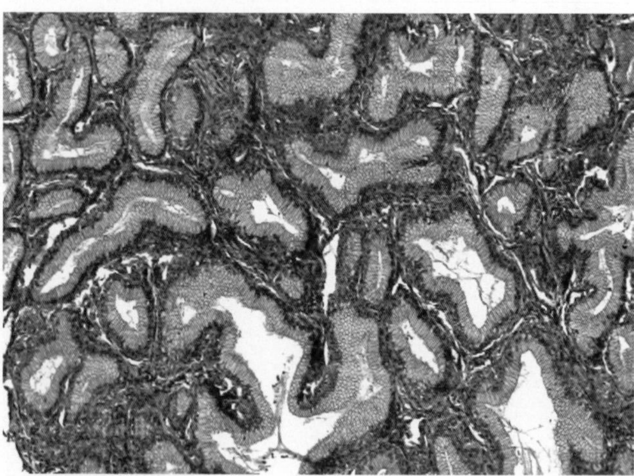

Figure 39.2 Uniformly distributed glandular spaces lined by monomorphic mucin-filled columnar cells with basally oriented nuclei.

40 Oncocytoma

Charles Leduc
Carlos Bedrossian*
Natasha Rekhtman

Pulmonary oncocytoma is an extremely rare benign neoplasm consisting of epithelial cells with classic oncocytic cytomorphologic and ultrastructural features. Its rarity has limited detailed understanding of this lesion; however, it is believed to likely originate from seromucinous glands of the bronchus, as it is morphologically identical to oncocytomas primary to the salivary glands. It is a well-circumscribed tumor composed of nests or trabeculae of uniform polygonal cells with abundant granular eosinophilic cytoplasm and round nuclei with discrete nucleoli. Occasional larger cells with more clear vacuolated cytoplasm or cells with pyknotic nuclei can be observed. The lesional cells are positive for broad-spectrum cytokeratins, and ultrastructurally they contain numerous mitochondria. The main entities in the differential are carcinoid tumor and metastatic oncocytic tumors of thyroid and renal origin. A concise immunohistochemical including neuroendocrine markers and the renal and thyroid marker PAX-8, along with close correlation with clinical and radiologic findings, can assist in separation of these entities.

CYTOLOGIC FEATURES

- Cells with uniform round nuclei and abundant granular cytoplasm.

HISTOLOGIC FEATURES

- Nested or trabecular arrangement of uniform oncocytic cells.

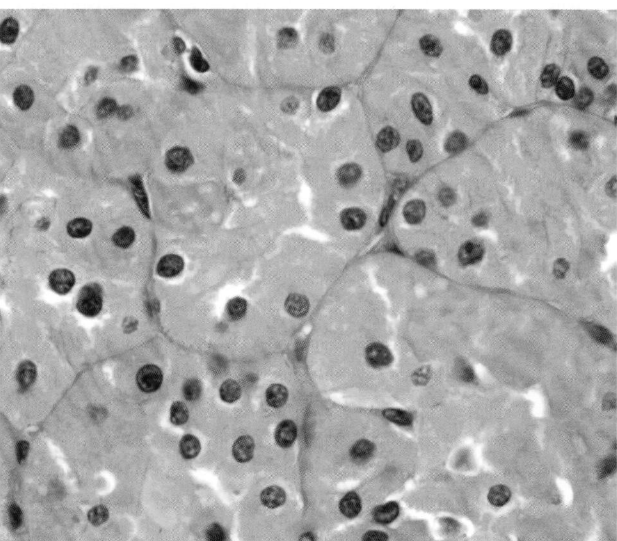

Figure 40.1 Polygonal tumor cells in a nested/organoid pattern, with typical oncocytic features including low nuclear to cytoplasm ratio, abundant granular cytoplasm, and rounded nuclei with discrete nucleoli.

*The authors would like to acknowledge the work of Dr. Bedrossian, who contributed to the previous edition.

41 Pleomorphic Adenoma

Charles Leduc
Natasha Rekhtman

Pleomorphic adenoma is a benign neoplasm believed to originate from the bronchial submucosal seromucinous glands. It is classified as a salivary gland–type tumor and is histologically indistinguishable from its counterpart in the salivary glands. Similar to other salivary gland–type tumors, it tends to occur centrally and has both epithelial and myoepithelial components. As its name implies, it is pleomorphic, displaying a variety of architectural patterns within a single tumor. On low power, typical cases form rounded to polypoid endobronchial masses with a generally prominent myxoid to chondromyxoid matrix and a cellular component that ranges from irregular biphasic gland and duct-like structures to loose sheets of myoepithelial cells with variable cytomorphology, including spindle, clear, and plasmacytoid appearances. Focal squamous differentiation is common. Peripheral tumors have been reported, in which case they tend to be well circumscribed but unencapsulated. Immunohistochemically, both the epithelial cells ("inner ductal cells") and myoepithelial cells are positive for broad-spectrum cytokeratins, whereas only the myoepithelial cells will variably coexpress S100 and/or smooth muscle markers such as SMA or calponin. In biopsy specimens, the distinctive architectural pleomorphism is not always apparent and thus the diagnosis should be considered in any tumor with a myoepithelial component. Malignant features and behavior have been documented (≥per 10 HPF, necrosis, and vascular invasion); however, malignant transformation is an extremely rare event and should raise the possibility of metastatic carcinoma ex pleomorphic adenoma of salivary gland origin. Other entities to exclude are pulmonary hamartoma, pulmonary blastoma, and primary or metastatic myoepithelial tumors. The correct diagnosis relies on careful histologic characterization of the individual tumor elements, exclusion of cytologic atypia and other malignant features, along with close clinical and radiologic correlation.

HISTOLOGIC FEATURES

- Epithelial and myoepithelial cells in ductal and/or loose sheet-like growth, without significant cytologic atypia.
- Highly variable matrix with myxoid, hyaline, or chondroid appearances most commonly.

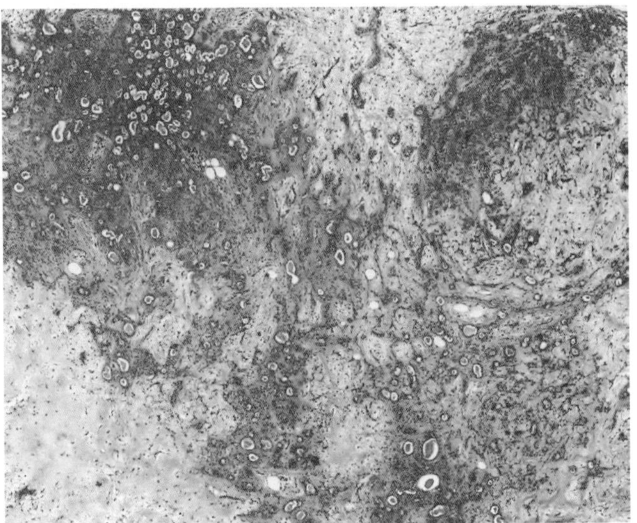

Figure 41.1 Aggregated ductal structures and focal solid clusters of neoplastic cells in an abundant myxoid to myxohyaline matrix.

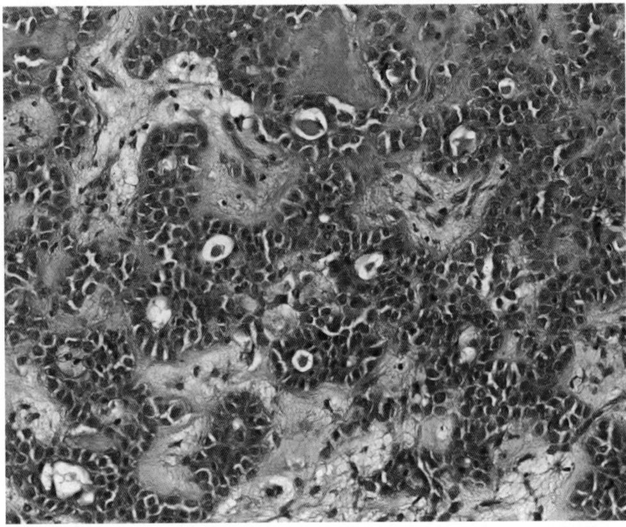

Figure 41.2 Focus of ductal differentiation showing bilayered ducts with inner ductal cells and outer myoepithelial cells and eosinophilic debris within the lumen, on a myxoid backdrop.

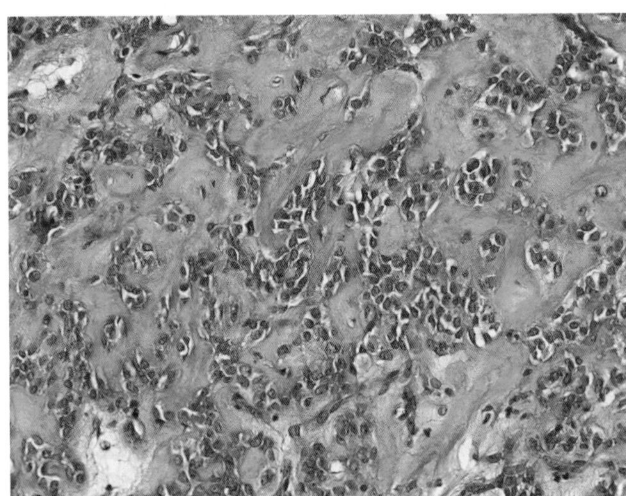

Figure 41.3 Focus of clear myoepithelial cells in a hyalinized matrix, without ductal elements.

Multifocal Multinodular Pneumocyte Hyperplasia

42

▶ Charles Leduc
▶ Philippe Romeo
▶ Natasha Rekhtman

Multifocal micronodular pneumocyte hyperplasia (MMPH) is a distinctive radiologic–pathologic entity that occurs exclusively in the context of tuberous sclerosis complex. Radiologically, the most common pattern is bilateral randomly distributed subcentimeric nodules, which can occasionally raise suspicion for metastatic disease or miliary tuberculosis. The histologic appearance is that of multiple well-demarcated, randomly located, small intraparenchymal lesions, which give the impression of patchy parenchymal atelectasis on low power. The lesions consist of mildly thickened interstitium with an increased number of enlarged reactive type II pneumocytes aggregated in a discontinuous fashion along thickened alveolar walls. Because of their association with tuberous sclerosis, they are often identified incidentally in the parenchyma of lungs resected for other lesions, such as lymphangioleiomyomatosis or PEComa. Immunohistochemically, the lesional cells are positive for CK7 and TTF-1 in keeping with their pneumocytic differentiation. Distinguishing these proliferations from multifocal atypical adenomatous hyperplasia (AAH) can be challenging and usually requires a combination of clinical context and subtle morphologic differences. Compared with AAH, MMPH tends to produce lesions that are well demar have slightly thicker alveolar septa, with pneumocytes having lower nuclear to cytoplasmic ratio and lacking significant nuclear hyperchromasia.

HISTOLOGIC FEATURES

- Nodular intraparenchymal lesion clearly demarcated from adjacent lung by interstitial thickening and increased number of pneumocytes.
- Discontinuous proliferation of reactive-appearing pneumocytes with preserved nuclear to cytoplasmic ratio and without significant nuclear hyperchromasia.

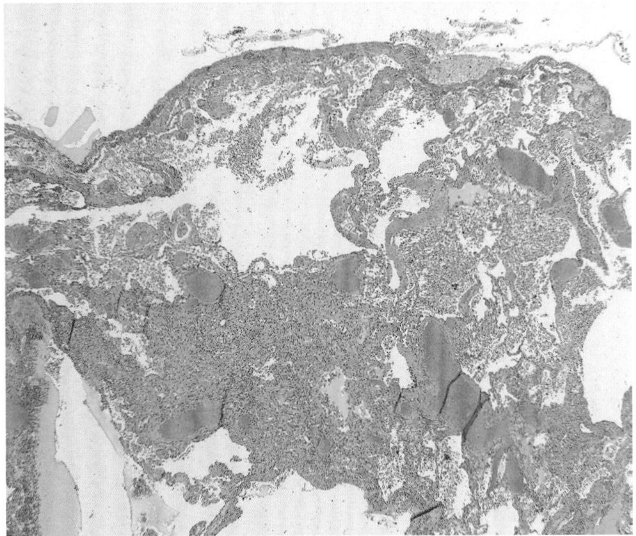

Figure 42.1 Irregular nodular proliferation simulating a zone of parenchymal atelectasis. Multiple cystic spaces are also present in the case pictured here, secondary to tuberous sclerosis–associated lymphangioleiomyomatosis.

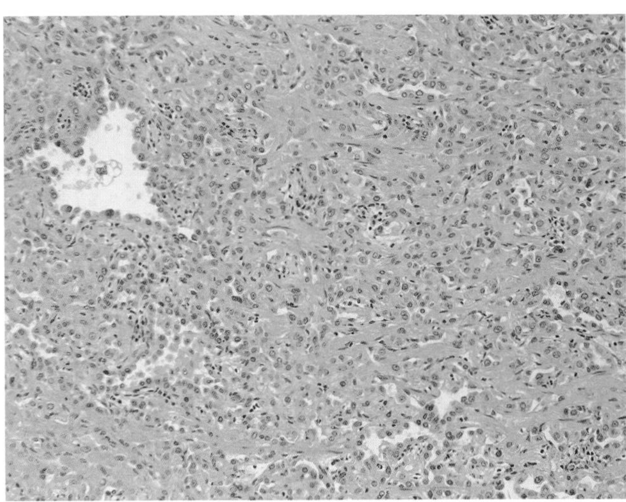

Figure 42.2 Thickened interstitium with compressed alveolar spaces lined by plump pneumocytes.

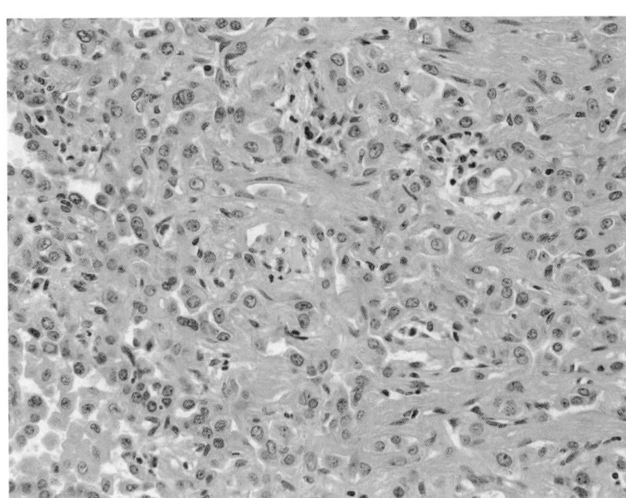

Figure 42.3 Numerous enlarged pneumocytes with mild cytologic atypia and preserved nuclear to cytoplasmic ratio, without significant nuclear hyperchromasia.

43

PEComa

Charles Leduc
Natasha Rekhtman

Clear cell sugar tumor of the lung is a benign proliferation of perivascular endothelial cells (PECs) and is often referred to by its synonym benign pulmonary PEComa. It is typically a solitary well-circumscribed peripheral lesion, consisting of irregular nests and sheets of tumor cells with interspersed thin-walled vessels. The lesional cells are medium to large, with abundant clear and/or pale eosinophilic cytoplasm, which can be vacuolated to slightly granular, and moderately pleomorphic nuclei with open chromatin and generally visible nucleoli. Large tumor cells and binucleation can be seen; however, significant nuclear atypia, mitotic activity, and necrosis are usually absent. As with other PEComatous tumors, such as lymphangioleiomyomatosis and angiomyolipoma, these tumors are associated with tuberous sclerosis and show myelomelanocytic differentiation by immunohistochemistry, being positive for both melanocytic (such as HMB45 and Melan-A) and myoid (such as desmin, SMA, and calponin) markers. Molecular studies specifically investigating primary pulmonary PEComas are lacking; however, molecular aberrations have been identified in extrapulmonary PEComas, including *TSC1* and *TSC2* gene mutations in both hereditary and sporadic cases, as well as *TFE3* gene fusions in a subset of cases. The differential diagnosis includes metastatic clear cell renal carcinoma, granular cell tumor, and metastatic malignant melanoma. Although the immunoprofile is relatively characteristic, differentiating from the latter can be occasionally challenging and exclusion of significant cytologic atypia and prior melanoma can be instrumental. Pulmonary metastases from extrathoracic PEComas (particularly uterine) have been documented; therefore close clinical correlation should be undertaken before a definitive diagnosis is rendered.

HISTOLOGIC CHARACTERISTICS

- Rounded tumor borders with solid growth of moderate to large round cells with abundant clear vacuolated to granular cytoplasm.
- Coexpression of melanocytic and myoid immunostains, while negative for cytokeratin.

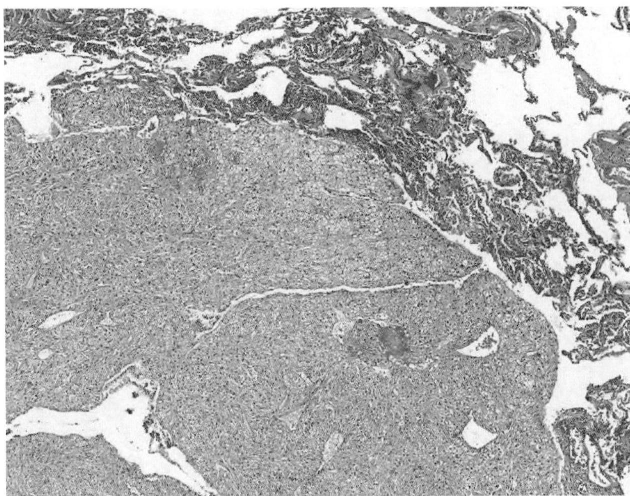

Figure 43.1 Well-circumscribed tumor border with solid growth pattern and scattered thin-walled and occasionally dilated vessels.

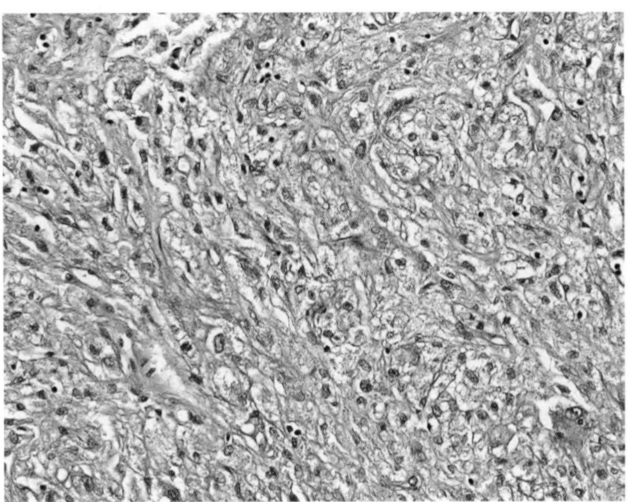

Figure 43.2 Sheets of rounded to irregular tumor cells with abundant clear vacuolated to granular cytoplasm. Moderate nuclear pleomorphism is not unusual.

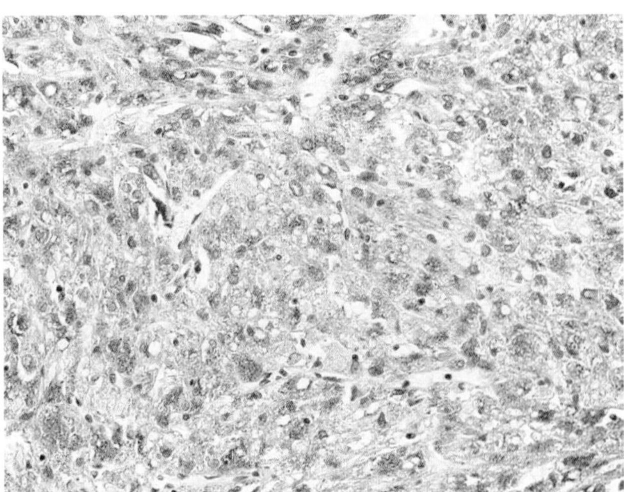

Figure 43.3 Diffuse immunoreactivity for the melanocytic marker HMB45.

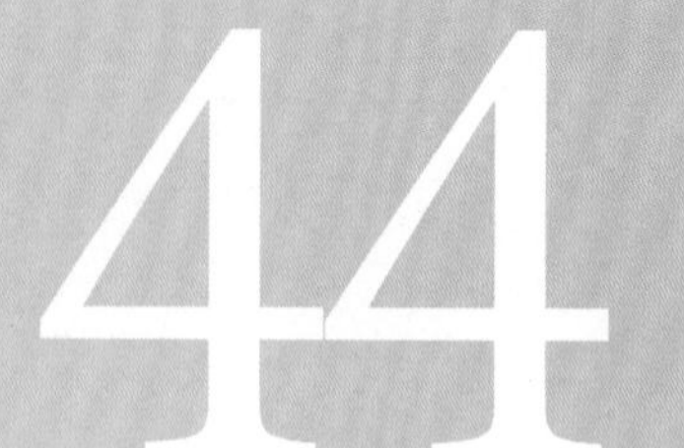

Glomus Tumor

▶ Charles Leduc
▶ Natasha Rekhtman

Glomus tumor of the lung is a rare benign neoplasm of perivascular (pericytic) cells, which is morphologically indistinguishable from its more common acral cutaneous counterpart. Its precise histogenesis is unclear, as native pulmonary glomus bodies are yet to be identified, although structures with similar appearance have been reported in the trachea. They can occur within both the proximal airways and the lung parenchyma, with hemoptysis as a possible presenting symptom in the former. They are generally well-circumscribed lesions, with a solid growth pattern, although an angiomatoid pattern with prominent dilated vessels can occur. The tumor is comprised of three components in varying amounts: uniform round glomus cells; spindle smooth muscle cells; dilated thin-walled vessels. Generally, the glomus cells predominate, giving rise to a relatively cellular, monomorphic-appearing solid lesion with scant foci of myxoid or hyalinized fibrotic stroma. Immunohistochemically, the glomus cells are uniformly positive for smooth muscle actin, while negative for epithelial markers and the vascular markers (such as ERG, CD31, CD34). The main entities in the differential diagnosis are carcinoid tumor and sclerosing pneumocytoma. The absence of an epithelial component as well as lack of immunoreactivity for pneumocytic or neuroendocrine markers renders distinction from these entities relatively straightforward.

HISTOLOGIC FEATURES

- Solid or angiomatoid growth pattern with scattered thin-walled blood vessels and areas of hyaline or myxoid matrix.
- Relatively monotonous population of round and occasionally epithelioid-appearing lesional cells, which are smooth muscle actin positive.

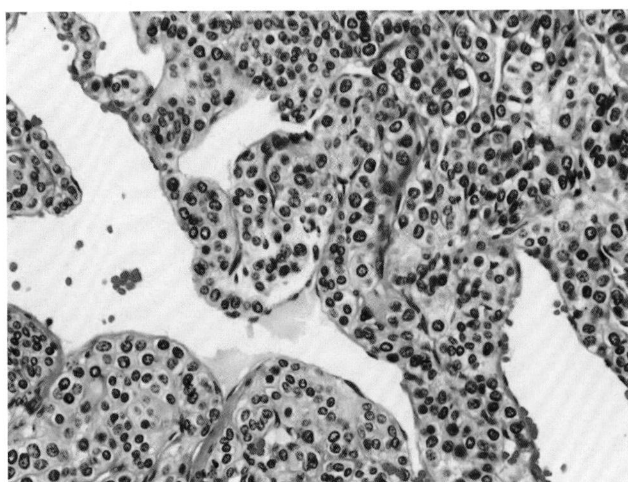

Figure 44.1 Angiomatoid glomus tumor with solid proliferation of monotonous round glomus cells in a focally hyalinized matrix, surrounding dilated vascular channels. (Image courtesy of Cristina Antonescu, MD.)

Giant Cell Tumor

45

▶ Charles Leduc
▶ Natasha Rekhtman

Giant cell tumor (GCT) of the lung is an exquisitely rare tumefactive proliferation of osteoclast-like histiocytes. Because of the morphologic similarity to its counterpart in the bone, it is presumed to be neoplastic, although detailed characterization of its histogenesis has been limited by its rarity. Both centrally and peripherally located cases have been reported. On low power, it is a relatively well-circumscribed (but unencapsulated), homogeneous, moderately to densely cellular mass. Foci of red cell extravasation and/or fresh hemorrhage are common. The lesional cell population is biphasic, consisting of scattered and aggregated osteoclast-like giant cells on a background of numerous plump round to spindled mononuclear stromal cells. The giant cells have abundant cytoplasm and numerous nuclei (not uncommonly >20). In typical cases, the nuclei of the giant cells are cytomorphologically similar to those of the mononuclear cells, with generally open chromatin and small visible nucleoli. Both the mononuclear and multinuclear components are positive for lysozyme and CD68 (KP-1). The primary differential diagnosis is metastatic extrapulmonary giant cell tumor (typically bone) and giant cell carcinoma. Excluding extrathoracic primary tumors is essential and requires close clinical and radiologic correlation. The lack of cellular atypia and cytokeratin reactivity distinguishes GCT from giant cell carcinoma. The morphology of the giant cells in GCT ("osteoclast-like") is relatively characteristic; however, polarization of tissue to exclude foreign bodies and special stains for microorganisms may be helpful in excluding reactive giant cell lesions.

HISTOLOGIC FEATURES

- Biphasic lesional cell population: scattered and aggregated osteoclast-like giant cells and round to spindled stromal mononuclear cells.
- Both lesional cell components have nuclei appearing similar and display cytoplasmic positivity for the histiocytic marker CD68.

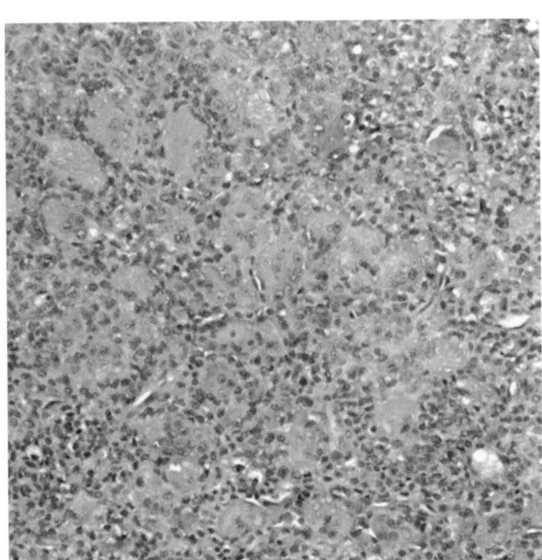

Figure 45.1 Isolated and aggregated osteoclast-like giant cells on a background of numerous interspersed monocular stromal cells with rare foci of red cell extravasation.

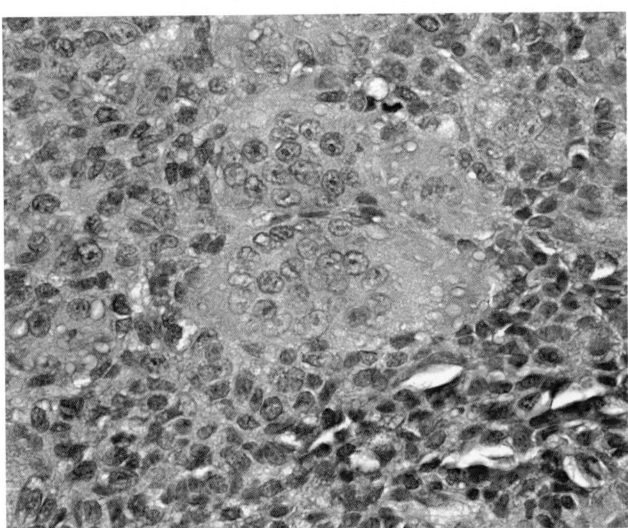

Figure 45.2 Giant cells are often clustered and can have more than 20 nuclei.

46 Meningioma

▶ Charles Leduc
▶ Natasha Rekhtman

Pulmonary meningioma (PM) is a neoplasm of meningothelial cells, which is morphologically identical to its more common counterpart involving the intracranial and extracranial dura mater. They most likely arise from pluripotent pulmonary stem cells, and while they share morphologic features of minute meningothelial nodules (MMNs), whether or not they are histogenetically and molecularly related to MMNs remains a topic of debate. Most cases present as an incidentally discovered solitary peripheral lung nodule, although central cases have been described and tend to be symptomatic. On low power, meningiomas are moderately cellular intraparenchymal tumors with well-circumscribed pushing borders. As with dural-based meningiomas, multiple architectural patterns can be seen, including meningothelial, fibroblastic, and psammomatous. The lesional cells are epithelioid to spindled, with generally eosinophilic cytoplasm, and round nuclei with occasional pseudoinclusions and/or grooves. Immunohistochemically, the lesional cells are positive for EMA, PR, and CD56. In core biopsy specimens, meningiomas are essentially indistinguishable from MMNs. Although there are no universally accepted size criteria to distinguish MMNs from PMs, the former are generally less than 5 mm and have an irregular or occasionally filiform growth pattern, whereas the latter are tumefactive and have expansile growth with mass effect on adjacent lung parenchyma. The other main entities in the differential diagnosis are metastatic meningioma and carcinoid tumor. Spindle cell lesions, such as schwannoma and solitary fibrous tumor, should also be considered if the architectural pattern in fibroblastic. Excluding primary intracranial or spinal meningioma on imaging is essential for the diagnosis of PM. PMs are generally negative for S100, cytokeratins, and the neuroendocrine markers chromogranin and synaptophysin, all of which can be useful in sorting out the differential diagnosis. As rare cases with aggressive behavior have been described, it is recommended to grade the tumors according to the WHO system for central nervous system meningiomas, as this can have prognostic relevance.

HISTOLOGIC FEATURES

- Well-circumscribed intraparenchymal nodule with a homogeneous population of epithelioid or spindle cells in whorls and short fascicles.
- Uniform nonatypical cells, positive for PR, EMA, and CD56.

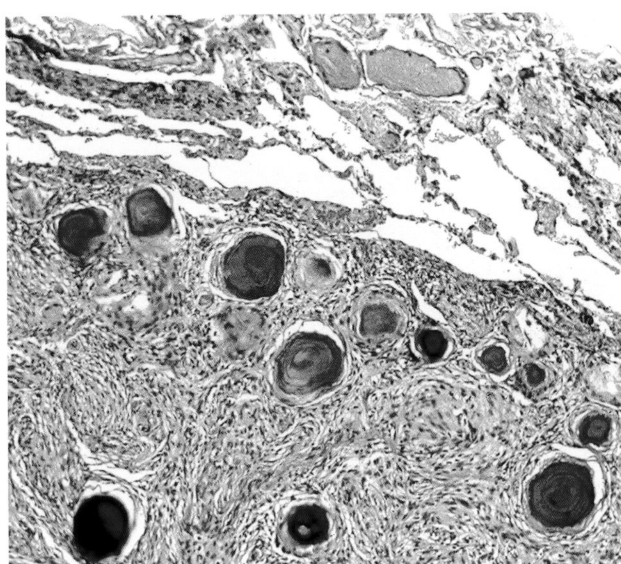

Figure 46.1 Well-circumscribed intraparenchymal mass with a pushing border. This case demonstrates a fibroblastic pattern with numerous psammomatous calcifications.

Section **5**

Pulmonary Histiocytic Proliferations

Anja C. Roden

Histiocytic disorders are rare diseases derived from macrophages or dendritic cells. In 2016, the Histiocyte Society revised the classification of histiocytoses to include (1) Langerhans-related histiocytoses, (2) cutaneous and mucocutaneous histiocytoses, (3) malignant histiocytoses, (4) Rosai–Dorfman disease, and (5) hemophagocytic lymphohistiocytosis and macrophage activation syndrome. The group of Langerhans-related histiocytoses is comprised of Langerhans-cell histiocytosis, Erdheim–Chester disease, and extracutaneous juvenile xanthogranuloma. Erdheim–Chester disease was added to the Langerhans-related histiocytoses, as it was found that nearly 20% of patients with that disease also have Langerhans-cell histiocytosis lesions. Furthermore, mutations of genes involved in the mitogen-activated protein kinase (MAPK) pathway, including *BRAF* and *MAP2K* mutations, have been identified in a subset of patients with both Langerhans-cell histiocytoses and Erdheim–Chester disease. For instance, *BRAF*^{V600E} mutations were found in 28% to 89% cases of pulmonary Langerhans-cell histiocytosis (PLCH) and 57.5% to 100% cases of Erdheim–Chester disease. *BRAF*^{V600E} mutations also recently have been identified in a subset ([intra]cranial) of juvenile xanthogranulomas. Other histiocytoses in which *BRAF*^{V600E} mutations were identified include Langerhans-cell sarcoma (17% to 100%), histiocytic sarcoma (0% to 62.5%), follicular dendritic cell sarcoma (18.5%), and giant-cell tumors (7%). However, this mutation has not been found in Rosai–Dorfman disease. *MAP2K1* (*MEK1*) mutations have also been identified in 46% of Langerhans-cell histiocytosis cases in one study. *MAP2K1* and *BRAF*^{V600E} mutations appear to be mutually exclusive in Langerhans-cell histiocytosis.

In the lung, although overall infrequent, the most common histiocytic disorder is PLCH, whereas involvement by Erdheim–Chester disease, Rosai–Dorfman disease, and other histiocytic proliferations is very rare. Morphologic, immunophenotypical, ultrastructural, and molecular features that might aid in the distinction of PLCH, Erdheim–Chester disease, and Rosai–Dorfman disease are summarized in Table 1.

Table 1. Morphologic, Immunophenotypical, Ultrastructural, and Molecular Features That Might Aid in the Distinction of the Most Common Histiocytic Proliferations in the Lung

	Pulmonary Langerhans-Cell Histiocytosis	Erdheim–Chester Disease	Rosai–Dorfman Disease
Disease distribution	Bronchiolocentric Upper lobe predominant	Lymphangitic	Lymphangitic
Characteristic cell	Medium to large epithelioid cells with ample pale to eosinophilic cytoplasm and folded or wrinkled nuclei with one to two conspicuous nucleoli	Foamy cytoplasm	Abundant pink or clear cytoplasm Emperipolesis
Morphologic features	Nodules comprised of Langerhans cells and various numbers of acute and chronic inflammatory cells including eosinophils Cyst formation Stellate scar in advanced disease	+/– Fibrosis	+/– Fibrosis
Immunophenotype			
CD1a/langerin (CD207)	+	–	–
S100	+	+/–	+
CD68	+/–	+	+
Factor XIIIa	–	+	+
Birbeck granule	Present	Absent	Absent
BRAF^{V600E} mutation	28%–40%	57%–100%	None

47

Pulmonary Langerhans-Cell Histiocytosis

Anja C. Roden

Pulmonary Langerhans-cell histiocytosis (PLCH) (formerly known as *histiocytosis X* or *eosinophilic granuloma*) is a disease of young adults and occurs in the second to fourth decades of life. There is no sex predilection. Smoking has been implicated in the pathogenesis of PLCH, as >90% of patients with the disease are current or former smokers. Moreover, smoking cessation is the most effective and important treatment in these patients.

On gross examination, PLCH is characterized by a fine nodular (in general up to 15 mm) infiltrate. In advanced disease the lungs will appear hyperinflated and reveal cystic changes in a predominantly upper lobe distribution. On microscopy, PLCH is characterized by nodules that comprise Langerhans cells and various numbers of chronic and acute inflammatory cells. These nodules are typically in a bronchiolocentric and upper lobe–predominant distribution. Eventually, the cellular infiltrates lead to destruction of small airways and adjacent alveolar structures and result in cyst formation. Therefore, it is not surprising that 15% to 25% of patients with PLCH present with recurrent spontaneous pneumothorax. PLCH should be in fact excluded in a patient who presents with spontaneous pneumothorax. As the disease progresses, the destructive bronchiolitis will result in progressive dilatation of the lumina of small airways. Eventually, the small airways will be surrounded by fibrous tissue forming stellate bronchiolocentric scars and irregular parenchymal cystic lesions while the number of Langerhans cells diminishes. While in most cases PLCH is reversible, especially with smoking cessation, in some cases the disease might only be suggested by centrilobular scars and cystic changes with an upper lobe–predominant pattern; however, Langerhans cells cannot be identified anymore.

Pulmonary hypertension is common in PLCH and can be severe, affecting 17% to 92% of these patients.

Usually, PLCH is limited to the lung. However, occasionally the lung can be involved by systemic Langerhans-cell histiocytosis. Although the histomorphologic features are similar, in contrast to PLCH, systemic Langerhans-cell histiocytosis is not associated with smoking and occurs in younger patients.

Although PLCH was considered a reactive process for a long time, recent evidence showed that 28% to 89% of PLCH harbor $BRAF^{V600E}$ mutation. *MAP2K1* mutations have also been identified in 18% of PLCH cases. These findings indicate that at least a subset of these cases represents a clonal process. These findings might also suggest that therapies targeting the MAPKinase pathway can be potentially useful in therapy-refractory patients with PLCH. While in many patients the disease resolves with smoking cessation, in some patients the disease progresses and patients might ultimately require lung transplantation.

HISTOLOGIC FEATURES

- Langerhans cells with interspersed chronic and/or acute inflammatory infiltrate, including a variable number of eosinophils, form nodules in the vicinity of small airways.
- Langerhans cells are characteristically large with abundant pale to eosinophilic cytoplasm; irregular nuclear borders; wrinkled, folded, or coffee bean- or kidney-shaped nuclei; and one to two conspicuous nucleoli.
- The nodules of Langerhans cells might lead to destruction of small airways and might be in the wall of cysts.
- Organizing pneumonia might be seen at the edge of the lesion, although extensive organizing pneumonia is not a typical feature of PLCH.
- Bronchiolocentric stellate scars are a characteristic of progressive disease. Typically, there are no or only few residual Langerhans cells present in late-stage disease. Honeycomb changes might occur.
- The background lung parenchyma typically shows other smoking-related changes, including emphysema, respiratory bronchiolitis, or desquamative interstitial pneumonia.
- Langerhans cells express S100, CD1a, and langerin (CD207) and are negative for CD68.
- In some cases, Langerhans cells are positive for the $\textit{BRAF}^{V600E}$ mutation–specific antibody by immunohistochemistry.
- The tennis-racket-shaped Birbeck granules are the hallmark of Langerhans-cell histiocytosis by ultrastructural analysis; however, this technique is not necessary for the diagnosis of PLCH.

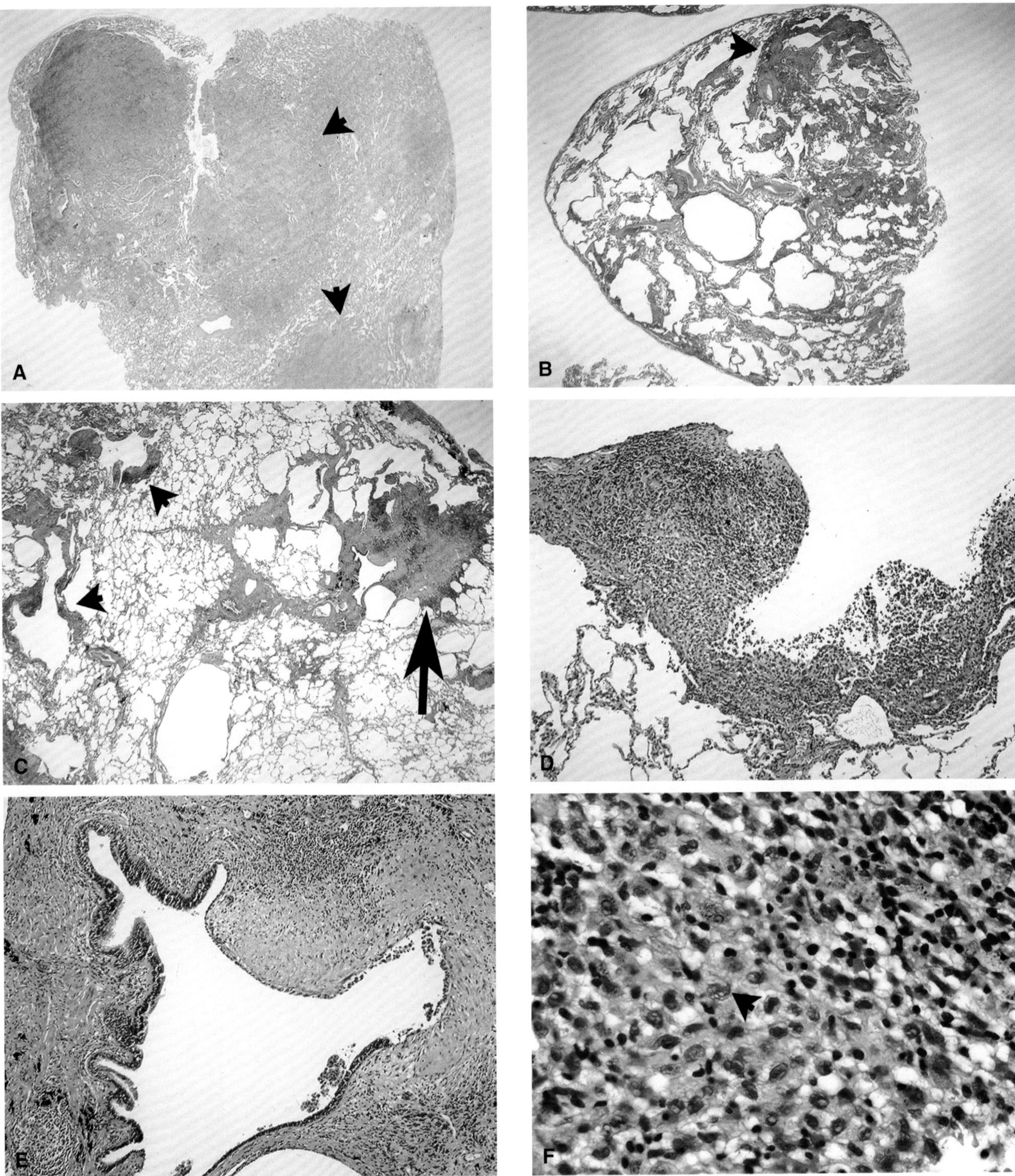

Figure 47.1 PLCH can present as large pulmonary nodular infiltrates (**A,** *arrows*), as vague bronchiolocentric nodules (**B,** *arrow*) in a background of emphysema (**B**), or as cellular (**C,** *short arrows,* **and D**) and fibrotic (**C,** *long arrow,* **and E**) nodules in the wall of cysts. The cellular nodules comprise large Langerhans cells (**F,** *arrow*) characterized by ample pale cytoplasm and irregular nuclei with conspicuous nucleoli and interspersed mixed inflammatory cells, including eosinophils, lymphocytes, and neutrophils (**G**). Focal organizing pneumonia might also be apparent (**H**). Langerhans cells express CD1a (**I**) and langerin (**J**), and in a subset of patients Langerhans cells mark with the $BRAF^{V600E}$ mutation–specific antibody (**K**). Some patients with PLCH present with spontaneous pneumothorax, which in this case was treated with talc pleurodesis (**L**, note nonnecrotizing granuloma with polarizable talc, *L inset*). The background lung parenchyma often shows smoking-related changes including intra-alveolar pigmented smoker's macrophages (**M**), which sometimes can also be found within the lesional nodules (**N,** *arrow*). **O:** These lung explants show upper lobe–predominant cystic changes characteristic of long-standing PLCH. Also note the peripheral lower lobe fibrosis with honeycomb changes in this case. These cases are characterized by extensive cystic changes with bronchiolocentric stellate scars (**P,** *arrow,* **Q, R**). Magnification: ×12.5 (**A–C and Q**), ×100 (**D, E, and R**), ×600 (**F, G, and N**), ×200 (**H and L**), ×400 (**I–K, L inset, and M**), scanned (**P**). (**O:** Reprinted from Roden AC, Yi ES. Pulmonary langerhans cell histiocytosis: an update from the pathologists' perspective. *Arch Pathol Lab Med.* 2016;140(3):230–240 with permission from *Archives of Pathology & Laboratory Medicine.* Copyright 2016 College of American Pathologists.)

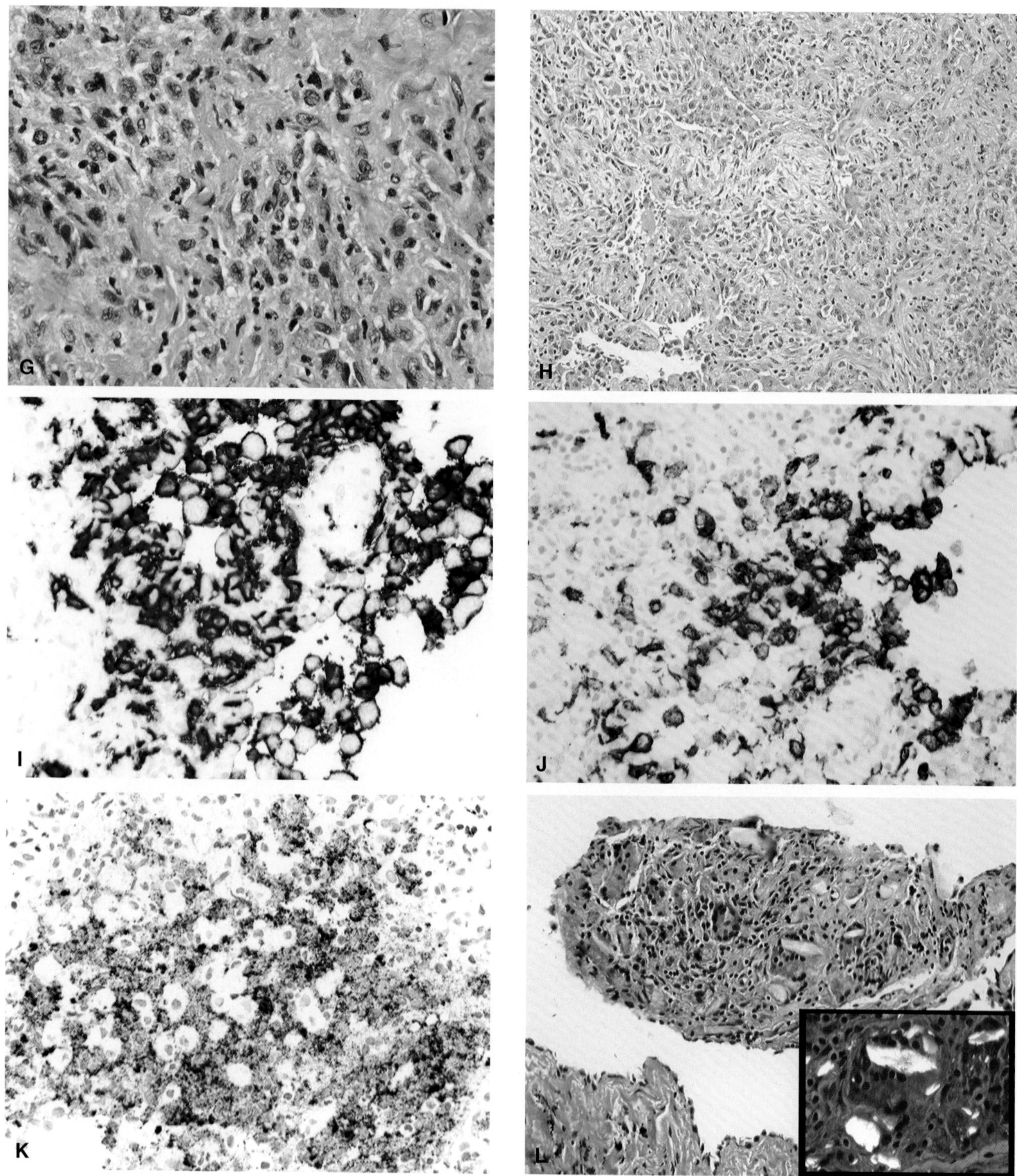

Figure 47.1 *(Continued)*

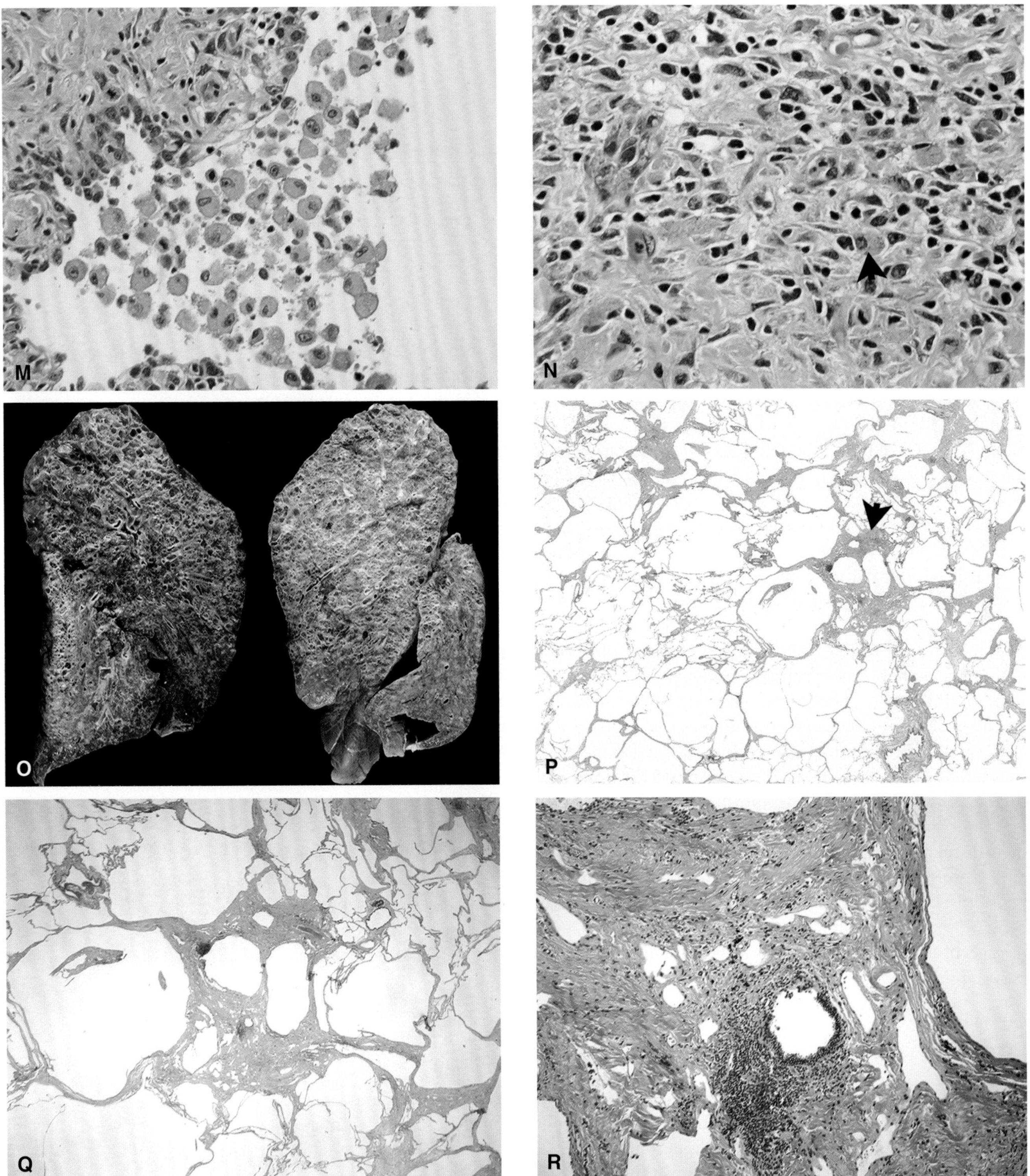

Figure 47.1 *(Continued)*

48 Erdheim–Chester Disease

Anja C. Roden

Erdheim–Chester disease (ECD) is an orphan disease, with only approximately 600 cases reported. ECD patients are more commonly male, are in general older than patients with pulmonary Langerhans-cell histiocytosis (PLCH), and are diagnosed in the fifth to seventh decades of life. This is a progressive disease with a mean or median time to death of only 1.6 to 2.3 years. ECD is a systemic disease that primarily involves the bone, in particular the femur and tibia, in 74% to >95% of cases. Neurologic symptoms occur in 25% to 50% of patients. The lungs are involved in 22% to 53% of patients; the pleura can also be involved in 20% to 41% of cases. Patients with pulmonary involvement usually present with nonspecific symptoms such as cough and dyspnea. In these patients, imaging studies may show mediastinal infiltration, pleural thickening and/or effusion, interlobular septal thickening, centrilobular nodular opacities, ground-glass opacities, and lung cysts.

Diagnostic criteria of ECD, as recently proposed by Haroche J et al. (2014), include "1. Characteristic histological findings [...]: foamy histiocyte infiltration of polymorphic granuloma and fibrosis or xanthogranulomatosis, with CD68-positive and CD1a-negative immunostaining; 2. Characteristic skeletal abnormalities: a) bilateral and symmetric cortical osteosclerosis of the diaphyseal and metaphyseal parts of the long bones on X-rays, and/or b) symmetric and abnormally intense labelling of the distal ends of the long bones of the legs, and in some cases arms, as revealed by 99Tc bone scintigraphy." Positron emission tomography–computed tomography has a high specificity for the disease.

While histiocytes in ECD can be distinguished from lesional cells in PLCH based on their distinct immunophenotypes, it has been shown that 20% of patients with ECD also have lesions of Langerhans-cell histiocytosis.

At least a subset of ECD cases have been shown to represent clonal processes, given that $BRAF^{V600E}$ mutations were identified in 57% to 100% of ECD cases. Clonality of histiocytes has also been shown in a few cases by the human androgene receptor (HUMARA) assay or karyotyping t(12;15;20)(q11;q24;p13.3).

HISTOLOGIC FEATURES

- Infiltration of clusters and nodules of large histiocytes with foamy cytoplasm and small nuclei. The lesional cells are often associated with lymphoplasmacytic infiltrate, interspersed multinucleated giant cells, and Touton cells.
- Histiocytes are forming vague nodules or xanthogranulomas.
- Histiocytes are distributed in a lymphangitic pattern (bronchovascular bundles, subpleural space, and interlobular septa).
- Eventually, fibrosis can occur, which will follow the lymphangitic distribution of the histiocytes.
- The lesional histiocytes mark with CD68 and sometimes with S100 and are negative for CD1a.

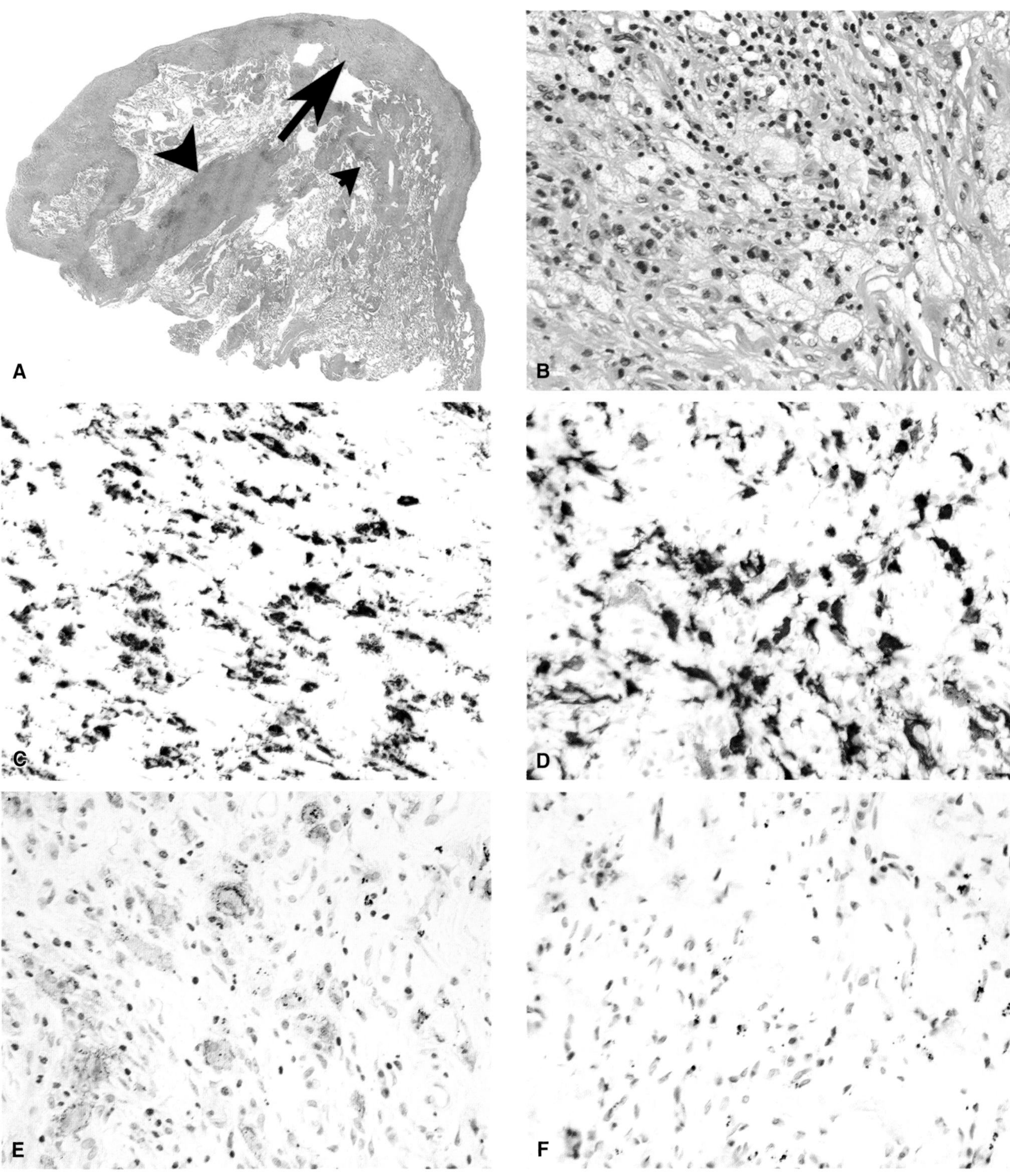

Figure 48.1 **A:** ECD is characterized by a histiocytic infiltrate with progressive fibrosis in a lymphangitic distribution involving areas around the broncho-vascular bundle *(short arrow)*, interlobular septa *(arrow head)*, and subpleural lung parenchyma *(long arrow)*. **B:** Cellular infiltrates are composed of large foamy histiocytes with small nuclei and interspersed lymphocytes. The lesional histiocytes express CD68 (**C**) and factor XIIIa (**D**), and in a few cases some of the histiocytes stain with S100 (**E**). They are negative for CD1a (**F**). **G:** In advanced cases, as in this autopsy case, the fibrosis can be extensive and diffuse with honeycomb changes. **H:** Nodules *(arrow)* composed of characteristic foamy histiocytes (**I**) might still be identified. Magnification scanned (**A**), ×400 (**B–F and I**), ×12.5 (**G and H**).

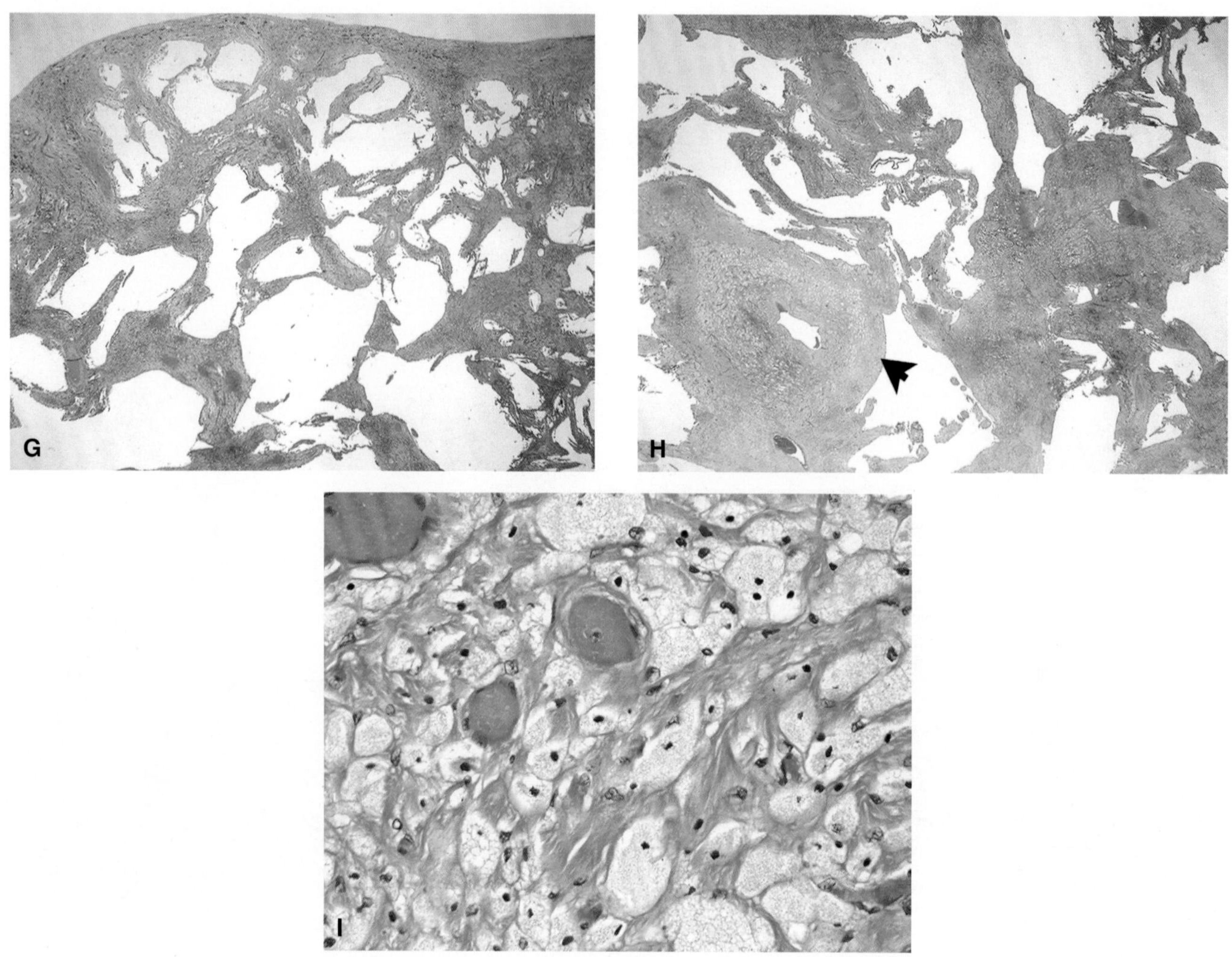

Figure 48.1 *(Continued)*

49

Rosai–Dorfman Disease

Anja C. Roden

Rosai–Dorfman disease (RDD) (synonym: sinus histiocytosis with massive lymphadenopathy) is primarily characterized by lymphadenopathy. There is a male predominance and the disease occurs usually in children and young adults. Patients most commonly present with fever, night sweats, fatigue, weight loss, and bilateral painless massive cervical lymphadenopathy. In patients with thoracic involvement, imaging studies will usually reveal mediastinal and hilar adenopathy. Cystic changes, parenchymal infiltrates, and airway disease might also be seen on imaging but are less common.

Large histiocytes with abundant pink to clear cytoplasm with engulfed erythrocytes, lymphocytes, plasma cells, and/or neutrophils (emperipolesis) are the hallmark of this disease. Nuclei are typically hypochromatic. Although other histiocytoses may also show emperipolesis, this is usually identified only in a few cells in contrast to RDD in which emperipolesis is a prominent finding. Abundant IgG4-positive plasma cells might be identified in RDD, which might make the distinction from IgG4-related disease sometimes difficult. *BRAF*^{V600E} mutations have not been identified in RDD cases.

Although RDD is usually a self-limited disease, occasionally patients may die because of the disease.

HISTOLOGIC FEATURES

- Nodular areas contain dense infiltrates of lymphocytes with intermixed large pale histiocytes, arranged both singly and in small clusters.
- The lesional histiocytes have abundant, eosinophilic to clear cytoplasm and round to oval nuclei with one or more prominent nucleoli.
- Nuclei may be multilobated and may exhibit mild atypia.
- Emperipolesis (engulfment of erythrocytes, lymphocytes, plasma cells, and/or neutrophils in the cytoplasm of the histiocytes) is the hallmark of the disease.
- Histiocytes infiltrate large airways; there can be a diffuse histiocytic infiltration of lung parenchyma in a lymphangitic distribution.
- Foamy alveolar macrophages, reactive type II pneumocytes, and admixed inflammatory cells are present in the background.
- Eventually fibrosis might occur, which will follow the lymphangitic distribution.
- The lesional cells mark with CD68 and S100 and lack staining with CD1a.

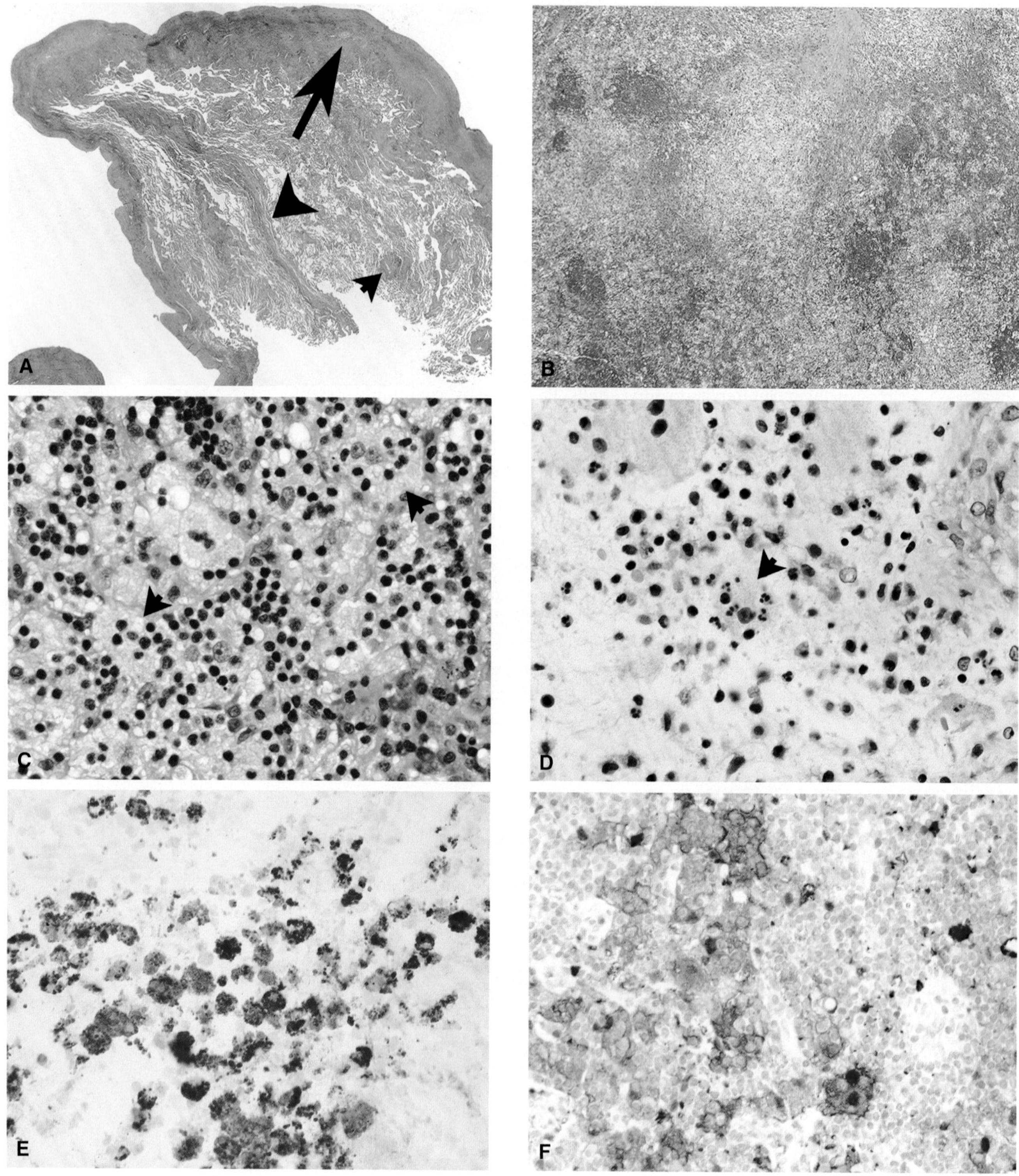

Figure 49.1 **A:** Cellular infiltrates and eventually fibrotic changes are often seen in a lymphangitic distribution around bronchovascular bundles *(short arrow)*, along the subpleural surface *(long arrow)*, or in interlobular septa *(arrow head)*. **B:** Cellular infiltrates are composed of large histiocytes with pale cytoplasm and varying numbers of inflammatory cells. Focal fibrosis is also present in the *upper part* of the picture. **C:** Emperipolesis is the hallmark of RDD and is characterized by the engulfment of lymphocytes *(***C***, arrows)*, neutrophils *(***D***, arrow)*, or other inflammatory cells by the histiocytes. The histiocytes are positive for CD68 (**E**) and S100 (**F**). Magnification: ×12.5 (**A**), ×40 (**B**), ×600 (**C and D**), and ×400 (**E and F**).

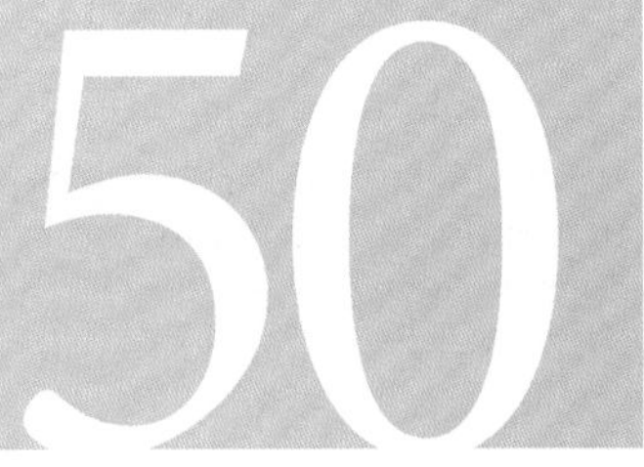

Other Pulmonary Histiocytic Proliferations

Anja C. Roden

Other histiocytic proliferations including follicular dendritic cell sarcomas and juvenile xanthogranulomas can occur in the lung but are extremely rare with only a few cases reported.

FOLLICULAR DENDRITIC CELL SARCOMAS

Follicular dendritic cell (FDC) sarcomas are intermediate-grade malignancies that usually occur in lymph nodes. FDCs are nonlymphoid antigen-presenting cells that form a meshwork in lymphoid follicles. They are also present extranodally where they are involved in the induction of immune responses. Ultrastructurally, they are characterized by long interwoven cell processes connected by well-developed desmosomes.

FDC sarcomas usually occur in young to middle-aged patients without gender predilection. Patients present with symptoms related to a mass lesion; systemic symptoms have also been described, including fevers, malaise, and weight loss. FDC sarcomas tend to recur (40%) and/or metastasize (25%) to lymph nodes, lungs, and liver. Necrosis, mitotic activity of more than 5/10 High Power Fields and significant nuclear atypia have been associated with metastasis and recurrence. FDC sarcomas are usually treated surgically although some patients undergo adjuvant therapy. Although other histiocytoses, such as pulmonary Langerhans-cell histiocytosis, Erdheim–Chester disease, or Rosai–Dorfman disease, usually do not enter the differential diagnosis because of sufficiently different morphologic appearances, the distinction of FDC sarcomas from interdigitating dendritic cell tumors/sarcomas (usually S100-positive, CD21-negative, lack desmosomes on electron microscopy), inflammatory myofibroblastic tumors (usually smooth muscle actin [SMA]-positive, can be ALK-positive, spindle cells have myofibroblastic features with more abundant eosinophilic cytoplasm and less cytologic atypia, more intermixed plasma cells), and sarcomatoid carcinomas (keratin-positive, negative for dendritic cell markers) can be challenging.

Histologic Features of Follicular Dendritic Cell Sarcoma

- Malignant spindle cells grow in fascicular, sheet-like, focally storiform or interlacing short fascicle patterns.
- Tumor cells have ill-defined cell borders, pale eosinophilic cytoplasm, and spindled to plump nuclei with vesicular chromatin and central, single nucleoli.
- Mitotic rates of the tumor cells vary.
- Fibrosis and necrosis can occur.
- Many lymphocytes and occasional plasma cells are interspersed with tumor cells.
- Neoplastic cells express clusterin and CD21; fascin is also usually expressed. CD23, CD35, and CD68 are also often expressed, whereas S100 is only expressed in a few such tumors. FDC sarcomas are negative for CD1a, CD45, and keratins.

JUVENILE XANTHOGRANULOMAS

Juvenile xanthogranulomas (JXGs) are usually encountered in children and adolescents; only approximately 15% of these cases occur in adults. JXGs present most commonly as cutaneous tumors with rapid growth and spontaneous regression within months or years. These lesions are rare in extracutaneous sites. If occurring at an extracutaneous site, a cutaneous JXG has usually been already diagnosed; however, on rare occasion, extracutaneous JXGs occur without a cutaneous component. The main tumor cells are thought to be dermal dendrocytes.

Histologic Features of Juvenile Xanthogranulomas

- Lesions are composed of a mixture of mononuclear and multinucleated cell types.
- JXTs consist of sheets of histiocytes. Although "early" lesions are composed of histiocytes with only little cytoplasmic lipid and homogeneous amphophilic or eosinophilic cytoplasm, older "classic" lesions consist of histiocytes with finely vacuolated or xanthomatous cytoplasm.
- Giant cells, including Touton giant cells, are typically interspersed with the histiocytes.
- Spindle-cell variants exist.
- A modest number of mixed inflammatory cells are usually present. Long-standing lesions might become fibrotic.
- Neoplastic cells express clusterin and CD21; fascin is usually also expressed. CD23, CD35, and CD68 are also often expressed while S100 is only expressed in a few such tumors. FDC sarcomas are negative for CD1a, CD45, and keratins.
- Ultrastructurally, bland fibrohistiocytic and/or xanthoma cells without Birbeck granules are identified. Nonspecific intracytoplasmic findings, such as dense bodies, worm-like bodies, and popcorn bodies, may be found.

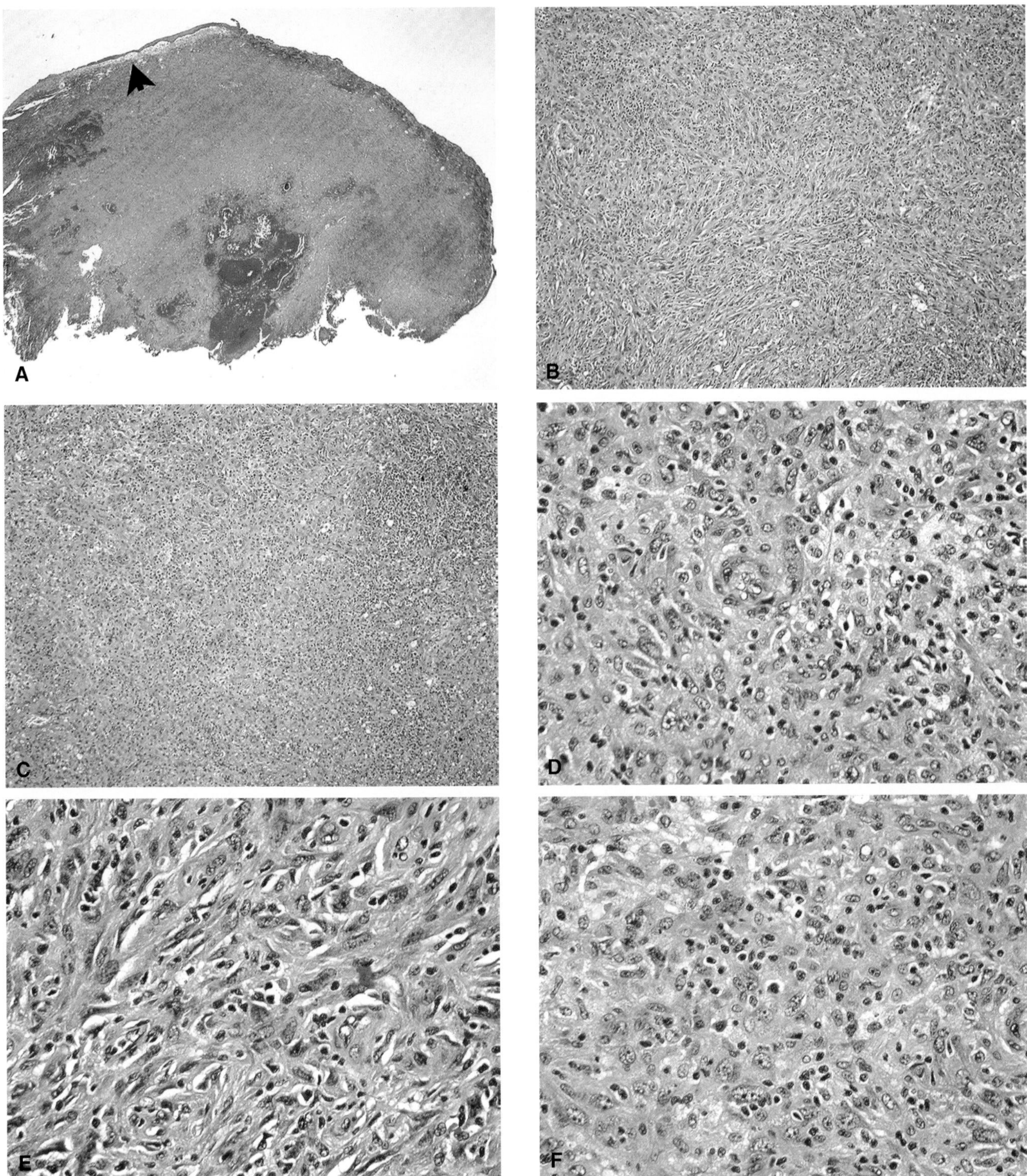

Figure 50.1 Follicular dendritic cell (FDC) sarcoma. **A:** This tumor presented clinically as an aggressive submucosal lesion in the right mainstem bronchus (note *arrow* pointing toward epithelium with squamous metaplasia). The neoplastic cells are arranged in a focally storiform (**B**) or haphazard (**C**) pattern. **D-F:** The neoplastic cells are elongated, spindled, or epithelioid with vesicular chromatin and prominent nucleoli. Focally chronic inflammatory cells, including lymphocytes, plasma cells, and eosinophils, are interspersed (**F**). The neoplastic cells are diffusely positive for clusterin (**G**), CD68 (**H**), and CD163 (**I**) and are negative for S100 (**J**), an immunophenotype characteristic for FDC sarcoma. Magnification: ×12.5 (**A**), ×100 (**B and C**), ×400 (**D–J**).

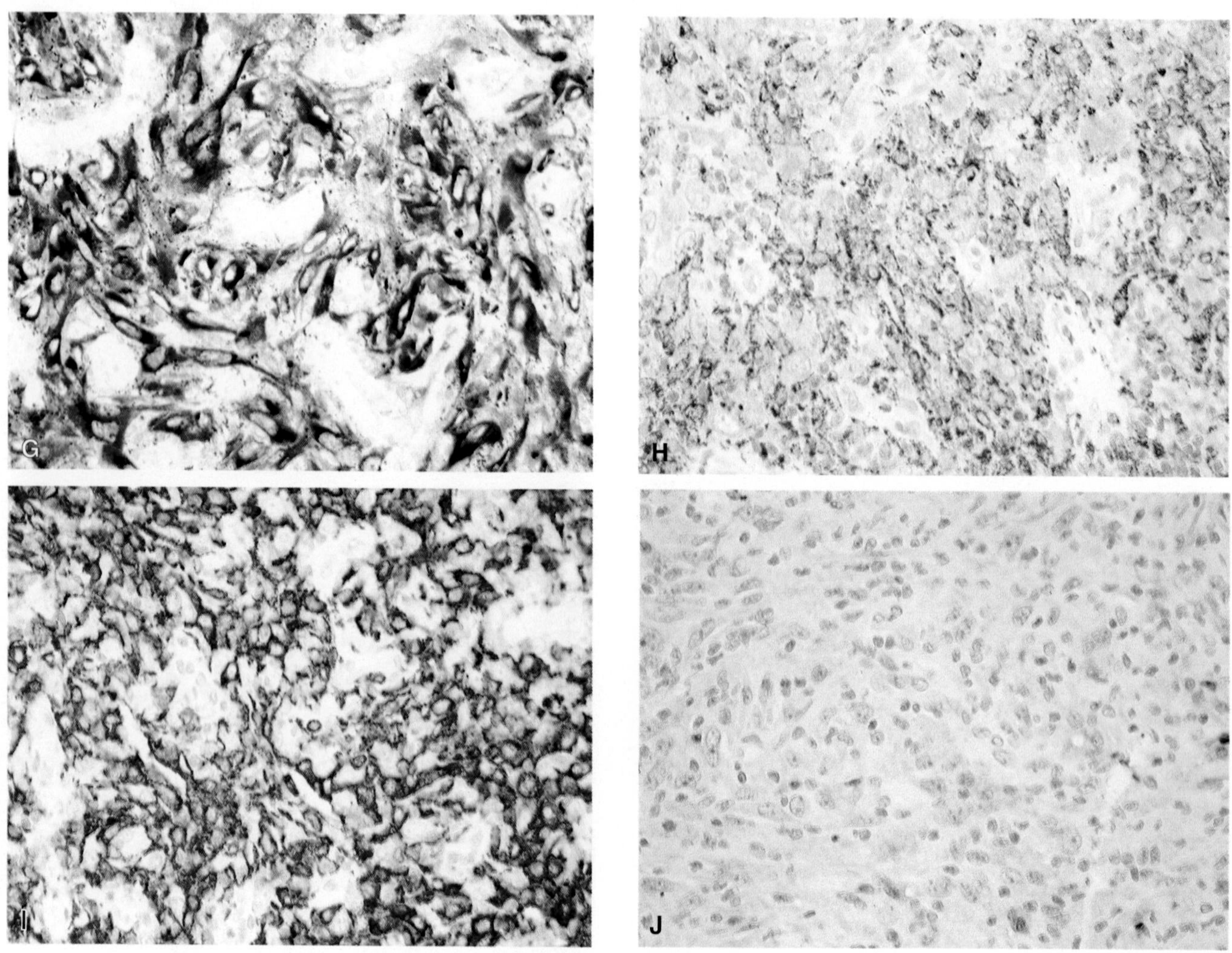

Figure 50.1 *(Continued)*

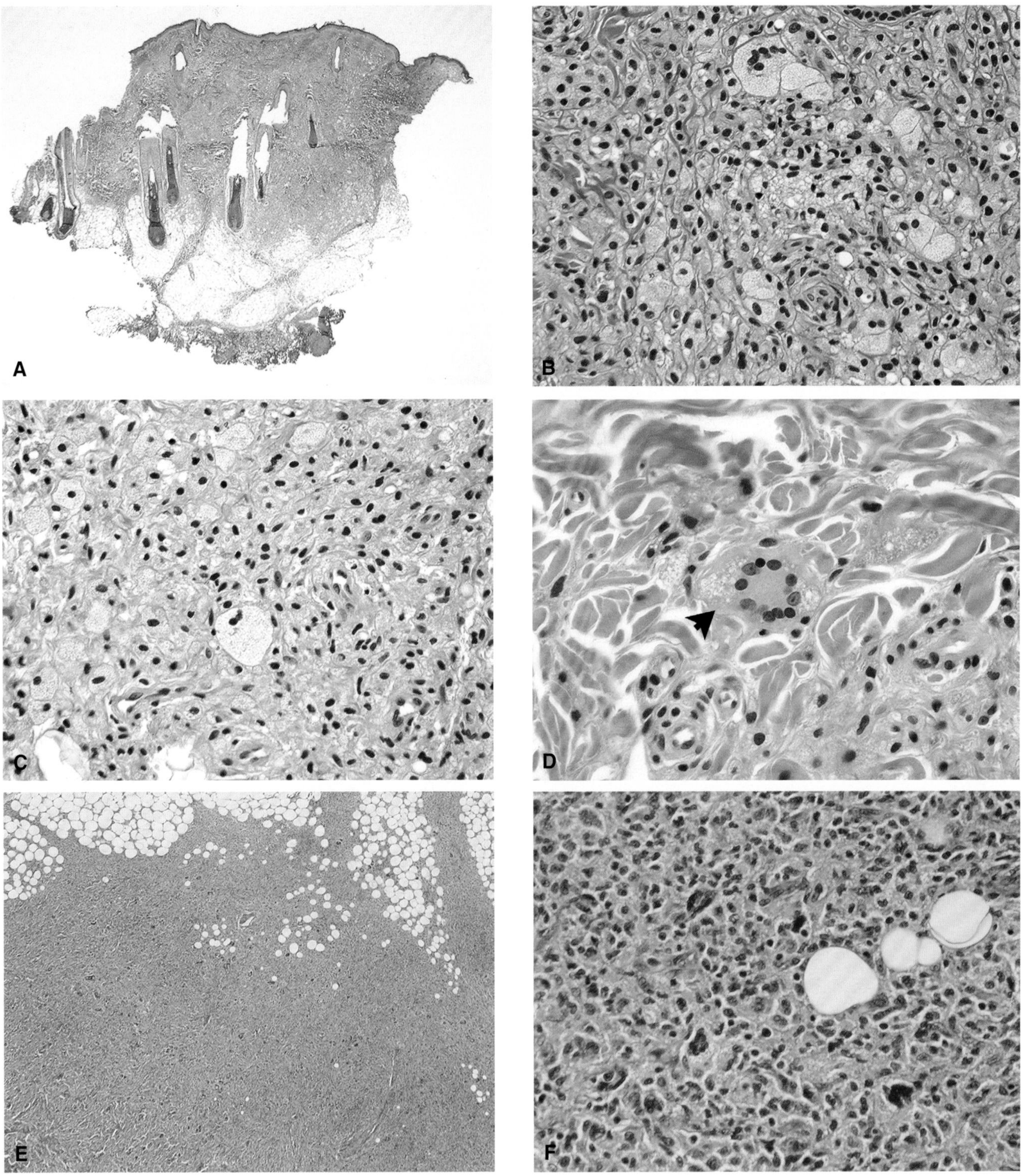

Figure 50.2 Juvenile xanthogranuloma (JXG). **A:** This epidermal and dermal infiltrate is composed of large lipid-rich histiocytes (**B and C**) that have one to multiple small nuclei. Touton giant cells (**D,** *arrow*) are also present. These morphologic features are typical of "classic" JXG. **E:** This thigh lesion is composed of an infiltrate of histiocytes that are characterized by a higher nuclear to cytoplasmic ratio than in the first case and more amphophilic and less lipid-laden cytoplasm. **F:** Numerous giant cells are present. These features are often seen in "early" JXG. Magnification: ×12.5 (**A**), ×400 (**B, C, and F**), ×600 (**D**), ×40 (**E**).

Section 6

Benign and Borderline Lymphoid Proliferations

▸ Kirtee Raparia

51 Follicular Bronchiolitis and Follicular Bronchitis

Kirtee Raparia

Follicular bronchiolitis and follicular bronchitis are polyclonal hyperplasia and expansion of the bronchus-associated lymphoid tissue from chronic antigen stimulation around peribronchiolar regions and distal bronchi at bronchial bifurcations. These hyperplastic lymphoid follicles are primarily composed of polytypic B cells, with minimal lymphocytic infiltration into the adjacent alveolar interstitium and bronchiolar epithelium. Patients usually present with follicular bronchiolitis and follicular bronchitis in their middle ages, although cases in children have been reported. It is slightly more common in males than females. It is often associated with collagen vascular diseases, particularly rheumatoid arthritis, congenital or acquired immunodeficiency disorders such as IgA deficiency, AIDS, and common variable immunodeficiency, hypersensitivity disorders associated with peripheral eosinophilia, and chronic obstructive pulmonary diseases. Symptoms include insidious onset of shortness of breath, dyspnea, cough, and weight loss. Follicular bronchiolitis involves the lung bilaterally and presents as centrilobular nodules, which can range from 3 to 12 mm in size and ground-glass opacities on computed tomography scan. Surgical lung biopsy is usually necessary to establish a diagnosis, especially in the absence of suggestive clinical history. These patients have overall good prognosis but can be variable in younger patients. Treatment involves management of the underlying disease, steroids, and immunosuppression.

HISTOLOGIC FEATURES

- It is difficult to appreciate these lesions grossly because they are small.
- Histologically, follicular bronchiolitis is characterized by eccentric peribronchiolar accumulation of hyperplastic lymphoid follicles primarily composed of polymorphous lymphoid cells, which has a tendency to distort and narrow the bronchiolar lumen.
- There is minimal interstitial involvement and the airspaces are not involved.
- Follicular bronchiolitis is composed of a mixture of B and T lymphocytes, which can be confirmed by CD20 and CD3 immunostains, respectively.
- The B cells in these lesions are polytypic, expressing both kappa and lambda light chains.

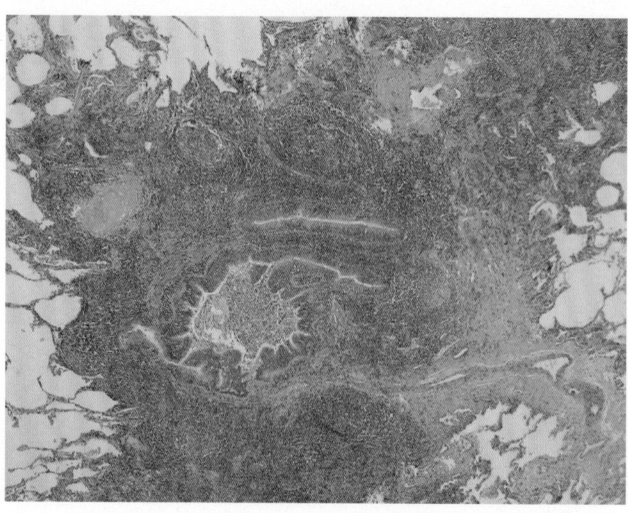

Figure 51.1 The bronchi and bronchioles are associated with hyperplastic polyclonal lymphoid follicles with reactive germinal centers compressing the lumens (hematoxylin–eosin, original magnification ×40).

Nodular Lymphoid Hyperplasia

52

Kirtee Raparia

Nodular lymphoid hyperplasia (NLH), referred to in the past as pseudolymphoma, is a rare reactive lymphoproliferative disorder presenting in middle age, although cases in children have been reported. NLH is associated with altered immune status (collagen vascular disease, acquired immune deficiency, dysgammaglobulinemia) but can also occur as an isolated finding in an asymptomatic individual. When symptoms are present, they include cough and dyspnea. NLH presents as a nodule, mass, or focal area of mass-like consolidation within the lung on chest radiographs and CT. Lesions are usually single but can be multiple. Air bronchograms are often present within the lesion on CT. Mediastinal and hilar lymphadenopathies, as well as pleural effusion, are absent. Treatment is surgical resection.

HISTOLOGIC FEATURES

- NLH presents as a nodule or mass-like lesion with relatively sharp demarcation from the surrounding normal lung parenchyma.
- NLH is composed of a polymorphous population of lymphoid cells (both B cells and T cells), lymphoid follicles with multiple germinal centers, and lymphoplasmacytosis in the interfollicular regions.
- Variable amounts of fibrosis may also be present in the lesion, and occasional giant cells and macrophages can be seen.
- Lesions typically lack lymphoepithelial lesions, which are seen commonly in lymphoma.
- NLH must be differentiated from MALT lymphoma, which is more common, and other rare types of lymphomas such as follicular lymphoma and mantle cell lymphoma.
- Immunohistochemical and flow cytometry studies are necessary to determine the polyclonal nature of the populations of lymphocytes and plasma cells, as well as molecular genetic analysis, to ensure that no rearrangements of the immunoglobulin light or heavy chains are present. Performing IgG and IgG4 stains to rule out IgG4-related disease is also recommended in nodules with increased plasma cells and the presence of storiform fibrosis.

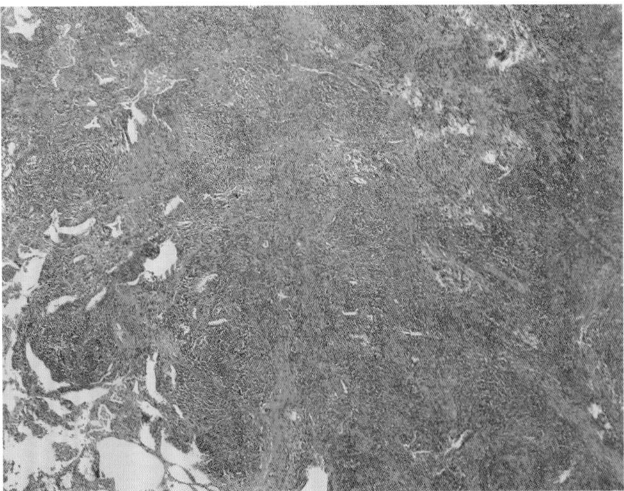

Figure 52.1 The nodule shows lymphocytes admixed with plasma cells and intervening fibrosis with relatively sharp demarcation (hematoxylin and eosin stain; original magnification 40×).

53 Lymphoid Interstitial Pneumonia

▸ Kirtee Raparia

Lymphoid interstitial pneumonia (LIP) is a rare benign polyclonal lymphoproliferative disorder of the lung parenchyma, presenting as extensive and diffuse disease. The updated 2013 American Thoracic Society–European Respiratory Society classification of the idiopathic interstitial pneumonias (IIPs) classifies idiopathic lymphoid interstitial pneumonia as a rare interstitial pneumonia. It occurs most commonly between the fourth and seventh decades of life, with slight predilection in women, and can arise in children as well. LIP has been associated with multiple diseases such as human immunodeficiency virus infection in pediatric population, common variable immunodeficiency, collagen vascular diseases such as Sjogren syndrome, and Castleman disease. LIP has been associated with chronic infections such as Ebstein–Barr virus, human herpes virus-8, and mycoplasma and is also a known complication of graft-versus-host disease in bone marrow transplantation patients. Patients with LIP present with symptoms including insidious onset of cough, dyspnea, and weight loss. Approximately 60% of patients with LIP have dysproteinemia, usually in the form of hypergammaglobulinemia and less often as hypogammaglobulinemia. Radiographic findings are nonspecific and range from nodular or reticular opacities in the lower lungs to no findings at all. CT shows ground-glass opacities, centrilobular nodules, bronchovascular bundle thickening, and peribronchovascular cysts, which predominately affect the lower lungs. Treatment involves corticosteroids as well as treatment of the underlying disease and outcome depends principally on the latter. Progression to lymphoma is seen in limited cases (~5% cases).

HISTOLOGIC FEATURES

- Diffuse infiltration of lymphocytes (predominately T cells intermixed with polytypic B cells) and plasma cells along the alveolar interstitium, resulting in expansion of the alveolar septa, with accentuation along bronchovascular bundles and lobular septa.
- Ill-defined granulomas and giant cells have been found in 20% to 50% of cases.
- Lymphoid follicles primarily composed of B cells, lymphoepithelial lesions, and cellular infiltrates around the vessels are variably present.
- Focal, microscopic honeycomb changes may be present.
- Immunohistochemical studies and flow cytometry studies are necessary to determine the polyclonal nature of the lymphocytes and distinguish LIP from low-grade lymphomas.
- Differential diagnosis is primarily from idiopathic cellular nonspecific interstitial pneumonia and mucosa-associated lymphoid tissue lymphomas.

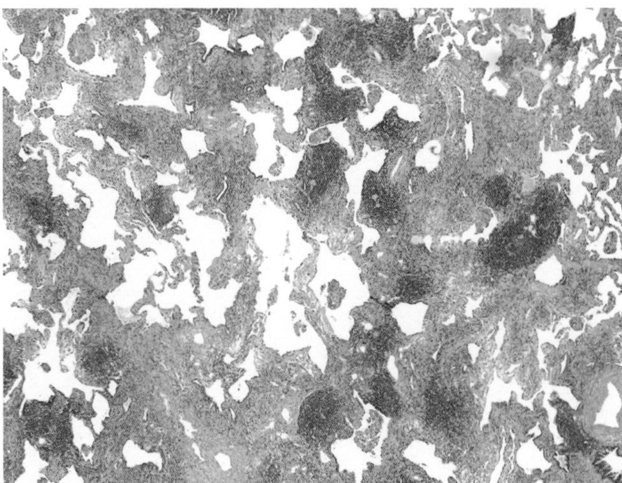

Figure 53.1 Lung parenchyma showing dominant interstitial pattern of distribution of lymphocytes mixed with plasma cells and formation of lymphoid follicles, commonly seen in adults and children with altered immune status (hematoxylin and eosin stain, original magnification 40×).

Section 7

Focal Lesions

▶ Ross A. Miller

Apical Caps

54

Ross A. Miller

Apical caps are scars that form in the apical aspect of the lung or superior segments of the lower lobes. They are typically found in older men and tend to be associated with a lower socioeconomic status. Early studies suggested tuberculosis was the underlying cause; however, the current belief is that the scarring results from a combination of chronic ischemia and infection. Findings include pyramidal to triangular-shaped gray–blue areas of elastotic scarring with adjacent emphysematous change occurring in the apices or superior aspects of the lower lung lobes. Reactive pneumocytes are often seen adjacent to the area of scar formation.

HISTOLOGIC FEATURES

- Pyramidal to triangle-shaped; the broad aspect or "base" is oriented along the pleura.
- Gray to blue elastotic scar formation.
- High power shows fragmented connective tissue fibers similar to solar elastotic change seen in the skin.
- Adjacent emphysematous change and reactive/hyperplastic pneumocytes.

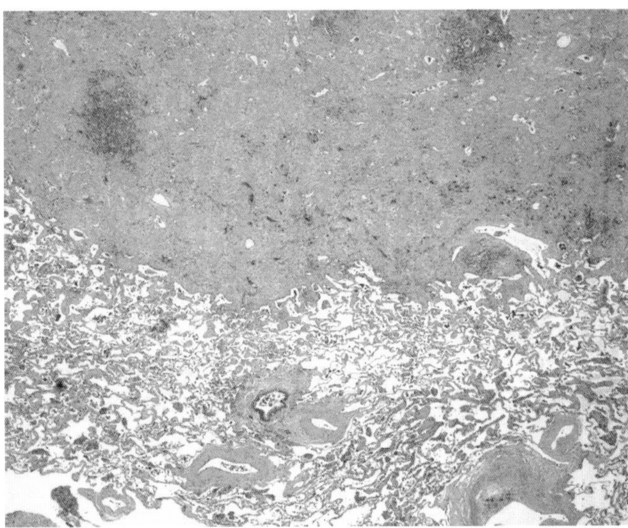

Figure 54.1 Subpleural fibrosis of an apical cap: the scar has a gray to blue hue and scattered lymphoid aggregates are seen.

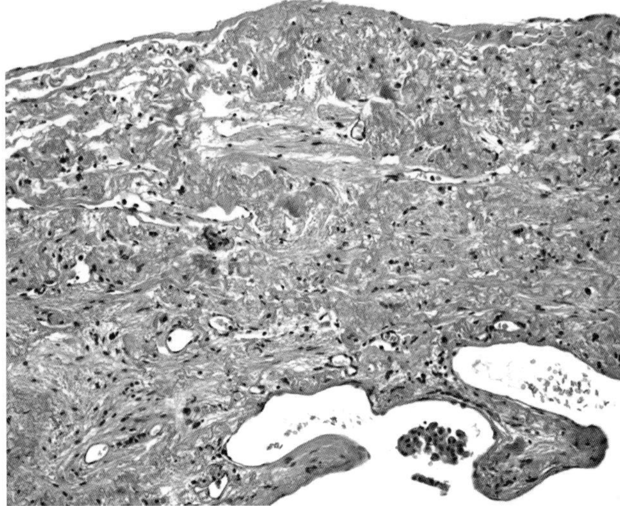

Figure 54.2 Gray to blue fibrosis of an apical cap: the connective tissue fibers are fragmented similar to the change seen in solar elastosis of the skin.

55

Focal Scars

Ross A. Miller

Localized fibrosis representing focal scar formation can occur secondary to a variety of conditions in the lung. Probably, the most frequent cause of localized scar formation is a healed infectious process. However, virtually any injurious process (for example, vascular insult or trauma) can potentially lead to focal fibrosis and scar as the lung has a finite number of ways to respond to injury.

Focal scars typically consist of fibrous and collagenous tissue forming a small nodular focus within the lung parenchyma. The adjacent alveolar septa may have a slightly wider interstitial space due to localized extensions of fibrosis. Associated findings can include chronic inflammation, smooth muscle hyperplasia, calcification, or ossification. Occasionally, an obliterated small- to medium-sized vessel can be seen adjacent to the process. The key feature for correct recognition is that the process is *localized*. Therefore, in a small biopsy specimen, it is essential to know if the intended biopsy target is from a localized lesion or if a diffuse interstitial process is being considered to avoid misclassification of the fibrosis. Without knowing the clinical or radiographic findings, the microscopic differential diagnosis may include a focal pulmonary scar, a fibrosing interstitial lung disease, or even a late lesion of pulmonary Langerhans cell histiocytosis (PLCH). It should be noted that the late lesions of PLCH can be almost exclusively composed of fibrous tissue and lack the characteristic Langerhans cells; the lesions are typically stellate in appearance and smoking-related changes are often seen in the adjacent lung. Of course, the identification of any residual Langerhans cells and/or eosinophils can aid in the diagnosis.

HISTOLOGIC FEATURES

- A *localized* nodular focus of fibrous tissue; often a nonspecific finding.
- Focal chronic inflammation, smooth muscle hyperplasia, calcification, or ossification may be seen.
- Sometimes, an obliterated small- to medium-sized vessels is associated with the scar.

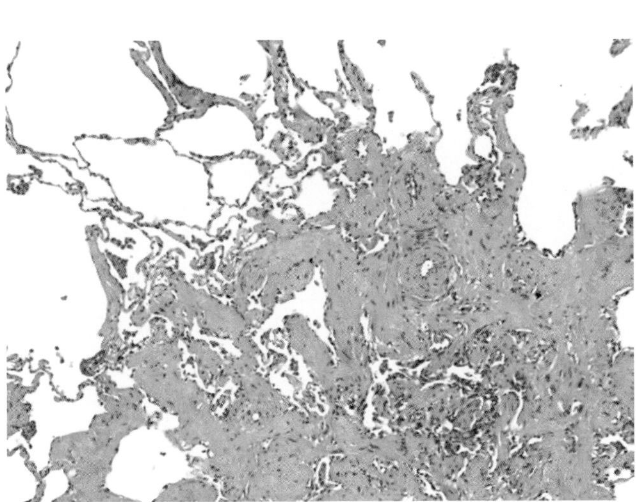

Figure 55.1 Focal scar in lung parenchyma.

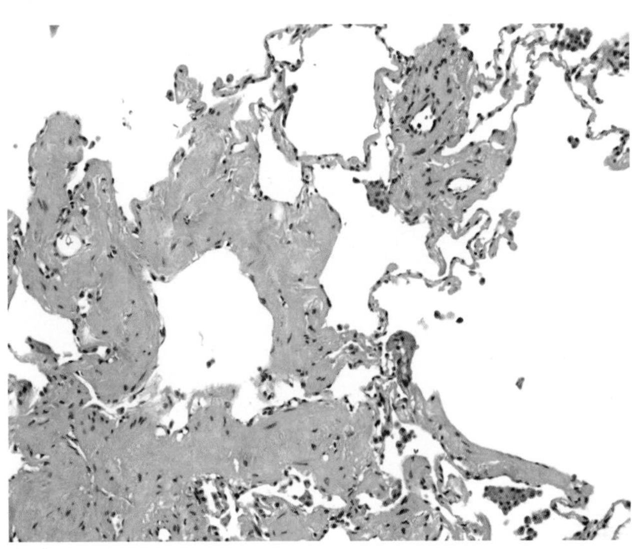

Figure 55.2 The scar is composed of dense fibrous tissue; small entrapped blood vessels can be seen.

56 Pulmonary Ossification

Ross A. Miller
Mary Beth Beasley

Metaplastic bone formation can occur in the lung; usually it is seen in branching or linear arrangements following the pulmonary interstitium. It is most commonly seen in long-standing fibrosis and often signifies a chronic fibrosing process. Occasionally, bone marrow elements can be identified within these metaplastic bone deposits.

In contrast to the linear or branching arrangements; nodules of metaplastic bone can be seen, which is termed nodular ossification. Nodular ossification is typically intra-alveolar in distribution. This type of metaplastic bone formation is associated with venous hypertension, and bone marrow elements are rarely observed.

HISTOLOGIC FEATURES

- Linear or branching metaplastic bone that tends to follow the interstitium; this type typically originates from long-standing fibrosis and signifies a chronic process.
- Ossified nodules are often intra-alveolar and have an association with pulmonary hypertension.

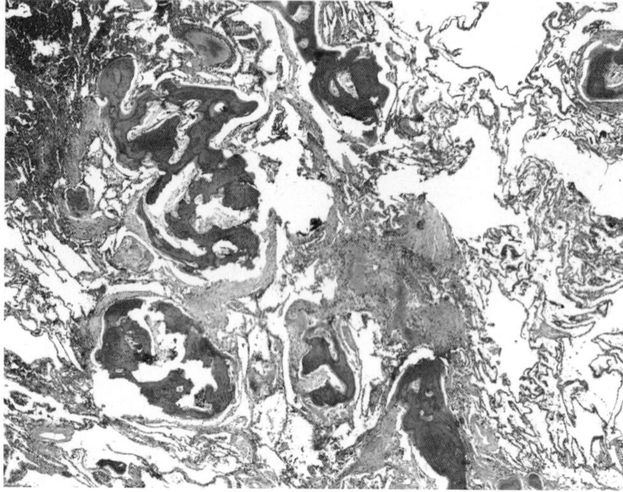

Figure 56.1 Low-power dendriform ossification shows linear and branching deposits of mature bone associated with fibrosis.

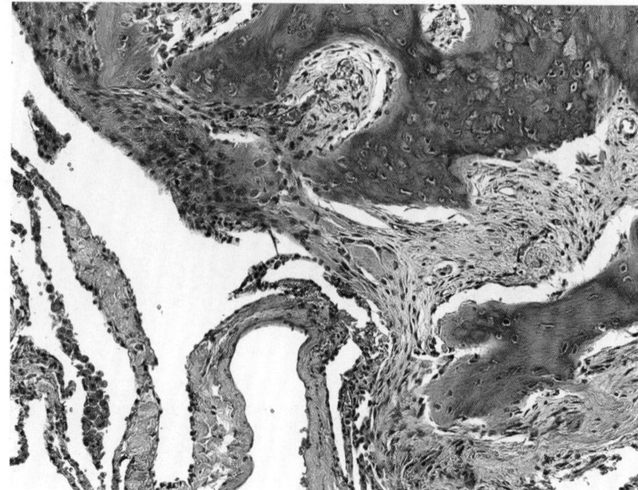

Figure 56.2 Higher power view shows the mature bone with fibrotic marrow.

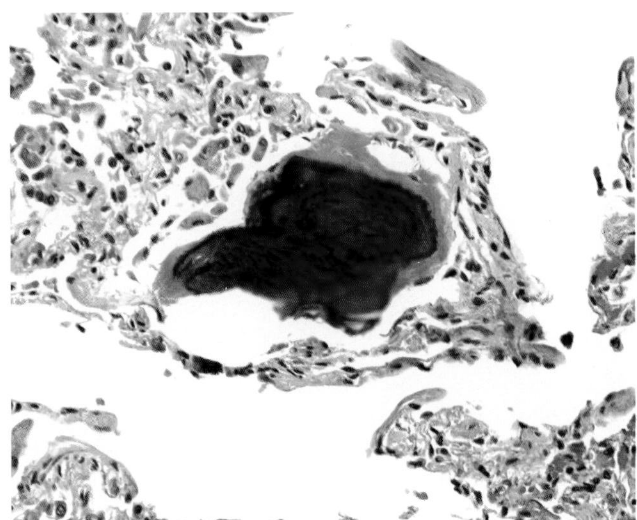

Figure 56.3 Nodular ossification shows irregular nodule of mature bone without marrow within an alveolar space.

Intrapulmonary Lymph Nodes

57

Ross A. Miller

Lymph nodes can be normally seen within lung parenchyma (termed *intrapulmonary lymph nodes*) and are often recognized on imaging studies. The typical distribution of intrapulmonary lymph nodes is peribronchial, septal, or subpleural. At times, they may be biopsied to rule out a neoplastic process, particularly in heavy smokers or in individuals who have a history of significant dust exposure, as the lymph nodes may become enlarged secondary to reactive change and/or an accumulation of pigmented histiocytes.

CYTOLOGIC FEATURES

- Benign intrapulmonary lymph nodes will have a polymorphous lymphoid population, scattered tingible body macrophages, and occasional follicular dendritic cells.
- Scattered pigmented macrophages may be present.

HISTOLOGIC FEATURES

- The excised lymph node will have an oval to round shape with a capsule, sinus, and normal constituents of a lymph node (cortex, paracortex, medulla, follicles).
- Sinus histiocytes, often containing pigment, is a common finding.

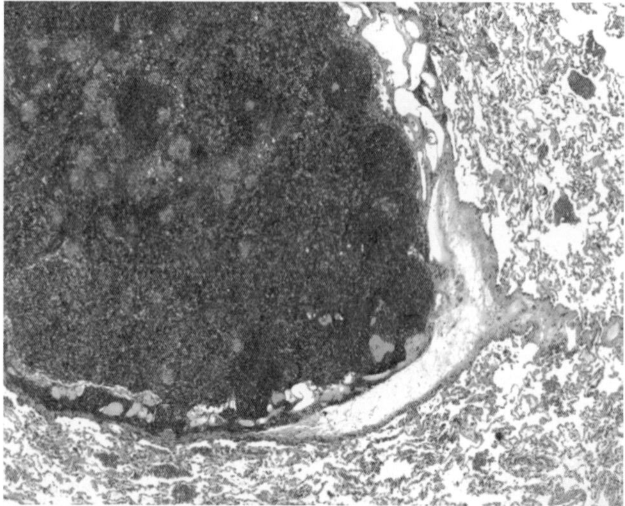

Figure 57.1 Intrapulmonary lymph node surrounded by normal lung parenchyma.

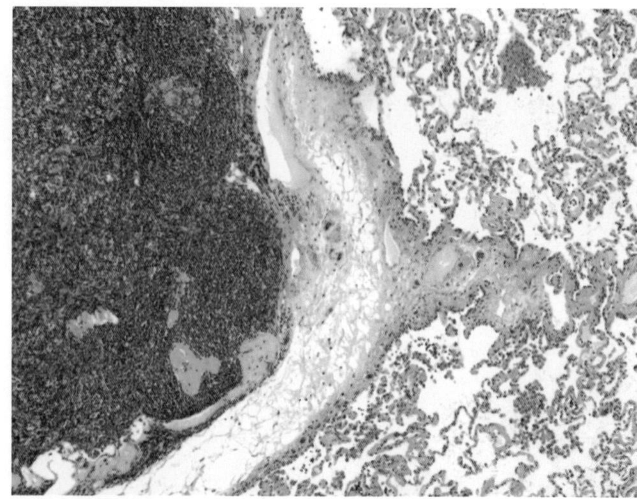

Figure 57.2 Higher power image of an intrapulmonary lymph node; the lymph node is surrounded by normal lung and has the normal constituents of a benign lymph node.

58

Rounded Atelectasis

▶ Ross A. Miller

When the pleura becomes scarred, the associated subpleural lung parenchyma can become atelectatic as a result of pleural folding and tension caused by the scar. This particular finding of scarred pleura and associated atelectatic change is termed rounded atelectasis. Around 50% of the time, rounded atelectasis is seen in the lower lobes; however, it can occur anywhere in the lung. Notable associations in the medical literature include asbestos exposure, postsurgery for coronary artery disease, and lymphangioleiomyomatosis. However, any process that can cause pleural scarring may result in the formation of rounded atelectasis. Imaging findings include a mass-like lesion forming along or adjacent to the pleura; as such, a neoplastic process may be a consideration.

HISTOLOGIC FEATURES

- Scarred and folded pleura with underlying atelectatic change of the lung parenchyma.
- A trichrome stain can highlight the folded and scarred pleura.

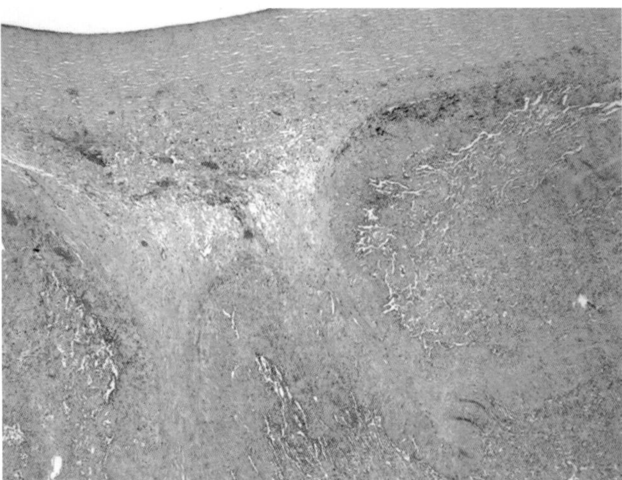

Figure 58.1 Rounded atelectasis: the pleura is scarred resulting in atelectatic change secondary to contraction. Note the infolding of scarred pleural tissue.

Amyloidosis (Nodular and Tracheobronchial)

59

▸ Ross A. Miller
▸ Sergio Pina-Oviedo

Nodular amyloidosis is a rare intrapulmonary lesion composed of extracellular amyloid material. When identified, the lesions are usually seen in adult patients and range in size from 1 to 4 cm. Often nodular amyloidosis is incidentally found on imaging studies as a mass-like lesion and a neoplasm may be suspected. Primary pulmonary amyloidosis is a localized form of amyloidosis that is confined to lung parenchyma and generally has a benign course, unlike systemic forms of amyloidosis. It is worth keeping in mind that patients with certain hematolymphoid processes (most often plasma cell neoplasms, others may include mucosa-associated lymphoid tissue lymphoma and lymphoplasmacytic lymphoma) can form amyloid deposits in the lung tissue. As such, correlating the histologic finding of amyloid with available clinical and imaging findings can help determine if it is a primary or secondary process.

Tracheobronchial amyloidosis is a form of amyloidosis confined to the tracheobronchial tree and can result in airway constriction and obstruction and result in associated pathologic sequelae (i.e., pneumonia, bronchiectasis).

CYTOLOGIC FEATURES

- Amorphous, acellular debris.
- Paucicellular background.

HISTOLOGIC FEATURES

- Amorphous sheets of eosinophilic extracellular material.
- Adjacent foreign body giant cell reaction may be seen.
- Often, lymphoplasmacytic inflammation is seen, usually at the periphery of amyloid material.
- Calcification, and even ossification, can occur.
- Congo red staining shows apple-green birefringence with polarized light.
- Nodular amyloidosis: intrapulmonary lesion.
- Tracheobronchial amyloidosis: amyloid deposition in the submucosa of the tracheobronchial tree.

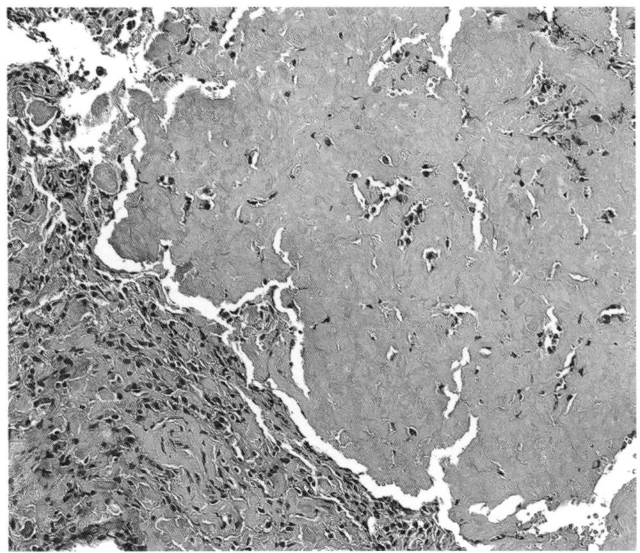

Figure 59.1 Amyloidosis seen on H and E stain; abundant amorphous eosinophilic material is seen.

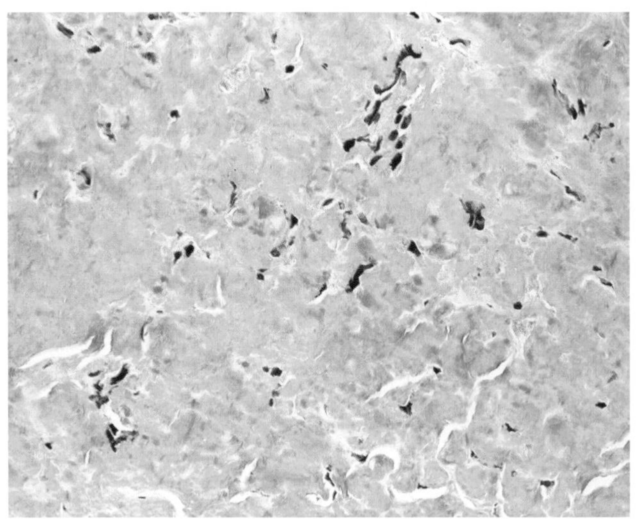

Figure 59.2 Amyloid material is light salmon pink on a Congo red stain.

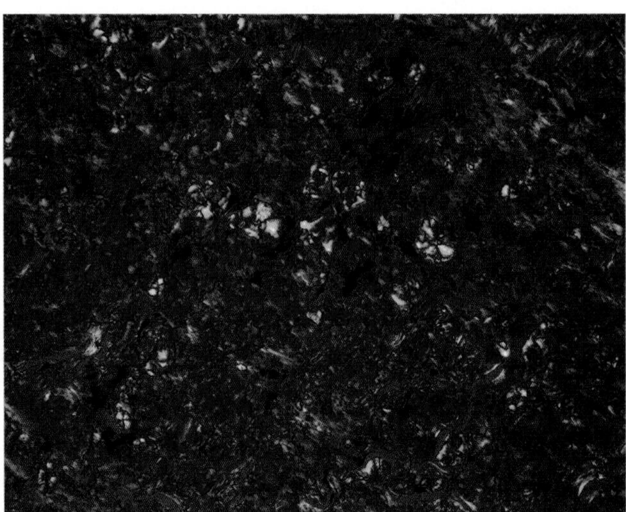

Figure 59.3 Apple-green birefringence is seen on Congo red staining with polarization.

Section 8

Granulomatous Diseases

► Yasmeen M. Butt

60

Infectious Granulomas

Infection is a common cause of both necrotizing and nonnecrotizing granulomas. Common infectious agents responsible for necrotizing granulomas are mycobacteria, *Aspergillus*, *Histoplasma capsulatum*, *Coccidioides immitis*, *Cryptococcus neoformans*, and *Blastomyces dermatitidis*. For details on specific infectious agents, please refer to Section 17: Specific Infectious Agents. This chapter will mainly serve as a brief overview of common infectious agents that can cause granulomas.

Part 1

Mycobacterium

▶ Yasmeen M. Butt

Mycobacterial infections of the lung can be broadly classified into those caused by *Mycobacterium tuberculosis,* being the most common worldwide, and nontuberculosis mycobacterium with *Mycobacterium avium* and *Mycobacterium intracellulare* (together called the *M. avium* complex or MAC), being more common in the United States.

HISTOLOGIC FEATURES

- Ziehl–Neelsen or auramine–rhodamine stains for acid-fast bacilli should be performed on up to three blocks in cases where a mycobacterium infection is suspected. Cultures should always be performed when possible, as bacilli may not always be seen on histology.
- Mycobacteria can be difficult to identify, and in many cases, only rare scattered bacilli are present. Careful screening on high power in areas of necrosis is recommended.
- Patients with *M. tuberculosis* often show a mixture of necrotizing and nonnecrotizing granulomas but rarely are purely nonnecrotizing.
- Granulomas may be airway centric or randomly distributed throughout the pulmonary parenchyma.
- Differentiation between *M. tuberculosis* and nontuberculosis mycobacterium cannot be realizably performed on histology; culture is required.

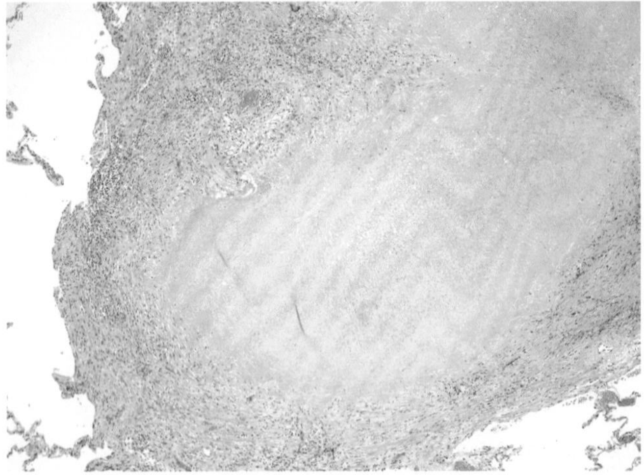

Figure 60.1 Low-power image of a necrotizing granuloma. The finding is not specific for a mycobacterial infection; however, special stains, including one for mycobacteria, should be performed. This patient had *M. tuberculosis* on culture.

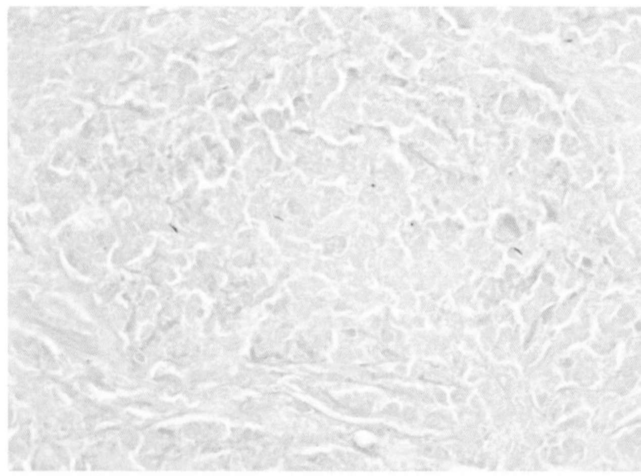

Figure 60.2 High-power image showing scattered acid-fast positive bacilli on an acid-fast stain. As in this case, bacilli are often rare and difficult to locate. Careful screening on high power is recommended.

Part 2

Fungi

▸ Yasmeen M. Butt

Fungal infections of the lung are most often seen in immunocompromised patients and the agents responsible are opportunistic fungi ubiquitous in the environment. Common agents include *Aspergillus*, *H. capsulatum*, *C. immitis*, *C. neoformans*, and *B. dermatitidis*.

HISTOLOGIC FEATURES

- Granulomas, when present, are often necrotizing and commonly contain multinucleated giant cells.
- Special stains can help highlight fungi and include Gomori methenamine silver (GMS) and/or periodic acid–Schiff (PAS).

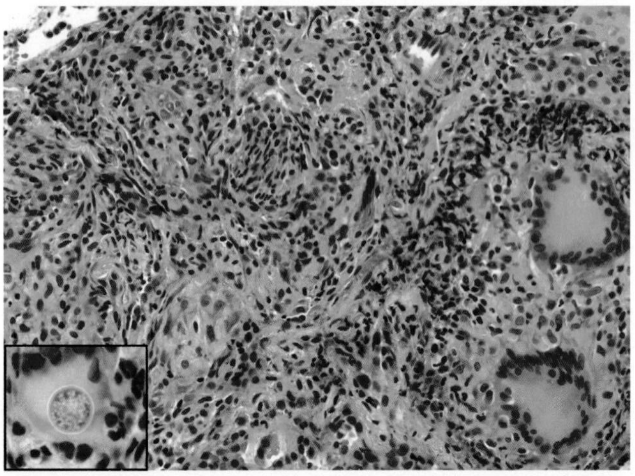

Figure 60.3 Low-power image showing a granuloma with giant cells in a patient with *C. immitis*. The *inset* shows a high-power image of a spherule with endospores.

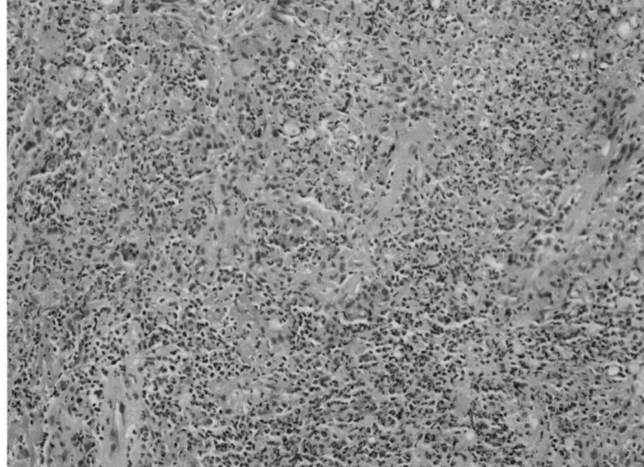

Figure 60.4 Low-power image showing the suppurative granulomatous inflammation characteristic of *B. dermatitidis*. Scattered single and budding yeast forms are present.

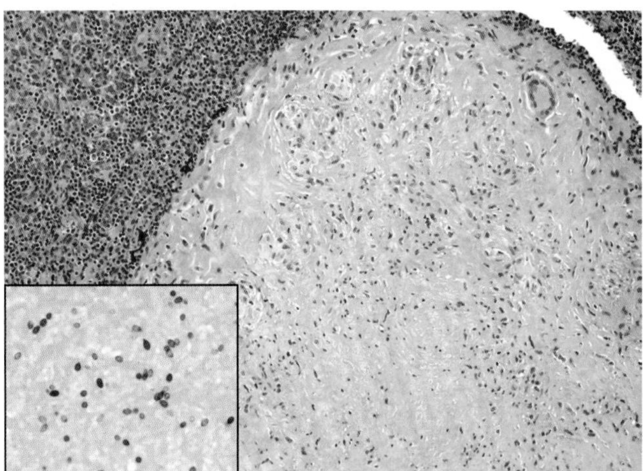

Figure 60.5 Low-power image showing an incidental granuloma with hyalinization in a hilar lymph node. The *inset* highlights fungal forms consistent with *Histoplasma*. This likely represents a remote infection.

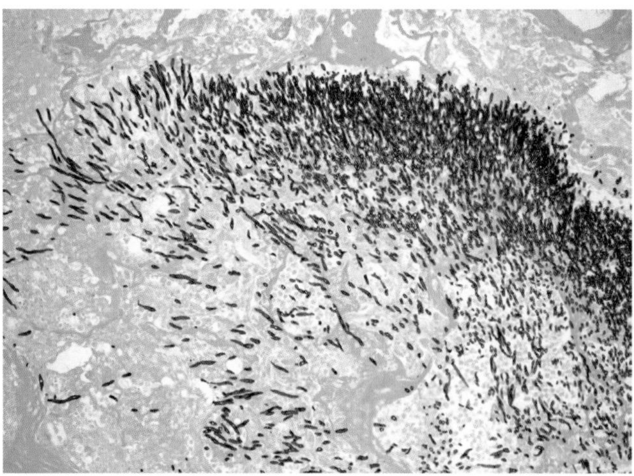

Figure 60.6 A GMS stain highlights septate hyphae in a lung section. It is recommended to offer a differential in cases such as this and defer to cultures for definitive speciation.

Part 3

Parasites

▸ Yasmeen M. Butt

There are a multitude of parasites that can make their way to the lungs and cause injury. A common example endemic in the eastern and midwestern United States is the dog heartworm *Dirofilaria immitis.* More than half of human patients are asymptomatic and detected as incidental findings on imaging. The typical lesion is a solitary nodule, which may be subpleural or centrally located. The parasite is transmitted to humans via mosquitoes that ingest the microfilaria from the blood of an infected dog. Humans are a dead-end host and the microfilarial forms fail to attain maturity in the right side of the human heart as they would in a dog's heart. Therefore, the immature adult worms subsequently die and embolize to the lungs causing necrosis that is often granulomatous.

HISTOLOGIC FEATURES

- Thrombosed artery with fragments of roundworm surrounded by a fibrous capsule and often with a rim of epithelioid histiocytes.
- Granulomas may contain eosinophils, macrophages, lymphocytes, plasma cells, and multinucleated giant cells.
- PAS will highlight fragments of dead worms.
- Movat (pentachrome) stains may be helpful in discerning remnants of vessels within necrotic lung parenchyma.

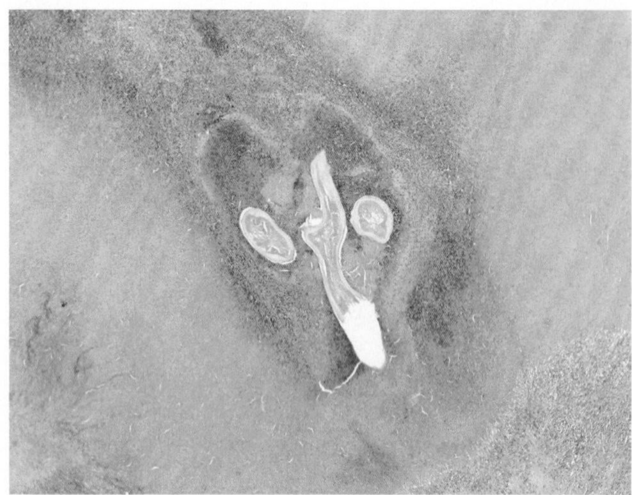

Figure 60.7 Low-power image showing nonviable worm fragments in a thrombosed vessel surrounded by bland necrosis with an appreciable rim of epithelioid histiocytes at the *bottom right corner*. (Courtesy of the *Mayo Clinic Pulmonary Pathology Study Set*. Rochester, MN.)

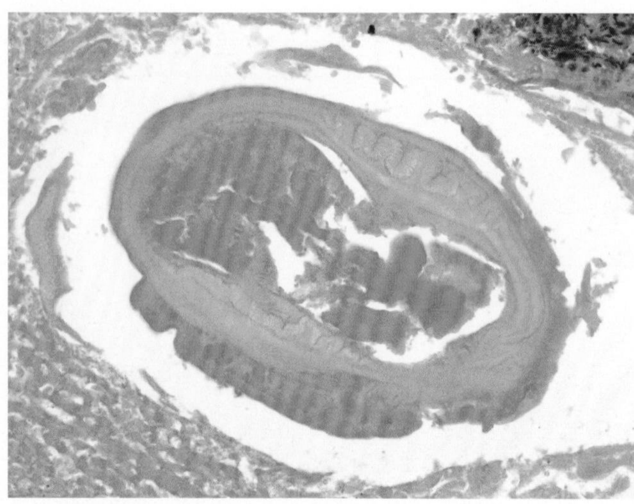

Figure 60.8 High-power image highlighting the cuticle of *D. immitis*. (Courtesy of the *Mayo Clinic Pulmonary Pathology Study Set*. Rochester, MN.)

Bronchocentric Granulomatosis

61

Yasmeen M. Butt

Historically, bronchocentric granulomatosis and allergic bronchopulmonary aspergillosis were essentially synonymous; however, since its initial description by Liebow in 1973, it has been described in a multitude of other settings including mycobacterial infections, rheumatoid arthritis, histoplasmosis, blastomycosis, echinococcosis, and granulomatosis with polyangiitis. Therefore, bronchocentric granulomatosis is more of a descriptive diagnosis than a unique disease. It consists of bronchiolocentric granulomatous inflammation, mucoid impaction of bronchi, and a prominent eosinophilic component consisting of necrotic eosinophilic material within the remains of bronchial lumens together with numerous eosinophils seen in the surrounding parenchyma. The classic example is that of an asthmatic patient with allergic bronchopulmonary fungal disease. In these cases, fungal elements are rare, located within the necrotic luminal contents, and not invasive.

HISTOLOGIC FEATURES

- Destruction of small bronchi and bronchioles by necrotizing granulomatous inflammation with surrounding uninvolved parenchyma away from bronchioles.
- All granulomas should be bronchiolocentric.
- Bronchial walls are variably involved, ranging from acute and chronic bronchiolitis to complete replacement of the airway walls with necrotizing granulomatous inflammation.
- Mucoid impaction of bronchi with mucin and cellular debris.
- A prominent eosinophilic component consisting of necrotic eosinophilic material within the remains of the bronchial lumens and numerous eosinophils in the surrounding parenchyma.
- Adjacent vessels may be secondarily involved by a chronic inflammatory infiltrate; however, a true vasculitis with necrosis or capillaritis should not be seen.
- In the setting of allergic bronchopulmonary fungal disease, a search for scattered hyphae within the necrotic areas should be performed. The hyphae are frequently rare and degenerated. Tissue invasion by fungal hyphae should not be present.
- Special stains for fungal hyphae as well as a search for other infectious causes should be performed.

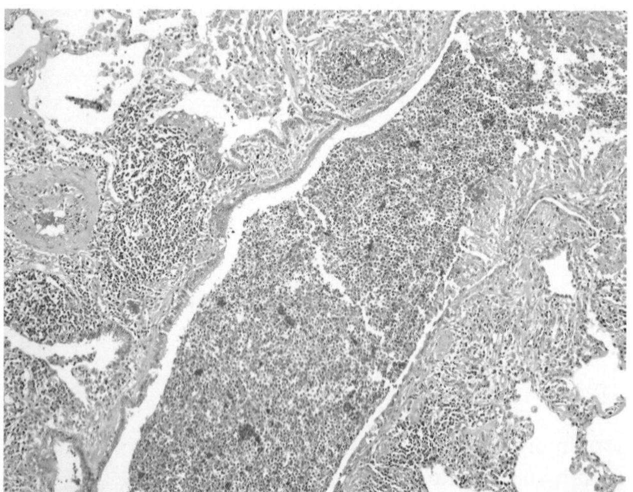

Figure 61.1 A bronchiole with partial replacement of the wall with necrotizing granulomatous inflammation. The lumen is filled with debris primarily consisting of eosinophils and eosinophilic breakdown products. The accompanying uninvolved pulmonary artery can be seen to the left of the bronchiole. An inflammatory infiltrate with a prominent eosinophilic component can be appreciated in the submucosa. (Case courtesy of the *Mayo Clinic Pulmonary Pathology Study Set.* Rochester, MN.)

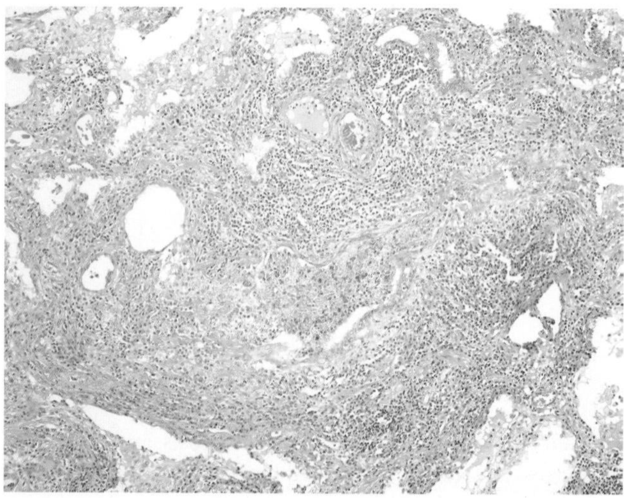

Figure 61.2 Only a small remnant of bronchial mucosa can be appreciated with the majority of the bronchial wall destroyed. There is a prominent eosinophilic infiltrate present within the lumen and in the surrounding parenchyma. (Courtesy of the *Mayo Clinic Pulmonary Pathology Study Set.* Rochester, MN.)

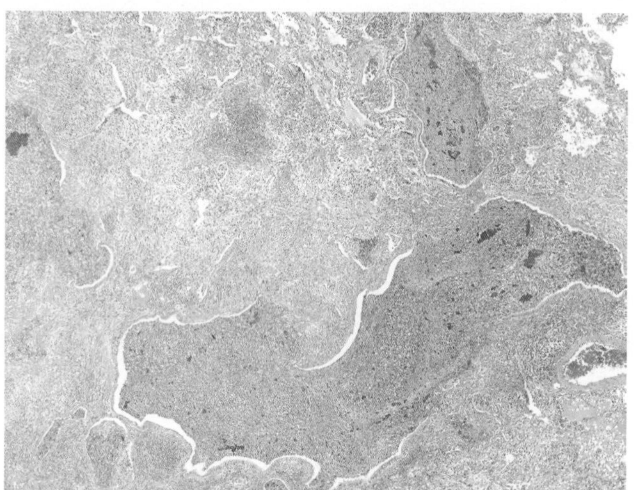

Figure 61.3 A low-power image shows necrotizing granulomatous inflammation tracking along a bronchiole with partial destruction of the wall and surrounding granulomatous inflammation. (Courtesy of the *Mayo Clinic Pulmonary Pathology Study Set.* Rochester, MN.)

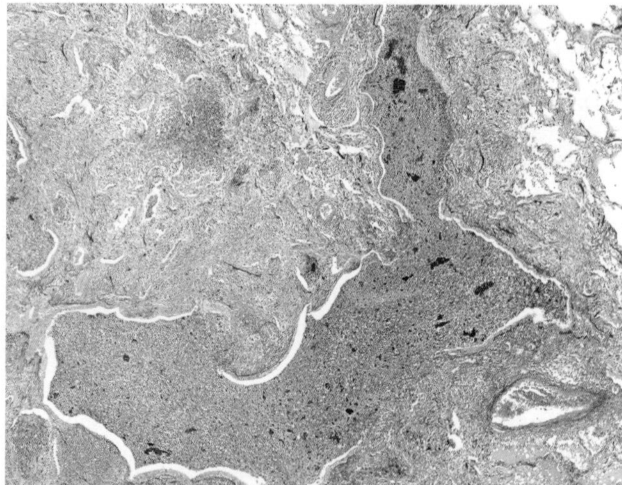

Figure 61.4 A Verhoeff–Van Gieson stain highlights the adjacent accompanying artery to the remaining intact portions of the bronchiole wall. (Courtesy of the *Mayo Clinic Pulmonary Pathology Study Set.* Rochester, MN.)

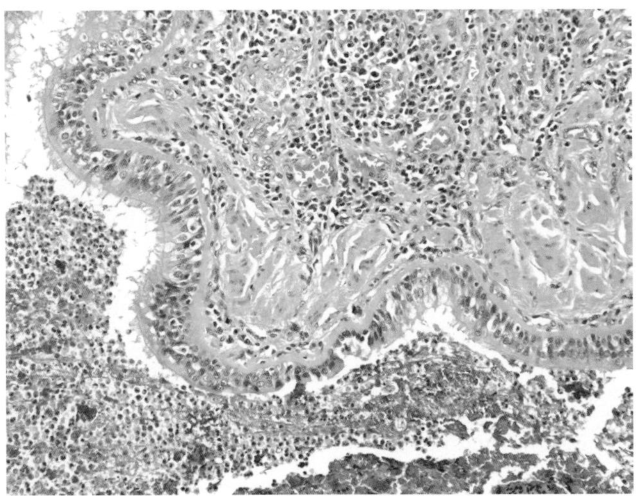

Figure 61.5 A higher power image shows a relatively intact portion of a bronchial wall in a case of bronchocentric granulomatosis. The lumen is filled with eosinophils and granular eosinophilic breakdown products. An inflammatory infiltrate with a prominent eosinophilic component can be appreciated in the submucosa. (Courtesy of the *Mayo Clinic Pulmonary Pathology Study Set.* Rochester, MN.)

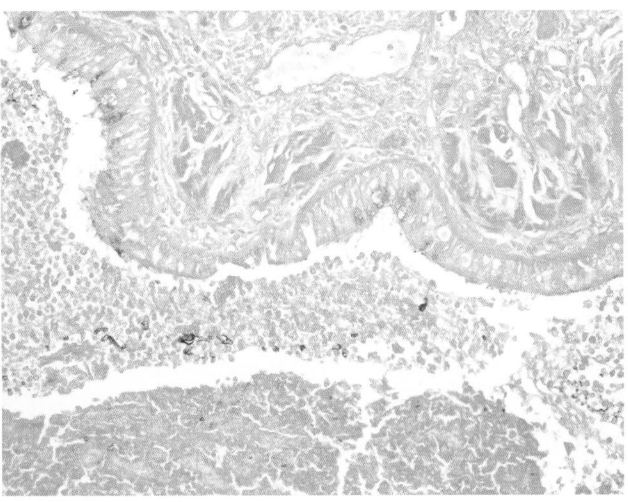

Figure 61.6 A Gomori methenamine silver stain highlights the rare scattered degenerated appearing fungal hyphae within the bronchiole lumen. No invasion is present. These were the only hyphae present in this specimen. (Courtesy of the *Mayo Clinic Pulmonary Pathology Study Set.* Rochester, MN.)

Pulmonary Hyalinizing Granuloma

Yasmeen M. Butt

Pulmonary hyalinizing granuloma (PHG) and its histologic correlates fibrosing mediastinitis and idiopathic retroperitoneal fibrosis are rare nonneoplastic fibroinflammatory diseases thought to be due to a variety of causes. PHG is most commonly attributed to an exaggerated immune response to a previous infection, most commonly histoplasmosis in the United States or less commonly tuberculosis or *Aspergillus*. PHG has been reported in association with a variety of immune-mediated conditions, including idiopathic thrombocytopenic purpura and idiopathic IgG4-related sclerosing disease. It is seen in young or middle-aged adults and consists of solitary or multiple slowly growing pulmonary nodules that can be mistaken for cancer on imaging. About 15% of patients with PHG also have or develop fibrosing mediastinitis.

Histologic examination reveals a well-circumscribed, but nonencapsulated, lesion consisting predominantly of dense, acellular, eosinophilic, keloid-like hyalinized collagen bundles. The collagen bundles are arranged in haphazard, lamellar, and/or whorled patterns, often with a vague pericellular orientation. Lesions usually contain loose aggregates of plasma cells, lymphocytes, and histiocytes in a perivascular distribution and/or scattered throughout the collagen bundles. This inflammatory infiltrate can also be appreciated at the interface with normal lung parenchyma. The amount of inflammation is variable and occasional examples with Russell bodies and eosinophils have been described. The infiltrate can be rich in CD20 positive B lymphocytes that, in the absence of cytologic atypia, are not indicative of a lymphoma. Necrotic foci can be present and are likely ischemic in nature. Calcification is rarely a feature. Despite its moniker, granulomatous inflammation should not be seen. Giant cells at the periphery have been rarely reported, but are not as common as they are in PHG's primary differential, nodular amyloidosis. Nodular amyloidosis has a more amorphous quality to the eosinophilic material and lacks the lamellar or whorled structures of the hyalinized collagen of PHG. Congo red will occasionally stain weakly with some cases of PHG but should not show strong apple-green birefringence as seen in nodular amyloidosis. Additional differentials include burned-out infectious granulomas, light chain deposition disease, solitary fibrous tumor, silicotic nodules, and inflammatory myofibroblastic tumor. In contrast to burned-out infectious granulomas, which can become hyalinized over time, PHG is not a burned-out remnant process. It is a slowly growing lesion of hyalinized collagen that creates its own scar as it extends outward.

HISTOLOGIC FEATURES

- Nodular arrangement of dense, acellular, eosinophilic, keloid-like collagen bundles arranged in haphazard, lamellar, and/or whorled patterns, often with a vague pericellular orientation.
- Sparse, variably sized aggregates of plasma cells, lymphocytes, and histiocytes interspersed throughout collagen bundles, some seen in a pericellular pattern and often prominent at the periphery of the lesion.
- Some cases can be weakly positive for Congo red stain.

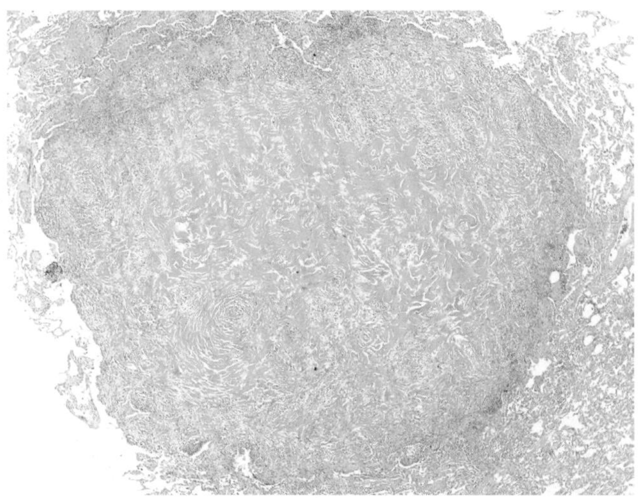

Figure 62.1 Low-power image showing a well-circumscribed, but nonencapsulated, PHG. (Courtesy of the *Mayo Clinic Pulmonary Pathology Study Set*. Rochester, MN.)

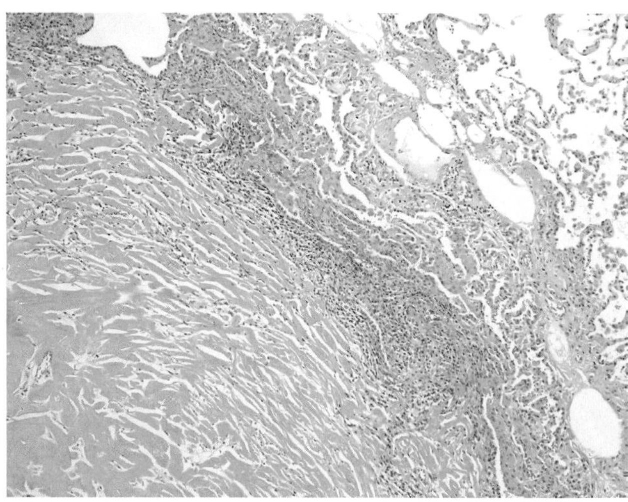

Figure 62.2 High-power image showing an inflammatory infiltrate of lymphocytes, plasma cells, and histiocytes at the interface of the lesion and normal lung parenchyma. (Courtesy of the *Mayo Clinic Pulmonary Pathology Study Set*. Rochester, MN.)

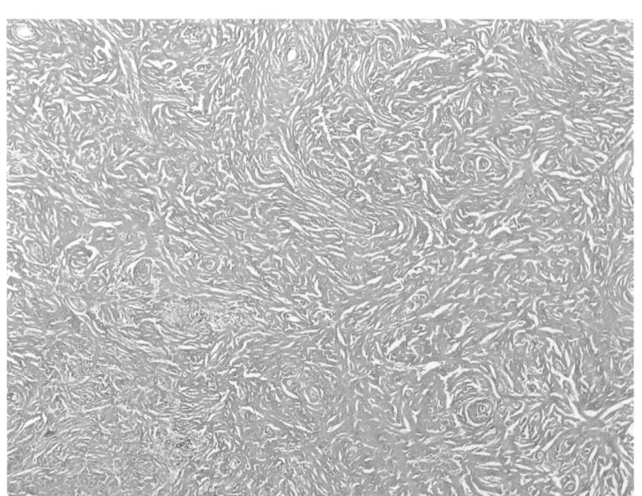

Figure 62.3 A PHG with characteristic dense, acellular collagen bundles in a haphazard arrangement with a vaguely pericellular whorling pattern. Small inflammatory aggregates can be appreciated around the vessels. (Courtesy of the *Mayo Clinic Pulmonary Pathology Study Set*. Rochester, MN.)

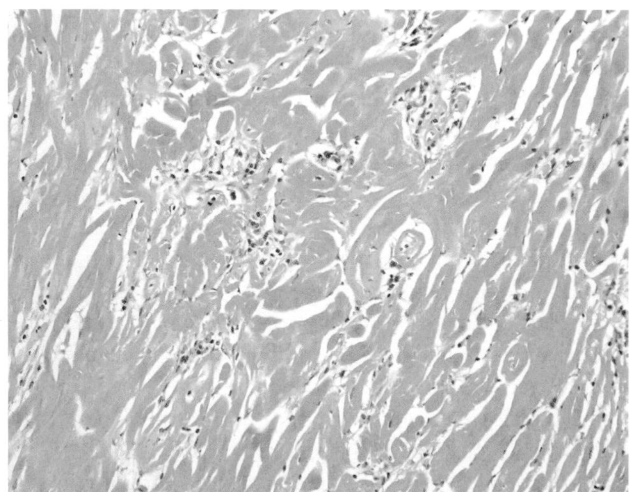

Figure 62.4 High-power image shows the characteristic dense, acellular keloid-like collagen bundles with scattered lymphoplasmacytic aggregates, some around small blood vessels. (Courtesy of the *Mayo Clinic Pulmonary Pathology Study Set*. Rochester, MN.)

63 Sarcoidosis

Yasmeen M. Butt

Sarcoidosis, a systemic disease of unknown etiology, is fundamentally a clinicopathologic diagnosis with pathology being indispensable. It can be suggested based on the findings seen on transbronchial biopsy, endobronchial biopsy, or biopsy of hilar or mediastinal lymph nodes.

In transbronchial and endobronchial biopsies, the granulomas of sarcoidosis can be seen in the superficial or deep submucosa and/or the peribronchiolar alveolar interstitium. The granulomas are nonnecrotizing, tightly formed, and predominantly composed of epithelioid histiocytes with scattered multinucleated giant cells that are typically bordered by a rim of lymphocytes, monocytes, and fibroblasts. The granulomas can become confluent forming large nodules. In early stages, the findings may only consist of small numbers of histiocytes and scattered multinucleated giant cells. Small foci of punctate necrosis can occasionally be appreciated; however, large amounts of necrosis, karyorrhectic debris, and neutrophils should not be present. In addition, these nonnecrotizing granulomas are often present within the adventitia and outer layers of the media of small- and medium-sized vessels (granulomatous vasculitis), with veins more often involved than arteries. A necrotizing vasculitis, however, should not be present and would suggest granulomatosis with polyangiitis. As the disease progresses, a characteristic hyalinized fibrosis can be seen surrounding and/or replacing the granulomas. In surgical wedge biopsies and explanted lung specimens, the distribution of sarcoidosis can be appreciated as along, but not in, the lymphatics of the subpleural space and interlobular septae.

Giant cells, while usually present, are not necessary for the diagnosis and can be of either the Langhan (nuclei arranged in horseshoe pattern along the periphery) or foreign body (nuclei clustered in the center) types. There are several nonspecific but characteristic inclusion bodies, consisting of endogenous breakdown products that can be seen within the giant cells, histiocytes, or less commonly in the extracellular space. None are pathognomonic though and may be seen in many other entities. Asteroid bodies are spider- or pinwheel-shaped bodies composed of cytoskeleton filaments and lipoproteins. Schaumann bodies, signs of a chronic granulomatous disease, are deeply basophilic to black concentrically laminated structures consisting of oxidized lipids, iron, and calcium carbonate. They are often compared to psammoma bodies. Clear polarizable fragments of birefringent calcium oxalate crystals can also be seen. Hamazaki-Wesenberg bodies, commonly found in the sinuses of the affected lymph nodes, are thought to be large lysosomes and consist of circular to oval-shaped light brown structures that stain positive with Gomori methenamine silver stain and resemble yeasts.

Sarcoidosis is a diagnosis of exclusion and it is important to evaluate for findings that would lead to a different diagnosis. Hypersensitivity pneumonitis is often found in the differential diagnosis and will show loose interstitial granulomas and an associated interstitial pneumonitis in contrast to sarcoidosis, which has more tightly formed and often confluent granulomas without an exuberant-associated inflammation. Infection is also found in the differential diagnosis of granulomas, especially if large amounts of necrosis or organizing pneumonia are present. Special stains always should be performed to rule out fungi and mycobacteria.

HISTOLOGIC FEATURES

- Nonnecrotizing tightly formed granulomas composed of epithelioid histiocytes with multinucleated giant cells with a rim of lymphocytes, monocytes, and fibroblasts.
- Granulomas follow a lymphangitic distribution in the subpleural spaces, along interlobular septae, in peribronchiolar alveolar interstitium, and in the submucosa.
- Granulomatous vasculitis of small- and medium-sized vessels is common; however, a necrotizing vasculitis should not be seen.
- Small foci of necrosis may be present, but large amounts should not be present.
- Infection must be ruled out in all cases by performing Gomori methenamine silver and Ziehl–Neelsen stains.
- Small biopsies in early stages of sarcoidosis may show only small aggregates of histiocytes and scattered giant cells. Clinical suspicion is key in these cases.
- Late-stage sarcoidosis can show progressive replacement of granulomas with hyalinized fibrosis.

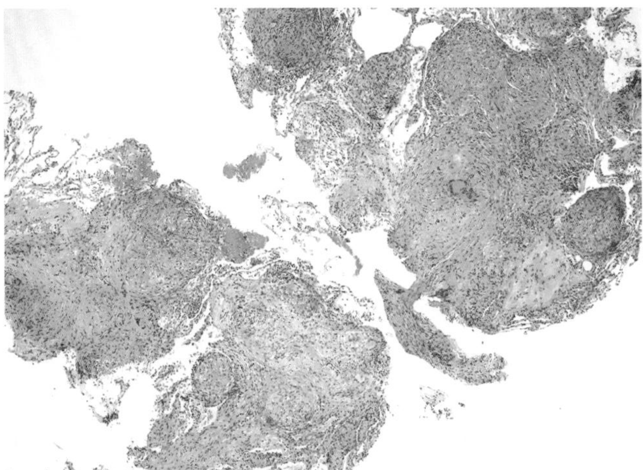

Figure 63.1 Low-power image of a transbronchial biopsy showing tightly formed confluent granulomas. A foreign body–type giant cell can be seen near the *top* of the image with a cluster of Langhan-type giant cells near the *center*.

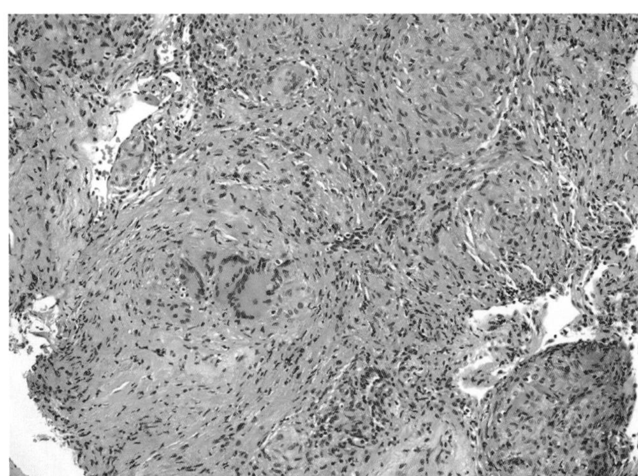

Figure 63.2 High-power image showing tightly formed confluent nonnecrotizing granulomas composed predominantly of epithelioid histiocytes with scattered giant cells. Lymphocytes can be appreciated at the *periphery*.

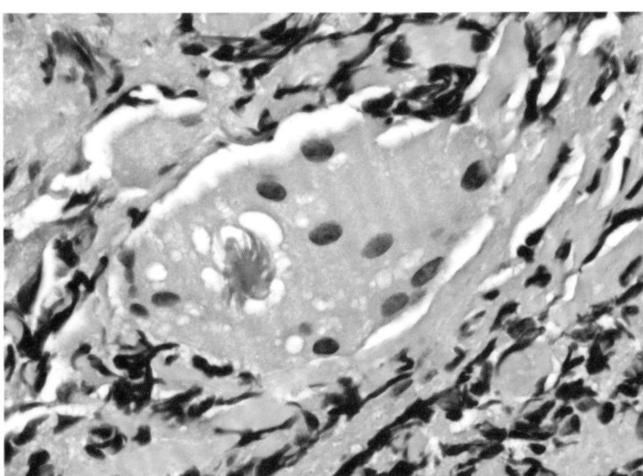

Figure 63.3 High-power image of a giant cell with an eosinophilic pinwheel-shaped asteroid body.

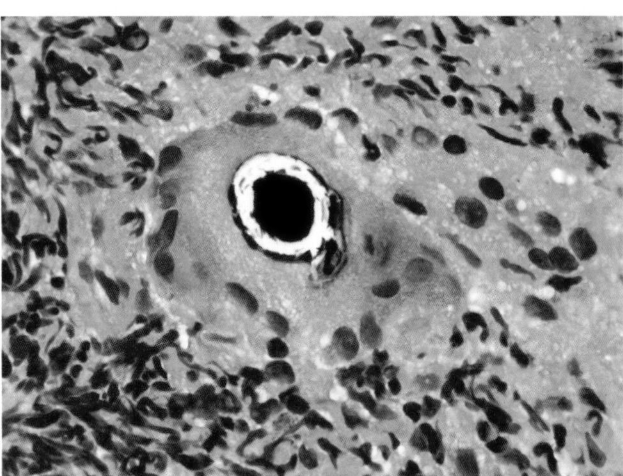

Figure 63.4 High-power image of a giant cell with a Schaumann body.

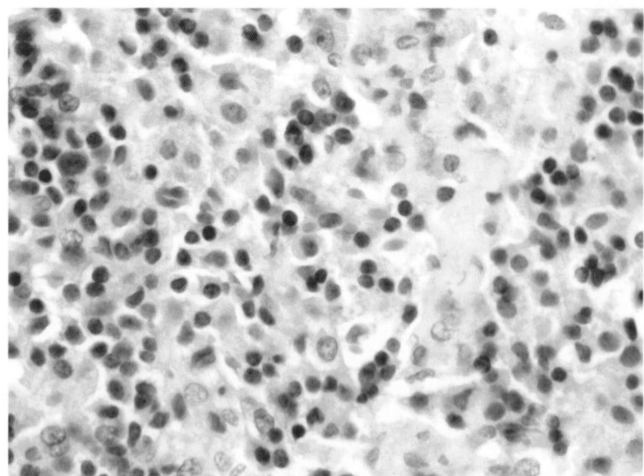

Figure 63.5 High-power image showing Hamazaki-Wesenberg bodies in the sinus of a lymph node in a patient with sarcoidosis. They can be appreciated as small light brown oval structures resembling yeasts.

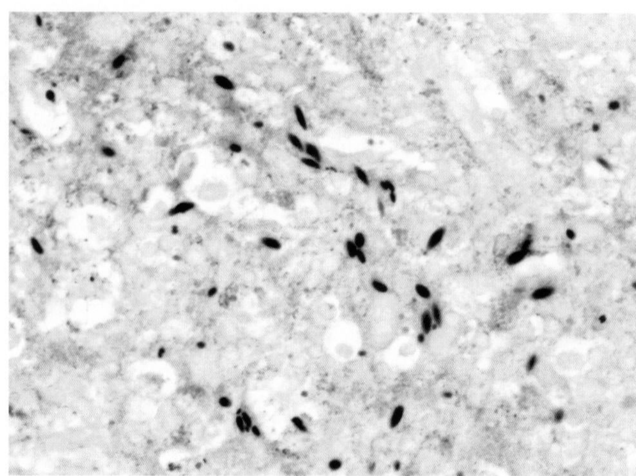

Figure 63.6 High-power image showing Hamazaki-Wesenberg bodies staining positive with a Gomori methenamine silver stain. Be cautious not to mistake these for fungi.

64

Berylliosis

Yasmeen M. Butt

Berylliosis is caused by exposure to beryllium and its alloys. This exposure typically occurs in industries where beryllium is utilized, which includes aerospace, electronics, and metal mining/production. Many of the early cases were described in association with the manufacture of fluorescent light bulbs, which contained beryllium prior to 1948. The Occupational Safety and Health Administration has currently set the exposure limit for beryllium at 0.2 $\mu g/m^3$ of air. Berylliosis can be either acute or chronic. Acute berylliosis yields a diffuse alveolar damage picture on histology. More commonly, although still exceedingly rare, the pathologist will encounter chronic beryllium disease on a transbronchial biopsy or wedge resection.

Histologically, although the findings in chronic berylliosis can be indistinguishable from sarcoidosis and consist of well-formed confluent nonnecrotizing granulomas with or without giant cells, the disease often shares more in common with hypersensitivity pneumonitis and demonstrates poorly formed loose granulomas with associated chronic inflammation. The chronic lymphocytic component may be relatively extensive and extend into the surrounding interstitial spaces. In addition to exposure history, this can be a helpful finding when distinguishing berylliosis from sarcoidosis. Necrosis should be absent. Nonspecific cytoplasmic inclusion bodies, such as asteroid or Schaumann bodies, may be present. Interstitial fibrosis may or may not be a feature. The distribution of the granulomas may be septal, subpleural, peribronchial, or perivascular. They do not necessarily follow the "lymphangitic" pattern of sarcoidosis. Unlike sarcoidosis, berylliosis lacks hilar lymphadenopathy. As with any of the granulomatous diseases in the lung, every effort to rule out infectious agents should be undertaken. While sarcoidosis and hypersensitivity pneumonitis remain the main differential diagnoses of berylliosis, differentiation should not be difficult with consideration of both the clinical history and abovementioned histologic features.

Confirmatory testing can be performed using the beryllium lymphocyte proliferation test.

HISTOLOGIC FEATURES

- Nonnecrotizing granulomas either loosely or tightly formed with or without giant cells.
- Interstitial inflammation associated with or distant from granulomas is often present.
- Asteroid or Schaumann bodies may be present.
- Special stains should be performed to rule out underlying infectious causes.

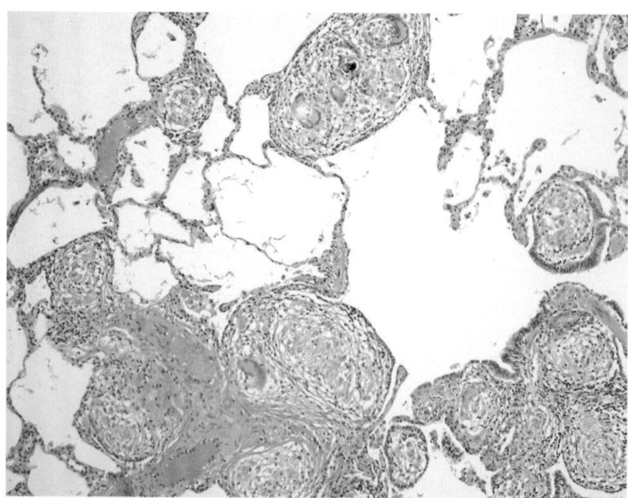

Figure 64.1 Several loosely formed granulomas, some with giant cells containing Schaumann bodies, can be seen in this case of the berylliosis. The granulomas are peribronchiolar and interstitial in distribution. (Courtesy of the *Mayo Clinic Pulmonary Pathology Study Set*. Rochester, MN.)

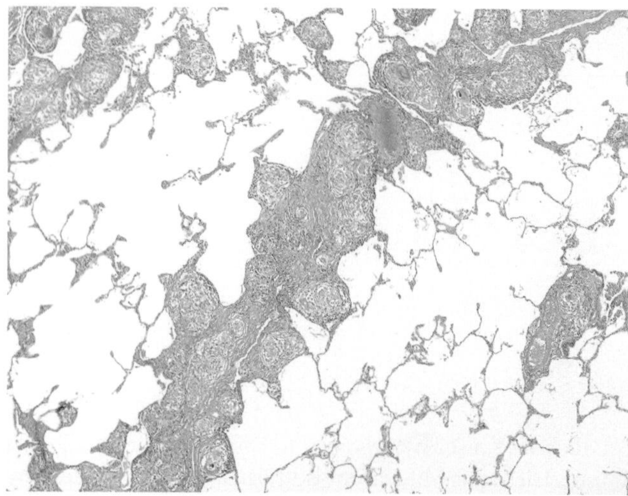

Figure 64.2 Low-power image demonstrating septal, peribronchiolar, and interstitial distribution of loosely to moderately well-formed confluent granulomas, many with giant cells containing Schaumann bodies. (Courtesy of the *Mayo Clinic Pulmonary Pathology Sstudy Set*. Rochester, MN.)

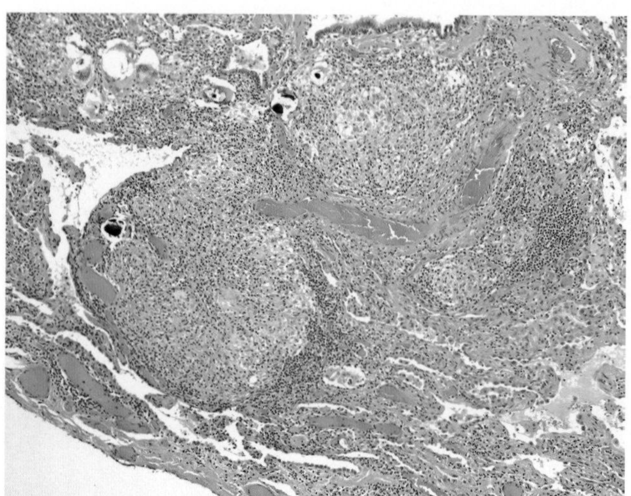

Figure 64.3 High-power image demonstrating several confluent nonnecrotizing granulomas with an associated lymphocytic infiltrate at the edges extending out into the adjacent parenchyma. Several Schaumann bodies can also be appreciated. (Courtesy of the *Mayo Clinic Pulmonary Pathology Study Set*. Rochester, MN.)

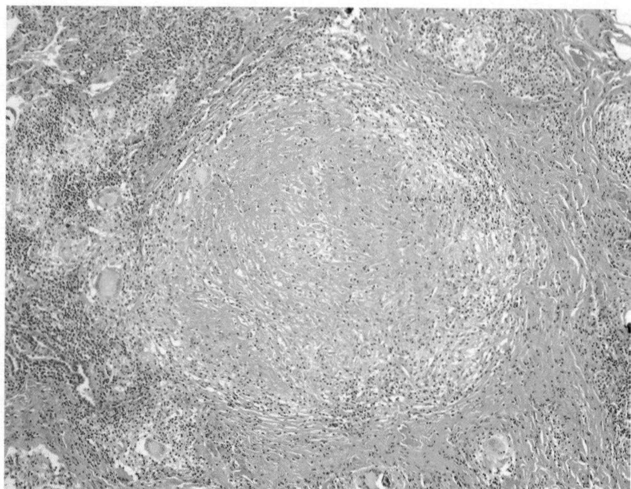

Figure 64.4 Large nonnecrotizing granuloma with giant cells containing Schaumann bodies with an associated lymphocytic infiltrate in the surrounding parenchyma. (Courtesy of the *Mayo Clinic Pulmonary Pathology Study Set*. Rochester, MN.)

65 Sarcoid-Like Reaction

Yasmeen M. Butt

Sarcoid-like epithelioid granulomas have been reported in association with primary lung carcinomas. The granulomas can be located in lymph nodes draining parenchyma containing a carcinoma, adjacent to the tumor, or in nonregional tissues. They can also be seen in association with lymphoproliferative disorders such as Hodgkin and non-Hodgkin lymphoma. It is postulated that they represent a reaction to soluble antigenic factors released from tumor cells. These granulomas can create a diagnostic pitfall in small biopsy specimens, as they are often identical to sarcoid-type granulomas. One should be careful not to precipitously diagnose sarcoidosis based on sarcoid-type granulomas when seen in association with a carcinoma or a lymphoproliferative disorder.

HISTOLOGIC FEATURES

- Sarcoid-type well-formed granulomas composed predominantly of epithelioid histiocytes with peripheral lymphocytes. Giant cells may or may not be present.
- Seen in association with a carcinoma or lymphoproliferative disorder.
- Clinical history and imaging are key to the correct diagnosis.

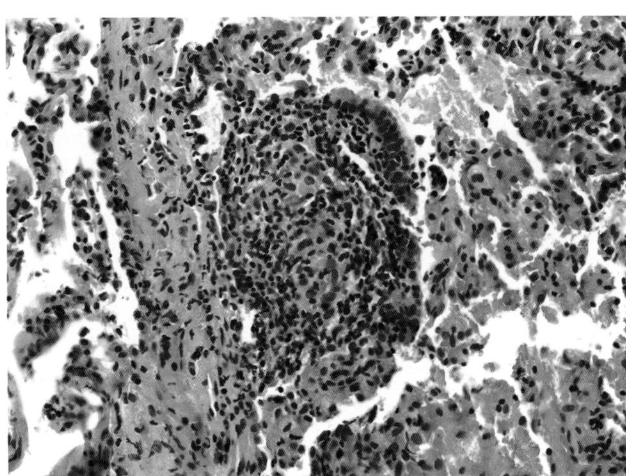

Figure 65.1 A small granuloma present in alveolar parenchyma adjacent to a primary lung adenocarcinoma.

66 Necrotizing Sarcoid Granulomatosis

Yasmeen M. Butt

Necrotizing sarcoid granulomatosis (NGS) was originally described by Liebow as a variant of granulomatosis with polyangiitis. It has since been recognized to be likely a variant of or exist on a continuum with nodular sarcoidosis. It has been suggested that the terminology *sarcoidosis with necrotizing sarcoid granulomatosis pattern* be used in place of NGS to reflect this entity as a form of sarcoidosis. The histologic findings are similar to sarcoidosis, consisting predominantly of nonnecrotizing tightly formed granulomas composed of epithelioid histiocytes with multinucleated giant cells with a rim of lymphocytes, monocytes, and fibroblasts following a lymphangitic distribution in the subpleural spaces, along interlobular septa, in peribronchiolar alveolar interstitium, and in the submucosa. The key addition is the presence of extensive granulomatous vasculitis and large foci of necrotic lung parenchyma. The presence of granulomatous vasculitis does not equal NGS by itself, as it can be seen in classical sarcoid, but should be more extensive in NGS. As with classical sarcoidosis, infection must be ruled out. Special stains should be performed along with cultures.

HISTOLOGIC FEATURES

- Large foci of necrotic lung parenchyma.
- Prominent granulomatous vasculitis component, typically nonnecrotizing.
- Nonnecrotizing tightly formed granulomas composed of epithelioid histiocytes with multinucleated giant cells with a rim of lymphocytes, monocytes, and fibroblasts.
- Granulomas follow a lymphangitic distribution in the subpleural spaces, along interlobular septa, in peribronchiolar alveolar interstitium, and in the submucosa.
- Infection must be ruled out in all cases by performing Gomori methenamine silver and Ziehl–Neelsen stains. Cultures should also be performed.

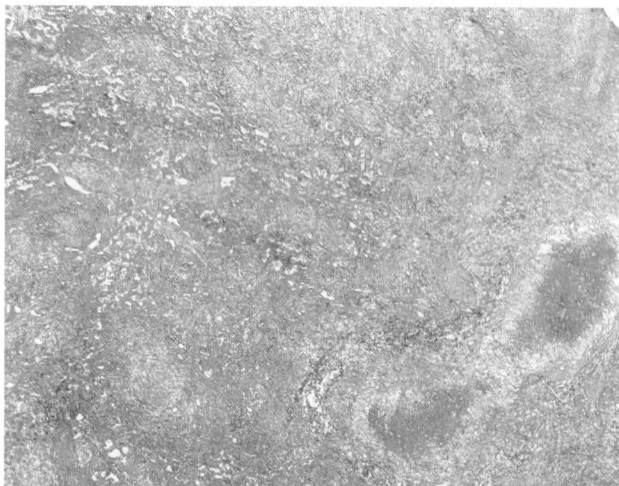

Figure 66.1 Low-power image of NGS with large foci of necrosis seen in the *lower right corner*. (Courtesy of the *Mayo Clinic Pulmonary Pathology Study Set.* Rochester, MN.)

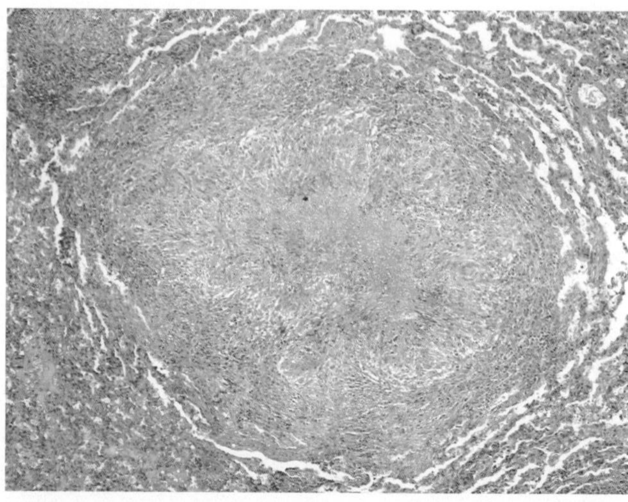

Figure 66.2 Epithelioid granuloma with central necrosis. (Courtesy of the *Mayo Clinic Pulmonary Pathology Study Set.* Rochester, MN.)

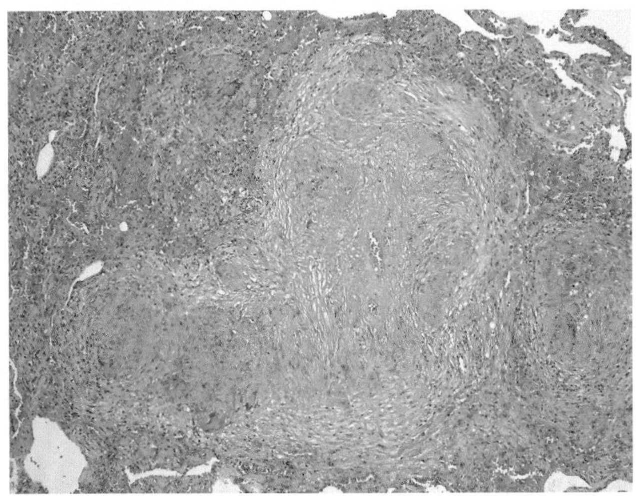

Figure 66.3 Granulomatous vasculitis in a pulmonary artery in NGS. (Courtesy of the *Mayo Clinic Pulmonary Pathology Study Set.* Rochester, MN.)

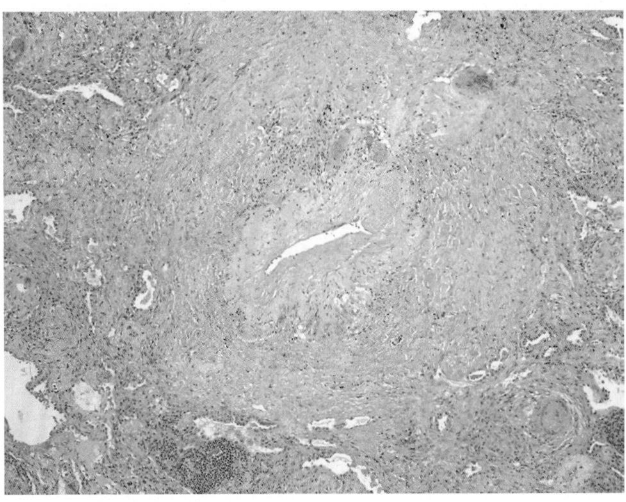

Figure 66.4 Granulomatous vasculitis in a vessel with surrounding confluent epithelioid granulomas. (Courtesy of the *Mayo Clinic Pulmonary Pathology Study Set.* Rochester, MN.)

67 Foreign-Body Granulomas

Yasmeen M. Butt

Foreign body–type granulomas or granulomatous reactions occur in the lung in multiple settings, including intravenous (IV) drug abuse and aspiration of food, pill particles, or mineral oils.

Part 1

Intravenous Drug Abuse

Yasmeen M. Butt

Lung damage in IV drug abusers' lung is due to IV administration of crushed oral pills. Pills meant to be taken orally, in addition to the pharmacologic agents, contain filler materials, such as microcrystalline cellulose, crospovidone, and talc. They do not dissolve in the blood and make their way to the lung through the right side of the heart and become lodged in small arteries, alveolar septal capillaries, and in the surrounding perivascular interstitium of the lung parenchyma.

A granulomatous response consisting of foreign body–type giant cells, histiocytes, and lymphocytes are seen in response to the filler particles. In chronic cases, changes of mild to moderate pulmonary hypertension can be present. The number and volume of particles can range from scant to numerous. Polarization can help in identification. Both talc and microcrystalline cellulose are clear particles, which polarize brightly under birefringent light. Talc particles are small and usually form sheet-like arrangements. Microcrystalline cellulose fragments are larger, elongated rod-like structures. If in question, a Movat (pentachrome) stain can differentiate between the two; talc stains blue and microcrystalline cellulose stains yellow. In addition, a Movat stain will help highlight blood vessels and therefore the location of the particles. Crospovidone is a deeply basophilic amorphous material that does not polarize.

In the past, talc served as the predominant filler in oral pills and the term *talc granulomatosis* is still used as a result; however, microcrystalline cellulose has replaced talc as the most commonly used filler.

The main differential diagnosis is typically aspiration pneumonia. A careful search for food particles, such as degenerating vegetable material and localization of the particles within the alveolar spaces, as opposed to small arteries, septal capillaries, and the perivascular interstitium, will lead to this diagnosis. The particles' mode of entry, either through the airways in aspiration or through the venous system in IV administration, dictates their final location within the lung parenchyma.

The granulomatous response can become extensive enough to mimic sarcoidosis; however, identification of the filler particles should rule this out.

HISTOLOGIC FEATURES

- Foreign-body granulomas with scant to numerous fragments of foreign material, both polarizable and nonpolarizable, are seen in small arteries, septal capillaries, and perivascular interstitium.
- Polarizable filler material most commonly consists of shard-like microcrystalline cellulose and sheet-like talc particles.
- Nonpolarizable filler material most commonly consists of crospovidone, a deeply basophilic amorphous substance.
- Mild to moderate pulmonary hypertensive changes in arteries may be present in chronic cases.

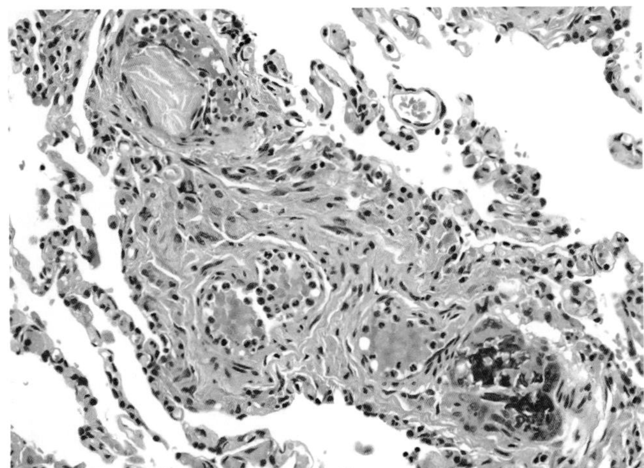

Figure 67.1 Fragments of microcrystalline cellulose *(upper left)* and crospovidone *(lower right)* can be seen here within a small artery.

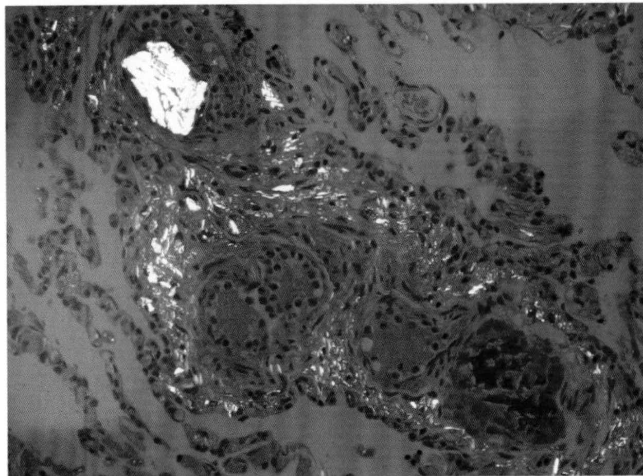

Figure 67.2 Polarization of Figure 67.1 highlights the microcrystalline cellulose in the *upper left*. Note that the crospovidone in the *lower right* does not polarize.

Part 2

Aspiration

Yasmeen M. Butt

Despite the perception that aspiration pneumonia can only occur in the right lower lobe in patients with severe clinical risk factors such as seizures, low-level chronic aspiration is often clinically overlooked and can occur in any lobe of the lung and often presents as nodular lung lesions. A wide variety of patients can be at risk including those who have limited motility, gastroesophageal reflux disease, are taking chronic pain medications, or have undergone a lung transplant. Finding the exogenous aspirated material is key to the diagnosis. Well-preserved skeletal muscle or vegetable particles can sometimes be appreciated; however, it is more common to find vegetable material in varying stages of degeneration. The degenerating particles can have many forms, but the most common are circular egg or "lentil"-like structures composed of amorphous pink material and serpentine, blood vessel–like structures. Aspirated pill filler fragments such as microcrystalline cellulose, crospovidone, and talc, as described in Part 1, can also be seen. The aspirated food particles and pill fragments are located in a peribronchiolar and alveolar distribution. Depending on the chronicity, the reaction can vary from minimal to an exuberant foreign-body granulomatous reaction with giant cells, lymphocytes, histiocytes, and even an airway-centered fibrosis in patients with chronic aspiration. Organizing pneumonia, consisting of fibroblastic plugs within alveoli, is often seen in association with aspiration pneumonia.

HISTOLOGIC FEATURES

- Exogenous material in the form of degenerating vegetable material, skeletal muscle, and pill filler fragments (microcrystalline cellulose, crospovidone, and/or talc) within airways and/or in a peribronchiolar location is key.
- Variable foreign-body granulomatous response around the foreign material is present.
- In severe chronic cases, bronchiolocentric fibrosis may be present.

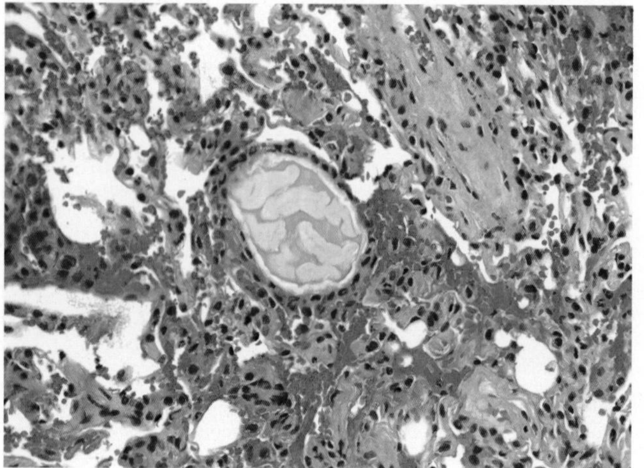

Figure 67.3 A degenerating vegetable particle can be seen in the *center* of the image within an alveolar space with a minimal inflammatory infiltrate surrounding it.

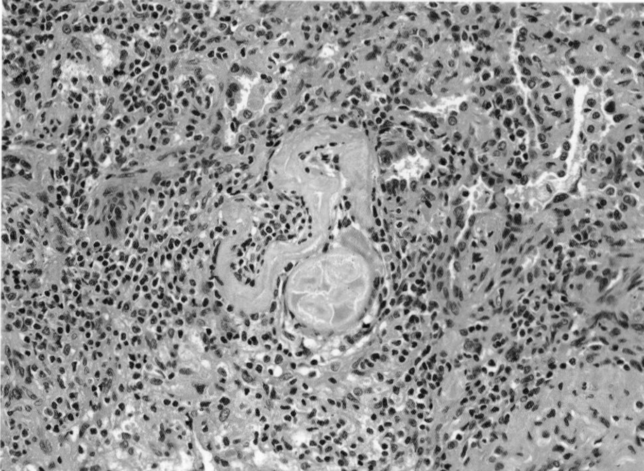

Figure 67.4 Rounded and more serpentine-shaped degenerating vegetable particles are seen here in the alveolar space with a brisk inflammatory reaction.

Part 3

Other Foreign-Body Reactions

Yasmeen M. Butt

Exogenous lipoid pneumonia is a type of aspiration pneumonia that occurs with exposure to exogenous oil or oil-containing substances, particularly aerosolized or ingested forms. Examples include cod liver oil, nose drops containing mineral oil, oils in cooking, exposures to burning fat, or hair sprays with mineral oil components. Treatment consists of identifying the relevant exposure and removing it.

Histologically, macrophages with large lipid-laden droplets are present, often with associated multinucleated giant cells and fibrosis if the exposure is chronic. They are most often present in the airways and can also be seen with in the interstitium in chronic cases. The macrophages should be differentiated from those seen in endogenous lipoid pneumonia, which contain smaller and almost granular-appearing vacuoles. As normal histologic processing techniques dissolve lipids, an oil red O stain can be performed on frozen tissue if this diagnosis is suspected.

HISTOLOGIC FEATURES

- Macrophages within airspaces and/or interstitium with large lipid-filled vacuoles are present.
- Multinucleated giant cells containing lipid droplets are often seen.
- Oil red O may be used to highlight lipids on frozen tissue if exogenous lipoid pneumonia is suspected.
- Fibrosis is often present in chronic cases.

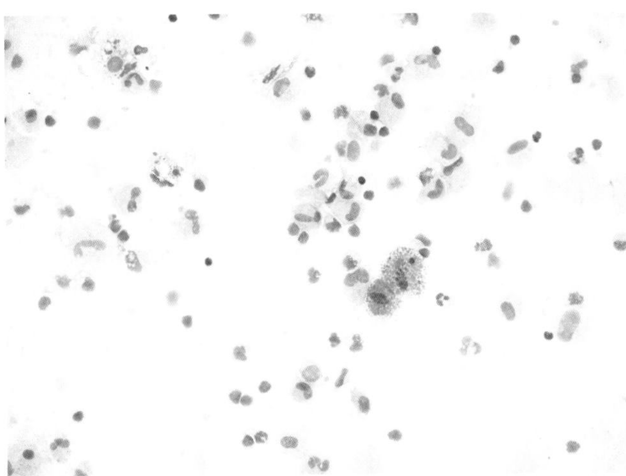

Figure 67.5 A bronchoalveolar lavage specimen stained with an oil red O preparation from a child with suspected lipoid pneumonia highlights lipid within macrophages in bright red.

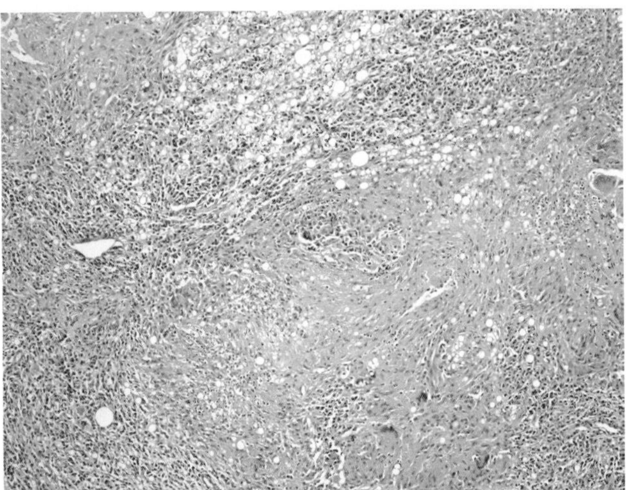

Figure 67.6 Low-power image showing exogenous lipoid pneumonia with numerous macrophages filled with large lipid inclusions and an associated foreign-body giant cell reaction with background fibrosis. (Courtesy of the *Mayo Clinic Pulmonary Pathology Study Set*. Rochester, MN.)

Nodules Resembling Granulomas

68

Certain lesions may enter into the differential of granulomas; these include rheumatoid nodules and malakoplakia.

Part 1

Rheumatoid Nodules

▸ Yasmeen M. Butt

Patients with rheumatoid arthritis can develop multiple different pulmonary manifestations throughout the course of their disease including, but not limited to, pleuritis, rheumatoid nodules, organizing pneumonia, interstitial pneumonia, vasculitis, lymphoid hyperplasia, usual interstitial pneumonia pattern fibrosis, and diffuse alveolar damage. Caplan syndrome, or rheumatoid pneumoconiosis, consists of multiple rheumatoid nodules together with coal worker's pneumoconiosis.

Rheumatoid nodules are most often bilateral and numerous. They are typically found in the pleura, subpleura, along the interlobular septae, and/or in the adjacent lung parenchyma. The nodules vary in size and can be up to several centimeters with a characteristic fibrinoid necrotic center and peripheral palisading by epithelioid histiocytes with irregular borders. There is often a dirty basophilic nature to the necrosis at the junction between the necrotic center and the epithelioid histiocytes that is primarily composed of neutrophil nuclear debris. The patient should have seropositive confirmed rheumatoid arthritis to make a diagnosis of a rheumatoid nodule and often also has rheumatoid nodules in nonpulmonary locations. The diagnosis is one of exclusion, and careful examination for infectious causes and necrotizing vasculitis to rule out granulomatosis with polyangiitis must be performed.

HISTOLOGIC FEATURES

- Rheumatoid nodules consist of granulomatous nodules with a core of central fibrinoid necrosis bordered by palisading histiocytes.
- "Dirty" basophilic necrosis is often present at the junction between the necrotic center and the epithelioid histiocytes.
- Multinucleated giant cells are rare and eosinophils should not be seen.
- Infectious causes must be ruled out by careful examination with special stains, such as Gomori methenamine silver for fungi and Ziehl–Neelsen or auramine–rhodamine stains for acid-fast bacilli.

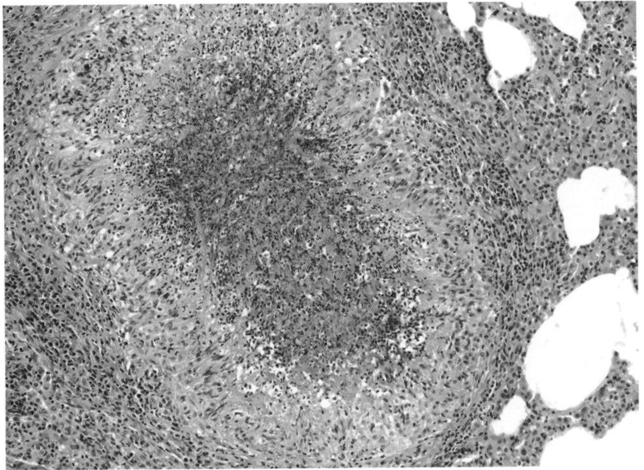

Figure 68.1 A small rheumatoid nodule with prominent palisading of epithelioid histiocytes, central necrosis, and intervening basophilic "dirty" necrosis.

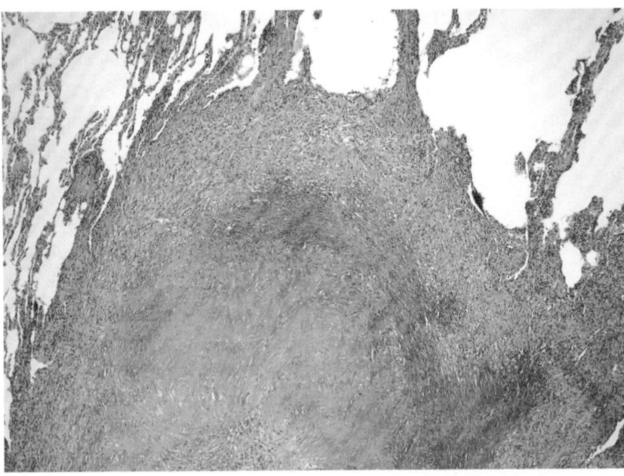

Figure 68.2 A large rheumatoid nodule with central fibrinoid necrosis, patchy peripheral palisading of epithelioid histiocytes, and foci of basophilic "dirty" necrosis at the junction between the central necrosis and peripheral histiocytes.

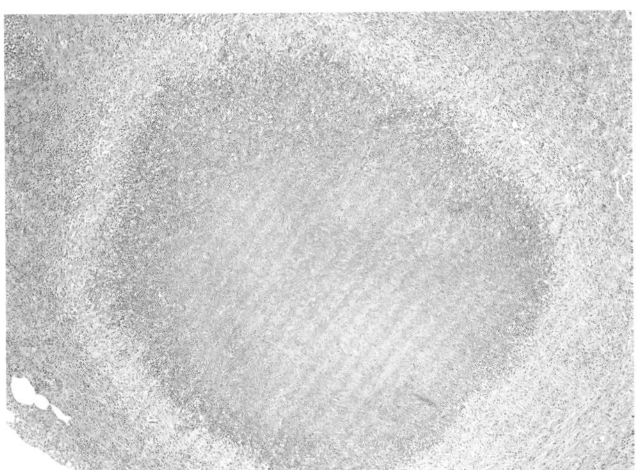

Figure 68.3 A large rheumatoid nodule showing central fibrinoid necrosis, prominent peripheral palisading of epithelioid histiocytes, and basophilic "dirty" necrosis at the junction between the central necrosis and peripheral histiocytes.

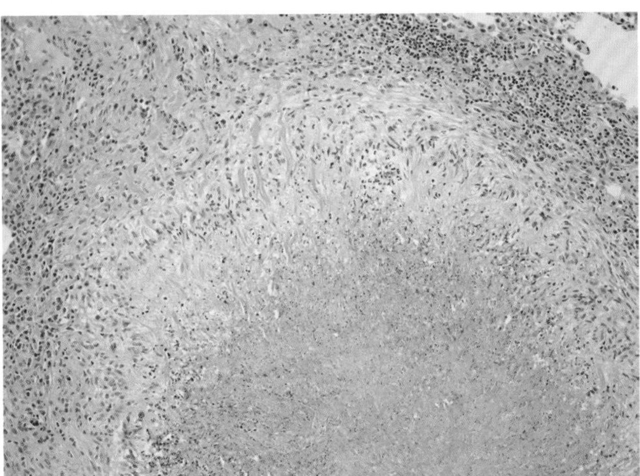

Figure 68.4 High-power image of the edge of a small rheumatoid nodule highlighting the "dirty" basophilic necrosis at the junction of central necrosis and peripheral epithelioid histiocytes. A lymphoplasmacytic component can be appreciated at the edge.

Part 2

Malakoplakia

▸ Yasmeen M. Butt

Malakoplakia is a rare exuberant histiocytic proliferation formed in response to an infection that is most often due to *Rhodococcus equi* pneumonia when seen in the lung. Affected patients are typically infected by human immunodeficiency virus (HIV) or are otherwise immunocompromised. *R. equi* is a weakly acid-fast gram-positive coccobacillus found in soil and animal feces. Patients usually present with a single upper lobe lesion, which, rather than consisting of discrete granulomas, shows sheets of histiocytes replacing lung tissue. The histiocytes have abundant eosinophilic to foamy cytoplasm with numerous intracellular coccobacilli seen on Gram stain. To diagnose malakoplakia, Michaelis–Gutmann bodies (MGBs) must be identified. MGBs can be seen on hematoxylin and eosin stains within histiocytes as small, round, weakly basophilic structures with targetoid concentric laminations. Ultrastructural studies of early MGBs reveal electron-dense cores containing *R. equi* bacteria. It has been hypothesized that an acquired macrophage dysfunction leading to the lack of intracellular digestion of phagocytized bacteria is responsible for malakoplakia with MGB formation, representing an alternative pathway for destruction of the bacteria, as older MGBs do not contain recognizable bacteria. They are highlighted by periodic acid–Schiff, von Kossa calcium, and Prussian blue iron special stains, as the MGBs are rich in calcium and iron from the degenerated bacterial fragments.

HISTOLOGIC FEATURES

- Present in upper lobes as a necrotizing bronchopneumonia, typically as a single lesion.
- Sheets of histiocytes with abundant eosinophilic to foamy cytoplasm.
- Gram stains highlight numerous intracellular coccobacilli.
- For a diagnosis of malakoplakia, MGBs, consisting of small, round, weakly basophilic structures with targetoid concentric laminations, should be present.
- MGBs can be highlighted with periodic acid–Schiff, von Kossa calcium, and Prussian blue iron special stains.

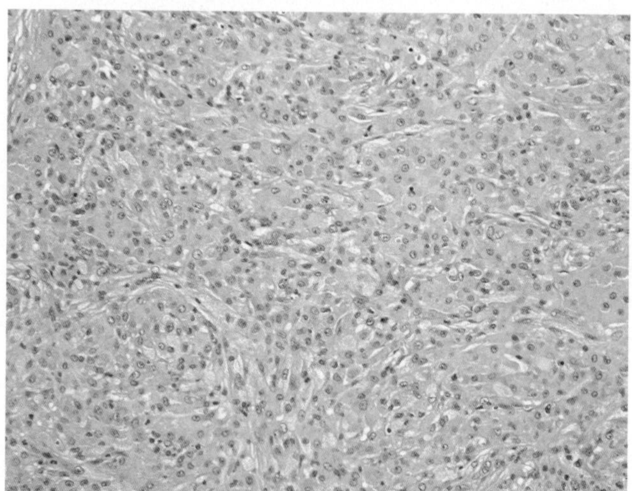

Figure 68.5 Sheets of histiocytes with eosinophilic and foamy cytoplasm replacing lung parenchyma in an HIV patient with *Rhodococcus equi* pneumonia.

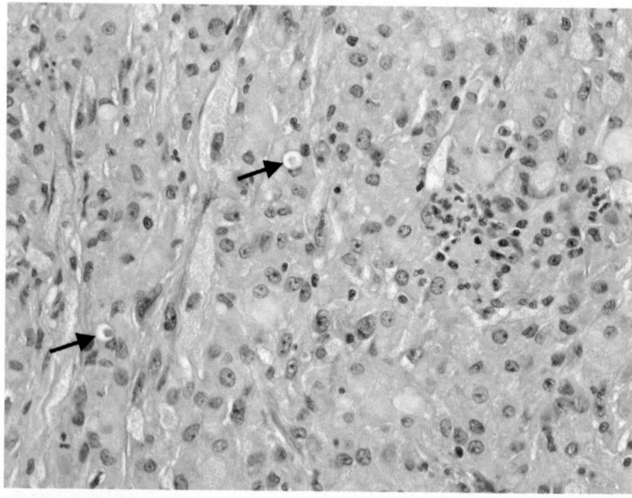

Figure 68.6 Higher power image of histiocytes with scattered Michaelis–Gutmann bodies *(arrows)*.

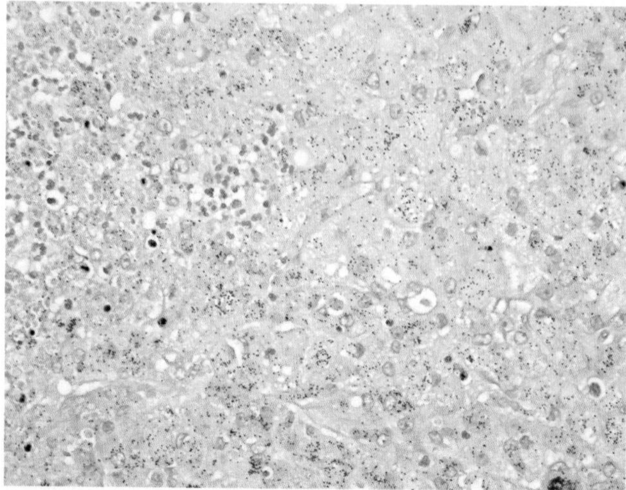

Figure 68.7 Gram stain demonstrating numerous intracellular coccobacilli.

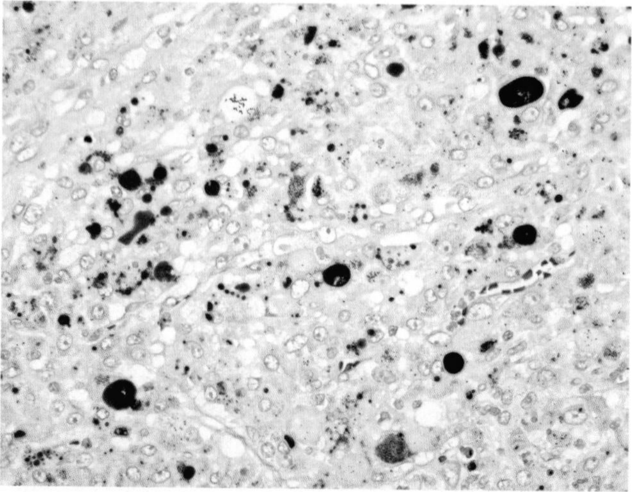

Figure 68.8 Higher power image of a Gram stain demonstrating numerous intracellular coccobacilli.

Section **9**

Diffuse Pulmonary Hemorrhage

▶ Lynette M. Sholl

69 Alveolar Hemorrhage without Vasculitis

Alveolar hemorrhage is a common finding in surgical lung specimens. In most circumstances, this reflects procedural hemorrhage as a result of iatrogenic injury to pulmonary vessels. However, hemorrhage may be seen in a variety of other settings, both as a manifestation of primary vascular injury, such as due to vasculitis, pulmonary thromboembolism, and pulmonary hypertensive changes, and as a secondary injury to a process affecting another compartment of the lung.

Clues are often present in the tissue, which may point to the cause of the bleeding, and typically the pathologist can discriminate between acute procedural hemorrhage and physiologic bleeding based on the absence or presence of hemosiderin deposition in the lung. In small biopsies and/or in patients with acute symptom onset, however, this may not always be possible and clinical correlation may be required.

Part 1

Artifactual (Procedural) Hemorrhage/ Hemorrhage in the Absence of Other Histologic Abnormalities

▸ Lynette M. Sholl

Hemorrhage in the absence of other histologic abnormalities may be seen most commonly in the setting of surgical or other interventional procedures (transthoracic or transbronchial core biopsies or fine needle aspirations). The findings here will be largely indistinguishable from other settings in which the lung is traumatized (e.g., motor vehicle accidents and lung puncture injuries). Patients with a coagulopathy will be more prone to pulmonary hemorrhage when undergoing a surgical procedure. Those with a preexisting coagulopathy will typically have hemosiderin-laden macrophages visible in the alveolar spaces; these are evidence for chronic bleeding and can help to discriminate between purely procedural hemorrhage and chronic or subacute hemorrhage. Blood from sources in the upper airways/sinonasal structures may track/be aspirated into the lungs, leading to a similar appearance of histologically normal lung with blood and hemosiderin-laden macrophages filling the airspaces.

HISTOLOGIC FEATURES

- Intra-alveolar or perivascular hemorrhage; fibrin and leukocytes may be visible.
- Histologically normal-appearing alveolar septa.
- Absence of hyaline membranes.
- Presence or absence of hemosiderin-laden macrophages, depending on chronicity.

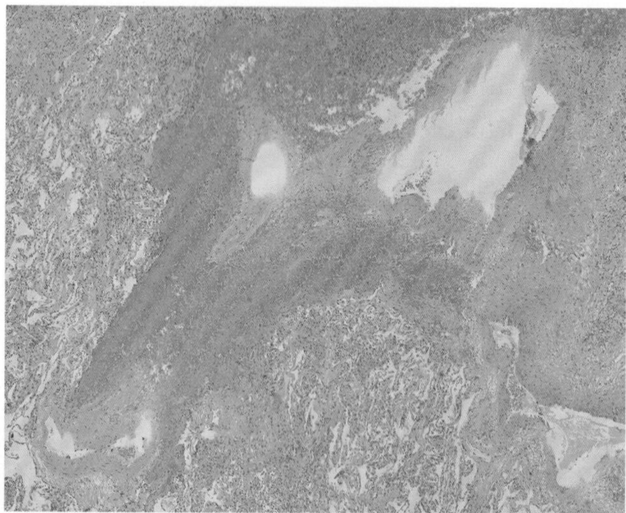

Figure 69.1 Procedural hemorrhage in a patient undergoing lobectomy for a lung mass. The hemorrhage in this case is tracking through the adventitia of a pulmonary vessel and has discrete boundaries.

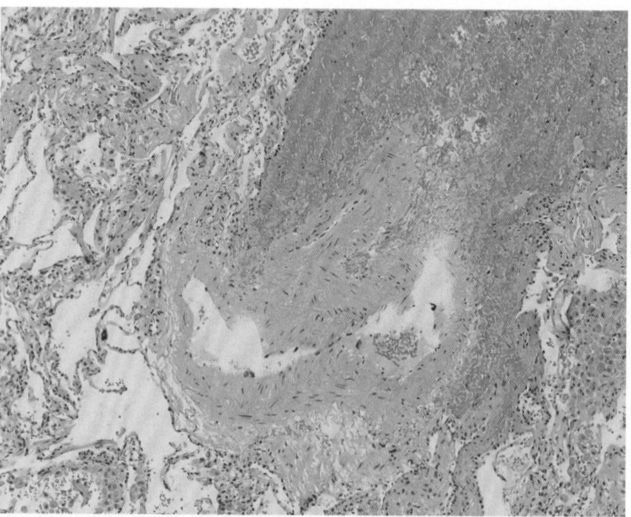

Figure 69.2 Hemosiderin-laden macrophages are absent in the surrounding tissue in the case of acute procedural hemorrhage.

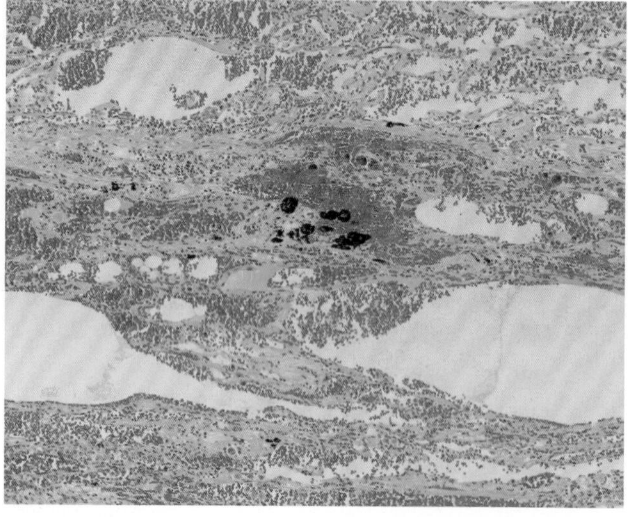

Figure 69.3 Alveolar hemorrhage with frequent hemosiderin-laden macrophages in a patient with an endobronchial salivary gland tumor as a source of bleeding.

Part 2

Hemorrhage as a Secondary Finding (Infection, Malignancy)

▶ Lynette M. Sholl

Hemorrhage due to localized infection or malignancy is common. Local injury to the capillaries and small pulmonary vessels may result in focal alveolar hemorrhage, whereas erosion into a large pulmonary vessel may lead to massive, fatal hemorrhage (as in tuberculosis, squamous-cell carcinoma).

Diffuse alveolar hemorrhage may be associated with a number of infectious etiologies that cause alveolar capillary injury. The implicated organisms vary based on the immune status of the host. In immunocompromised patients, diffuse alveolar hemorrhage is most often associated with *Aspergillus*, cytomegalovirus, adenovirus, legionella, and mycoplasma. In immunocompetent hosts, it is most commonly seen with *Staphylococcus aureus* and influenza A infections, as well as dengue, malaria, and leptospirosis. Patients typically, but not universally, present with hemoptysis. Increasing red blood cell content in sequential bronchoalveolar lavage specimens can confirm a clinical or radiographic suspicion of diffuse alveolar hemorrhage.

HISTOLOGIC FEATURES

- Intra-alveolar red blood cells and fibrin will be adjacent to a mass lesion when present as a focal finding or throughout the sample airspaces when present as a diffuse process.
- Hemosiderin-laden macrophages should be identifiable in the setting of subacute to chronic disease.
- Hyaline membranes may be identified in the context of diffuse alveolar hemorrhage due to infectious causes (see Chapter 93).

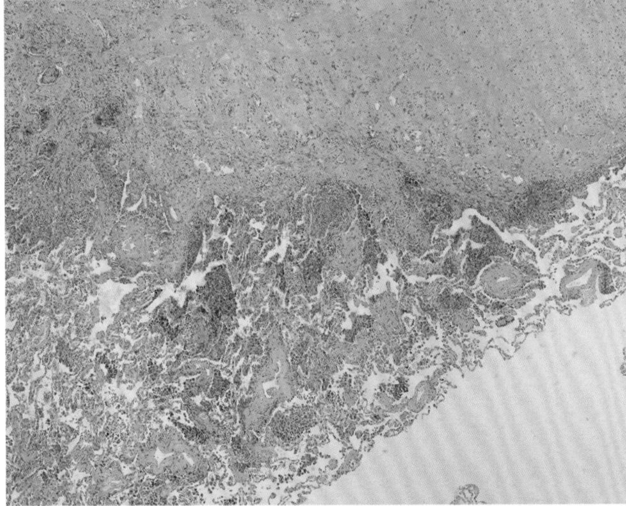

Figure 69.4 Localized alveolar hemorrhage with abundant hemosiderin-laden macrophages adjacent to a nodule of epithelioid hemangioendothelioma in the lung.

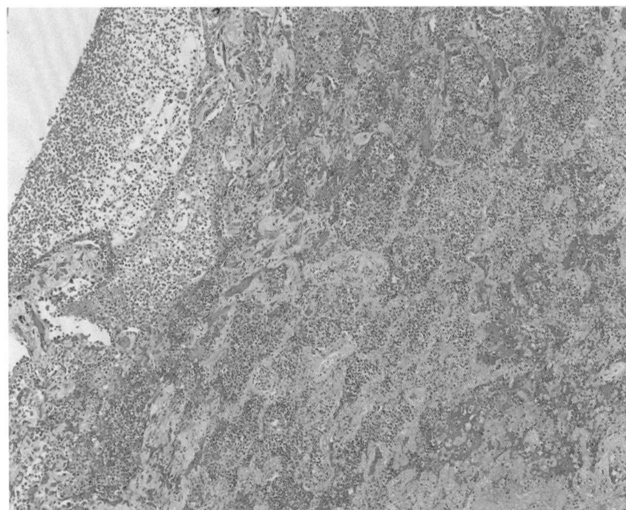

Figure 69.5 Acute hemorrhage in the setting of a necrotizing pneumonia due to a nosocomial gram-negative rod (*Chryseobacterium gleum*). Sheets of neutrophils are also visible.

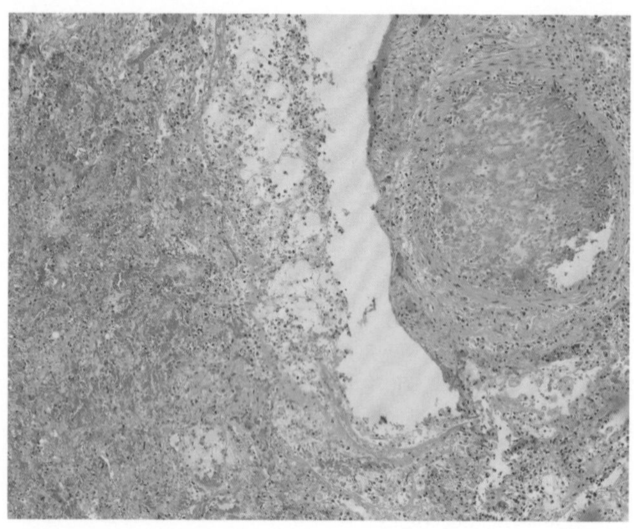

Figure 69.6 Lung infarction, diffuse alveolar hemorrhage, and necrosis in the setting of angioinvasive *Aspergillus* infection in an immunocompromised host. Fungal forms are visible in the dilated vessel at the *right* of the image.

Part 3

Hemorrhage with Diffuse Alveolar Damage

▶ Lynette M. Sholl

Intra-alveolar hemorrhage occurs in the exudative phase of diffuse alveolar damage, defined as the first 1 to 7 days following injury, and is accompanied by edema, neutrophilic infiltrates, and hyaline membrane formation. During the proliferative and organizing phases of diffuse alveolar damage, the red cells will be consumed by macrophages and the resulting hemosiderin-laden macrophages will serve as evidence of earlier hemorrhage. However, patients with iterative injury to the lung, as is common in diffuse alveolar damage, may show a combination of fresh hemorrhage and organizing lung injury. Identification of hemorrhage in the context of diffuse alveolar damage does not point to a specific etiology. See Chapter 93 for further discussion of diffuse alveolar damage.

HISTOLOGIC FEATURES

- Hyaline membranes line the surfaces of the alveolar ducts and sacs.
- Capillaries appear engorged.
- Red blood cells fill the alveolar spaces.
- Alveolar septa are widened by proliferating fibroblasts/myofibroblasts in the organizing phase of diffuse alveolar damage, and hemosiderin-laden macrophages may be prominent.

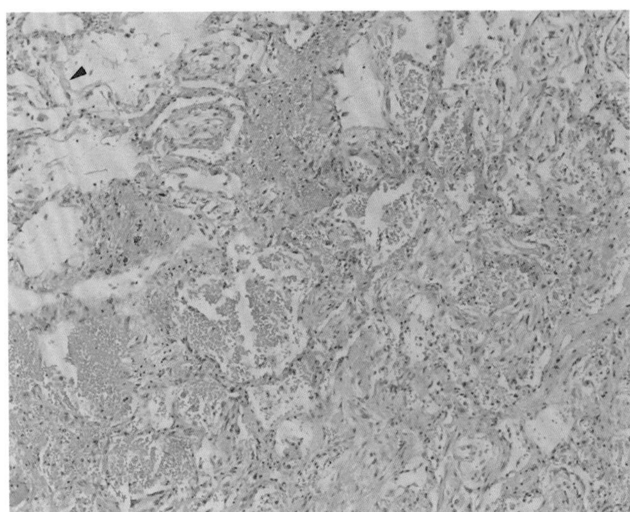

Figure 69.7 Alveolar hemorrhage in a patient with acute and organizing diffuse alveolar damage. Hyaline membranes are visible *(arrowhead)* along with abundant intra-alveolar red blood cells. Organization of the diffuse alveolar damage is evident in the *right half* of the image.

Part 4

Passive Congestion

Lynette M. Sholl

Passive congestion in the lung is most commonly a manifestation of chronic pulmonary venous hypertension. This results from aberrations of the left side of the heart, pulmonary veins or aorta that obstruct blood flow. Changes can be seen across the pulmonary vascular bed as a result of the elevated pressures (see Section 10: Pulmonary Hypertension and Emboli). Alveolar hemorrhage results from increased pressure ("stress failure") at the level of the pulmonary capillaries. The capillaries will appear distended and may become displaced deeper into the wall of the alveolar septum in the context of long-standing venous hypertension. Patients characteristically present with episodic hemoptysis. Lung biopsy specimens will show hemosiderosis.

Acute right-sided heart failure in the setting of congenital heart disease, pulmonary hypertension, thromboembolic disease, or cardiac surgery can lead to pulmonary hemorrhage and hemoptysis. Patients present with acute onset of shortness of breath. Echocardiography or autopsy studies will demonstrate enlargement of the right ventricle and pulmonary artery.

HISTOLOGIC FEATURES

- Pulmonary alveolar capillaries appear distended and may or may not appear engorged.
- Capillaries appear displaced into the center of the alveolar structures, and increased collagen deposition leads to a widened septal profile.
- Hemosiderosis manifests as intra-alveolar pigmented macrophages and iron encrustation of elastic fibers.
- Hemosiderosis may not be apparent in the setting of acute right-sided heart failure.

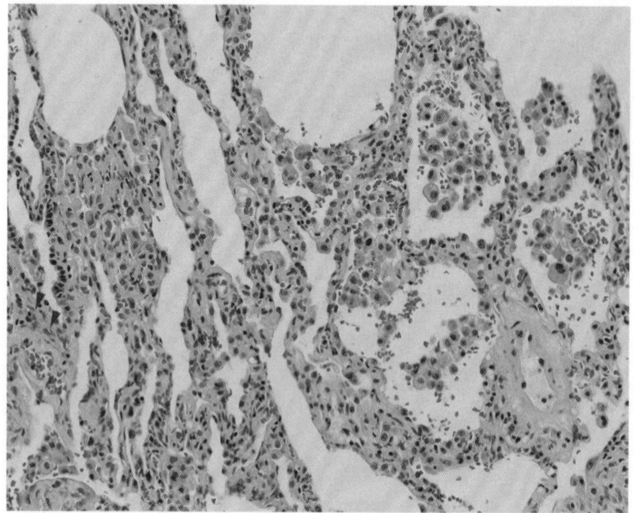

Figure 69.8 Alveolar capillaries are distended and engorged, hemosiderin-laden macrophages are prominent in the airspaces, and iron encrustation of elastic fibers is evident in the supporting tissues *(arrowheads)*.

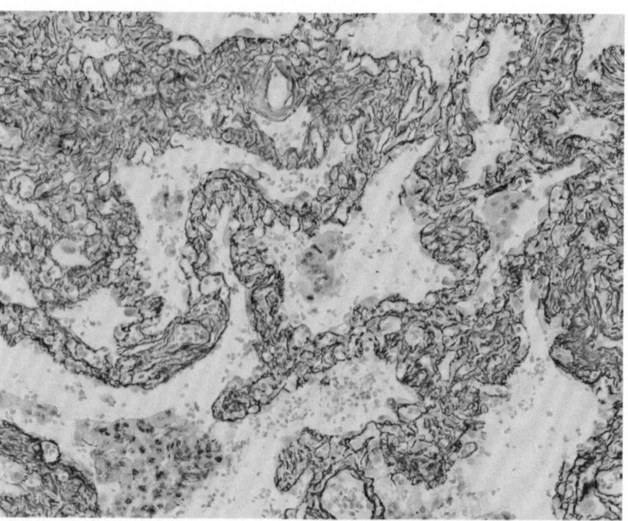

Figure 69.9 A reticulin stain highlights the prominent, dilated alveolar capillaries. Prominent iron deposition can be seen, decorating the elastic fibers of a small vessel at the *top left*.

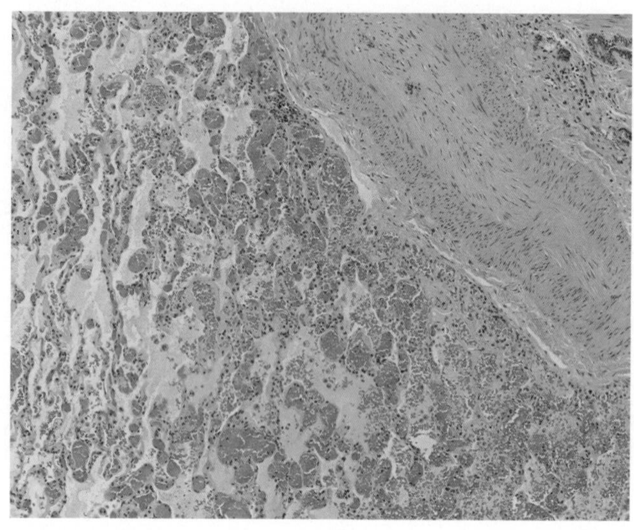

Figure 69.10 Acute capillary engorgement with alveolar filling by edema fluid and red blood cells in a patient with peripartum right-sided heart failure and a history of primary arterial hypertension. An occluded artery is evident in the *top right* of the image.

Part 5

Arteriovenous Malformations

Lynette M. Sholl and Keith M. Kerr

The most common malformations of the pulmonary vasculature occur as communications between the pulmonary arterial and venous systems. Most cases are congenital. More than half of the patients with pulmonary arteriovenous malformations have the autosomal-dominant disorder hereditary hemorrhagic telangiectasia, also known as *Rendu–Osler–Weber disease*. Symptomatic pulmonary arteriovenous malformations are more commonly associated with hereditary hemorrhagic telangiectasia-1, resulting from mutations in the gene encoding endoglin (*ENG*). The lesions are found in the subpleura of the lower lobes and are most commonly unifocal. The vast majority are considered to be "simple," with a single feeding artery and draining vein. Physiologically, these create an extracardiac right-to-left shunt, leading to dyspnea and cyanosis. Disruption of the malformation can trigger hemoptysis or hemothorax. Acquired pulmonary arteriovenous malformations may result from surgery to repair congenital cardiac defects and have been reported rarely in adults secondary to cancer, cirrhosis, or trauma.

HISTOLOGIC FEATURES

- Arteriovenous malformations show aneurysmal dilatation of thin-walled vessels containing blood or organized thrombus.
- These are typically located in the subpleura.
- Vessel walls show variable admixtures of collagen, elastic tissue, and smooth muscle.

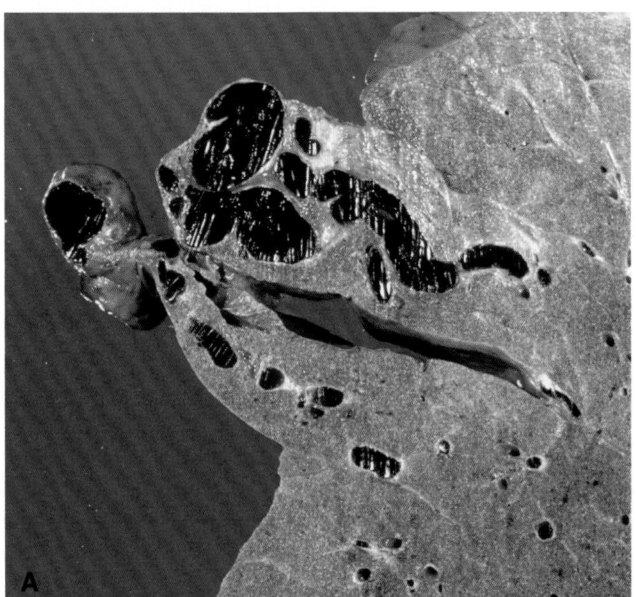

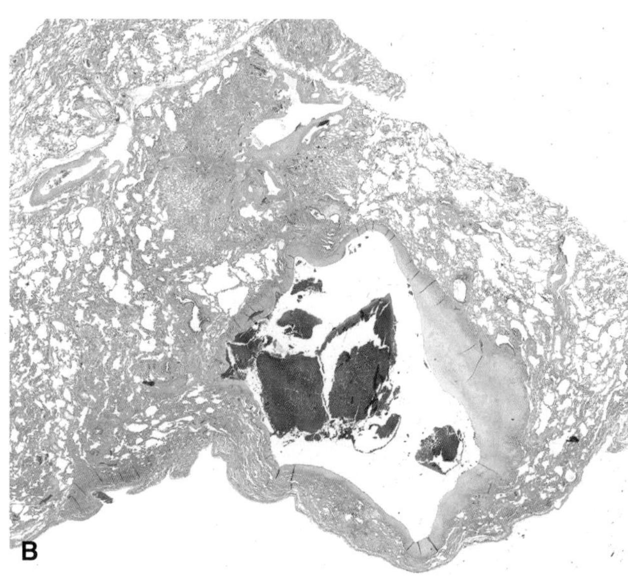

Figure 69.11 **A:** Gross figure of arteriovenous malformation shows group of dilated blood vessels filled with thrombus. **B:** Aneurysmal dilatation of a subpleural vessel with variable thickening of the wall by collagen and smooth muscle and containing blood. Feeding/draining vessels are evident at the top and at the left of the dilated vessel.

Part 6

Idiopathic Pulmonary Hemosiderosis

Sara O. Vargas and Lynette M. Sholl

Idiopathic pulmonary hemosiderosis is a form of diffuse pulmonary hemorrhage; about 80% of cases are reported in the pediatric population. It is a diagnosis of exclusion, made only after known causes of upper and lower respiratory tract bleeding have been ruled out. The disease is thought to arise from chronic pulmonary microhemorrhage; reports of association with antineutrophilic cytoplasmic antibodies (ANCAs) and antinuclear antibodies, celiac disease, and Down syndrome point to a role for autoimmunity and genetic predisposition. Idiopathic pulmonary hemosiderosis is excluded in the setting of a more specific cause of diffuse pulmonary hemorrhage, such as capillaritis (associated with connective tissue disease, drug reaction, and other immune and idiopathic causes), granulomatosis with polyangiitis, cardiovascular disease (such as pulmonary arterial hypertension, pulmonary veno-occlusive disease, and mitral valve disease), bone marrow transplantation, and others. Truly idiopathic cases are rare.

Patients present with hemoptysis, iron-deficiency anemia, and pulmonary opacities on chest imaging. Detection of hemosiderin-laden macrophages in bronchoalveolar lavage fluid is helpful in confirming the diagnosis; in many settings, lung biopsy can be useful to exclude histologically evident causes of hemorrhage. Of note, capillaritis in particular can be difficult to confirm in a lung biopsy because active capillaritis can be exquisitely localized and healed capillaritis can be unrecognizable as such. Therefore, the distinction between, for example, "ANCA-associated pulmonary capillaritis" and "idiopathic pulmonary hemosiderosis in a patient with ANCA" may rely on the serendipity of biopsy sampling. Patients are treated with supportive care and immunosuppression. Pediatric patients tend to have more severe disease and worse clinical outcomes, including pulmonary fibrosis and death. The disease tends to be milder in adults.

HISTOLOGIC FEATURES

- Red blood cells seen in the interstitium and alveolar spaces may be difficult to distinguish from procedural artifact.
- Hemosiderin-laden macrophages are visible in the airspaces; they may be numerous or sparse.
- Interstitial fibrosis may be prominent in patients with persistent disease.
- Capillaritis/vasculitis, vasculopathy, infection, tumor, infarct, or other known cause of hemorrhage and hemosiderosis are absent.

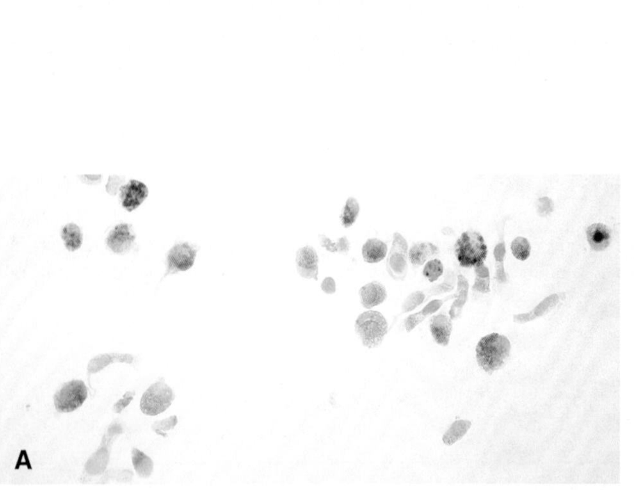

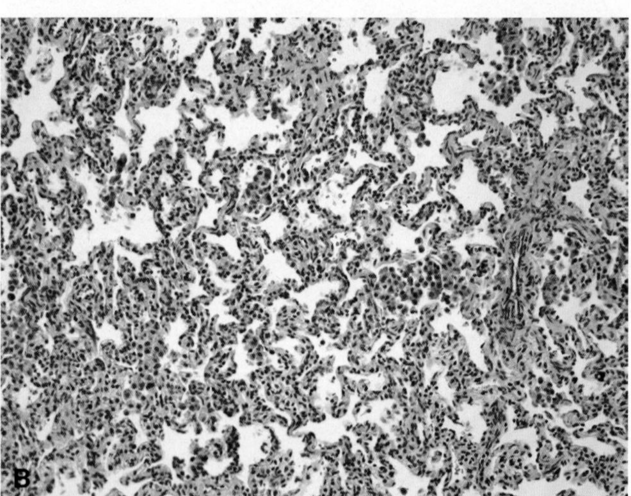

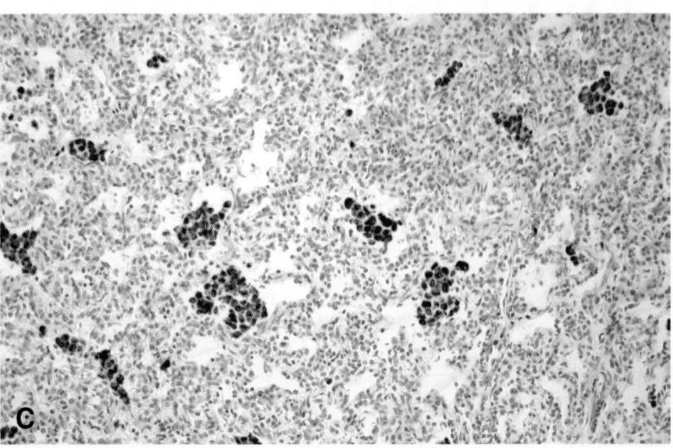

Figure 69.12 A–C: Idiopathic pulmonary hemosiderosis in a 2-month-old boy with recurrent respiratory distress, hemoptysis, anemia, and bibasilar lung infiltrates. Bronchoalveolar lavage fluid (**A**) demonstrated numerous hemosiderin-laden macrophages. Lung biopsy (**B**), including an iron stain (**C**), confirmed the hemosiderosis and helped to rule out more specific causes of pulmonary bleeding.

Alveolar Hemorrhage with Vasculitis

70

Alveolar hemorrhage in the context of vasculitis results from immune-mediated injury to the pulmonary vasculature. The vasculitides are characterized by the nature of the inflammation affecting the vessels, the caliber of the affected vessels, and the associated serologic markers. The nature of the clinical presentation similarly reflects the types of vessels affected, including the vessels in extrapulmonary organs.

In this context, diffuse alveolar hemorrhage results from pulmonary capillaritis and is most commonly associated with microscopic polyangiitis and granulomatosis with polyangiitis (formerly Wegener granulomatosis). Clinically, patients present with progressive dyspnea and declining hemoglobin in the absence of other sources of hemorrhage or hemolysis; hemoptysis is often absent. Radiology studies reveal diffuse pulmonary ground-glass infiltrates. Bronchoalveolar lavage fluid appears bright red. Over half of patients will require mechanical ventilation. Treatment should be aimed at the underlying etiology and typically involves immunosuppression.

Alveolar hemorrhage is a rare manifestation of autoimmune disorders such as systemic lupus erythematosus (SLE) and antiphospholipid syndrome and vasculitides such as eosinophilic granulomatosis with polyangiitis (formerly Churg–Strauss disease). A variety of distinctive clinical presentations can be seen in vasculitides lacking an alveolar hemorrhage component.

Part 1

Vasculitis in Collagen Vascular Diseases

▶ Lynette M. Sholl

Among patients with connective tissue disorders, and outside of the systemic vasculitides, alveolar hemorrhage is observed most commonly with SLE. While alveolar hemorrhage is rare in this context—occurring in 1% to 5% of SLE patients according to some studies—it may be the presenting sign of the underlying connective tissue disease. Alveolar hemorrhage in SLE is most commonly observed in women in the third to fifth decades and appears to be associated with more severe forms of the disease, with patients experiencing significant extrapulmonary involvement, including nephritis, pleuritis/pericarditis, arthritis, and constitutional symptoms. Alveolar hemorrhage may also be seen in pediatric patients with SLE.

Alveolar hemorrhage, likely resulting from pulmonary capillaritis, is reported in a variety of other connective tissue and autoimmune disorders, including rheumatoid arthritis, Behçet disease, Sjogren syndrome, and mixed connective tissue disease.

SLE-associated alveolar hemorrhage presents abruptly with dyspnea and fever, along with the classic features of dropping hemoglobin, hemoptysis, and new infiltrates on chest radiograph. In the absence of aggressive immunosuppressive therapy (glucocorticoids and cytotoxic agents), alveolar hemorrhage can lead to respiratory failure and rapid death in this context.

HISTOLOGIC FEATURES

- Red blood cells and hemosiderin-laden macrophages are visible in the alveolar spaces.
- Intra-alveolar fibrin deposition.
- Capillary infiltration by neutrophils.
- Reactive hyperplasia of type II pneumocytes.

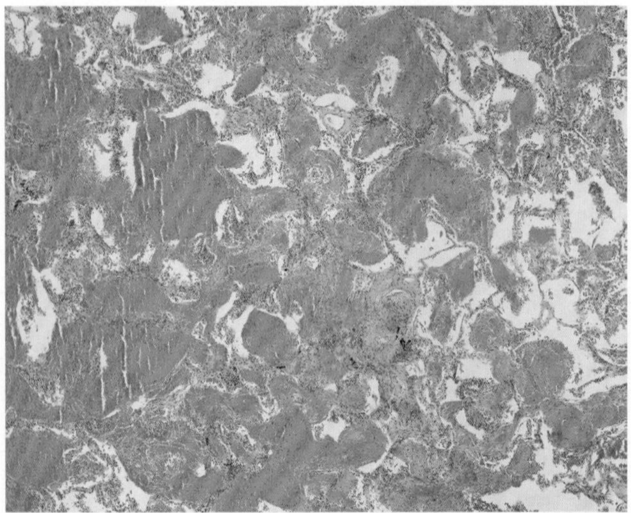

Figure 70.1 Filling and distension of the alveolar spaces by fresh blood and fibrin in a patient with acute alveolar hemorrhage in the setting of rheumatoid arthritis.

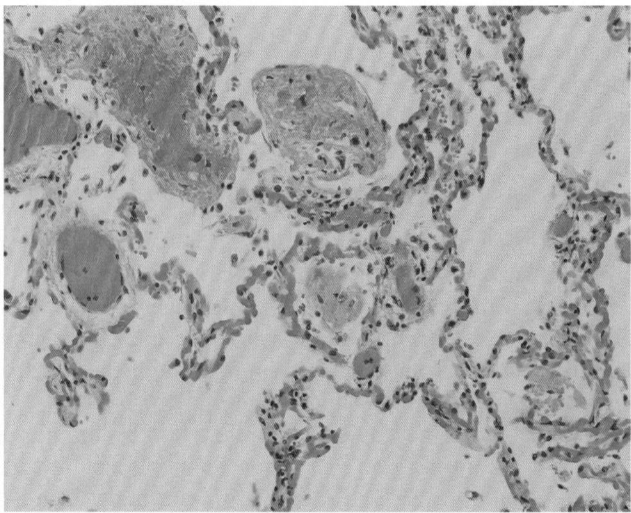

Figure 70.2 Fresh blood and fibrin admixed in airspaces, with capillary engorgement. Scattered interstitial neutrophils are visible suggestive of partially treated capillaritis.

Part 2

Anti–Glomerular Basement Membrane Antibody Disease (Goodpasture Syndrome)

▸ Lynette M. Sholl

Anti–glomerular basement membrane (anti-GBM) antibody disease, also known as *Goodpasture syndrome*, is mediated by antibodies to the glomerular basement membrane. It clinically manifests as rapidly progressive crescentic glomerulonephritis with acute renal failure, pulmonary hemorrhage, and autoimmune inner ear disease. Anti-GBM antibodies target the noncollagenous-1 domain of the alpha 3 chain of type IV collagen. Immunofluorescence studies reveal linear deposition of IgG along the alveolar basement membrane. Anti-GBM antibodies can be detected in the circulation. Up to a third of patients will have detectable p-antineutrophilic cytoplasmic antibody (ANCA) antibodies in the serum with associated symptoms of systemic vasculitis. Immunosuppression is the mainstay of therapy; plasmapheresis has been suggested in patients with alveolar hemorrhage, but controlled trials demonstrating a benefit to this approach are lacking.

HISTOLOGIC FEATURES

- Alveolar spaces are filled with red blood cells and hemosiderin-laden macrophages.
- Neutrophilic capillaritis may be seen.
- Features of diffuse alveolar damage including hyaline membranes may be seen.

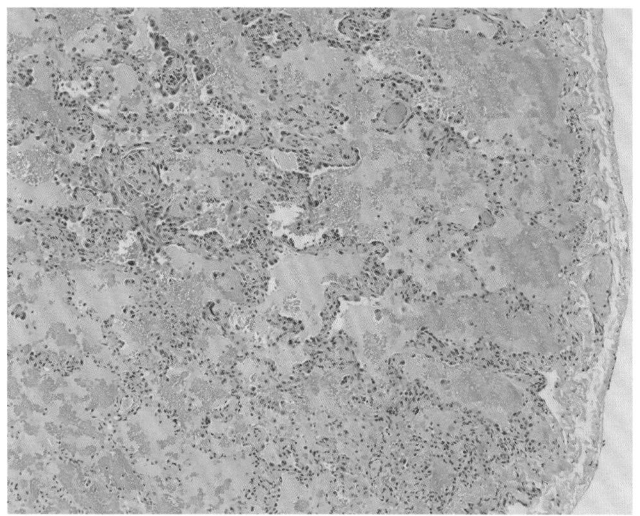

Figure 70.3 Acute hemorrhage in a patient presenting with diffuse alveolar hemorrhage in the context of Goodpasture syndrome. The airspaces are filled with proteinaceous fluid and red blood cells. Type II pneumocytes show reactive hyperplasia and atypia. Focal fibroblastic proliferation and myxoid matrix deposition is consistent with organizing pneumonia.

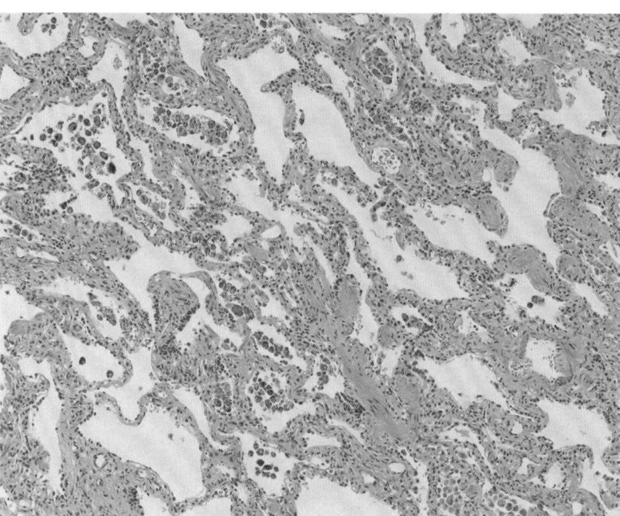

Figure 70.4 Diffuse interstitial fibrosis in a patient with a long-standing history of Goodpasture syndrome and systemic mixed connective tissue disorder. The alveolar septa are uniformly thickened by increased collagen deposition, and hemosiderin-laden macrophages are prominent in the airspaces.

Part 3

Granulomatosis with Polyangiitis (Formerly Wegener Granulomatosis)

Lynette M. Sholl

Granulomatosis with polyangiitis (GPA) is a form of ANCA-associated vasculitis affecting small vessels and capillaries. GPA most commonly manifests as granulomatous vasculitis in the lung and upper respiratory tract and pauci-immune necrotizing glomerulonephritis but may affect multiple other organ systems, including skin and central nervous system. It preferentially affects middle-aged adults of Northern European descent and has been associated with polymorphisms in immune-related genes HLA-DP and CTLA4 and in SERPINA1, the gene encoding alpha 1 antitrypsin.

Patients may initially present with granulomatous inflammation limited to the respiratory tract or lung; the clinical and radiographic differential in this latter setting may be broad and include infection or malignancy. Among the ANCA-associated vasculitides, GPA is most likely to give rise to constitutional symptoms, including fever and arthralgias. GPA is associated with autoantibodies to the neutrophil glycoproteins proteinase 3 (PR-3) in two-thirds of cases and myeloperoxidase (MPO) in about a quarter of cases; immunofluorescence staining of neutrophils shows diffuse cytoplasmic distribution of PR3-ANCA (C-ANCA) compared with perinuclear distribution of MPO-ANCA (P-ANCA). Untreated, GPA can be fatal. Rituximab is the preferred treatment.

HISTOLOGIC FEATURES

- "Geographic necrosis" characterized by serpiginous bands and islands of basophilic necrotic debris.
- Palisading histiocytes and frequent giant cells.
- Fibrinoid necrosis of the vascular media.
- Abundant necrotic neutrophils.
- Alveolar hemorrhage may be prominent.

Figure 70.5 Lung tissue with geographic necrosis and associated necrotic neutrophils, abundant histiocytes and giant cells, and hemorrhage.

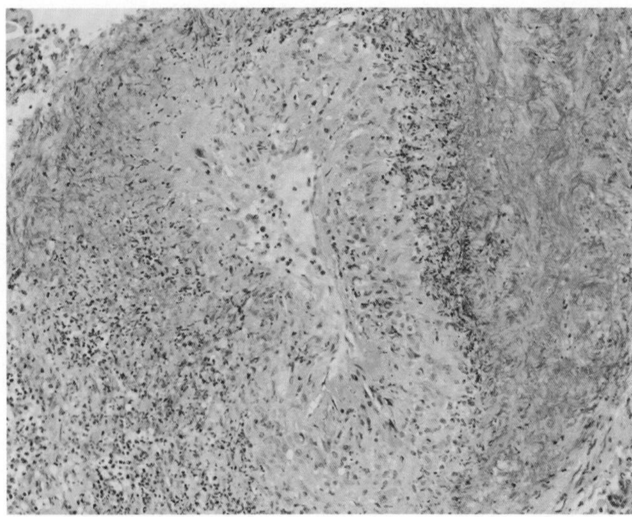

Figure 70.6 Fibrinoid necrosis of a small pulmonary vessel with adjacent necrotic neutrophils and basophilic necrosis.

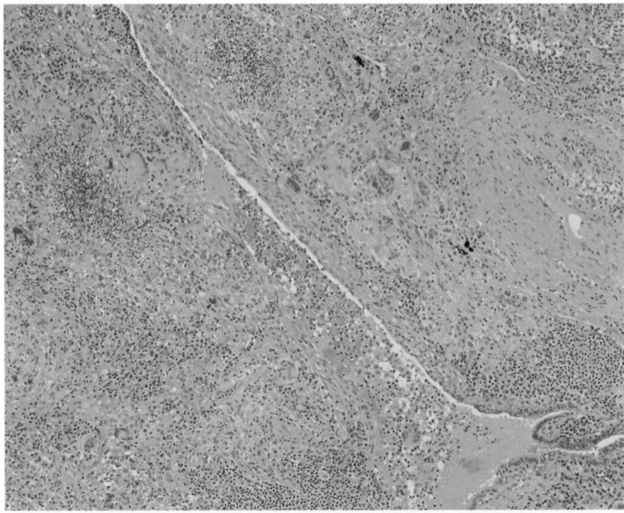

Figure 70.7 Airway destruction in a rare case of GPA with extensive airway involvement. Giant cells are prominent. Multiple neutrophilic abscesses are visible in the field.

Part 4

Eosinophilic Granulomatosis with Polyangiitis (Formerly Churg–Strauss Syndrome)

Lynette M. Sholl

Eosinophilic granulomatosis with polyangiitis (EGPA) is the least common of the ANCA-associated vasculitides. EGPA affects small- and medium-sized vessels and is associated with asthma and tissue and blood eosinophilia. Asthma symptoms almost always precede the diagnosis of EGPA, typically by several years, and are often poorly controlled. The clinical manifestations overlap with a variety of other processes, including *Toxocara* or *Strongyloides* infections, allergic bronchopulmonary aspergillosis, chronic eosinophilic pneumonia, and hypereosinophilic syndrome. Features pointing to a diagnosis of EGPA include migratory lung infiltrates by high-resolution computed tomography scanning, nasal polyps, glomerulonephritis, and granulomatous inflammation in biopsies of affected tissues. Disease involvement may be restricted to the respiratory tract in some patients. Nerve and cardiac involvement may be prominent in EGPA; eosinophilic infiltration of the heart muscle with resulting fibrosis leads to ventricular dysfunction and is associated with poor prognosis.

Perinuclear anti-MPO ANCA (p-ANCA) antibodies predominate in EGPA but are detected in fewer than half of patients who otherwise meet diagnostic criteria. Genetic association studies have identified an increased risk of EGPA and other forms of MPO-ANCA in patients with *HLA-DQ*. A Th2 pattern of T-cell response predominates in EGPA.

Alveolar hemorrhage is seen less commonly here than in other forms of ANCA-associated vasculitis but is considered a life-threatening manifestation of EGPA and requires prompt intervention with glucocorticoids and other immunosuppressants. EGPA must be distinguished from hypereosinophilic syndrome resulting from *FIP1L1-PDGFRA*-driven myeloproliferative neoplasm; this latter entity is highly responsive to therapy with the imatinib mesylate tyrosine kinase inhibitor.

HISTOLOGIC FEATURES

- Extravascular tissue infiltration by eosinophils, including eosinophilic abscesses.
- Inflammatory involvement of small- to medium-sized vessels, including by eosinophils.
- Necrotizing vasculitis may be seen but is not required.
- Alveolar hemorrhage, when present, appears as fresh blood and hemosiderin-laden macrophages in the alveolar spaces.

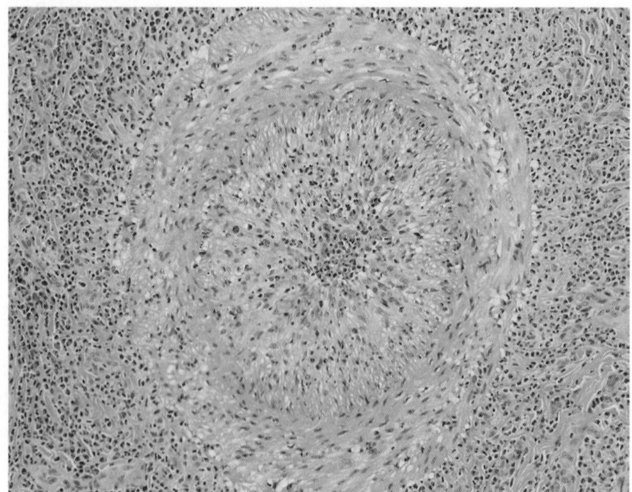

Figure 70.8 A medium-sized muscular artery with eosinophilic infiltration and marked reactive intimal proliferation. Pronounced extravascular eosinophil-rich infiltrates can be seen around the vessel in association with scar formation and airspace obliteration.

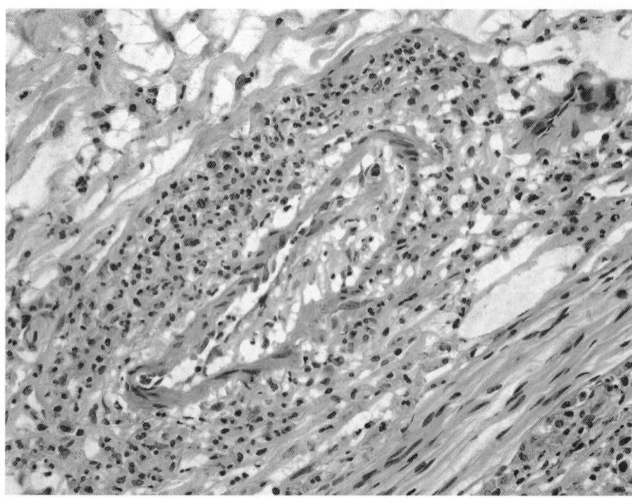

Figure 70.9 Small pulmonary vessel infiltrated by eosinophils with fibrinous necrosis and obliteration of the vascular lumen.

Part 5

Antiphospholipid Syndrome

Lynette M. Sholl

Antiphospholipid syndrome is a thrombotic microangiopathy characterized by arterial, venous, or small-vessel thrombosis and evidence for serum anticardiolipin, anti–beta 2 microglobulin, or lupus anticoagulant antibodies. In the classic clinical syndrome, a young woman presents with recurrent miscarriages; however, men and older individuals, particularly those with a history of lupus, are also affected. Antiphospholipid syndrome is commonly implicated in venous thromboses and stroke episodes in individuals below the ages of 70 and 50 years, respectively. Antiphospholipid syndrome is associated with elevated plasma levels of oxidized beta 2 microglobulin, and this is proposed to serve as a nidus for endothelial cell injury and thrombosis. Antiphospholipid syndrome may arise secondarily in patients with SLE.

Pulmonary hemorrhage is a rare complication of antiphospholipid syndrome and can occur without evidence of coexisting pulmonary vessel thrombosis. Although antiphospholipid antibody–mediated neutrophil recruitment and capillaritis has been implicated as the cause of hemorrhage in these cases, the hemorrhage is commonly bland and its etiology only determined based on clinical and serologic correlation. Alveolar hemorrhage in the setting of antiphospholipid syndrome is consider a rheumatologic emergency and may be refractory to immunosuppressive therapies. Alveolar hemorrhage is fatal in up to a quarter of patients in this setting.

HISTOLOGIC FEATURES

- Blood and fibrin-filled alveolar spaces.
- In cases with evident capillaritis, neutrophils decorate the alveolar interstitium.
- Vascular thrombosis is typically not evident in the context of alveolar hemorrhage.

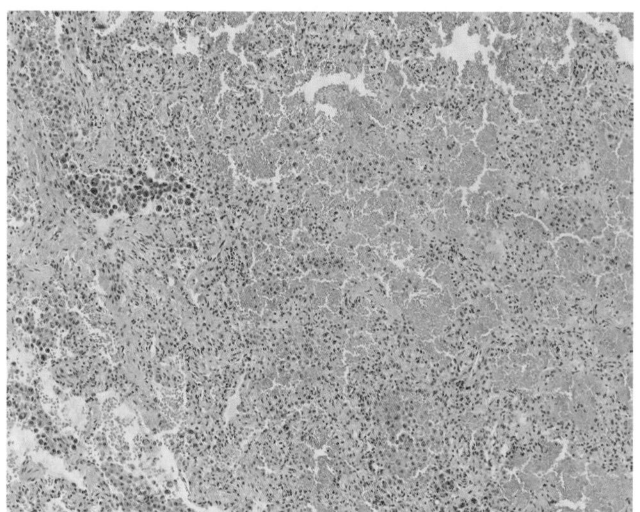

Figure 70.10 Diffuse alveolar hemorrhage in a patient with antiphospholipid syndrome based on serologic criteria. Diffuse airspace filling by fresh blood and hemosiderin-laden macrophages can be seen.

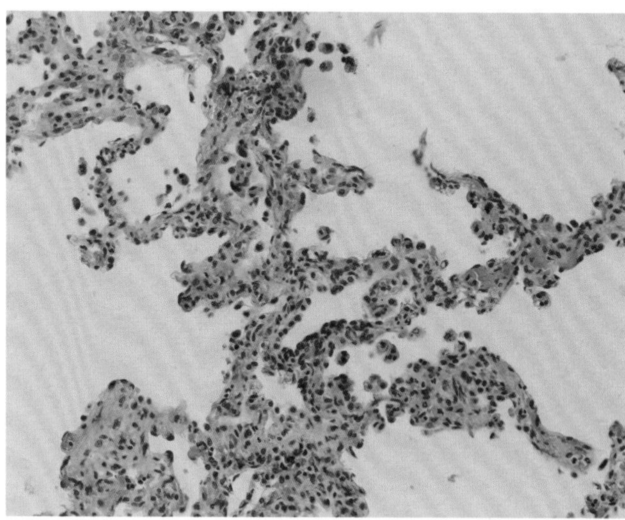

Figure 70.11 Higher magnification shows alveolar interstitium thickened by neutrophil-rich inflammatory infiltrates, mild collagen deposition, and reactive pneumocyte hyperplasia. Vascular thrombosis was not evident in this pulmonary wedge resection specimen.

Part 6

Microscopic Polyangiitis

▸ Lynette M. Sholl

The clinical features of microscopic polyangiitis (MPA) overlap with that of GPA and polyarteritis nodosa (PAN) and include capillaritis and small-vessel vasculitis predominantly affecting the kidney and lung. In contrast to GPA, MPA lacks the granulomatous inflammation, affecting the lung and upper respiratory tract. Rather, alveolar hemorrhage is the principle manifestation in the lung, occurring in about a third to half of patients. Detection of antineutrophilic cytoplasmic antibodies (anti-MPO-ANCA > anti-PR3-ANCA) will distinguish MPA from PAN. MPA is the most common ANCA-associated vasculitis in Asian populations. Clinically, patients present with nonspecific complaints, including fever and weight loss, and the diagnosis may not become evident before the kidney, lungs, or other organs suffer irreversible damage. In the lung, a clinical diagnosis of fibrosing interstitial lung disease may precede the recognition of ANCA vasculitis, a relationship that appears particularly striking in the context of Japanese patients with MPA.

Alveolar hemorrhage in patients with MPA tends to occur bilaterally and affects the upper and lower lung zones; however, about a third of patients have hemorrhage restricted to the upper lungs. Significant alveolar hemorrhage is a major contributor to disease morbidity and mortality. Immunosuppressive therapies improve outcomes; treatment regimens are similar to those used in other ANCA-associated vasculitides, including glucocorticoids, steroid-sparing agents, and rituximab.

HISTOLOGIC FEATURES

- Fresh blood in alveolar spaces.
- Hemosiderin-laden macrophages in alveolar spaces.
- Neutrophils decorating the interstitial capillaries with fibrinoid necrosis of capillary walls.
- Established interstitial fibrosis may be evident in a subset of patients.

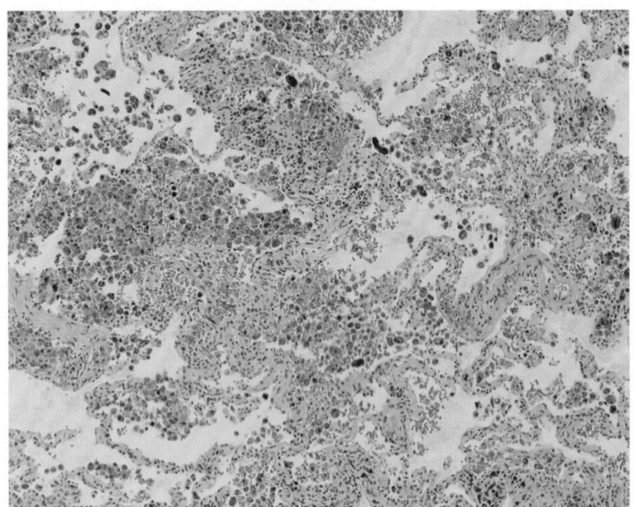

Figure 70.12 The alveolar septa are diffusely thickened by collagen and interstitial hemosiderin deposition. Fresh blood and hemosiderin-laden macrophages fill the airspaces.

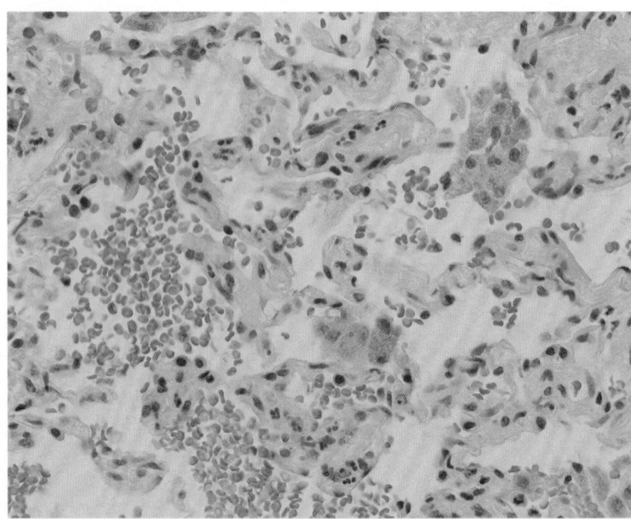

Figure 70.13 Neutrophils and occasional eosinophils are evident in the alveolar septa; this finding may be relatively focal and subtle, as in this example, particularly if the patient has received immunosuppression prior to the biopsy. The airspaces are filled with fresh red blood cells and frequent hemosiderin-laden macrophages.

Section 10

Pulmonary Hypertension and Embolic Disease

▸ Alain Borczuk

Pulmonary hypertension is a pathophysiologic state defined hemodynamically by elevations in mean pulmonary arterial pressures (≥25 mmHg) and refined into categories by additional hemodynamic factors, such as pulmonary arterial wedge pressure and measurement of pulmonary vascular resistance. These hemodynamic differences stem in part from the portion of the vascular bed involved, the size of the vascular channel involved, and the mechanism of the occlusion (e.g., vasoconstrictive or fixed obstruction). Although this is a definition that is both useful and reproducibly measurable, the set of diseases that can result in pulmonary vascular changes are quite diverse. For a pathologist, these associated vascular changes can be quite distinctive, but when encountered they are not invariably associated with hemodynamic changes. This may be due to the extent and distribution of the pathologic changes within the lung. The consequence of this observation is that pulmonary hypertension, while potentially suggested by vascular findings, is generally classified by a combination of hemodynamic findings and clinical scenarios than by specific pathologic findings.

Nevertheless, the current clinical classification of pulmonary hypertension has useful gross and histopathologic correlates. This classification divides pulmonary hypertension into five groups: (1) pulmonary arterial hypertension (with a 1′ group including pulmonary veno-occlusive disease and pulmonary capillary hemangiomatosis); (2) pulmonary hypertension due to left-sided heart disease; (3) pulmonary hypertension due to lung disease and/or hypoxia; (4) chronic thromboembolic disease and other pulmonary artery obstructions; and (5) pulmonary hypertension with unclear and/or multifactorial mechanisms.

Although many of the categories represent multiorgan diseases that have pulmonary hypertension as one outcome, a subset, especially in category 1, represent diseases in which pulmonary hypertension is the primary manifestation. In a remarkable expansion of molecular knowledge of these entities, mutations have been identified that play a causative role in subgroups of patients with pulmonary hypertension. The expanding list includes mutations in *BMPR2, BMPR1B, ACVRL1, CAV1, ENG, KCNK3, NOTCH3, SMAD1, SMAD4, SMAD8/9,* and *EIF2AK4*. These represent familial forms of pulmonary hypertension for which the corresponding pathology can be seen in both familial and sporadic forms.

71 Pulmonary Arterial Hypertension

Alain Borczuk

Pulmonary arterial hypertension, or Class 1, has a hemodynamic definition of mean pulmonary arterial pressure greater than 25 mmHg. This group consists of idiopathic and heritable pulmonary hypertension, as well as known associations that include certain medications and toxins, connective tissue disease, human immunodeficiency virus infection, and cirrhosis (portal hypertension, schistosomiasis). This group can have a wide number of arterial changes that range from medial and intimal thickening to complex-appearing vascular profiles that have been termed *plexiform arteriopathy*. These changes include vascular channels with marked cellular proliferation that can partially or completely fill the lumen of the vessel. These proliferations form secondary vascular spaces that are often collapsed and sieve-like. Other findings can include necrosis of the vascular wall in the most severe cases and, in some vessels, the appearance of secondary aneurysmal dilatations in arterial walls with secondary vascular channel formation.

Pulmonary hypertension secondary to left-sided heart disease, or Class 2, can have pathologic features that overlap with Class 1, in that arteries can show medial thickening and intimal proliferation. However, plexiform arteriopathy is not generally a feature of Class 2 with the exception of uncorrected congenital heart disease. While venous changes are likely a feature of left-sided heart disease–associated pulmonary hypertension, these changes are, in most instances, less dramatic than the venous changes of pulmonary veno-occlusive disease (PVOD); as a result, these subtle histopathologic venous changes should be interpreted with caution, as they can be seen in isolation—that is not associated with left-sided heart disease.

HISTOLOGIC FINDINGS

- Progressive vascular changes include intimal proliferation and medial thickening.
- Plexiform arteriopathy consists of a proliferation of cells with complex neolumen formation.
- Some arteries show aneurysmal dilation and secondary thrombosis with recanalization.
- High pressures can lead to fibrinoid necrosis without neutrophilic vasculitis.

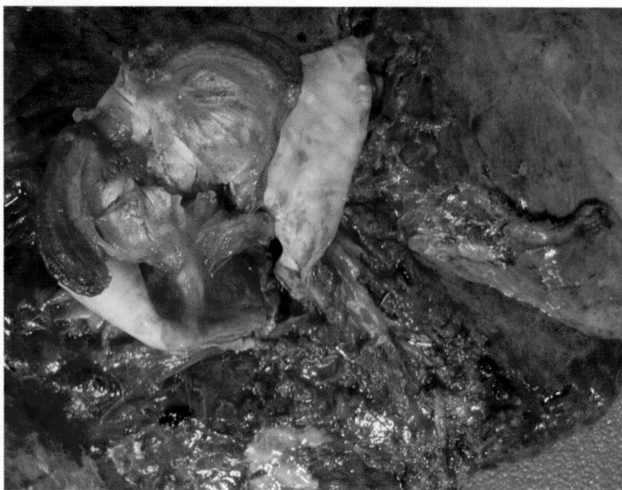

Figure 71.1 The opened pulmonary artery shows atheroma, which is a consequence of chronic elevation of pulmonary pressure.

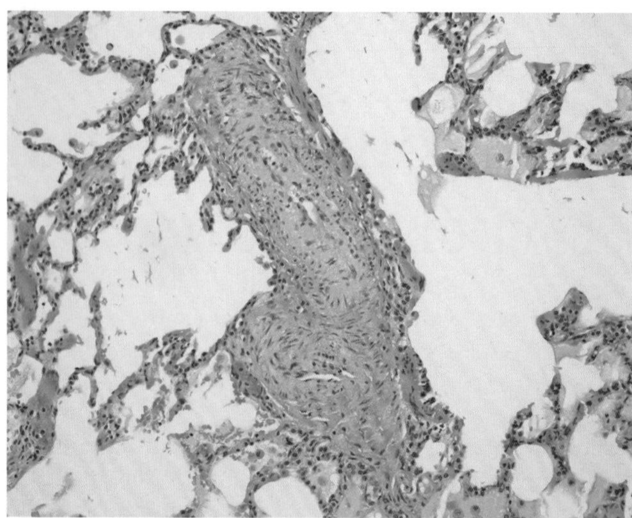

Figure 71.2 A pulmonary artery branch showing medial thickening and intimal proliferation from a patient with uncorrected congenital heart disease.

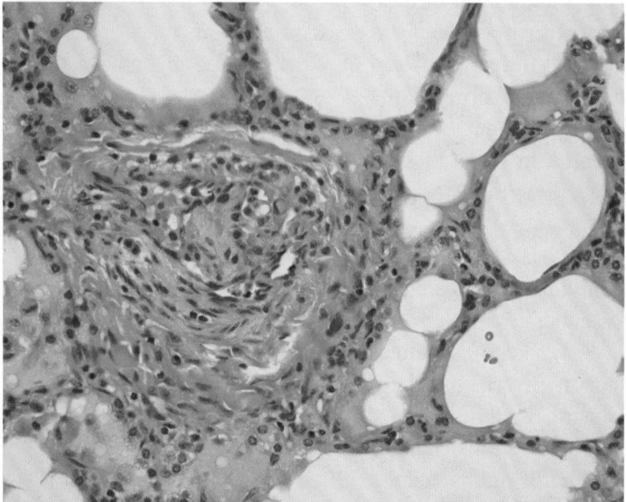

Figure 71.3 This small pulmonary artery shows a cellular proliferation with spindle-cell and endothelial proliferation and neolumen formation. This plexiform lesion was seen in a patient with uncorrected congenital heart disease.

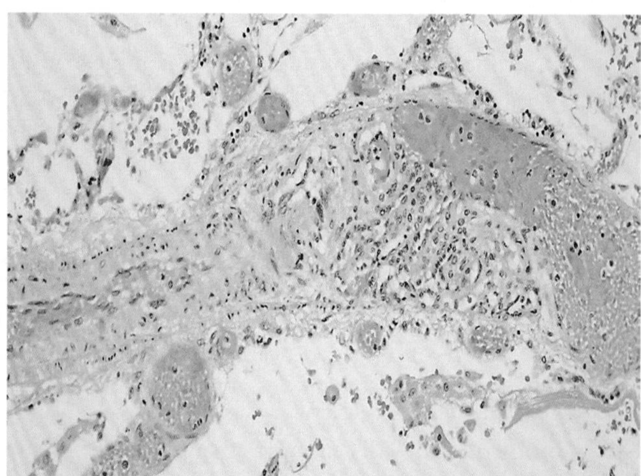

Figure 71.4 This artery shows dilatation associated with a marked endothelial proliferation with neolumen formation seen longitudinally within the vascular channel. This plexiform lesion was seen in a patient after the use of the medication fenfluramine–phentermine.

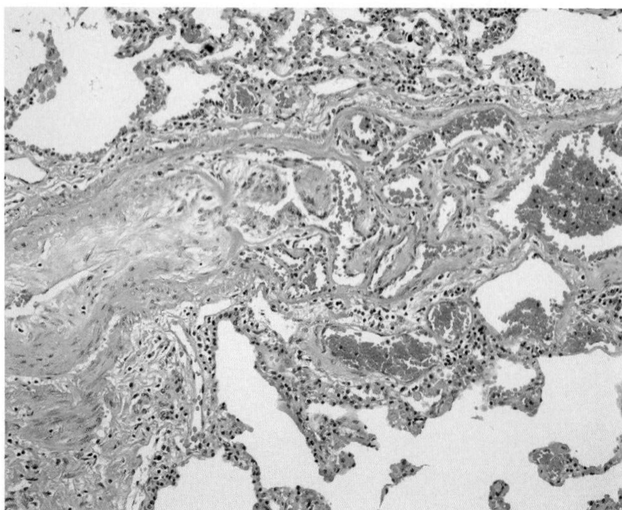

Figure 71.5 This artery shows an area of aneurysmal dilation that has experienced secondary thrombosis with recanalization, which has been described as an angiomatoid lesion of pulmonary hypertension.

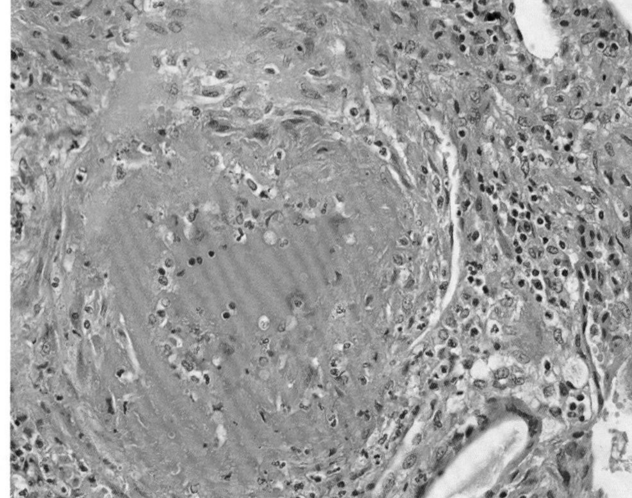

Figure 71.6 Severe pulmonary hypertension can lead to fibrinous necrosis in the wall of arteries.

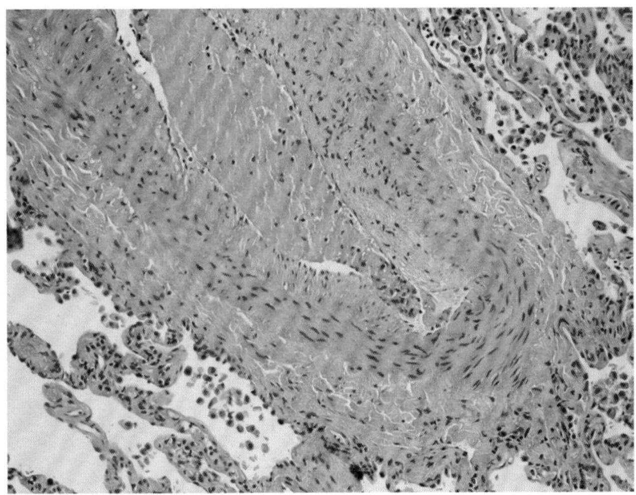

Figure 71.7 This artery has a relatively normal media but shows intimal proliferation in a patient with left-sided heart disease.

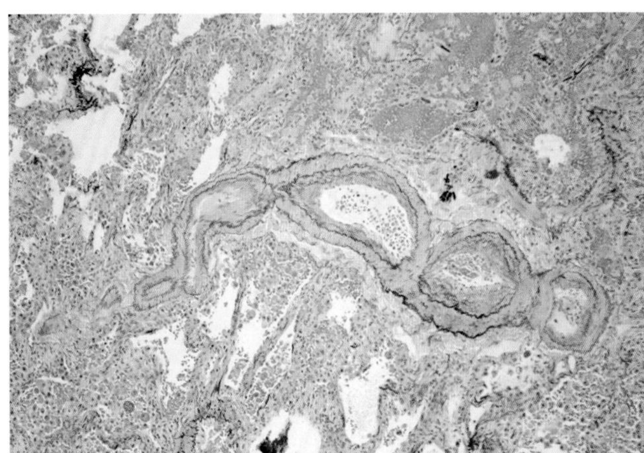

Figure 71.8 A pentachrome (Movat) stain highlights a pulmonary artery with medial thickening and intimal proliferation from a patient with left-sided heart disease.

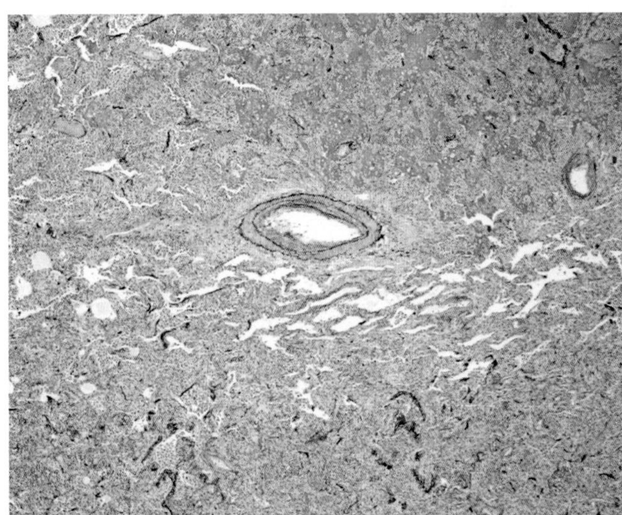

Figure 71.9 This vein, within an interlobular septum, shows adventitial thickening and some medial thickening. Such changes can be seen in left-sided heart disease but lack the more extensive dilatation and thrombosis seen in PVOD.

Pulmonary Veno-Occlusive Disease

72

Alain Borczuk

Pulmonary veno-occlusive disease (PVOD) and pulmonary capillary hemangiomatosis are part of "Class 1" and are pathologically distinct from Class 1 in that they involve veins and the capillary bed. While there is significant overlap between these two processes and they can be seen in the same patient, the process can involve large veins along the pleura and interlobular septa with prominent secondary thrombosis and recanalization as well as arterialization of the veins. This arterialization is often associated with marked vascular enlargement and adventitial thickening. Lung parenchyma can have associated interstitial widening, and alveoli may contain hemorrhage and hemosiderin-laden macrophages. PVOD can be associated with hypercoagulability, medications, stem cell transplantation, autoimmune disease, or infection, or can be idiopathic. Recently, genetic causes have been identified, including mutation in EIF2AK4.

HISTOLOGIC FEATURES

- Pulmonary veins are dilated with intimal proliferation and adventitial thickening.
- Pulmonary veins can show thrombosis and some with recanalization.
- Pulmonary veins in the interlobular septa and pleura can become arterialized.
- Complete obliteration of veins can mimic areas of pulmonary scarring.
- Hemosiderin can be prominent with iron encrustation of elastic tissue. These iron encrusted bodies can be confused with foreign material.

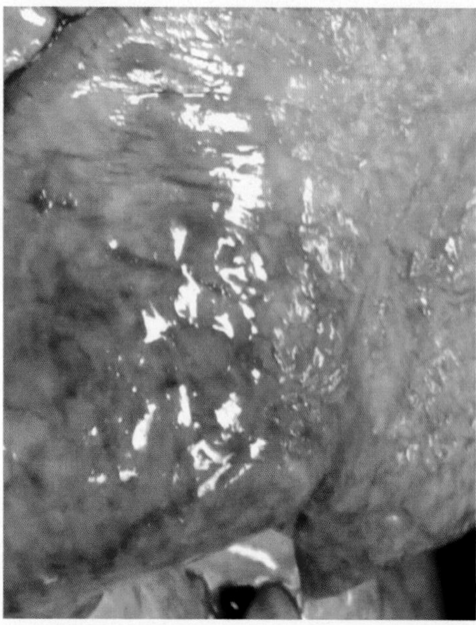

Figure 72.1 The surface of the lung shows prominent enlarged and dilated veins in a patient with PVOD.

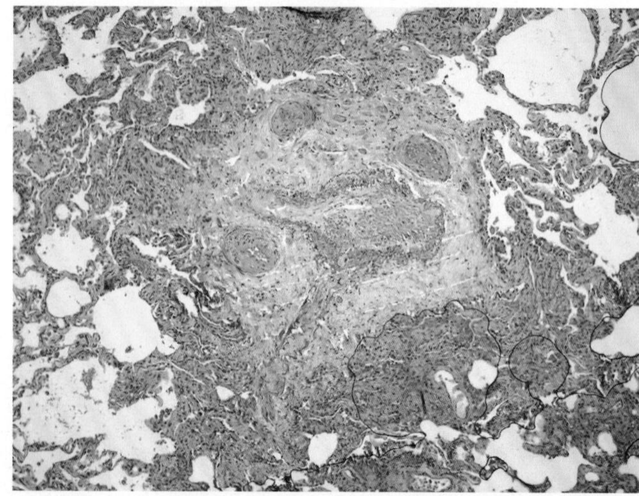

Figure 72.2 A pulmonary vein, on pentachrome stains, shows luminal occlusion and recanalization. The vein is enlarged and is associated with marked adventitial thickening.

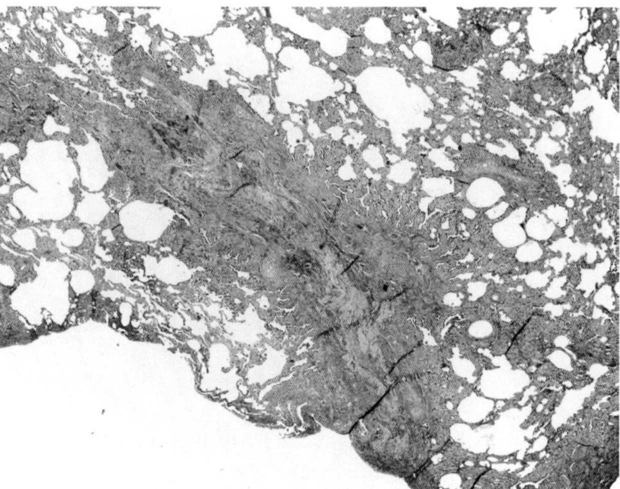

Figure 72.3 A pulmonary vein, on trichrome stain, is completely obliterated and as a result can be confused with an area of scarring on hematoxylin and eosin stain. Some fibrosis in the interstitium directly surrounding the vessel may give the mistaken impression of a fibrotic interstitial disease.

Pulmonary Capillary Hemangiomatosis

73

Alain Borczuk

In contrast to larger vein involvement in pulmonary veno-occlusive disease, some pulmonary hypertension patients in "Class 1" have involvement of only small venules with a marked capillary proliferation (pulmonary capillary hemangiomatosis) without the larger venous involvement. The gross pathology consists of fairly distinct hemorrhage nodules. These nodules correspond to microscopic areas of capillary proliferation and engorgement. The capillaries in these lesions are tortuous and appear more numerous. The tortuosity of the capillaries gives the impression of capillaries on either side of the alveolar wall, and these capillaries are visible within the walls of other structures, such as small airways. Within these areas of capillary proliferation, there are visible, small, more muscularized channels that represent venules.

HISTOLOGIC FEATURES

- Nodular areas of alveolar wall thickening by proliferating capillaries, with distinct transition to normal lung.
- Capillaries in the alveolar wall are tortuous and seen on both sides of the alveolar wall.
- The capillaries are seen in the walls of airways and blood vessels.
- Small, thick-walled venules can be seen in areas of capillary proliferation.

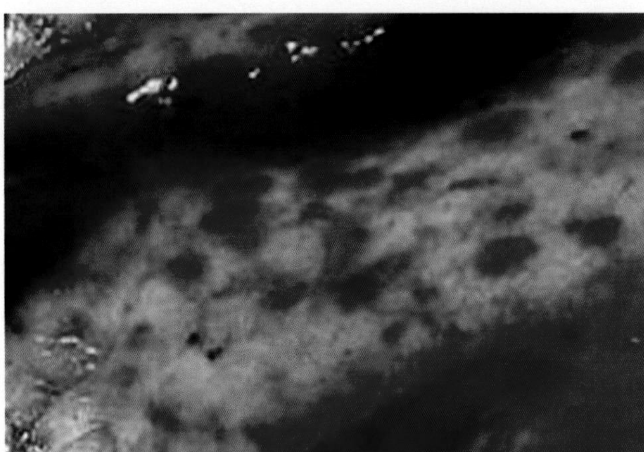

Figure 73.1 Hemorrhagic nodules are seen in pulmonary capillary hemangiomatosis, on the pleural surface. These are also seen in the lung parenchyma.

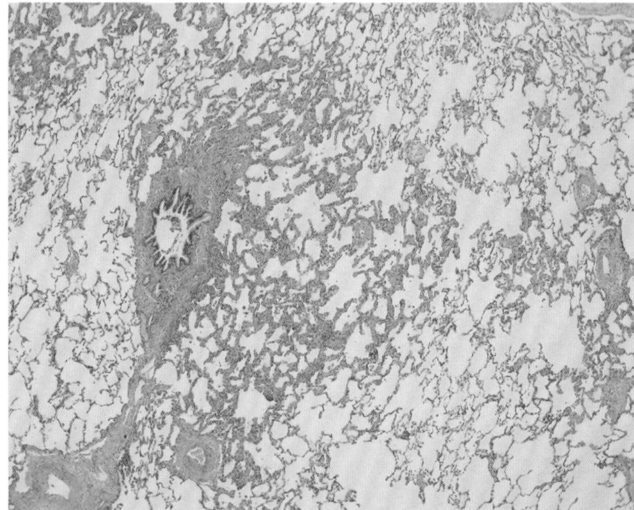

Figure 73.2 This lower power photomicrograph demonstrates the relatively demarcated area of alveolar wall thickening corresponding to the grossly visible nodules.

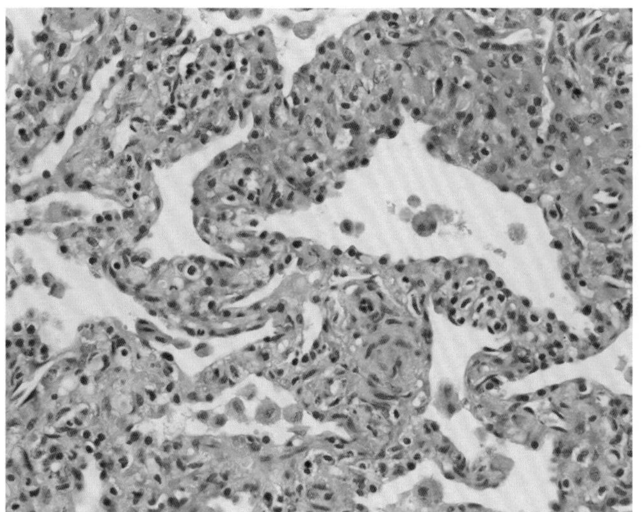

Figure 73.3 The alveolar walls show tortuous capillaries that appear to be on both sides of the alveolar wall. An abnormal muscularized channel is also seen in the interstitium.

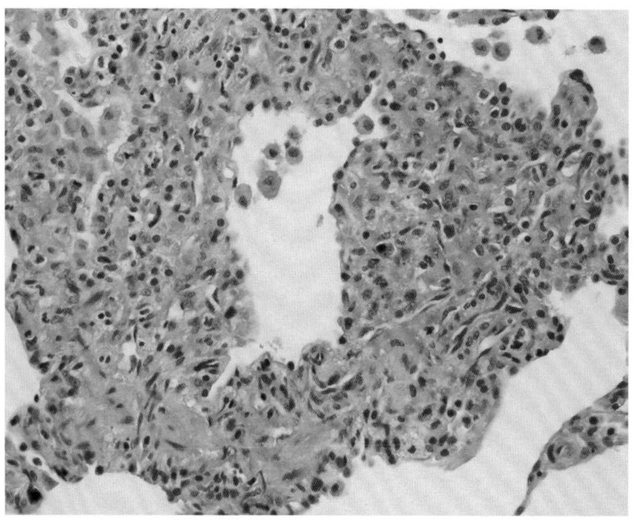

Figure 73.4 The capillary channels appear to be increased in number and to involve the wall of a small airway.

Pulmonary Hypertension Associated with Lung Disease and/or Hypoxemia

74

Alain Borczuk

This type of pulmonary hypertension, Class 3, is associated with lung diseases such as chronic obstructive lung disease or interstitial lung disease such as pulmonary fibrosis. It can also be the result of other causes of hypoxemia such as sleep apnea and living at high altitude. In interstitial lung disease, some patients have vascular changes that seem to be out of proportion to the degree of interstitial disease, and treating the associated pulmonary hypertension in these conditions may help improve patient lung function. These changes are usually limited to medial thickening and intimal hyperplasia, so that plexiform arteriopathy is not a feature in this setting.

HISTOLOGIC FEATURES

- Arterial medial hypertrophy and intimal proliferation.
- Underlying lung disease—for example, emphysema or fibrosis—is evident.

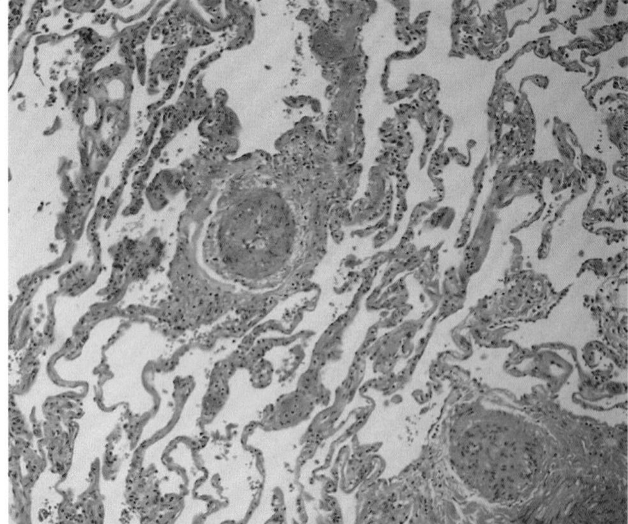

Figure 74.1 Two pulmonary arteries show marked medial thickening in a patient with usual interstitial pneumonia. This wedge showed prominent vascular changes despite relatively spared alveolar lung parenchyma and interstitium.

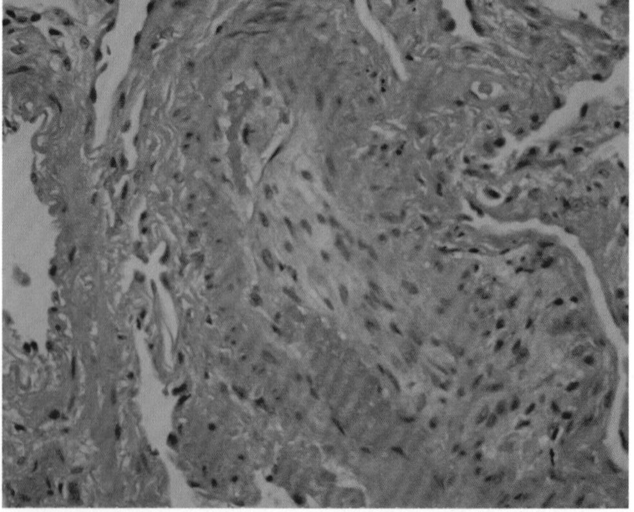

Figure 74.2 In addition to medial thickening, some arteries showed marked intimal proliferation.

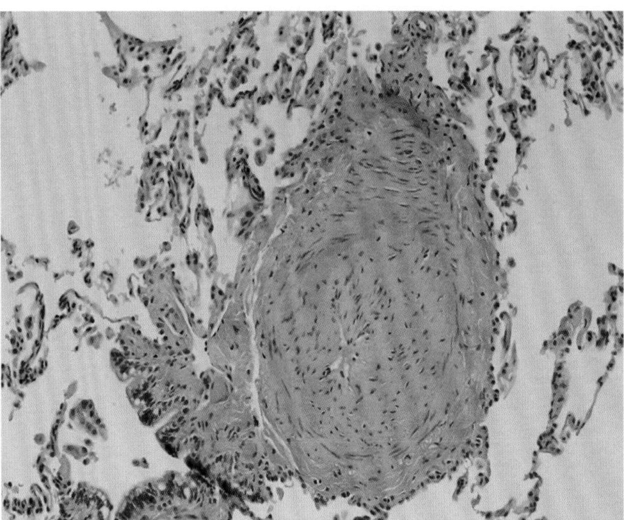

Figure 74.3 A clue that vascular disease may be present is the disparity in size of the artery relative to the airway within the bronchovascular bundle. These structures are normally of equal diameter. In this image, the artery is larger than its paired airway, in addition to showing medial thickening and intimal proliferation.

Thromboembolic Disease—Acute and Chronic

75

Part 1

Thromboemboli

Alain Borczuk

Acute thromboemboli can result in sudden changes in respiratory function as well as in sudden death. These can be small or large; large emboli can lodge into the main pulmonary artery and at its bifurcation ("saddle embolus") or can be seen in pulmonary artery branches.

Large pulmonary emboli generally arise from the deep veins of the lower extremity and pelvis. As a result, they have the shape of the vein they arose in, with a twisted irregular appearance that can have the depressions of valve markings. Their cut surface is multilamellated and not separated into two distinct zones of red and pale material (red gelatinous appearance and "chicken fat"). In some instances, thrombi will form in situ that can extend from existing thromboemboli.

Chronic thromboemboli will eventually become fibrotic and the channel will recanalize, forming a band or web.

HISTOLOGIC FEATURES

- The thrombi will initially induce a neutrophilic response, but with time they will become adherent to the vessel wall.
- Ultimately, these can have endothelial overgrowth and fibroblast infiltration. Eventually, these can become fibrotic and recanalized.

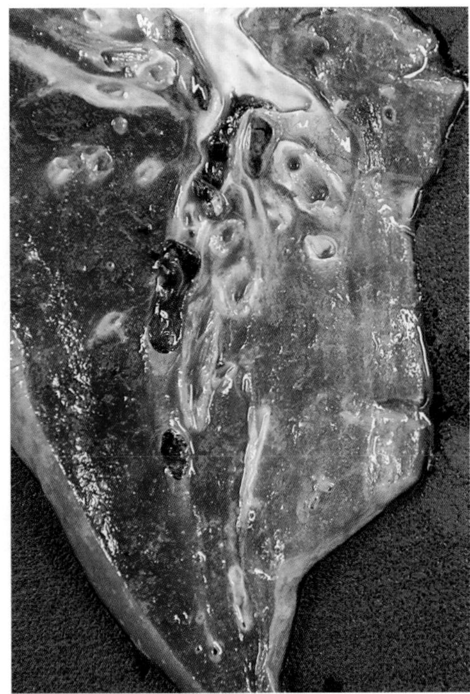

Figure 75.1 Pulmonary artery branch with large thromboembolus.

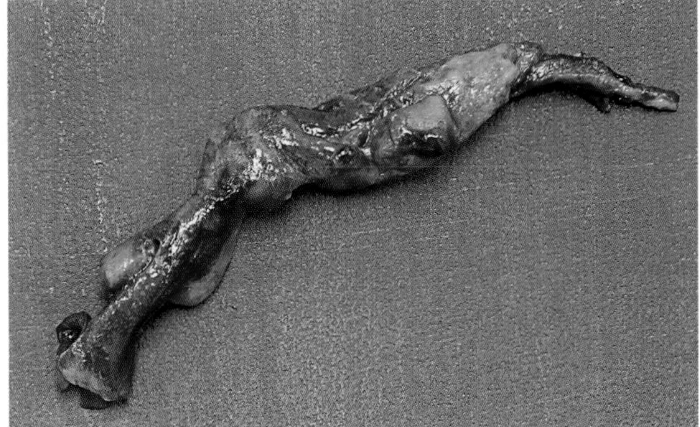

Figure 75.2 A thromboembolus removed from the main pulmonary artery bifurcation shows the irregular contour, areas narrowing (putatively from venous valve indentation), twisted appearance, and multilayered appearance.

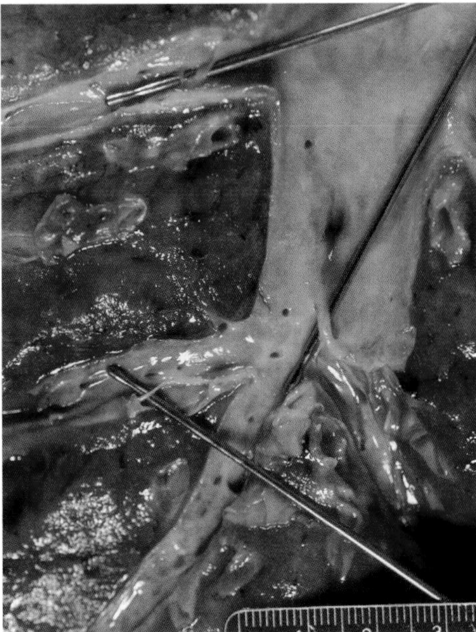

Figure 75.3 Gross image showing a dilated pulmonary artery with atheromatous plaque. The probes demonstrate webs and bands that are evidence of previous organized thromboemboli.

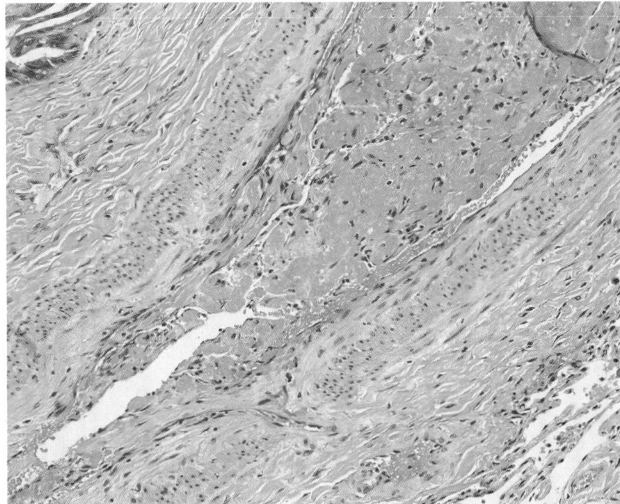

Figure 75.4 Thrombus with organization showing fibrin with intermixed spindle cells and endothelial ingrowth.

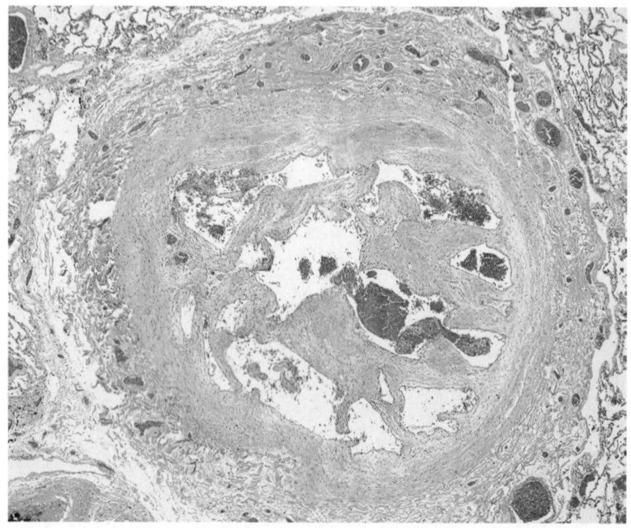

Figure 75.5 After a period of time, thrombi will organize and demonstrate recanalization.

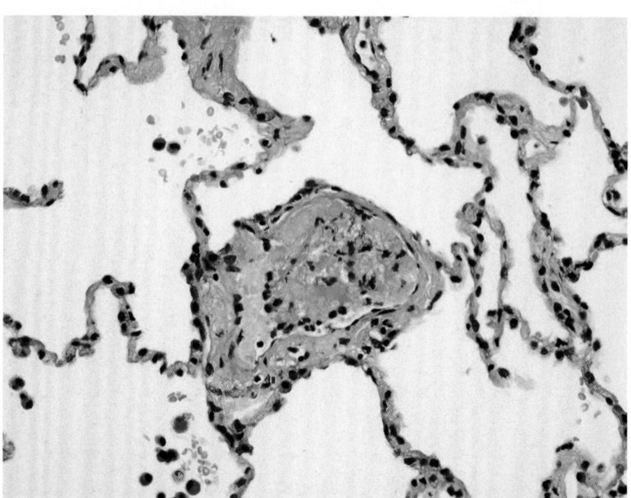

Figure 75.6 Lung biopsy from a patient with antiphospholipid antibody syndrome. Such a thrombus may have formed in situ, rather than representing a thromboembolic disease.

Part 2

Foreign-Body Emboli

▶ Alain Borczuk

Intravenous injection of foreign material will become trapped in the pulmonary arterial circulation and induce a tissue reaction characteristic of foreign-body reaction—giant cells and fibrosis. This has been described with materials, such as talc and microcrystalline cellulose, which are the consequence of intravenous injections of medications intended for oral use. In such samples, material can be seen in the lumen of small vessels and in the wall of the vessel. Over time, these will cause sufficient damage to the vascular wall that these granulomas and fibrosis can appear perivascular as well as endovascular.

HISTOLOGIC FEATURES

- Foreign material induces giant-cell reaction in vessels, vessel walls, and perivascular tissue.
- Polarized light can highlight foreign material such as talc, suture, and microcrystalline cellulose.

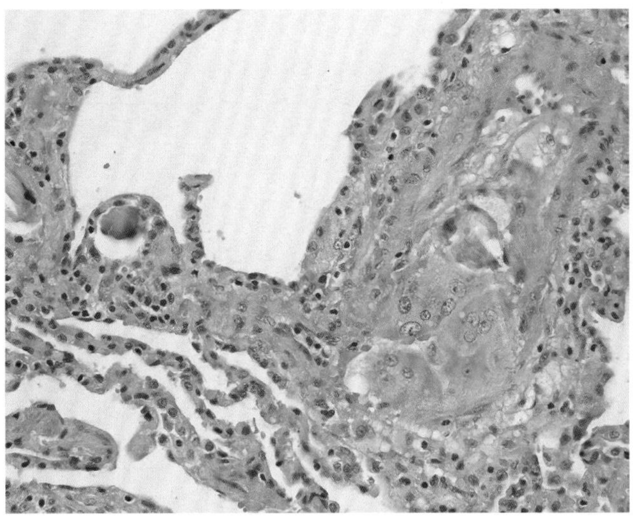

Figure 75.7 Pulmonary artery with foreign-body giant-cell reaction with refractile material in the vessel and in the capillary bed.

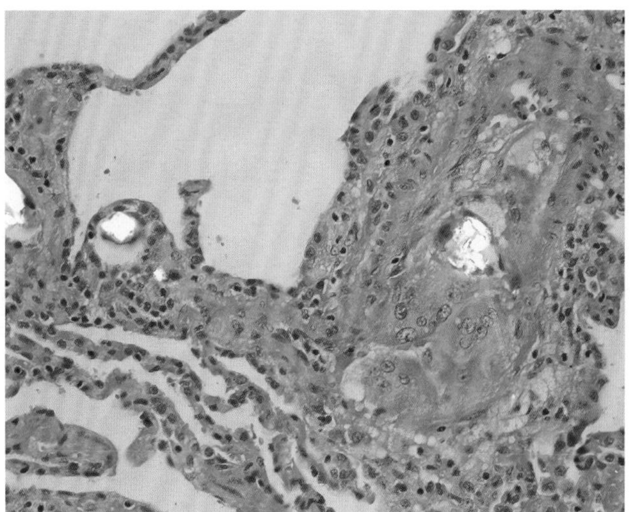

Figure 75.8 Polarized light in the same field highlights the polarizable foreign material.

Part 3

Fat Emboli

Alain Borczuk

Fat can enter the circulation from a variety of causes, but the most common is blunt force trauma to long bones, to adipose tissue, or rarely to a fatty liver. Other associations include pancreatitis, diabetes, and bone infection. The fat may cause physical plugging but may also induce a toxic injury to the endothelium. It can induce severe hypoxemia and tachypnea and can result in acute respiratory distress syndrome.

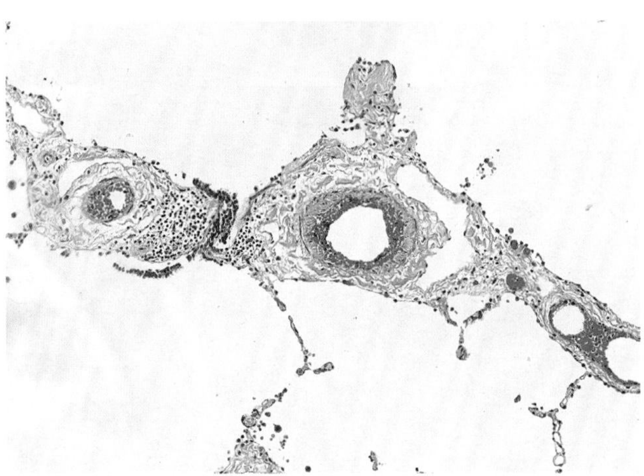

Figure 75.9 After processing, fat globules can be seen as a round dilated area in the vascular channel.

Part 4

Amniotic Fluid Embolism

Alain Borczuk and Jason K. Graham

Pulmonary amniotic fluid embolism is an uncommon complication of delivery that can cause respiratory distress. It remains a significant cause of maternal morbidity and mortality. Although it can be associated with difficult labor, it remains an unpredictable complication.

HISTOLOGIC FEATURES

- Pulmonary artery branches and small vessels can contain squamous epithelial cells, lanugo hair, and mucin.

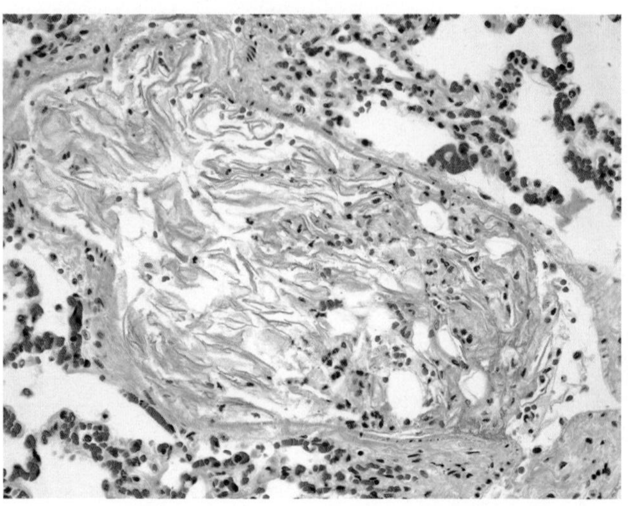

Figure 75.10 Anucleated squames are seen filling a thin-walled artery.

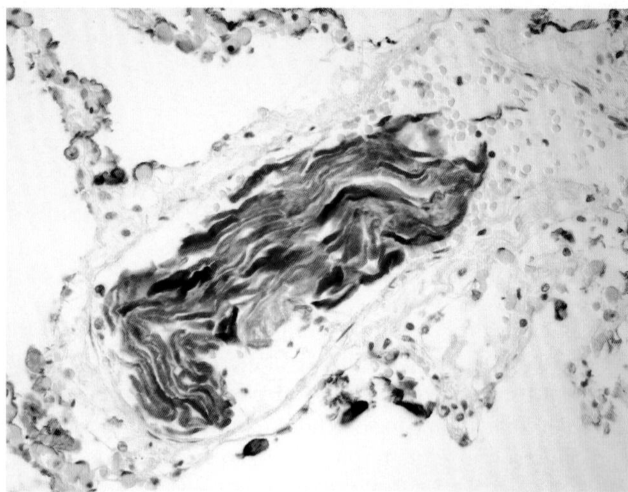

Figure 75.11 Immunohistochemistry for cytokeratin highlights the anucleated squamous.

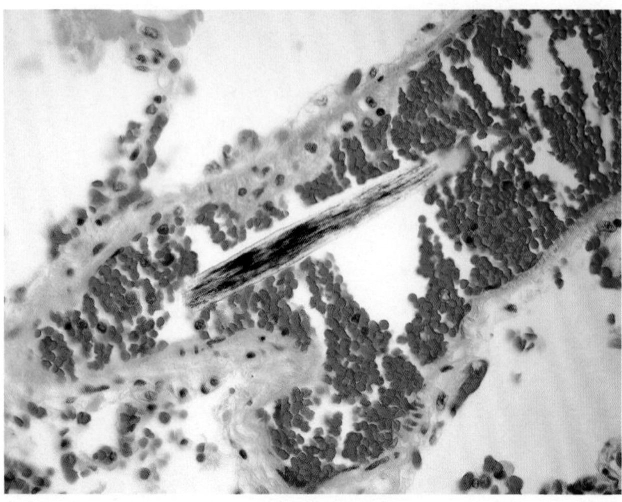

Figure 75.12 Fragment of hair (lanugo) in a pulmonary artery branch.

Part 5

Tumor Emboli

Alain Borczuk

Tumor can enter the venous circulation and travel via the flow of blood into the pulmonary arterial bed. This can occur in renal cell carcinoma through renal vein invasion into the inferior vena cava and can also be seen in liver tumors (primary or metastatic), which erode into large veins such as the hepatic veins. However, some tumors will invade smaller channels and lodge in the pulmonary microcirculation. Angiosarcomas, while potentially primary in the lung, can manifest as endovascular metastatic disease from cardiac or hepatic angiosarcoma; some cases result in diffuse pulmonary hemorrhage.

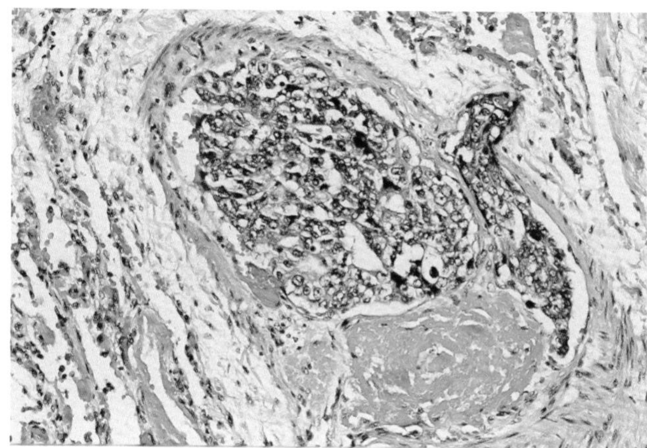

Figure 75.13 Breast carcinoma tumor embolus is seen in a pulmonary artery with associated thrombus from a patient with massive liver metastasis.

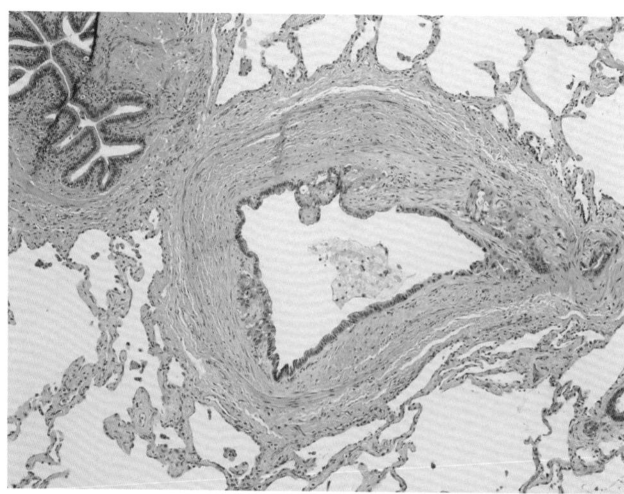

Figure 75.14 A pancreatic cancer invaded the inferior vena cava with pulmonary tumor emboli.

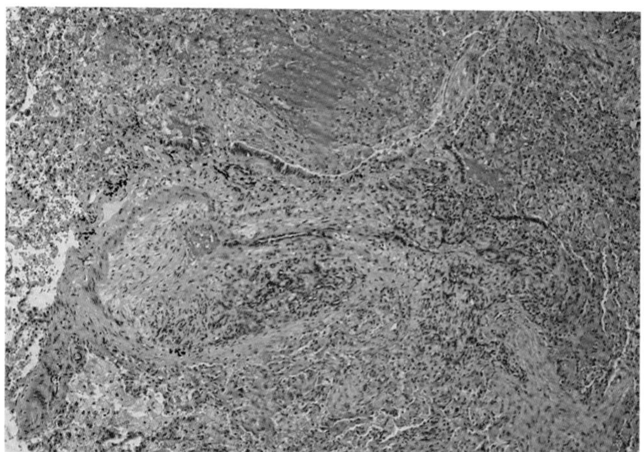

Figure 75.15 A low-power view of a pulmonary artery shows a proliferation that can resemble an organized thrombus but is metastatic angiosarcoma.

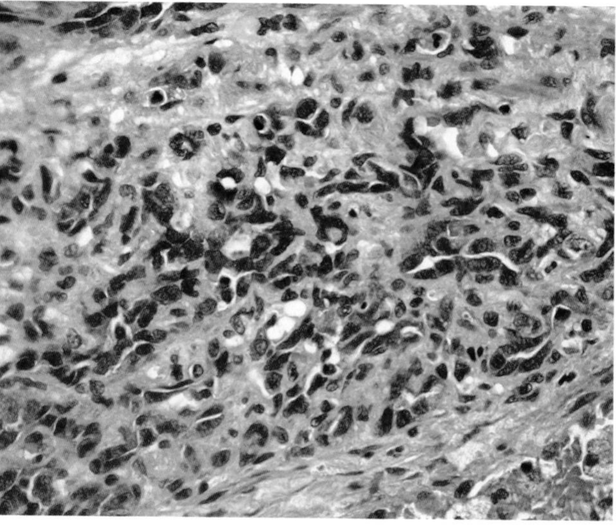

Figure 75.16 At higher magnification the vascular channels are interanastomosing and lined by atypical endothelial cells of angiosarcoma.

Part 6

Parasitic Emboli

▶ Alain Borczuk

Parasitic emboli, an uncommon phenomenon, has been described with *Dirofilaria immitis* in the United States and *Dirofilaria repens* in Europe. The life cycle of the dog heartworm in humans is characterized by the death of the roundworm, as humans are not a definitive host for the organism. This results in embolization of the worm fragments into the lungs and causes granulomatous coin lesions and sometimes infarcts. In rare instances, hepatic echinococcal cysts can rupture into hepatic veins and embolize into the pulmonary circulation.

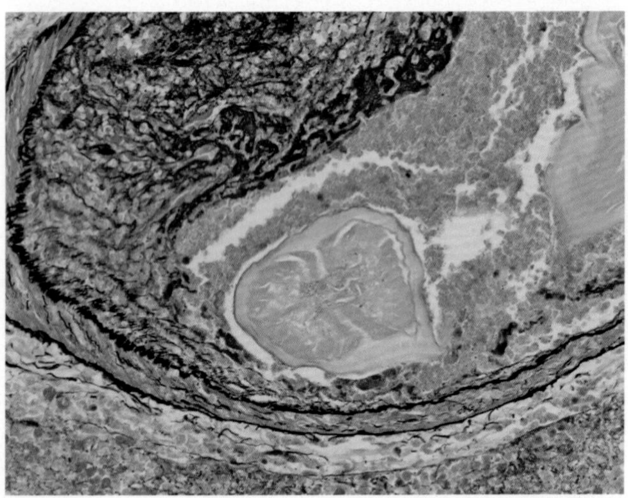

Figure 75.17 A cross section of a *D. immitis* fragment. An elastic stain highlights the arterial wall.

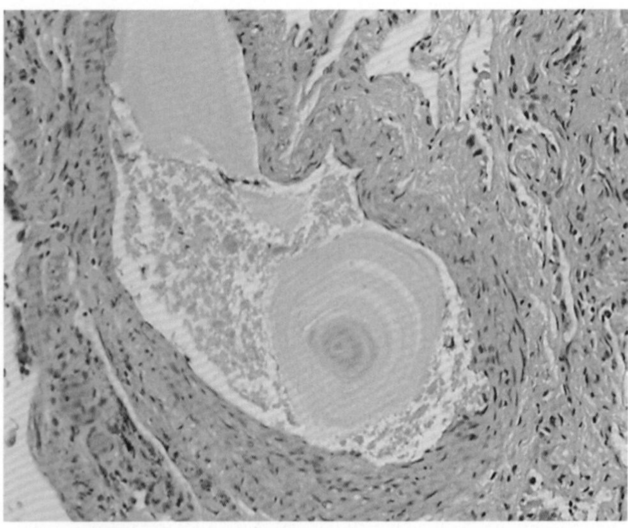

Figure 75.18 Fragments of a lamellated echinococcal cyst wall are seen in a pulmonary artery.

Part 7

Bone Marrow Emboli

▶ Alain Borczuk

These are observed most frequently after vigorous cardiopulmonary resuscitation, although they have also been described in sickle-cell disease.

HISTOLOGIC FEATURES

- Small pulmonary arteries will have adipose tissue intermixed with hematopoietic elements.

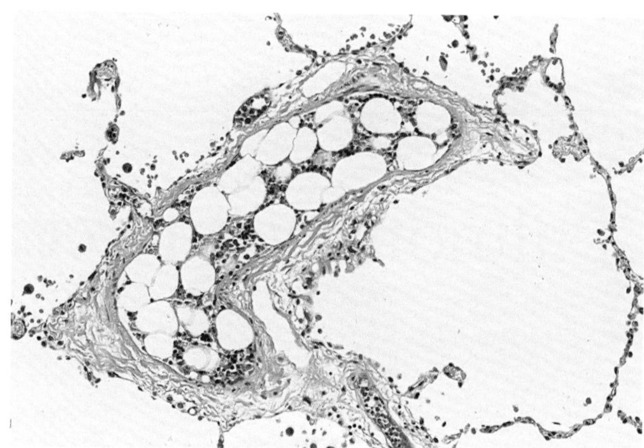

Figure 75.19 A pulmonary artery filled with adipose tissue and bone marrow elements.

76 Pulmonary Infarct

▶ Alain Borczuk

The lung receives blood through two circulations—pulmonary artery circulation from the right side of the heart and bronchial circulation from the aorta. As a result, occlusion of the pulmonary artery circulation by thrombi does not cause infarction in most cases. In roughly 10% of cases in which infarction occurs, the majority are hemorrhagic rather than bland infarcts. Infarcts are usually peripheral and pleural-based and described as wedged-shaped. However, depending on the plane of view, they can look more ovoid or circular.

HISTOLOGIC FEATURES

- Early infarcts go through stages of coagulative necrosis, starting with hemorrhage and with progressive neutrophil influx at the edges of the infarct.
- Infarcts will complete coagulative necrosis with ghosts of preexisting alveolar architecture.
- Infarcts will become progressively fibrotic over time with eventual scar formation.

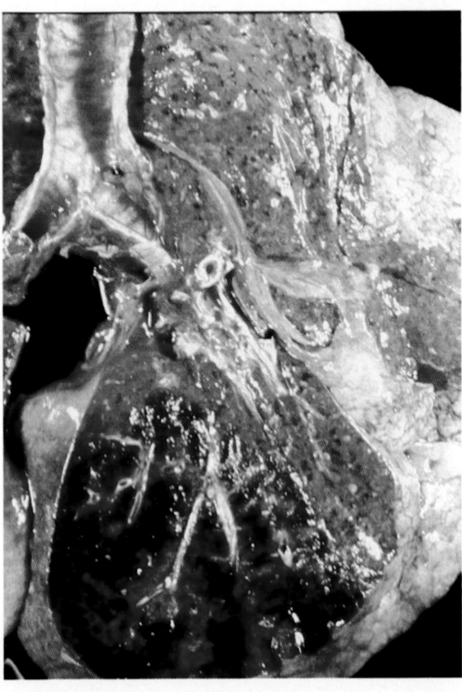

Figure 76.1 A pulmonary infarct is hemorrhagic, pleural-based, and roughly wedged-shaped.

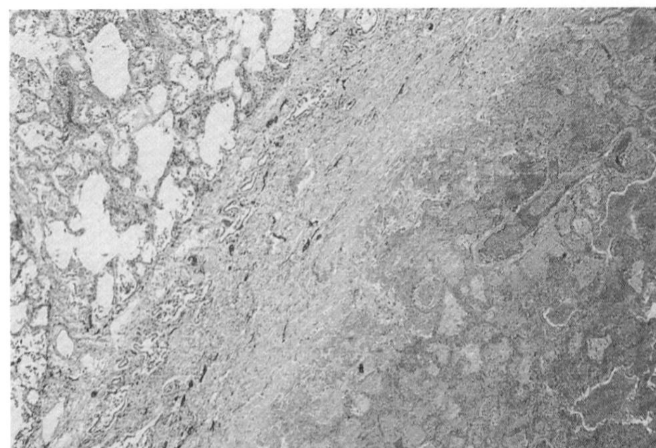

Figure 76.2 An area of infarction shows coagulative necrosis with the ghosts of alveolar architecture. Over time, the area around the infarct shows fibrosis and eventually the infarct becomes organized and fibrotic.

Pulmonary Hypertension with Unclear or Multifactorial Mechanisms

77

Alain Borczuk

This last group of mechanisms is a heterogeneous and consists of entities that may cause physical obstruction or plugging, vascular proliferation, or production of prothrombotic molecules. In some instances, causes are multifactorial. For example, sarcoidosis can cause compression of venous outflow but may also cause pulmonary fibrosis with associated hypoxemic pulmonary hypertension.

Entities in this category include chronic hemolytic anemia, sickle-cell anemia, thalassemia, myeloproliferative disorders, thyroid disease, glycogen storage disease, Gaucher disease, sarcoidosis, Langerhans cell histiocytosis, lymphangioleiomyomatosis, and fibrosing mediastinitis.

Some tumors will induce the relatively sudden onset of pulmonary hypertension; this has been attributed to the production of vascular endothelial growth factor and tissue factor by the tumor and has been described in adenocarcinoma, most often gastric adenocarcinoma. This is termed *pulmonary tumor thrombotic microangiopathy* (PTTM) and portends a poor prognosis. Importantly, these patients will not show evidence of large vascular occlusion as might be seen in thromboemboli or larger tumor thrombi.

HISTOLOGIC FEATURES

- In patients with chronic myeloproliferative disorders, especially in myelofibrosis, pulmonary hypertension will be associated with vascular proliferation and lung vessels will be expanded by extramedullary hematopoiesis.
- The associated disease may be evident in tissue sampling, such as nonnecrotizing granulomas of sarcoid, Gaucher cells, Langerhans cell, or cells of lymphangioleiomyomatosis.
- In PTTM, vessels will show tumor plugs in small channels, often with thrombosis or dramatic intimal reaction.

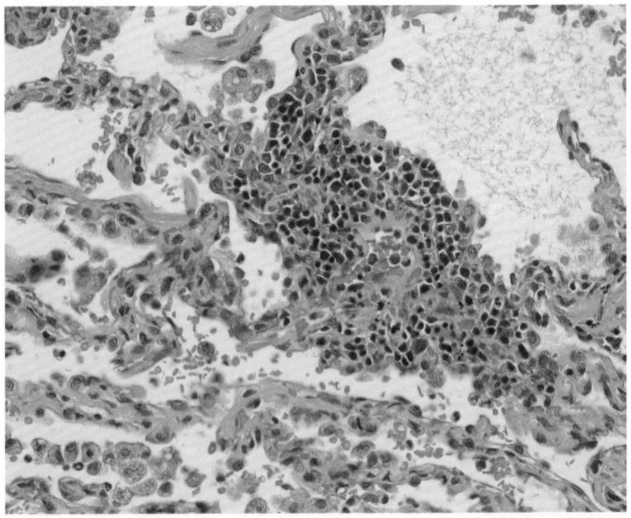

Figure 77.1 New onset pulmonary hypertension was seen in this patient with myelofibrosis in which there was extensive extramedullary hematopoiesis, here with red cell precursors.

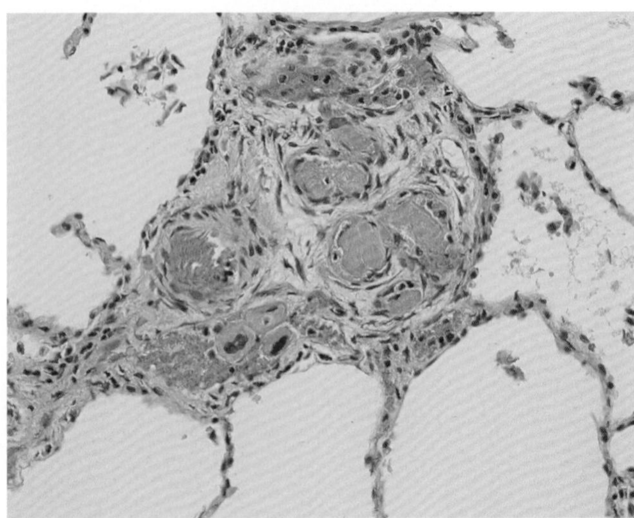

Figure 77.2 In Gaucher disease, thrombi and Gaucher cell are seen within the vascular channel.

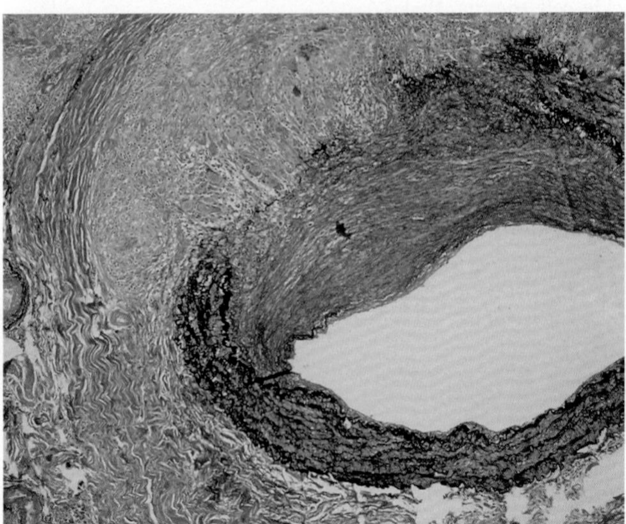

Figure 77.3 Nonnecrotizing granulomas in a mass lesion of sarcoidosis causes compression of venous structures, highlighted here by elastic stain.

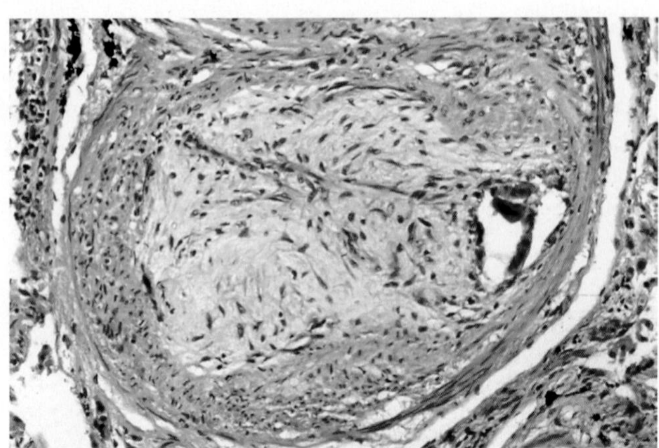

Figure 77.4 Adenocarcinoma cells are seen amidst a dramatic intimal proliferation in PTTM.

Section 11

Large Airways

▶ Ross A. Miller

78 Bronchiectasis

Ross A. Miller

Chronic inflammation and fibrosis can result in irreversible dilation of the bronchi known as *bronchiectasis*. Downstream bronchioles may also be affected, which is referred to as *bronchiolectasis*. Most often, the lower lobes are involved and these changes often arises in the setting of a chronic infectious process. However, there are numerous conditions that seemingly predispose one to developing bronchiectasis, including airway obstructive processes, cystic fibrosis, immune deficiency syndromes, and ciliary dyskinesia.

HISTOLOGIC FEATURES

- Dilated bronchi; often variable amounts of inflammation, erosion/ulceration, and squamous metaplasia of the bronchiolar epithelium can be seen.
- Lymphoid follicles may be present in the bronchial walls.
- Fibrosis of the bronchial wall and surrounding tissues; destruction of bronchial wall structures.
- Similar changes often seen in downstream bronchioles (bronchiolectasis).
- Often associated with other pathologic processes (e.g., acute and chronic pneumonia, organizing pneumonia, and fibrosing conditions).

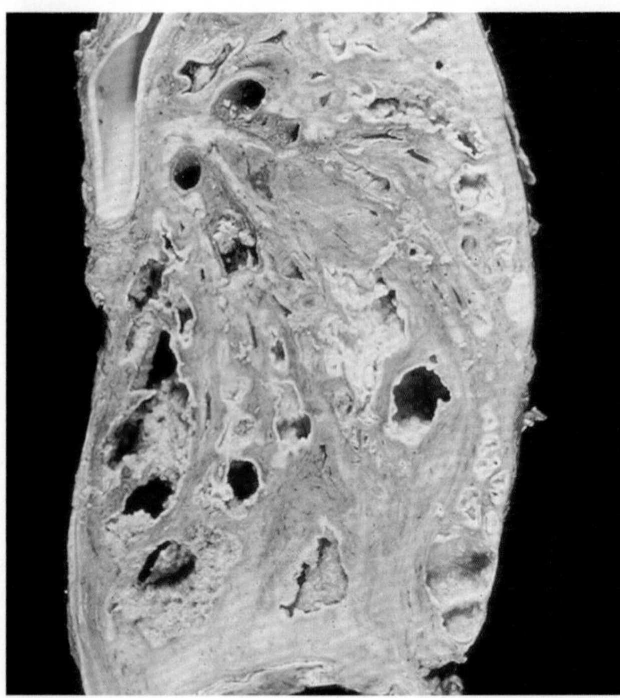

Figure 78.1 Gross image of bronchiectasis showing dilated segmental bronchi and surrounding parenchymal fibrosis.

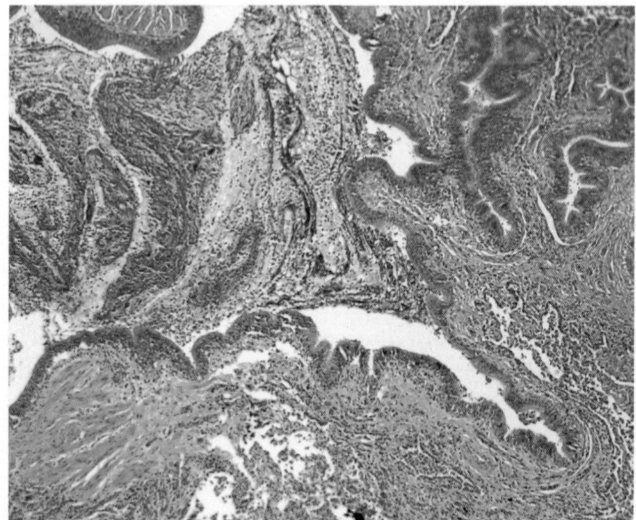

Figure 78.2 A large dilated cystic space lined by ciliated respiratory epithelium and containing mucin with admixed acute inflammatory cells. Surrounding fibrosis can be seen.

79

Middle Lobe Syndrome

▸ Ross A. Miller
▸ Timothy C. Allen

The right middle lobe and lingula tend to have reduced collateral ventilation compared with other areas of the lung; the bronchi feeding the right middle lobe and lingula are relatively long and narrow and have a sharp take off from the bronchial tree. If there is surrounding lymphadenopathy and/or a mass-forming process, extraluminal compression or intraluminal obstruction can potentially occur and result in middle lobe syndrome. Findings include those expected from a postobstructive pathologic process and include atelectasis, infections, organizing pneumonia, lipid pneumonia, and the development of bronchiectasis. Middle lobe syndrome is most often seen in adults. When it does occur in children, it is often seen in asthmatic patients and spontaneous recovery has been described. Lady Windermere syndrome is a classically described rare form of middle lobe syndrome occurring in seemingly healthy middle-aged to elderly women. *Mycobacterium avium* complex has been isolated in these patients and there seems to be a correlation with intentional, long-term, cough suppression.

HISTOLOGIC FEATURES

- Bronchiectasis, bronchiolectasis, variable inflammation.
- Organizing pneumonia is often seen; abscess formation can occur.
- The presence of granulomas and/or granulomatous inflammation may suggest a mycobacterial or fungal infection; one should meticulously look for possible fungal or acid-fast organisms with special stains at high magnification and correlate with cultures (if available).

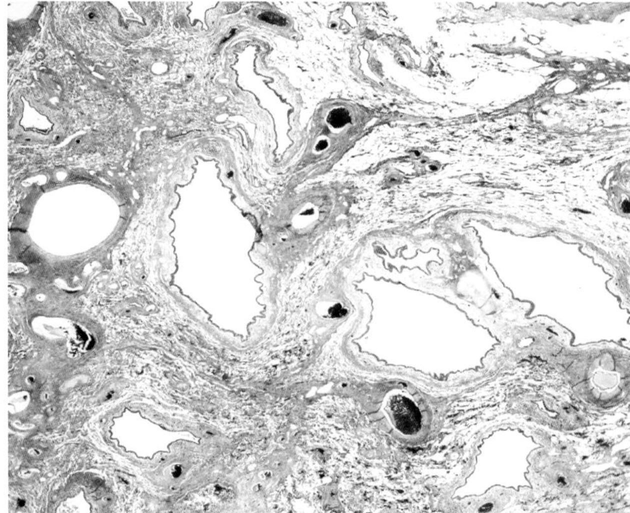

Figure 79.1 Middle lobe syndrome low-power view shows multiple dilated bronchi with surrounding fibrosis and collapsed lung parenchyma.

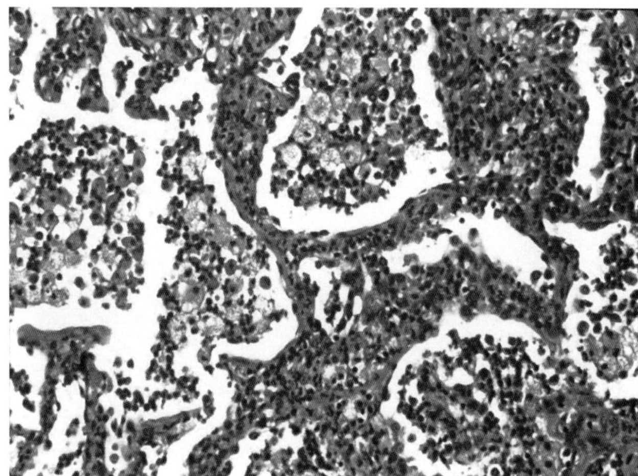

Figure 79.2 Postobstructive pneumonia consists of collapsed lung with intra-alveolar lipid-filled macrophages mixed with neutrophils and interstitial acute and chronic inflammation.

Tracheobronchopathia Osteochondroplastica

▶ Ross A. Miller
▶ Roberto Barrios*

Tracheobronchopathia osteochondroplastica (TBO) is an extremely rare condition of unknown etiology causing bronchial obstruction and recurrent pneumonia. Numerous nodules composed of bone and cartilage involve the submucosa of the tracheobronchial tree, sparring the membranous portion of the trachea. The overlying epithelium can have squamous metaplastic change and/or show areas of erosion/ulceration.

The condition is typically seen in adult patients and tends to affect males more often than females. Usually, the condition is incidentally detected by a chest x-ray or during bronchoscopy; some patients may have nonspecific symptoms such as dyspnea or hemoptysis. Bronchoscopic biopsy is typically diagnostic where multiple submucosal 2- to 5-mm nodules are seen involving the tracheobronchial tree. The nodules tend to have a propensity for the lower two-thirds of the trachea and often a communication between the nodules and the trachea and/or bronchial cartilage can be found.

HISTOLOGIC FEATURES

- Tracheal and bronchial submucosal nodules are composed of bone and cartilage; the nodules tend to be situated between the epithelium and normal cartilage.
- Overlying epithelium can have erosion/ulceration or metaplasia change.
- Some bone marrow elements can be seen in areas of bone formation.
- The bone and cartilage is cytologic benign.

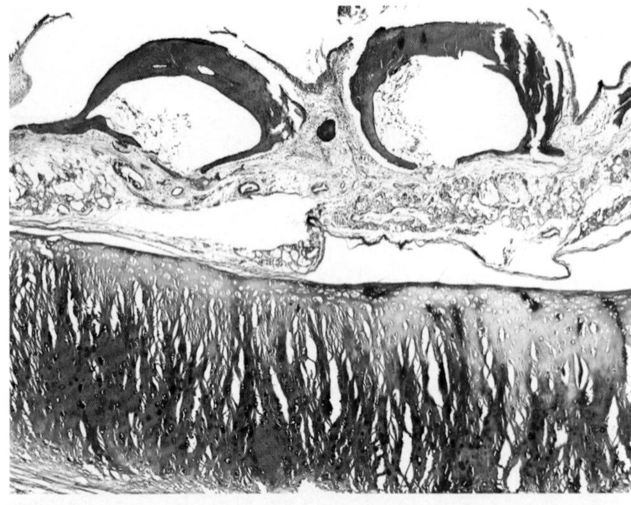

Figure 80.1 Low-power view showing the round areas of ossification partially covered by columnar epithelium. Tracheal cartilage plate can also be seen.

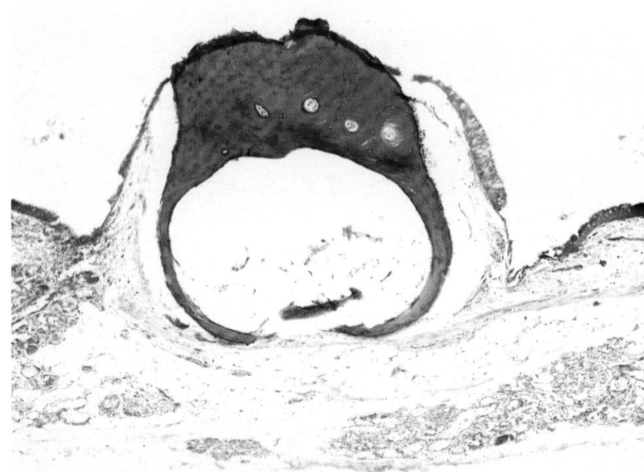

Figure 80.2 High-power view of an area of ossification between the epithelium and the tracheal glands.

*The author would like to acknowledge the work of Dr. Barrios, who contributed to the previous edition.

81 Asthma

Ross A. Miller
Philip T. Cagle

Asthma can occur from a variety of allergic and nonallergic stimuli. Regardless of the inciting stimulus, the symptomatology results from increased airway irritability, resulting in acute or episodic airway narrowing. The airway narrowing can resolve spontaneously; however, many patients require some type of pharmacologic intervention. Various conditions, including eosinophilic esophagitis and Churg–Strauss syndrome, are associated with the condition.

CYTOLOGIC FEATURES

- Findings are not specific for asthma; however, abundant mucus, eosinophils and Charcot–Leyden crystals, Creola bodies, and Curschmann's spirals can be seen.

HISTOLOGIC FEATURES

- Bronchial and bronchiolar smooth muscle hyperplasia.
- Bronchial mucus gland hyperplasia.
- Goblet-cell metaplasia.
- Mixed inflammation of the bronchial wall typically with abundant eosinophils can be seen.
- Basement membrane thickening and abundant mucous or mucin plugs in bronchi.

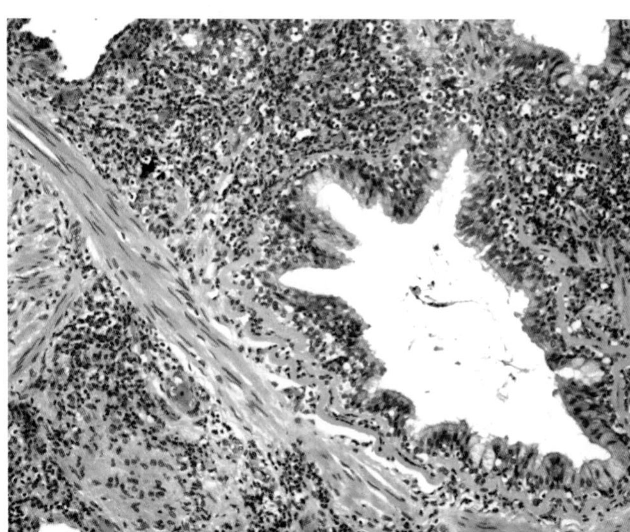

Figure 81.1 A bronchiole with focal goblet-cell metaplasia and surrounding smooth muscle hyperplasia. A mixed inflammatory infiltrate is seen within the wall, and numerous eosinophils are present.

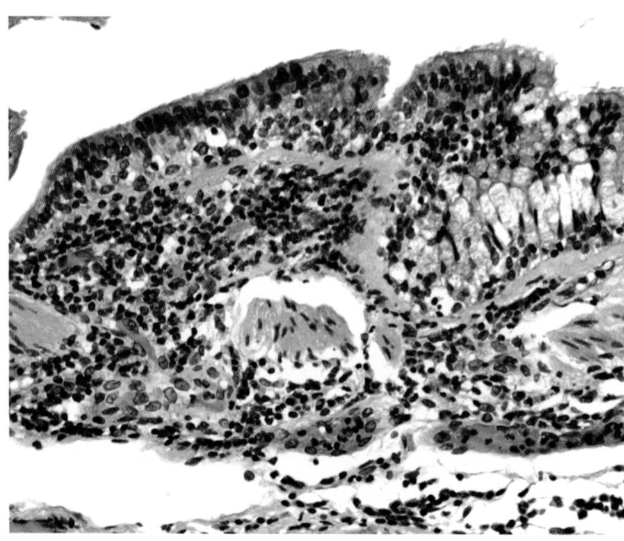

Figure 81.2 Focal goblet-cell metaplasia is seen along with numerous eosinophils.

Allergic Bronchopulmonary Aspergillosis

82

Ross A. Miller

Allergic bronchopulmonary aspergillosis (ABPA) occurs when the bronchial tree becomes colonized with *Aspergillus* species or other fungal organisms in susceptible individuals. ABPA is a hypersensitivity reaction to colonizing fungal elements rather than an invasive fungal infectious process. The token finding is the presence of "allergic mucin," which is characterized by mucin admixed with numerous eosinophils and eosinophil cytoplasmic granular material, similar to the allergic mucin seen in fungal hypersensitivity processes that can occur in the sinuses. Occasionally, calcium oxalate crystals can even be seen. Special stains for fungal elements can help identify fungal elements within the mucin; however, many times definitive organisms are not seen as they are often fragmented and degenerated or may not be in the plane of section examined. Patients affected are typically asthmatics or those who have some other lung pathologic process (cystic fibrosis, etc.). Additional findings that often occur and are associated with ABPA include mucoid impaction, bronchocentric granuloma formation, eosinophilic pneumonias, and even bronchiectasis. The presence of these other findings depends on the severity of disease and associated comorbid conditions.

HISTOLOGIC FEATURES

- Mucus with large numbers of eosinophils; many of the eosinophils are shrunken; degranulation and Charcot–Leyden crystals can be seen.
- Sometimes calcium oxalate crystals will be present.
- Occasionally, fungal elements can be identified in the mucus. Special stains can be helpful.
- Desquamated epithelial cells and mixed inflammatory cells can be seen.
- The bronchi often show findings compatible with asthma.
- Mucoid impaction, bronchocentric granulomas, eosinophilic pneumonia, and even bronchiectasis can be seen.

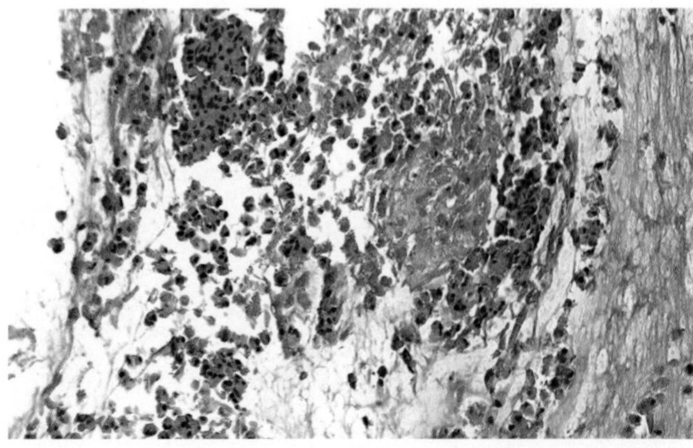

Figure 82.1 ABPA shows mucus containing a dense eosinophilic infiltrate and occasional fungal hyphae.

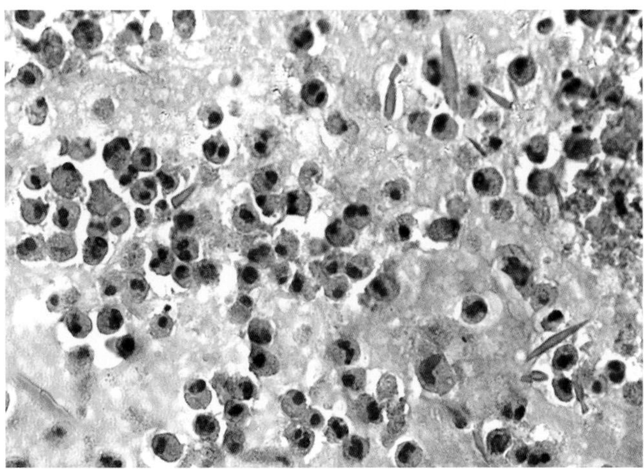

Figure 82.2 Higher power image showing eosinophils and scattered Charcot–Leyden crystals within a background of mucus.

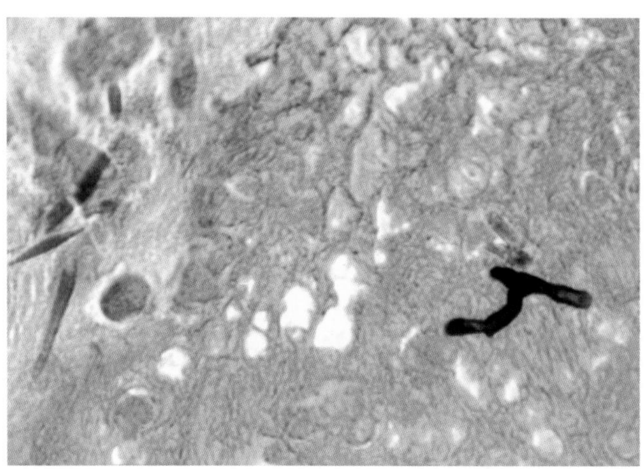

Figure 82.3 Gomori methenamine silver stain showing acute branching hyphae consistent with *Aspergillus* sp. and a Charcot–Leyden crystal.

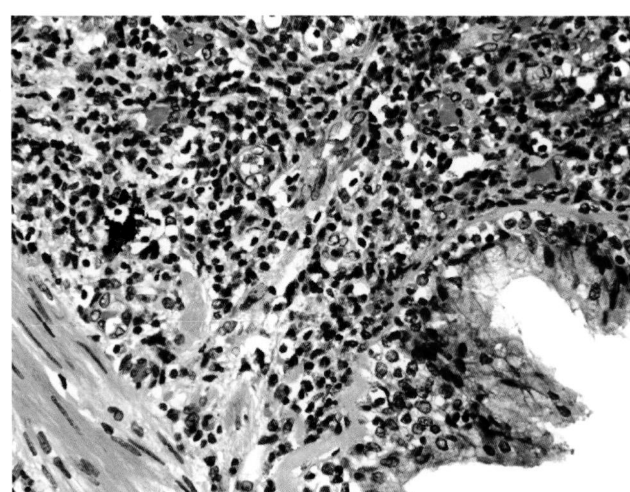

Figure 82.4 Underlying bronchiolar mucosa showing features of asthma, including a dense chronic inflammatory infiltrate rich in eosinophils, a thickened basement membrane, and smooth muscle hyperplasia.

Section 12

Small Airways

Sanja Dacic

Bronchiolar and Peribronchiolar Inflammation, Fibrosis, and Metaplasia

83

Sanja Dacic

Small airways may be involved by inflammation and scarring either as an isolated or focal condition (e.g., a scarred bronchiole from a prior focal infection) or as a widespread or diffuse process. Inflammation and scarring of bronchiolar walls and the adjacent alveolar septa may be accompanied by metaplasia of the bronchiolar or alveolar epithelium. The bronchiolar epithelium may undergo goblet-cell metaplasia or squamous metaplasia. The appearance of bronchiolar-type epithelium on the surface of fibrotic alveoli next to a scarred bronchiole is sometimes called *lambertosis*, which refers to an older concept that this epithelium grew onto the alveolar surface from the bronchiolar lumen via the canals of Lambert. Small airways may be a primary site of disease, or most frequently the scarring and inflammation are the result of secondary involvement such as in bronchiectasis or bronchopneumonia.

HISTOLOGIC FEATURES

- Inflammation and scarring in the walls of bronchioles and in the alveolar septa adjacent to the bronchioles.
- Goblet-cell metaplasia or squamous metaplasia of the bronchiolar epithelium.
- Bronchiolar metaplasia, goblet-cell metaplasia, or squamous metaplasia of the surface lining of adjacent scarred alveolar septa (lambertosis).

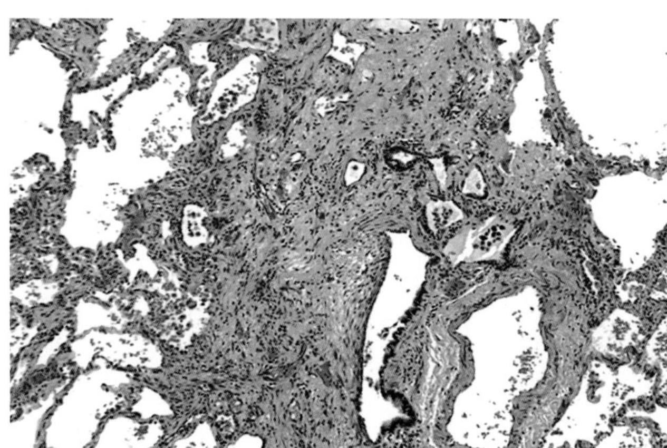

Figure 83.1 Small airway scarring extending into adjacent alveolar septa lined by metaplastic bronchiolar-type epithelium.

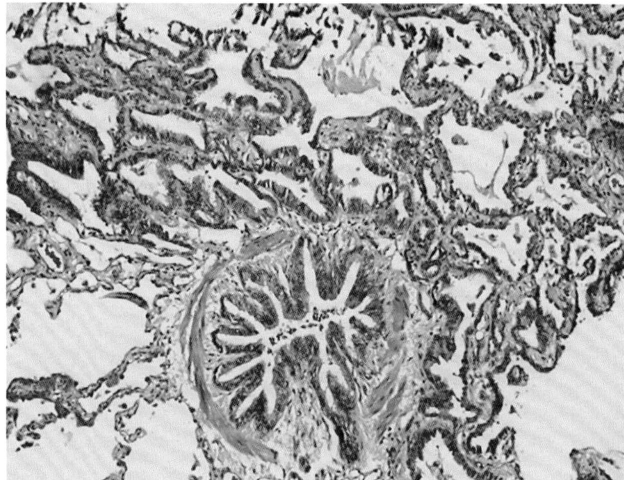

Figure 83.2 Small airway submucosal scarring and prominent bronchiolar metaplasia (lambertosis) in the adjacent lung parenchyma.

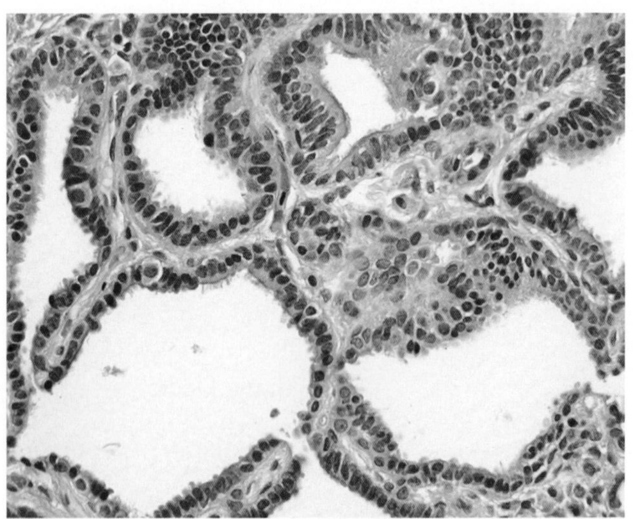

Figure 83.3 High-power magnification of bronchiolar metaplasia.

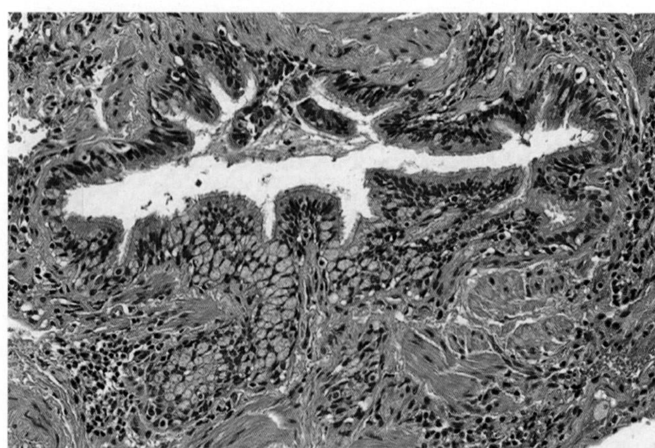

Figure 83.4 Small airways with lymphocytic inflammation and goblet-cell metaplasia.

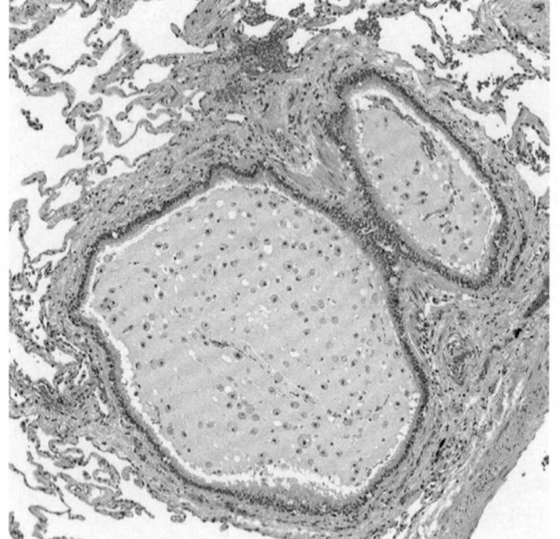

Figure 83.5 Mucostasis, a finding frequently seen in lungs with impaired small airway function.

84

Lobular Pneumonia

▸ Philip T. Cagle

In lobular pneumonia, also called *bronchopneumonia* or *focal pneumonia*, acute inflammation fills the respiratory bronchioles and adjacent alveolar ducts and alveoli in the center of the lobule. This is in contrast to lobar pneumonia, which involves an entire lobe. Generally, lobular pneumonia is caused by an infectious organism. Specific organisms that can cause pneumonias are discussed in Chapters 120 to 123.

HISTOLOGIC FEATURES

- Acute inflammation comprising neutrophils fills respiratory bronchioles and spills into adjacent alveolar ducts and alveoli.

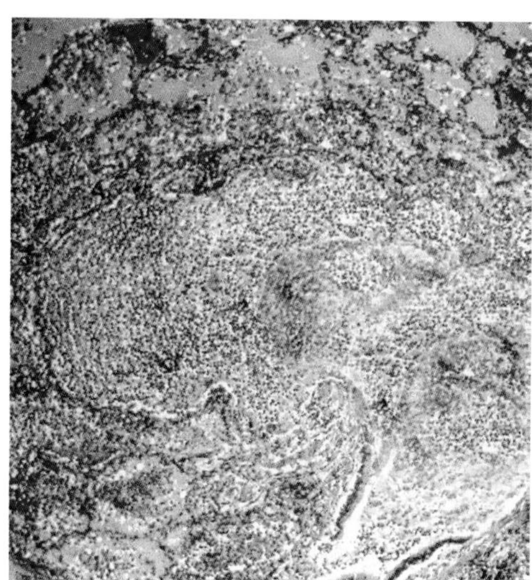

Figure 84.1 Low-power view shows neutrophils filling a bronchiole *(lower right)* and expanding into the adjacent alveoli. Other nearby alveoli are filled with pink edema fluid.

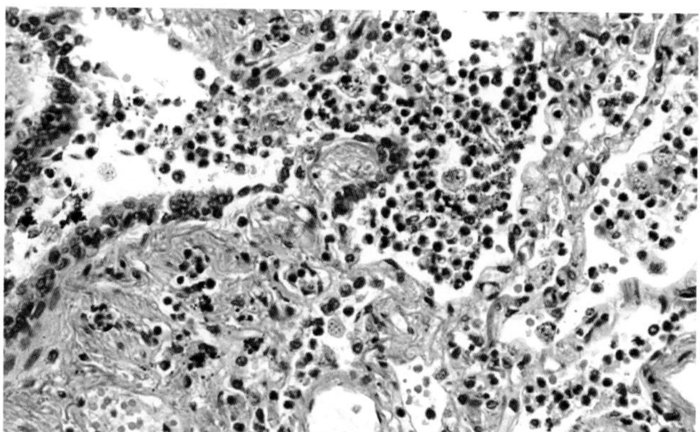

Figure 84.2 Higher power view shows bronchiole and adjacent alveoli filled with neutrophils.

85 Organizing Pneumonia

▶ Sanja Dacic

Organizing pneumonia (OP) is a nonspecific manifestation of a variety of lung injuries and as a component of several specific lung diseases. The same histologic pattern occurs as an idiopathic clinical syndrome called *cryptogenic organizing pneumonia* (COP; formerly referred to as *idiopathic bronchiolitis obliterans organizing pneumonia*), classified with the *idiopathic interstitial pneumonias* (see Section 16: Idiopathic Interstitial Pneumonias). OP may be a primary manifestation of infections, drug reactions including reaction to chemotherapy/radiation, bronchiolar obstruction, inhalation of toxic fumes, and aspiration. This pattern can also be a minor component of other specific lung diseases, such as hypersensitivity pneumonitis, eosinophilic pneumonia, or collagen vascular diseases involving the lungs. OP may also be a nonspecific reaction to unrelated pathologic processes, such as neoplasms, granulomas, or infarcts. The morphologic hallmark of OP is the presence of distinct plugs of granulation tissue (fibroblasts in an edematous or myxoid stroma) in the bronchiolar lumens and peribronchiolar airspaces. Rounded nodules of granulation tissue in alveolar spaces are called *Masson bodies*. There may be accompanying interstitial lymphocytes or other inflammation. Transbronchial biopsy may fail to sample small airways, and the only finding may be the granulation tissue in the alveoli. Histopathologic clues to the etiology of OP may not be present, and clinical correlation is often necessary to determine the underlying cause. If an identifiable etiology is excluded, then the diagnosis is COP. The OP may resolve with or without residual scarring.

HISTOLOGIC FEATURES

- Plugs of granulation tissue (fibroblasts in an edematous or myxoid stroma) in the lumens of bronchioles, alveolar ducts, and adjacent alveoli.
- Rounded nodules of granulation tissue in alveolar spaces (Masson bodies).
- There may be accompanying interstitial lymphocytes or other inflammation.
- Transbronchial biopsy may sample only alveoli with granulation tissue and may not sample involved bronchioles.
- Intra-alveolar collections of foamy macrophages indicate bronchiolar obstruction.

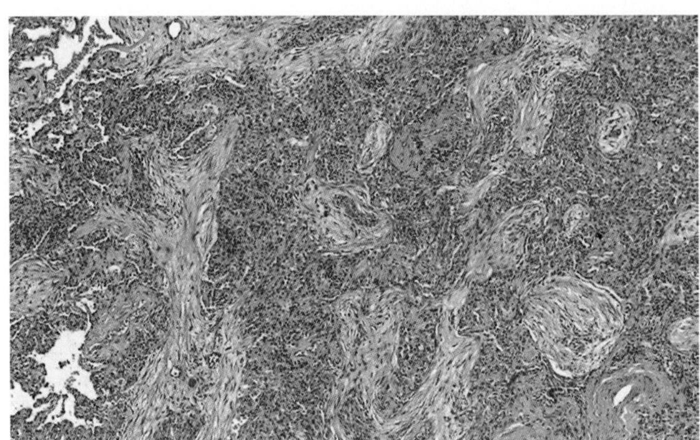

Figure 85.1 OP with granulation-like tissue proliferation filling airspaces and associated with mild lymphocytic inflammation. The *right lower corner* demonstrates similarly appearing tissue filling the small airway lumen.

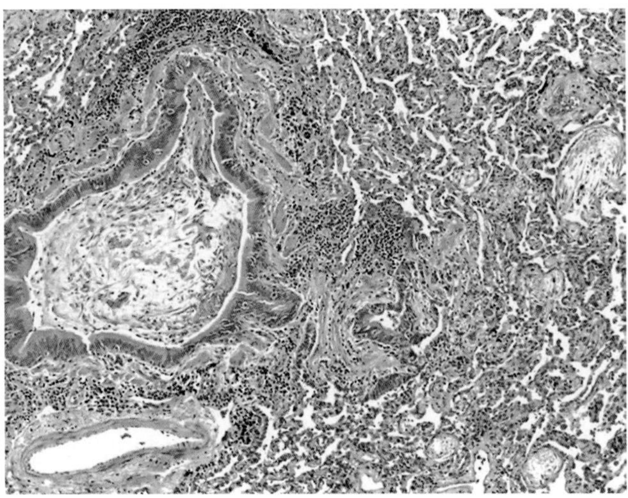

Figure 85.2 Higher magnification of a small airway filled with granulation-like tissue.

Constrictive Bronchiolitis

86

Sanja Dacic

Constrictive bronchiolitis is a condition in which the bronchiolar lumens are narrowed by concentric submucosal fibrosis. Constrictive bronchiolitis may be caused by infection (particularly viral and mycoplasma), collagen vascular diseases involving the lungs (particularly rheumatoid arthritis), drug reactions (gold and penicillamine), and exposures to fumes and toxins. It is most often encountered following lung or heart–lung transplantation or bone marrow transplantation when considered to represent a manifestation of chronic allograft rejection or graft-versus-host disease, respectively. Constrictive bronchiolitis can also be seen in patients with bronchiectasis, asthma, or inflammatory bowel disease. Rapidly progressive dyspnea with cough is the most common clinical presentation. Prognosis is usually poor, and steroid therapy is less beneficial. Fully developed constrictive bronchiolitis showed bronchiolar lumens narrowed and surrounded by concentric fibrous tissue. Often, only a scar is seen, and elastic stains may be helpful in demonstrating the remnants of bronchiole elastica surrounding the fibrosis. Similarly, trichrome stains may highlight small airway muscle surrounding fibrosis. In less advanced cases, narrowing of the bronchiolar lumen may be subtle, and clinical symptoms may be disproportionate to the morphologic narrowing. Fibrosis does not extend into adjacent alveolar septa or airspaces. Inflammation may be present, or it may be minimal or absent.

HISTOLOGIC FEATURES

- Bronchiolar lumen is narrowed by submucosal fibrous tissue.
- Bronchiolar lumens may be completely obliterated, leaving only a scar; trichrome stain may help identify obliterated bronchioles by highlighting their smooth muscle. Elastic stains help to highlight bronchiole elastica surrounding the fibrosis.
- Inflammation may be present, or it may be minimal or absent.

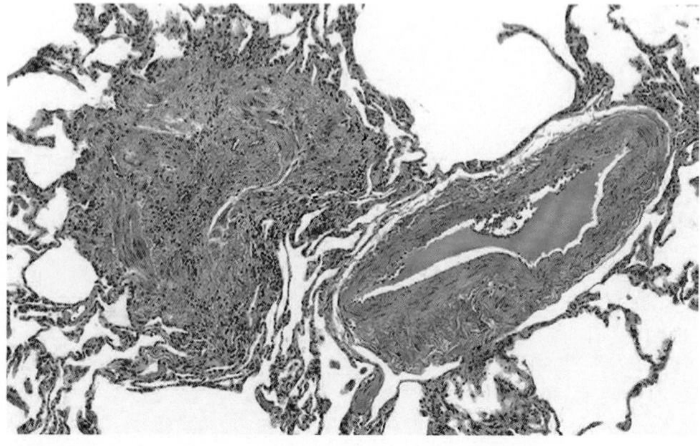

Figure 86.1 Bronchovascular bundle demonstrating a complete obliteration of the small airway lumen by scar tissue associated with mild lymphocytic inflammation in a patient with rheumatoid arthritis.

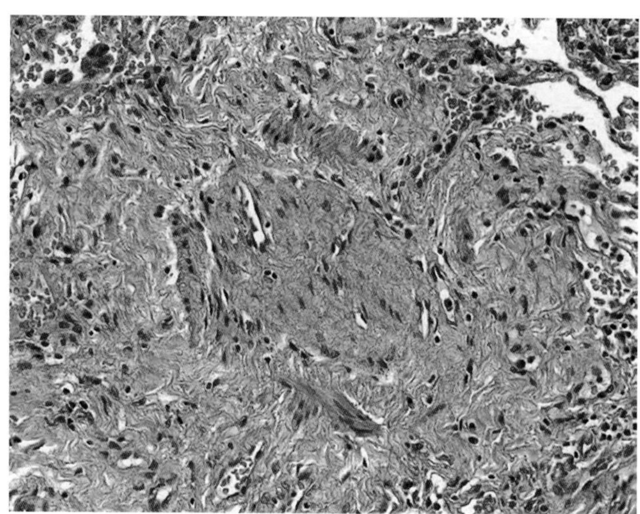

Figure 86.2 High magnification of complete obliteration of a bronchiolar lumen.

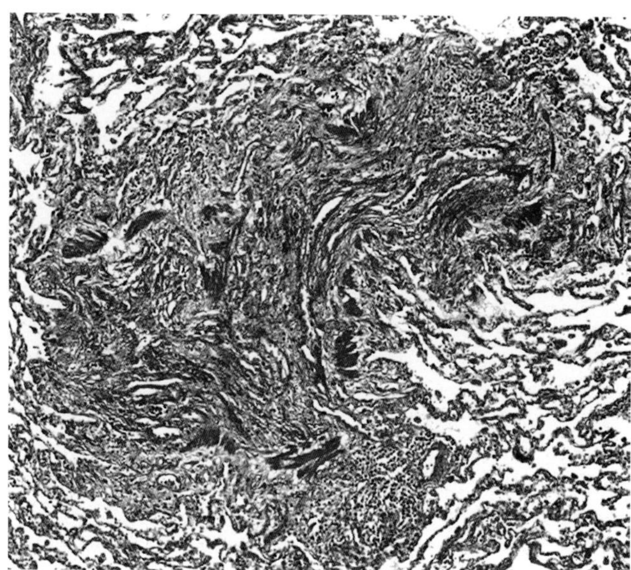

Figure 86.3 Trichrome stain highlights bronchiolar smooth muscle *(purple)* surrounding luminal scar *(blue)*.

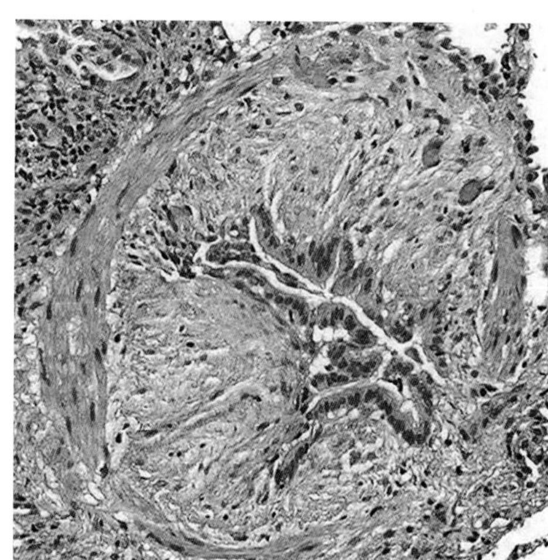

Figure 86.4 Incomplete obliteration of a bronchiolar lumen by submucosal fibrosis as a manifestation of chronic allograft rejection in a lung transplant patient.

Respiratory Bronchiolitis and Membranous Bronchiolitis

87

Sanja Dacic

Tobacco smoking results in inflammatory, sometimes fibrotic, lesions of the membranous (terminal) bronchioles and respiratory bronchioles, referred to as *membranous bronchiolitis* and *respiratory bronchiolitis,* respectively. If a patient has evidence of interstitial lung disease, the term used for the same lesion is *respiratory bronchiolitis–associated interstitial lung disease* (RB-ILD) or *desquamative interstitial pneumonia.* Histologically, respiratory bronchiolitis and RB-ILD are identical. Mild restrictive defects are usually found on pulmonary function tests. The process tends to be stable and may improve, particularly with cessation of cigarette smoking.

HISTOLOGIC FEATURES

Respiratory Bronchiolitis

- Respiratory bronchioles and adjacent airspaces filled with macrophages containing a finely granular brown cytoplasmic pigment.
- Mild to moderate infiltrates of lymphocytes and/or histiocytes in the bronchiolar wall; histiocytes may contain black anthracotic pigment or the same finely granular brown cytoplasmic pigment as the macrophages.
- Minimal to mild fibrosis in the bronchiolar wall and first tiers of adjacent alveolar septa, which may be lined by hyperplastic type II pneumocytes or metaplastic bronchiolar epithelium.

Membranous Bronchiolitis

- Lesions may be seen involving occasional membranous bronchioles of smokers or may be more extensive and accompanied by respiratory bronchiolitis or other smoking-related changes, such as emphysema and/or desquamative interstitial pneumonia.
- Collections of macrophages containing a finely granular brown cytoplasmic pigment within lumens of membranous bronchioles and often in lumens of respiratory bronchioles, alveolar ducts, and alveoli.
- Mild to moderate infiltrates of lymphocytes and/or histiocytes in the bronchiolar wall, smooth muscle hyperplasia, adventitial fibrosis, and/or hyperplasia or metaplasia of the bronchiolar epithelium.

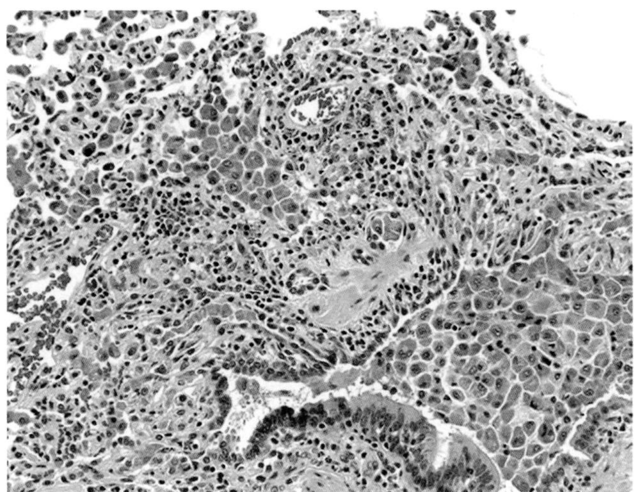

Figure 87.1 Respiratory bronchiolitis showing clusters of pigmented macrophages filling the respiratory bronchiole lumen and surrounding airspaces.

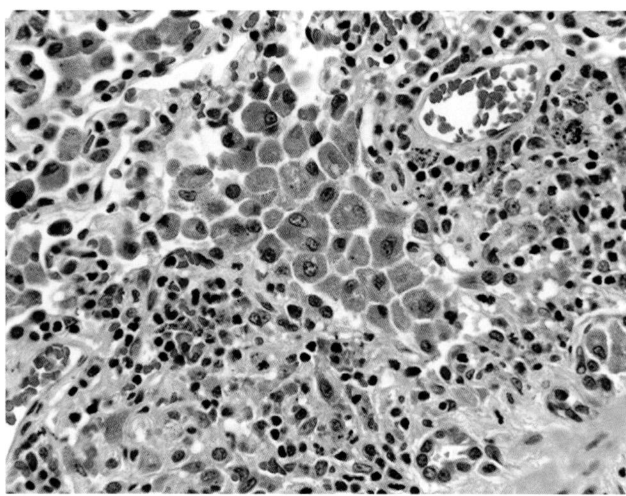

Figure 87.2 High magnification demonstrating the granular appearance of the macrophage cytoplasm.

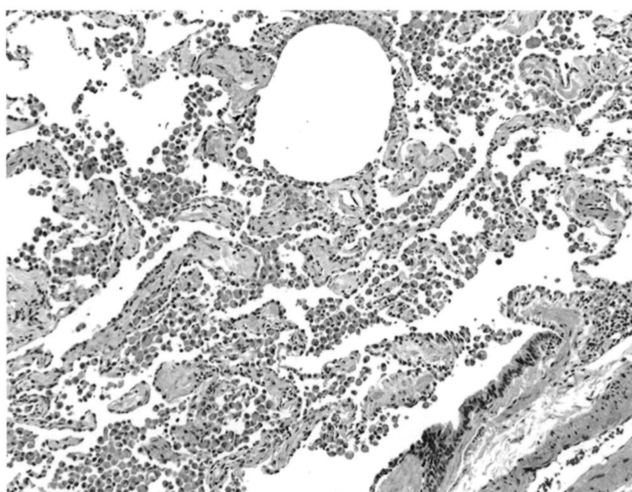

Figure 87.3 Smoker's macrophages filling the respiratory bronchiole lumen and adjacent airspaces.

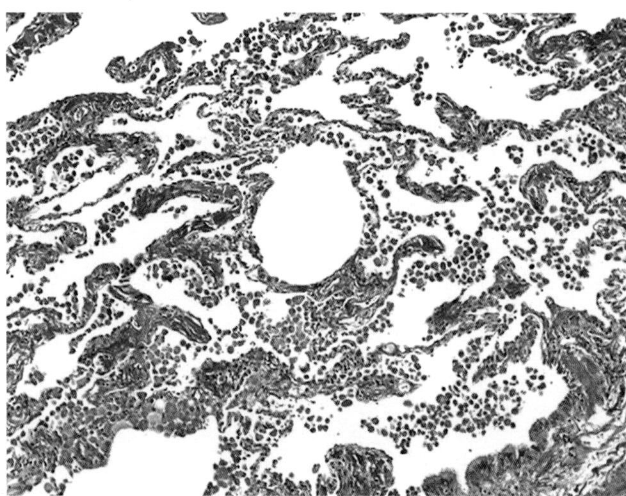

Figure 87.4 Trichrome stain highlights mild fibrosis in the bronchiolar wall and first tiers of adjacent alveolar septa.

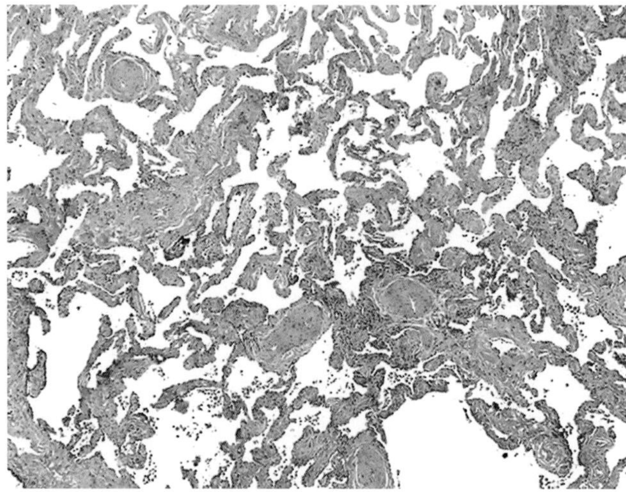

Figure 87.5 Smoking-related lung fibrosis demonstrates glassy, eosino philic thickening of the alveolar septa in the area of emphysematous change.

88 Follicular Bronchiolitis

▶ Sanja Dacic

Follicular bronchiolitis is characterized by hyperplasia of the bronchus-associated lymphoid tissue (BALT) often containing germinal centers that is confined to bronchioles. It occurs in a large spectrum of diseases including collagen vascular diseases involving the lungs (particularly rheumatoid arthritis and Sjögren syndrome), in bronchiectasis, in immunodeficiency states (congenital and acquired). It may also be a manifestation of viral infections, particularly in children, or a hypersensitivity reaction. Some cases are idiopathic. It may also be seen in association with lymphoma of the BALT.

HISTOLOGIC FEATURES

- Prominent lymphoid tissue with follicles and germinal centers surrounding airways.

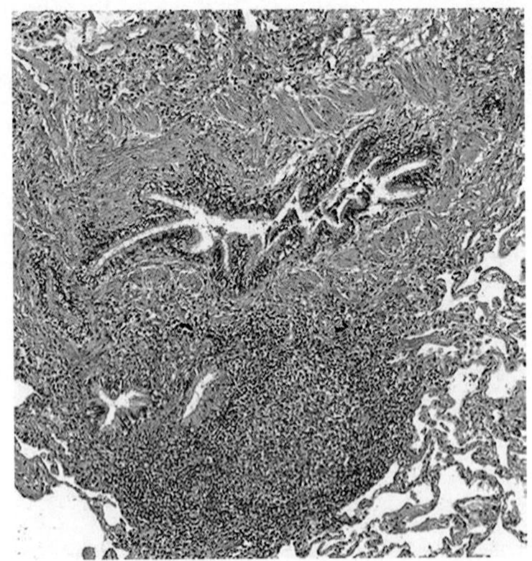

Figure 88.1 Follicular bronchiolitis showing prominent lymphoid aggregate with germinal center slightly narrowing the lumen of the terminal bronchiole.

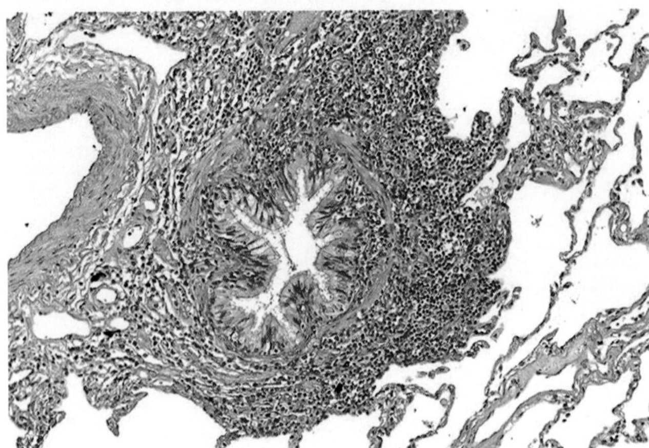

Figure 88.2 Follicular bronchiolitis showing dense lymphoid infiltrate surrounding the terminal bronchiole.

89 Diffuse Panbronchiolitis

Sanja Dacic
Philip T. Cagle

Diffuse panbronchiolitis is a progressive obstructive small airway disease associated with sinusitis that occurs primarily in adults of Japanese heritage. The disease is typically complicated by infections and, when untreated, leads to bronchiectasis and eventually death. An association with rheumatoid arthritis in Japan has been reported. Grossly, bronchiolocentric yellow 1- to 3-mm nodules are present. Histologically, the bronchiolar interstitium in diffuse panbronchiolitis is infiltrated by foamy macrophages, lymphocytes, and plasma cells. Follicular bronchiolitis may be present, and there may be histopathologic findings of superimposed acute or organizing pneumonia.

HISTOLOGIC FEATURES

- Respiratory bronchioles, terminal (membranous) bronchioles, and alveolar ducts may be involved; membranous (terminal) bronchioles may be ectatic.
- Transmural infiltration of bronchiolar interstitium and peribronchiolar tissue by foamy macrophages, lymphocytes, and plasma cells.
- Follicular bronchiolitis may be present.
- Acute inflammation may be present in bronchiolar lumens.
- Histopathologic findings of superimposed acute or organizing pneumonia and bronchiectasis may be present.

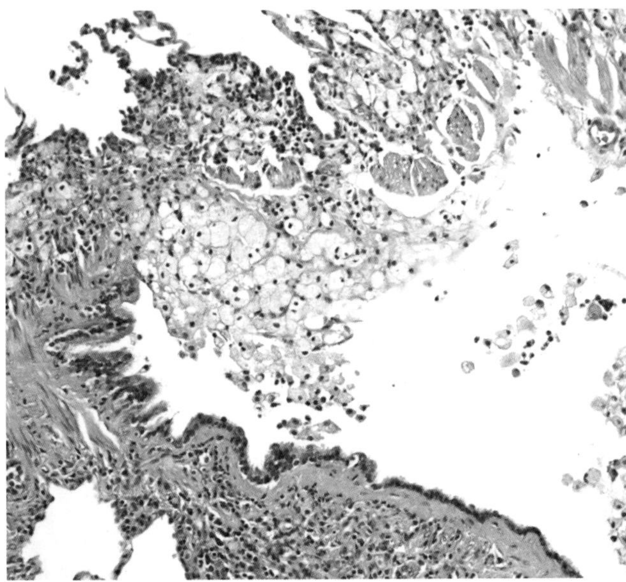

Figure 89.1 Bronchiolar wall is infiltrated by chronic inflammatory infil trates and foamy macrophages that have spilled into the lumen.

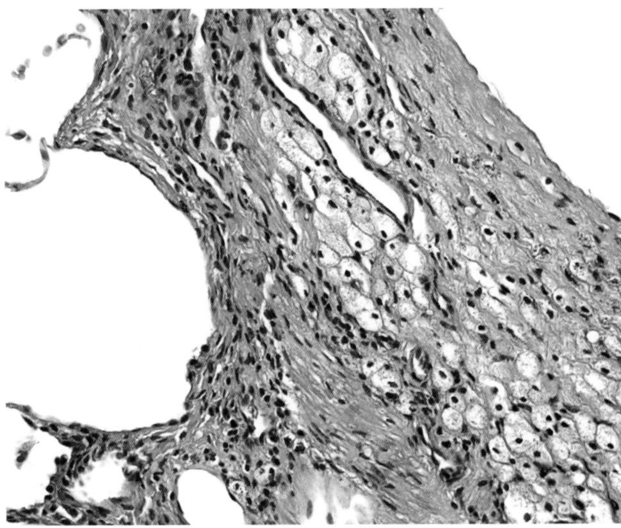

Figure 89.2 Foamy macrophages and lymphocytes in the interstitium in a Japanese patient.

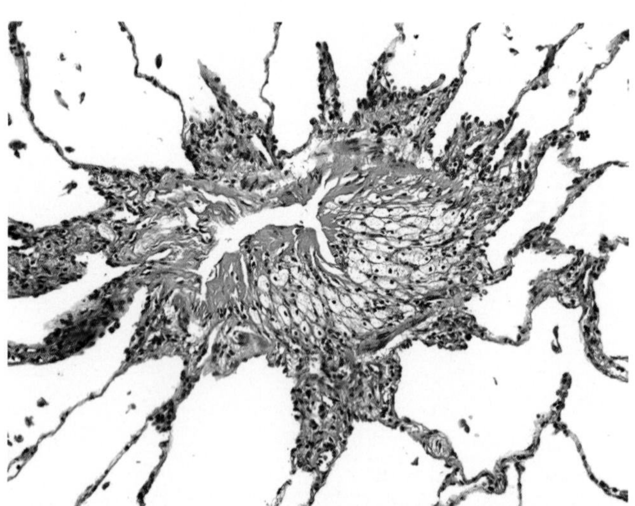

Figure 89.3 Lumen of small bronchiole is narrowed by foamy macro phages and lymphocytes in its wall in a North American patient. This patient had a xanthomatous bronchiolitis obliterans with some features resembling diffuse panbronchiolitis in Japanese patients and required lung transplantation.

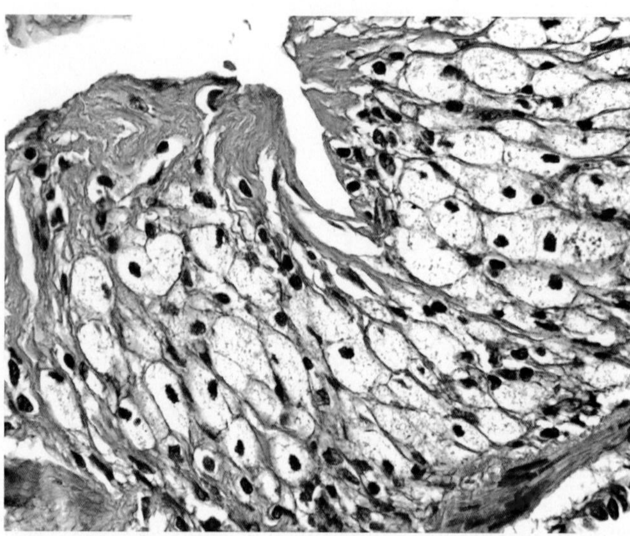

Figure 89.4 Higher power view of Figure 89.3 shows foamy macrophages in the bronchiolar wall.

Small Airways and Inorganic Dust

Sanja Dacic

Small airways (terminal or membranous bronchioles, respiratory bronchioles, and alveolar ducts) may be affected by exposure to both fibrogenic and inert mineral particles, including silica, silicates, coal dust, asbestos, iron, and mixed dusts. Small airways are often involved by macules and nodules of various dust exposures (see Section 21: Pneumoconioses, Chapters 143 to 150). The term *mineral dust-associated small airway disease* has been coined to describe fibrosis of small airways that evolves from nonfibrotic dust macules. There is deposition of mineral dusts and minimal fibrosis in the walls of the membranous bronchioles, respiratory bronchioles, and alveolar ducts. With time, the lesions may progress, with fibrotic distortion of the airways and focal emphysema of the adjacent parenchyma.

HISTOLOGIC FEATURES

- Small airways are often involved by macules and nodules of various dust exposures.
- In mineral dust-associated small airway disease, there are deposits of dust and dust-laden macrophages in the walls of terminal (membranous) bronchioles, respiratory bronchioles, and alveolar ducts associated initially with minimal fibrosis.
- Mineral dust-associated small airway disease may progress into more severe fibrosis of the walls of small airways, with distortion and potentially focal emphysema of parenchyma around the affected airways.

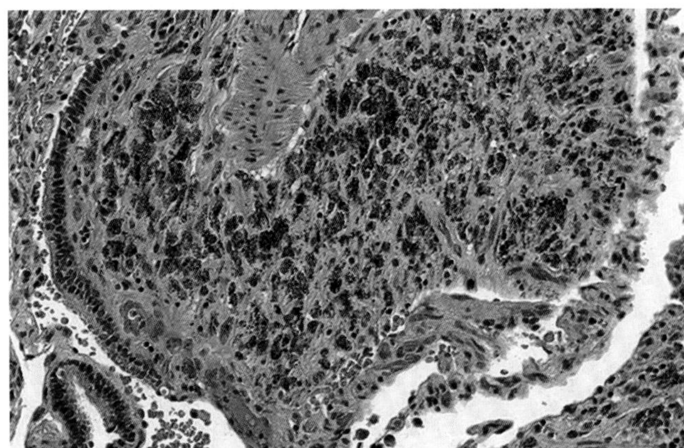

Figure 90.1 Respiratory bronchiole with numerous macrophages with iron oxides/welder's pigment.

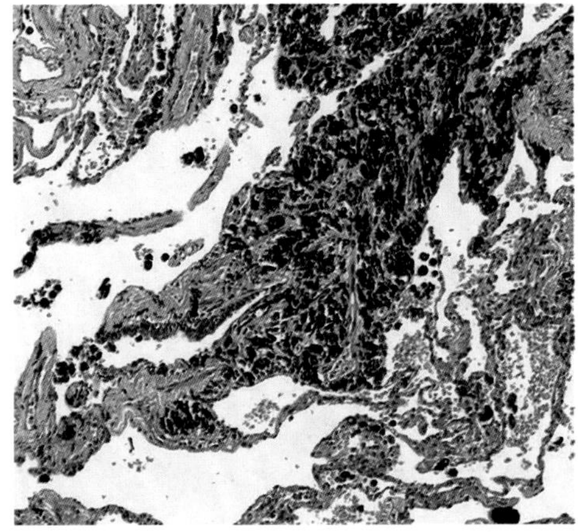

Figure 90.2 Dust macule located around small airways and associated with focal emphysema.

Section 13

Alveolar Infiltrates

Mary Beth Beasley

91

Acute Pneumonia

Mary Beth Beasley

Acute pneumonia is characterized by the accumulation of neutrophils within alveolar spaces. Classically associated with a variety of bacterial infections (*Streptococcus* sp., *Staphylococcus* sp., *Klebsiella* sp., *Pseudomonas* sp., *Haemophilus* sp., and others), accumulation of neutrophils may also occur secondary to aspiration or other inhalational injuries.

Acute pneumonia has been classically divided into "bronchopneumonia" and "lobar pneumonia." The histologic findings are the same in both processes, and the designation refers to the distribution of disease. Bronchopneumonia is classically a patchy process centered around airways (see also Chapter 84), whereas lobar pneumonia refers to involvement of an entire lobe. The term *necrotizing pneumonia* refers to acute pneumonia associated with a significant amount of tissue necrosis and is often caused by a particularly virulent bacterial strain.

Abscess formation may be a complication of acute pneumonia. By definition, an abscess is a localized collection of pus, and in the lung this manifests as an area of necrotic lung with marked neutrophilic infiltrates typically walled off from the surrounding lung parenchyma in attempt to contain the process.

Acute pneumonia may evolve into organizing pneumonia, in which the alveolar exudate organizes by the ingrowth of fibroblastic tissue. Ultimately, the acute exudate is replaced by fibroblastic tissue. This finding should be distinguished from organizing pneumonia pattern/cryptogenic organizing pneumonia discussed in Chapter 85.

Acute pneumonia may be caused by aspiration of gastric contents. This may result in significant tissue necrosis. Helpful clues are giant cells within small airways and alveolar spaces or the finding of definitive foreign material, such as vegetable material, skeletal muscle, or pill fragments.

HISTOLOGIC FEATURES

- Neutrophilic exudates within alveolar spaces.
- Necrosis may be present, particularly in the setting of virulent bacteria or aspiration.
- Abscess formation may be a complication of acute pneumonia.
- Acute pneumonia may evolve into organizing pneumonia characterized by organizing fibroblastic tissue within alveolar spaces.

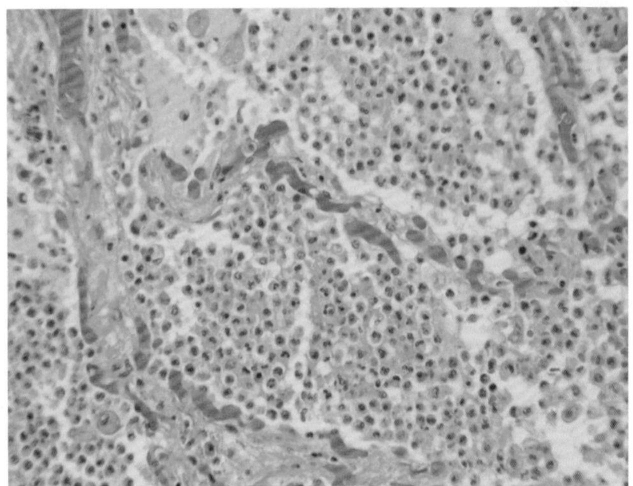

Figure 91.1 Acute pneumonia is characterized by the filling of alveolar spaces with neutrophils (hematoxylin and eosin [H&E] stain, 200×).

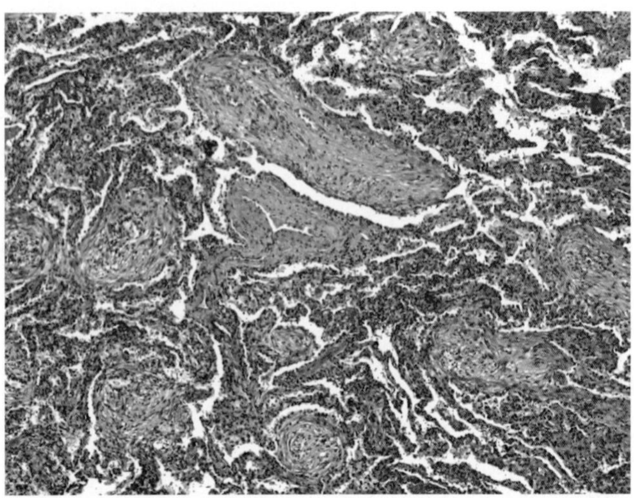

Figure 91.2 Organizing pneumonia is characterized by organizing fibroblastic tissue within alveolar spaces (H&E stain, 200×).

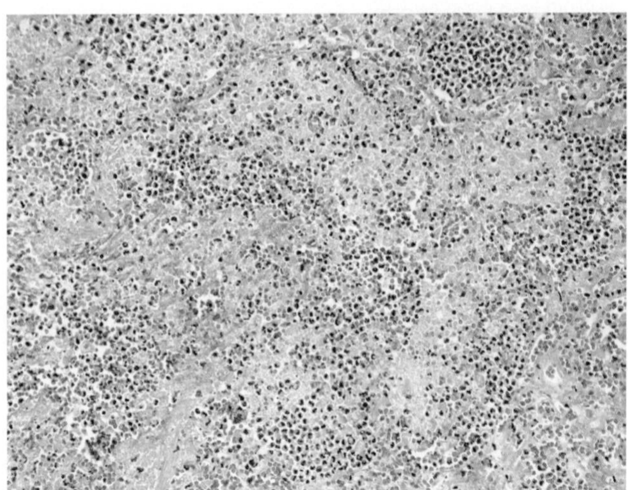

Figure 91.3 Necrotizing pneumonia is typically encountered in association with especially virulent organisms or with aspiration of gastric contents. In this example, neutrophilic infiltrates are present and there is destruction of the alveolar walls (H&E stain, 100×).

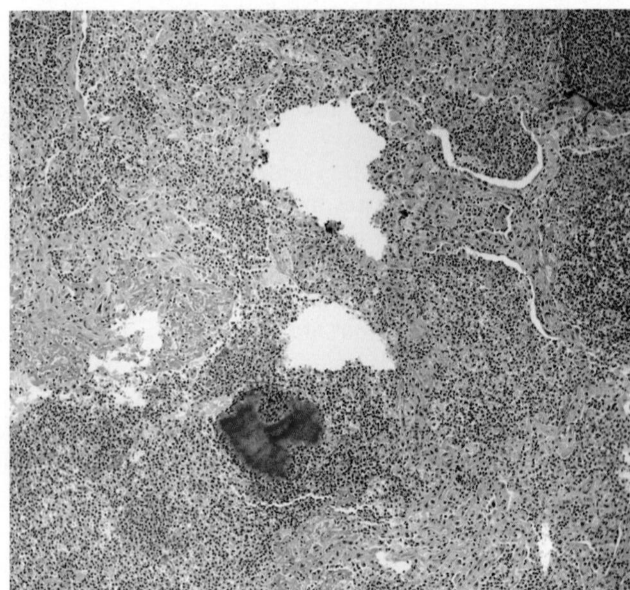

Figure 91.4 Abscess formation is characterized by a localized collection of neutrophils within an area of destroyed parenchyma. In this example, a cluster of bacteria surrounded by Splendore–Hoeppli phenomenon is present (H&E stain, 200×).

92 Pulmonary Edema

Mary Beth Beasley

Edema refers to the accumulation of fluid in the extravascular space. Pulmonary edema is a manifestation of increased perfusion pressure within the pulmonary capillaries, lack of effective drainage of the interstitial space by the lymphatics, increased permeability of the cellular junctions between capillary endothelial cells, or a combination of one or more of the above. Pulmonary edema may result from a variety of underlying conditions, most commonly arising from hemodynamic alterations in the heart that result in increased perfusion pressure in the pulmonary capillaries and/or block effective lymphatic draining. Left ventricular failure, mitral stenosis, and mitral valve insufficiency are among the most common underlying conditions associated with pulmonary edema. In these scenarios, a rise in pressure on the venous side of the pulmonary capillaries results in increased amount of fluid leaving the vessels, which cannot be reabsorbed by the capillaries or effectively cleared by the pulmonary lymphatics. Noncardiac causes of pulmonary edema include exposure to toxic gases, uremia, hypoproteinemia, fluid overload, drug reactions, drug overdose (especially heroin), and infections. Other, rarer etiologies include high-altitude pulmonary edema and cerebral injury (neurogenic pulmonary edema). Edema is also the earliest light microscopic feature seen in diffuse alveolar damage, discussed in Chapter 93.

Regardless of etiology, the microscopic manifestations are similar. Initially, fluid accumulates in the interstitium, resulting in swelling of the interlobular septa and perivascular connective tissue. Ultimately, fluid fills the alveolar spaces and consists of homogenous, proteinaceous eosinophilic material filling the airspaces. Small amounts of fibrin may be present, and entrapped air bubbles may be seen.

The differential diagnosis includes primarily *Pneumocystis jirovecii* pneumonia and pulmonary alveolar proteinosis (PAP). In pneumocystis pneumonia, the eosinophilic alveolar material has a frothy, bubbly appearance and organisms can be demonstrated on Gomori methenamine silver stains. In PAP, the material is dense, coarsely granular and may contain cholesterol clefts.

HISTOLOGIC FEATURES

- Homogenous, proteinaceous eosinophilic material filling alveolar spaces.
- Differential diagnosis—*P. jirovecii* pneumonia and PAP.

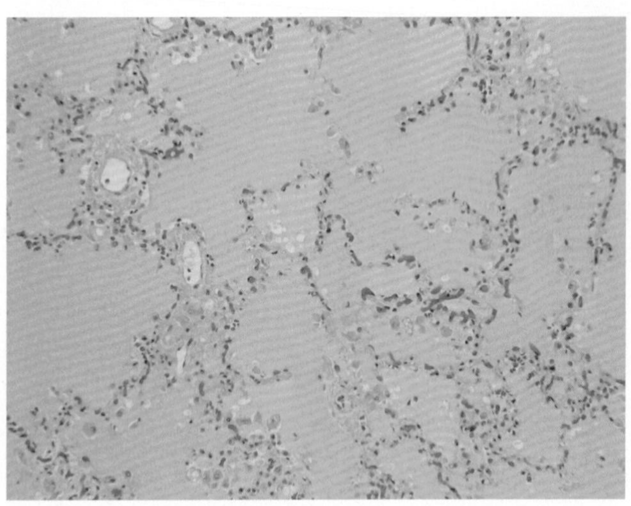

Figure 92.1 Pulmonary edema. The alveolar spaces are filled with homogenous eosinophilic material. Alveolar septa show mild congestion. The eosinophilic alveolar material lacks coarse granularity or a frothy, bubbly appearance (hematoxylin and eosin stain, 200×).

93

Diffuse Alveolar Damage

Mary Beth Beasley

Diffuse alveolar damage (DAD) is a histologic pattern, which may occur secondary to myriad underlying causes (infection, drug reaction, collagen vascular disease, ingestants, inhalants, trauma/shock, sepsis, radiation, numerous others) or may rarely be idiopathic in origin. Idiopathic DAD is referred to as *acute interstitial pneumonia* clinically. Patients with histologic DAD typically correspond to patients with acute respiratory distress syndrome clinically. DAD is thought to result from a pulmonary insult occurring at a single point in time and progresses through acute/exudative and organizing/proliferative phases, culminating in a final fibrotic phase. Regardless of etiology, the initial injury results in damage to both the epithelial and endothelial components of the alveolar wall. The acute phase generally comprises the first week following injury. The earliest changes consist of interstitial edema and fibrin deposition. Hyaline membranes, a classic feature of the acute phase of DAD, are most prevalent between days 3 and 5 of the first week and become gradually resorbed. The organizing phase, which commences toward the end of the first week, is characterized by marked type II pneumocyte hyperplasia, often with pronounced cytologic atypia and interstitial fibrosis. The fibrosis consists of loose, myxoid fibroblastic tissue in contrast to dense collagenous fibrosis seen in many other fibrotic lung diseases. Immature squamous metaplasia may also be present. Significant inflammation is typically lacking unless a coexisting acute pneumonia is present. Intravascular thrombi may be present in all phases of DAD and are secondary to localized alterations in the coagulation cascade and do not indicate underlying embolic disease, even if small infarcts are present.

The differential diagnosis of the acute phase includes acute fibrinous and organizing pneumonia (AFOP) and acute eosinophilic pneumonia (AEP). AFOP is characterized by organizing intra-alveolar fibrin balls and lacks hyaline membranes. AEP may have hyaline membranes but is characterized by the presence of numerous eosinophils. Unlike DAD, AEP is exquisitely responsive to steroids, so this distinction is of particular clinical importance. The differential diagnosis of the proliferative phase of DAD is primarily with the fibrotic variant of nonspecific interstitial pneumonia (NSIP). Fibrotic NSIP is characterized by dense collagenous fibrosis in contrast to the loose myxoid fibrosis and marked pneumocyte hyperplasia present in organizing DAD.

HISTOLOGIC FEATURES

Acute/Exudative Phase

- Hyaline membranes.
- Interstitial congestion and edema.

Organizing/Proliferative Phase

- Interstitial fibrosis—loose, myxoid; not collagenous.
- Marked type II pneumocyte hyperplasia, often with atypia.
- Squamous metaplasia and organizing thrombi may be seen.

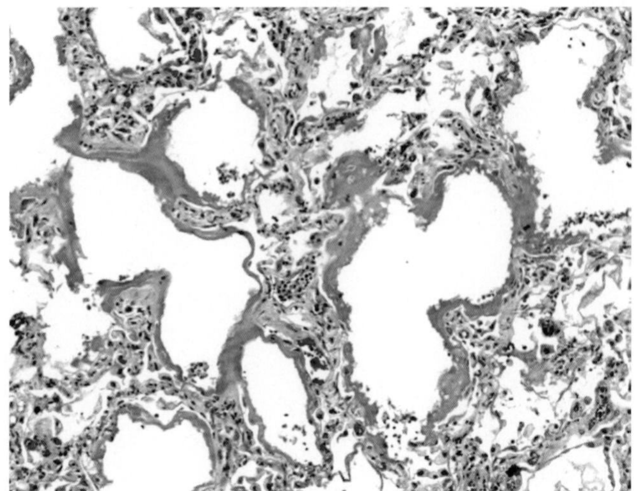

Figure 93.1 Acute DAD is characterized by hyaline membranes—eosinophilic structures composed of protein and cellular material, which line alveolar spaces and alveolar ducts (hematoxylin and eosin [H&E] stain, 100×).

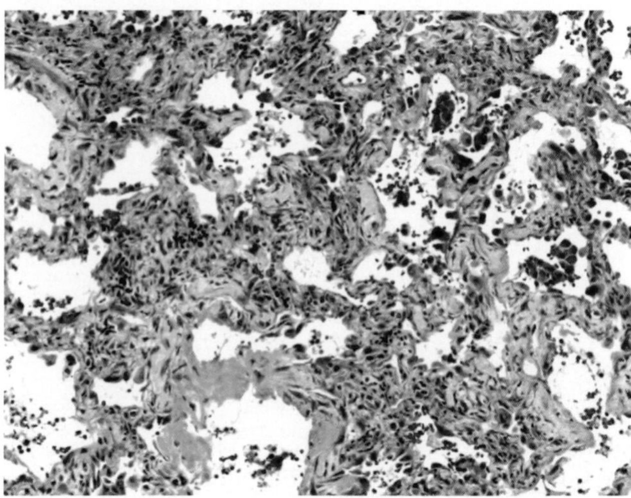

Figure 93.2 Organizing DAD is characterized by myxoid interstitial fibrosis and marked type II pneumocyte hyperplasia. A residual hyaline membrane is present in this example (H&E stain, 100×).

94 Acute Fibrinous and Organizing Pneumonia

Mary Beth Beasley

Acute fibrinous and organizing pneumonia (AFOP) is a histologic pattern of acute lung injury characterized by organizing intra-alveolar fibrin balls and lacking hyaline membrane formation or significant eosinophils or neutrophils. While the overall mortality is similar to that of diffuse alveolar damage (DAD), the reported cases of AFOP fall into one of two clinical categories, those with fulminate respiratory failure and a poor prognosis and one with a subacute presentation with generally good recovery, although often experiencing a higher relapse rate than cryptogenic organizing pneumonia. No histologic feature has been correlated with outcome to date, although a greater extent of radiographic disease has been correlated with a worse outcome. Like DAD, reported cases of AFOP have been attributed to a variety of underlying etiologies, including infection, acute hypersensitivity pneumonia, collagen vascular disease, drug reaction, and as a complication of hematopoietic stem cell transplant, whereas some cases appear to be idiopathic in origin.

AFOP is characterized by the presence of intra-alveolar fibrin balls associated with varying degrees of organizing fibroblastic tissue, although the fibrin is the dominant finding. The distribution may be patchy or relatively diffuse, and the adjacent alveolar walls may show mild lymphocytic inflammation, edematous expansion, and type II pneumocyte hyperplasia. The lung parenchyma between involved areas is relatively unremarkable. Hyaline membranes and significant eosinophils or neutrophils are absent. A definitive diagnosis of AFOP should not be made on a small sample, as organizing intra-alveolar fibrin may be seen adjacent to or as a component of a variety of processes, including vasculitides, necrotizing granulomas, necrotizing pneumonia, and malignancies.

The differential diagnosis of AFOP includes DAD and eosinophilic pneumonia. DAD may have areas of organizing fibrin, but the presence of classic hyaline membranes discriminates DAD from AFOP. Eosinophilic pneumonia may greatly resemble AFOP, given that both may have prominent intra-alveolar fibrin; however, eosinophilic pneumonia is characterized by the presence of significant eosinophils. Partially treated eosinophilic pneumonia should be considered clinically if sparse eosinophils are present in a case otherwise consistent with AFOP if steroids have been administered prior to biopsy.

HISTOLOGIC FEATURES

- Dominant finding of intra-alveolar organizing fibrin.
- Variable amounts of associated organizing pneumonia.
- Mild interstitial lymphocytes, edematous/myxoid interstitial expansion, and prominent pneumocyte hyperplasia may be present.
- Hyaline membranes, significant eosinophils or neutrophils, and vasculitis are absent.
- Patchy distribution is typical although some cases may be relatively diffuse.

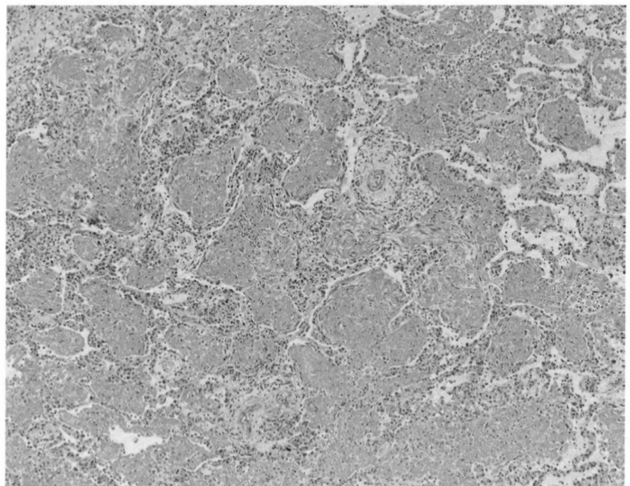

Figure 94.1 AFOP is characterized by patchy to relatively diffuse filling of alveolar spaces by organizing fibrin balls (hematoxylin and eosin [H&E] stain, 100×).

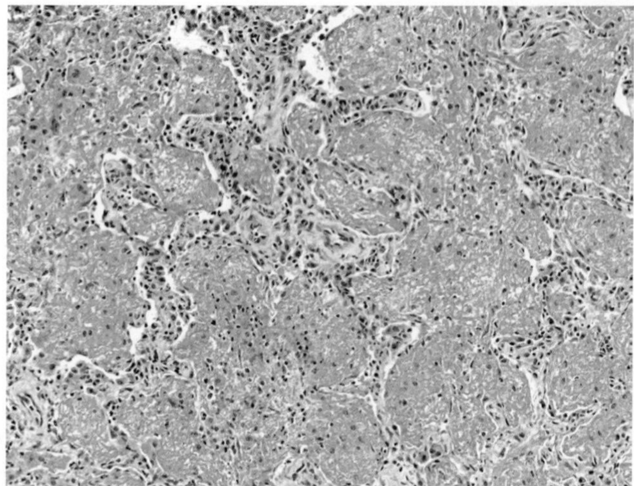

Figure 94.2 Acute fibrinous and organizing pneumonia. Intra-alveolar fibrin balls are the dominant finding. Interstitial changes are relatively minimal and hyaline membranes, significant eosinophils or neutrophils are absent (H&E stain, 200×).

95 Lipoid Pneumonia

Mary Beth Beasley

Lipoid pneumonia can be divided into two types, endogenous and exogenous, depending on the origin of the lipid in the lesion.

Endogenous lipoid pneumonia is often referred to as *postobstructive pneumonia*, as it is always found distal to an area of airway obstruction (i.e., secondary to foreign body, malignancy, inflammation, etc.). Endogenous lipoid pneumonia is characterized by the accumulation of foamy, finely vacuolated macrophages within the alveolar spaces and to a lesser extent in the interstitium. The term *golden pneumonia* refers to the gross appearance of endogenous lipid pneumonia, as the lipids produce a golden color.

Exogenous lipoid pneumonia results from inhalation or aspiration of small quantities of mineral oil or similar substances over time. In contrast to the fine vacuoles of endogenous lipoid pneumonia, exogenous lipoid pneumonia is characterized by the presence of variably sized lipid droplets within both macrophages and the interstitium. A foreign-body giant-cell reaction may occur around the lipid droplets, and fibrosis typically develops over time.

HISTOLOGIC FEATURES

Endogenous Lipoid Pneumonia

- Finely vacuolated macrophages predominantly within alveolar spaces.
- Cholesterol clefts may be present.
- Fibrosis typically absent.

Exogenous Lipoid Pneumonia

- Variably sized lipid vacuoles.
- Foreign-body giant-cell reaction.
- Fibrosis often present.

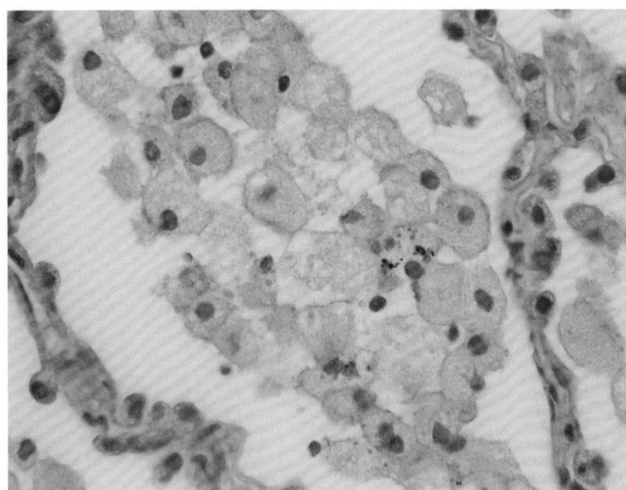

Figure 95.1 Endogenous lipoid pneumonia is characterized by lipid-laden macrophages with fine, relatively uniform vacuoles (hematoxylin and eosin [H&E] stain, 400×).

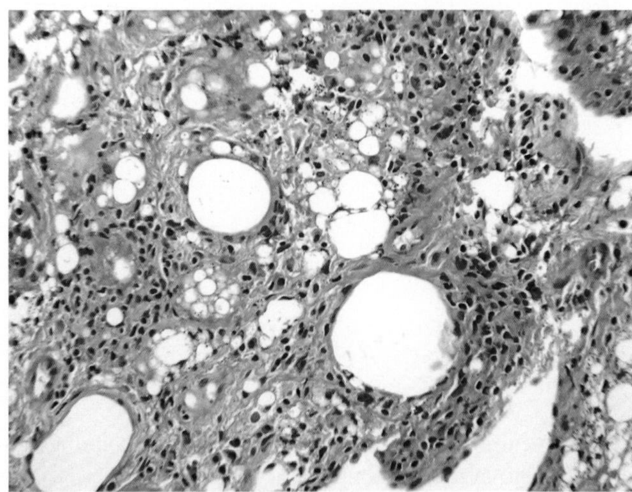

Figure 95.2 Exogenous lipoid pneumonia is characterized by variably sized lipid droplets within both the interstitium and macrophages. Fibrosis and a foreign-body giant-cell reaction may be present (H&E stain, 400×).

96 Eosinophilic Pneumonia

Mary Beth Beasley

Eosinophilic pneumonia (EP), as the name implies, is characterized by an alveolar exudate containing large numbers of eosinophils. EP may occur as a component of systemic disease such as Churg–Strauss syndrome (eosinophilic angiitis and granulomatosis), but this chapter will focus on EP as a primary disease process. Broadly, EP can be divided into acute and chronic forms. Both are characterized by increased eosinophils in bronchioloalveolar lavage fluid of over 25%. Chronic EP is characterized by a subacute presentation and typically occurs in a patient with a history of asthma, and patients have a peripheral blood eosinophilia. Acute EP presents with acute disease, often with fulminate respiratory failure. Patients with acute EP do not typically have a history of asthma, and peripheral blood eosinophilia is absent in most cases. Both chronic and acute EP are usually idiopathic in origin; however, cases may be attributable to drug reactions or infections, particularly parasites or fungi. An interesting association also occurs with cigarette smoking, particularly in patients who have recently initiated smoking, restarted smoking, or changed smoking habits.

Chronic EP is characterized by variable amounts of organizing intra-alveolar fibrin, macrophages and organizing fibroblastic tissue admixed with numerous eosinophils. Acute EP may have similar features but additionally has hyaline membranes similar to those seen in diffuse alveolar damage. Both acute and chronic EP are sensitive to steroid therapy although relapse is more common with chronic EP.

HISTOLOGIC FEATURES

- Prominent eosinophils.
- Intra-alveolar fibrin, macrophages, +/– organizing pneumonia.
- Eosinophilic microabscesses may be present.
- Hyaline membranes in acute EP.
- Granulomas absent.
- Vasculitis absent.

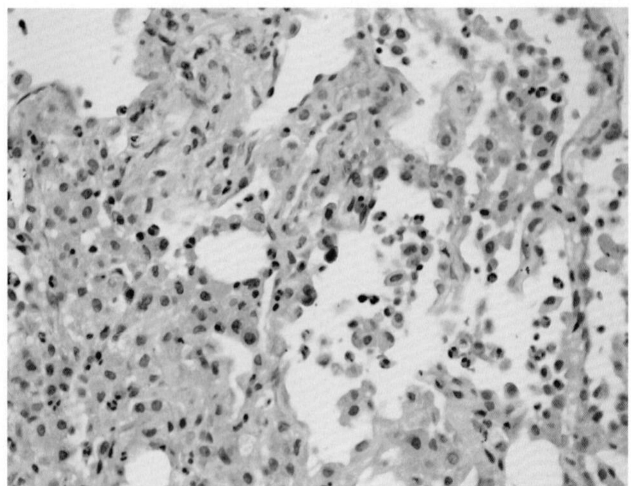

Figure 96.1 Eosinophilic pneumonia is characterized by prominent eosinophilic infiltrates within the alveolar spaces and interstitium. Intra-alveolar macrophages may be present, as in this case, and intra-alveolar fibrin may also be present (hematoxylin and eosin [H&E] stain; 200×).

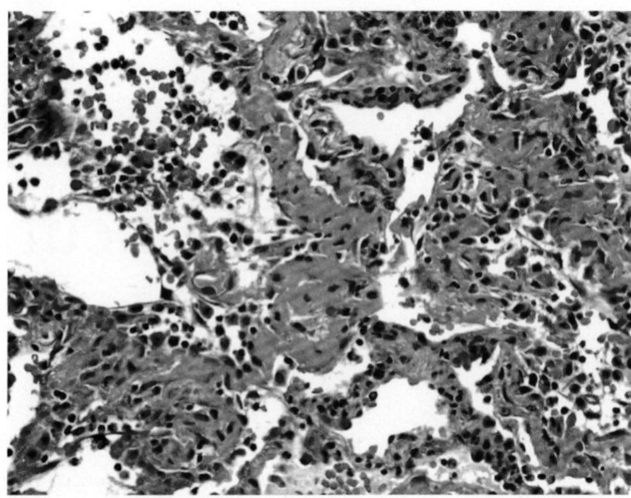

Figure 96.2 Acute eosinophilic pneumonia may have features similar to those in Figure 96.1, but will additionally have hyaline membrane formation similar to that seen in diffuse alveolar damage admixed with eosinophils (H&E stain; 200×).

Desquamative Interstitial Pneumonia (DIP)-Like Pattern

97

Mary Beth Beasley

Desquamative interstitial pneumonia (DIP) is a rare form of interstitial lung disease seen almost exclusively in cigarette smokers and characterized by diffuse filling of alveolar spaces by macrophages containing finely granular brown pigment (smoker's type macrophages). Although glassy, hyaline fibrosis associated with cigarette smoking may be present, significant fibrosis is typically absent in cases of DIP. A diagnosis of DIP should be made only in the appropriate setting of a clinical interstitial lung disease. DIP is discussed in Chapter 102.

True cases of DIP are rare. The finely granular pigmented macrophages characteristic of DIP may be encountered in lung tissue from virtually any cigarette smoker and may remain in the lung after cessation of smoking, up to several years in some studies. As such, the finding of extensive accumulation of smoker's type macrophages does not automatically indicate a diagnosis of DIP and must be interpreted in the context of the totality of findings in a given biopsy. The finding of accumulation of smoker's type macrophages in the lungs of a patient with another underlying process has been termed *DIP-like reaction*. As might be expected, this finding is frequently encountered in the lungs of patients with other disorders often encountered in cigarette smokers. A DIP-like reaction is frequently seen in patients who otherwise have Langerhans cell histiocytosis (LCH), another lung disease classically seen in smokers. Similarly, a DIP-like reaction may be seen in patients who otherwise have usual interstitial pneumonia (UIP) or occasionally nonspecific interstitial pneumonia. In biopsy specimens for clinical interstitial lung disease, evaluation of the background lung for features of LCH, UIP, or other fibrotic lung diseases and correlation with clinical and radiographic findings should distinguish DIP-like reactions from true cases of DIP. Substantial accumulation of smoker's type macrophages may be seen in the nonneoplastic lung in reactions for lung cancer. Again, unless the patient is known to have a clinical interstitial lung disease, such findings generally constitute a DIP-like reaction as opposed to true DIP.

HISTOLOGIC FEATURES

- Intra-alveolar macrophages with finely granular pigment (smoker's type macrophages).
- DIP-like reaction occurs in the setting of another underlying disorder, such as LCH or UIP, as opposed to cases of true DIP.
- Smoker's type macrophages may be seen in the tissue of any smoker and should be interpreted in the context of any background findings.

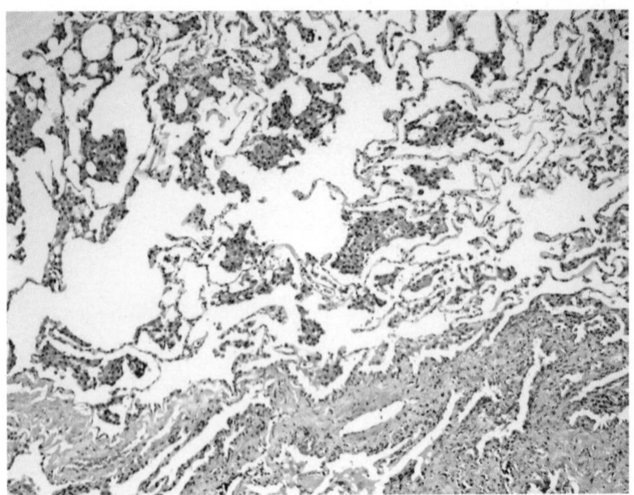

Figure 97.1 Macrophages with finely granular brown pigment fill the alveolar spaces in this section. This section is taken adjacent to a lesion of Langerhans cell histiocytosis, which is just in view at the *bottom* of the image (hematoxylin and eosin stain; 40×).

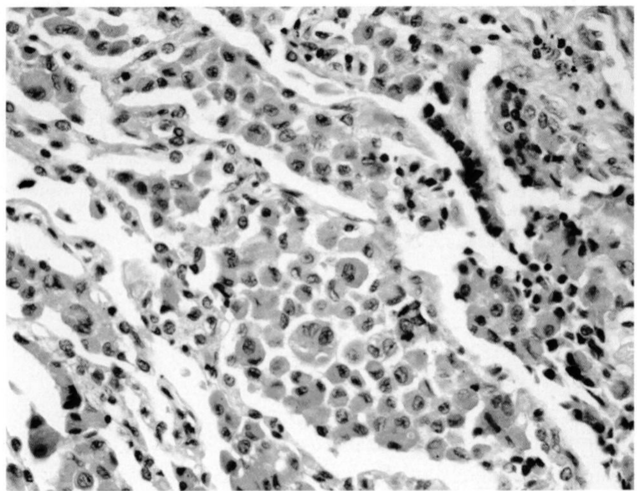

Figure 97.2 The macrophages in DIP-like reactions, like those in DIP itself, are characterized by intracytoplasmic finely granular brown pigment (hematoxylin and eosin stain; 400×).

98 Pulmonary Alveolar Proteinosis

Mary Beth Beasley

Pulmonary alveolar proteinosis (PAP) is a diffuse lung process characterized by the presence of amorphous eosinophilic material within the alveolar spaces. Previously thought to be a deficit in surfactant clearance by alveolar macrophages, it is now known that most patients develop PAP because of an autoimmune process secondary to the presence of anti-granulocyte macrophage colony stimulating factor, which is responsible for the impaired macrophage function. Other patients may develop PAP secondary to heavy exposure to dusts, especially silica, and some patients will have an underlying leukemia, lymphoma, or other diseases resulting in an impaired immune system. PAP has also been reported following lung transplantation.

Histologically, the alveoli are filled with granular eosinophilic material, which is composed of lipid and protein. Foamy macrophages, large granules, and cholesterol clefts may also be present. The material is typically positive with periodic acid–Schiff (PAS) staining due to the large amounts of surfactant apoprotein. The material is also positive with stains for surfactant apoprotein B. Electron microscopy demonstrates that the alveolar material consists of osmiophilic lamellar bodies consistent with denatured surfactant. The surrounding alveolar walls are generally histologically unremarkable, although rare cases with intersttial fibrosis have been reported. Opportunistic infections may occur, particularly *Nocardia*, although fungal and, less frequently, mycobacterial infections may occur.

The differential diagnosis includes *Pneumocystis jirovecii* pneumonia and pulmonary edema. The alveolar material in PAP is coarse and granular in contrast to the homogenous nature of pulmonary edema. *Pneumocystis* pneumonia is characterized by frothy, bubbly appearance, and organisms can be demonstrated on GMS stains.

HISTOLOGIC FEATURES

- Intra-alveolar accumulation of granular eosinophilic material.
- Large granules, foamy macrophages, and cholesterol clefts may be seen.
- Intra-alveolar material is typically PAS positive and stains for surfactant apoprotein B.
- Alveolar walls are usually unremarkable and only show fibrosis in rare cases.
- Infections with *Nocardia* and other organisms may be a complication.

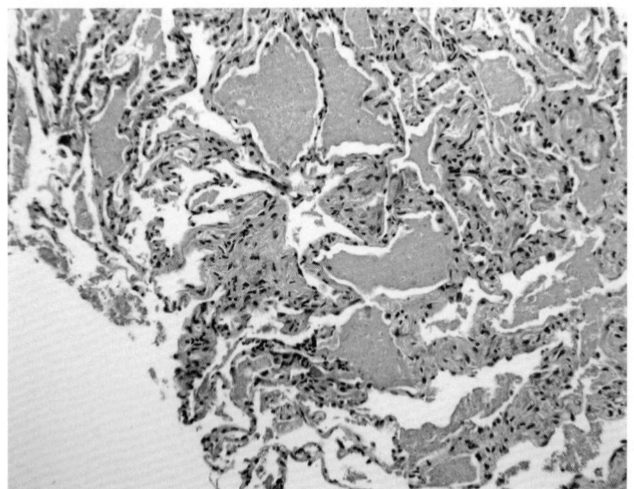

Figure 98.1 Pulmonary alveolar proteinosis is characterized by alveolar spaces filled with coarsely granular material (hematoxylin and eosin stain; 100×).

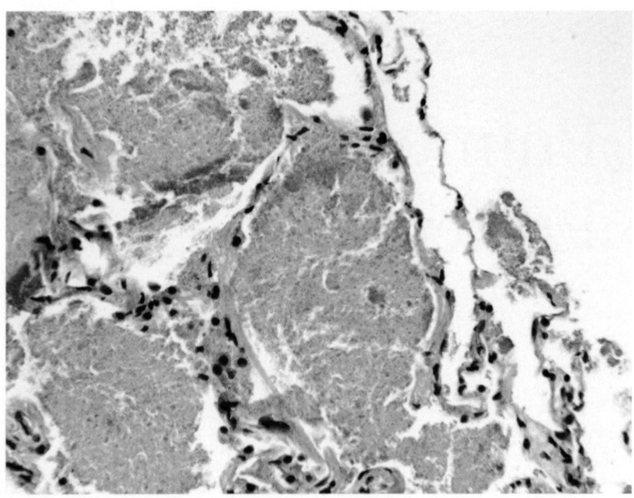

Figure 98.2 PAP with larger granules in the intra-alveolar material. The alveolar walls are relatively unremarkable (hematoxylin and eosin stain; 200×).

Section 14

Tobacco-Related Diseases

▸ Lynette M. Sholl

99

Emphysema

Lynette M. Sholl

Emphysema results from the destruction of the alveolar septal structures; the subtypes of emphysema are defined by the pattern of destruction relative to the architecture of the pulmonary lobule and include centrilobular, panacinar, paraseptal, and paracicatricial or scar emphysema. In smokers, the predominant pattern of emphysema is centrilobular (or proximal acinar destruction), which results from chronic deposition of irritants at the level of the terminal airways in the center of each pulmonary lobule. Chemical compounds in cigarette smoke promote local inflammation with release of tissue-destructive proteases while directly inhibiting the activity of alpha-1-antitrypsin; this combination of actions ultimately tips the protease–antiprotease balance in the lung tissue toward breakdown of the delicate alveolar structures. Destruction of the alveolar capillary bed leads to the loss of the available surface area for gas exchange.

Emphysema tends to co-occur with chronic bronchitis and asthma and represents a core contributor to chronic obstructive pulmonary disease. The clinical presentation of emphysema is modified by the contribution of the aforementioned airways diseases, but in general it is characterized by poor exercise tolerance due to shortness of breath. Emphysema patients maintain relatively normal oxygen levels in the blood by hyperventilating; the extra work of breathing seen in these patients gives rise to what is termed *pink puffer*. Radiographically, emphysema appears as increased tissue lucency and should be distinguished from other cystic lung diseases by the *absence* of thin walls surrounding the areas of lucency. In smokers, emphysema shows an upper lobe predominance.

The tissue damage that characterizes emphysema is irreversible. Therapy involves symptomatic management, including oxygen supplementation. Patients with concomitant asthma require inhaled corticosteroids and long-acting bronchodilators. Patients with upper lobe–predominant emphysema may benefit from lung volume reduction surgery. Pleural bleb formation as a result of air trapping in areas of peripheral lung destruction may lead to recurrent pneumothorax requiring surgical bleb removal.

HISTOLOGIC FEATURES

- Enlarged airspaces with simplification of the acinar unit with reduced numbers of alveolar sacs.
- Irregular destruction of alveolar septal structures; in smokers the damage tends to center around the terminal airways in the center of the pulmonary lobules.
- Variable degree of interstitial fibrosis can be present in association with airspace destruction but is generally only microscopically apparent.
- Grading of severity of emphysematous change can be difficult in tissue sections and is best evaluated on well-fixed gross specimens (or, historically, paper-mounted sections) or on computed tomography images.

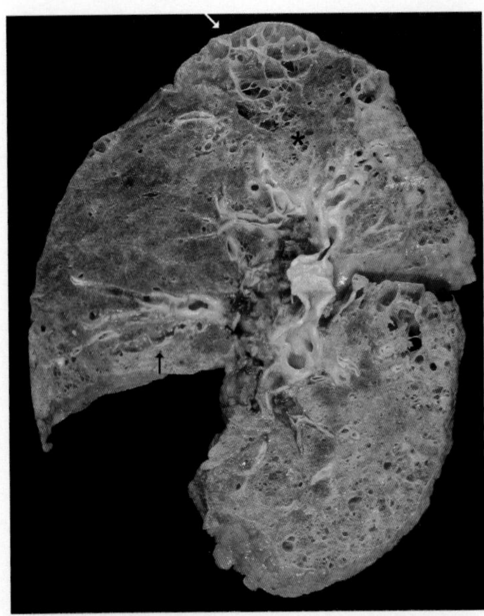

Figure 99.1 Gross image of an explanted lung with combined emphysema and pulmonary fibrosis. Emphysematous changes are most pronounced in the apex of the upper lobe *(white arrow)* and superior segment of the lower lobe; small subpleural bullae are evident at both sites. The centrilobular distribution of emphysematous destruction is most evident in the upper lobe *(asterisk)*. The lower lobe and inferior aspect of the upper lobe both show increased tissue density and traction bronchiectasis *(black arrow)* due to excess collagen deposition consistent with a concomitant fibrosing process.

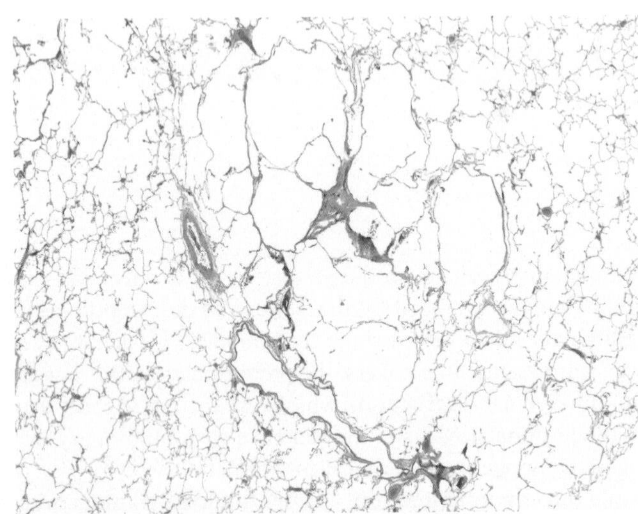

Figure 99.2 Enlarged peribronchiolar airspaces due to tissue destruction in a patient with smoking-related centrilobular emphysema. There is mildly increased collagen deposition in the residual airway structure. Areas of relatively preserved acinar structures can be seen in the tissue surrounding the emphysema.

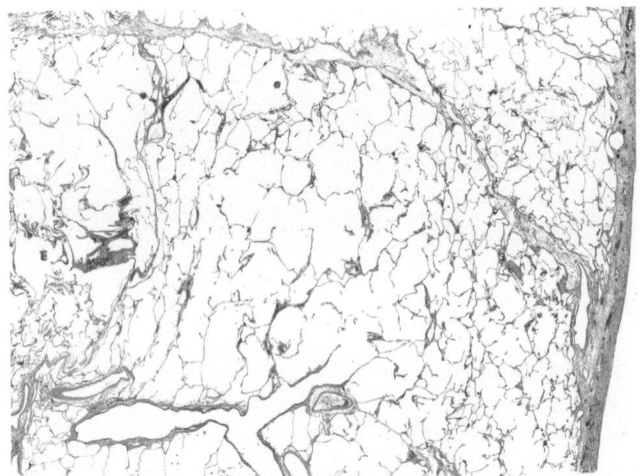

Figure 99.3 Diffuse airspace enlargement throughout the pulmonary lobule in a smoker with centrilobular and panacinar emphysema. Panacinar emphysema is associated with alpha-1-antitrypsin deficiency, but may be observed in some smokers without known deficiency of this enzyme.

Part 1

Placental Transmogrification of the Lung

▸ Lynette M. Sholl

Placental transmogrification of the lung is an exceptionally rare cystic lesion that resembles placental villi morphologically. This has also been described as "placentoid bullous lesion" and represents the pathologic correlate of idiopathic giant bullous emphysema. This disorder has been described in individual case reports and small case series predominantly in young adults and has a variable association with smoking. Some authors have speculated that this represents a congenital lesion; however, it is rare in pediatric populations. Others have suggested that this process represents a clonal proliferation of a poorly defined population of interstitial mesenchymal cells. It occurs unilaterally. Presenting signs include pneumothorax, exertional dyspnea, and obstructive physiology. Clinical management includes surgery to remove the involved area of lung.

HISTOLOGIC FEATURES

- Proliferation of papillary structures lined by TTF-1 positive epithelial cells.
- Papillary structures are supported by fibrovascular cores containing variable amounts of inflammatory and stromal cells. Adipose or smooth muscle metaplasia within the cores may be apparent.
- Papillary cores may contain a proliferation of ovoid cells with abundant clear cytoplasm that have been reported to express CD10 and lack differentiation on ultrastructural examination.
- Airway structures are preserved.
- Adjacent normal lung is collapsed.

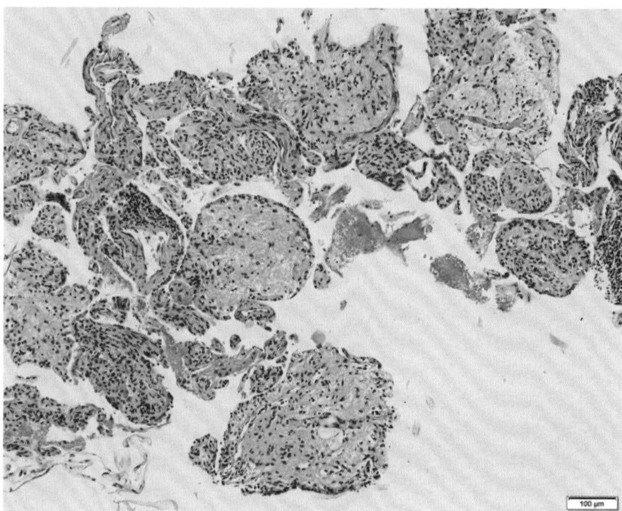

Figure 99.4 Core biopsy of placental transmogrification of the lung. Papillary structures are lined by attenuated pneumocyte epithelium and the papillary cores are filled with large, foamy cells with bland ovoid nuclei, delicate lymphovascular structures, and frequent lymphocytes.

Chronic Bronchitis

100

▶ Ross A. Miller

Chronic bronchitis is clinically defined by persistent couch and sputum production for a minimum duration of 3 months in at least two consecutive years. The two major factors of pathogenesis include infection and chronic irritation secondary to some inhalational exposure. Heavy exposure to various dust particles and fumes are contributing factors; however, the primary cause of chronic inhalational irritation is cigarette smoking. Typical features include bronchial mucus gland hyperplasia, goblet-cell metaplasia, increased inflammation, bronchial smooth muscle hyperplasia, and increased mucus. Associated fibrosis can occur along with squamous metaplasia and the development of dysplasia.

HISTOLOGIC FEATURES

- Bronchial mucous gland hyperplasia.
- Smooth muscle hyperplasia and even fibrosis around bronchi.
- Increased chronic inflammation in the bronchial wall.
- Goblet-cell metaplasia.
- Increased mucus with associated inflammatory cells.
- Squamous metaplasia and dysplasia can be seen.

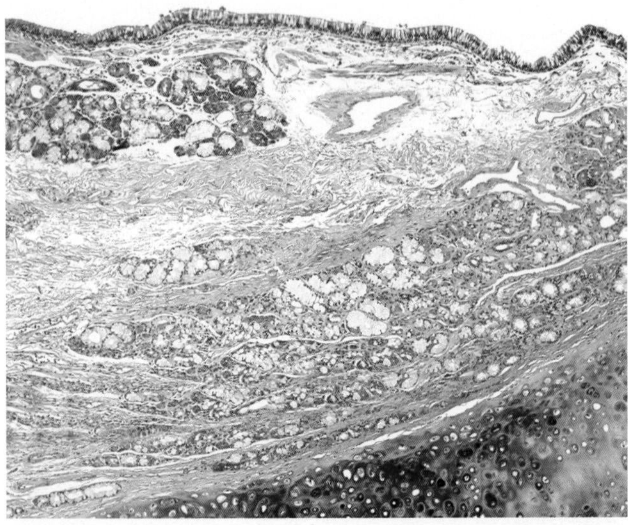

Figure 100.1 Bronchial wall shows increased numbers of bronchial glands characteristic of chronic bronchitis.

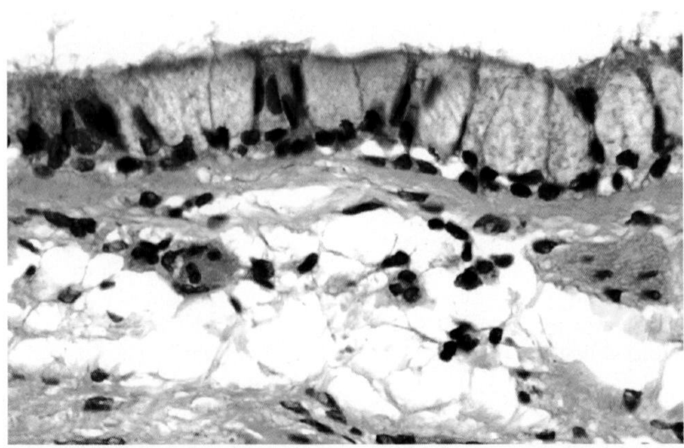

Figure 100.2 Chronic bronchitis shows bronchial surface epithelium with goblet-cell metaplasia.

Respiratory Bronchiolitis

101

Lynette M. Sholl

Respiratory bronchiolitis is defined by the presence of finely pigmented macrophages located in the airspaces around the terminal airways and is frequently associated with mild inflammatory infiltrates and fibrosis in the walls of the respiratory bronchiole. Respiratory bronchiolitis is an essentially universal finding in smokers; in nonsmokers it may rarely occur as a result of other inhalational exposures. The characteristic pigmented macrophages, which contain particulates carried within the inhaled smoke, are frequently referred to as *smoker's macrophages.*

Respiratory bronchiolitis is often clinically and radiographically silent. Computed tomography imaging shows poorly defined centrilobular nodules and upper lobe–predominant ground glass opacities; however, many patients will have no appreciable radiographic abnormalities. Pulmonary function tests most commonly reveal obstructive physiology.

The pathologic changes associated with respiratory bronchiolitis can persist for years following smoking cessation. The physiologic changes also may be irreversible; however, it is not clear that any adverse clinical outcomes can be independently attributed to respiratory bronchiolitis. Respiratory bronchiolitis frequently coexists with chronic obstructive pulmonary disease, which likely confounds the study of its clinical implications.

HISTOLOGIC FEATURES

- Small clusters of macrophages containing pale yellow to brown fine pigment are visible in the airspaces and are enriched in the terminal airway lumen, alveolar duct, and surrounding alveolar sacs of the respiratory bronchiole.
- Inflammatory cells with a lymphocytic predominance may be visible in the walls of the terminal respiratory unit.
- Mild, hyalinized fibrosis of the respiratory bronchiole wall may be seen.

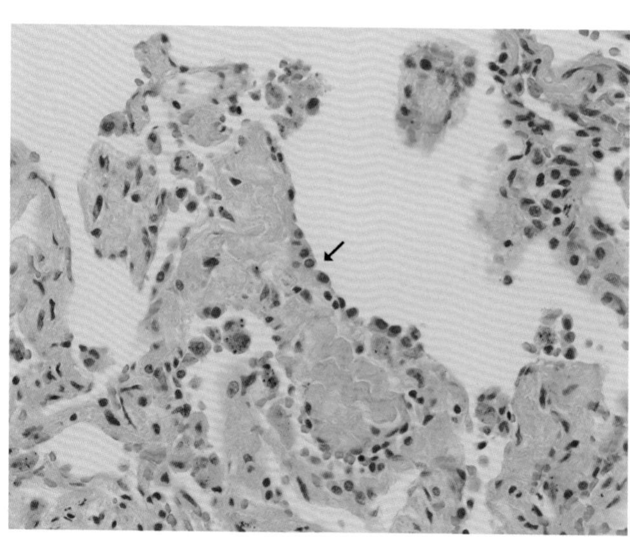

Figure 101.1 A terminal airway structure is seen with partially denuded epithelium *(arrow)* and mild, hyalinized collagen depositions in the wall. The characteristic pigmented macrophages are present singly and as small clusters in the airspaces. In this case the macrophages contain a combination of fine, pale tan to yellow pigment as well as larger gray to black particulates, which may result from smoking with an unfiltered device or another environmental exposure.

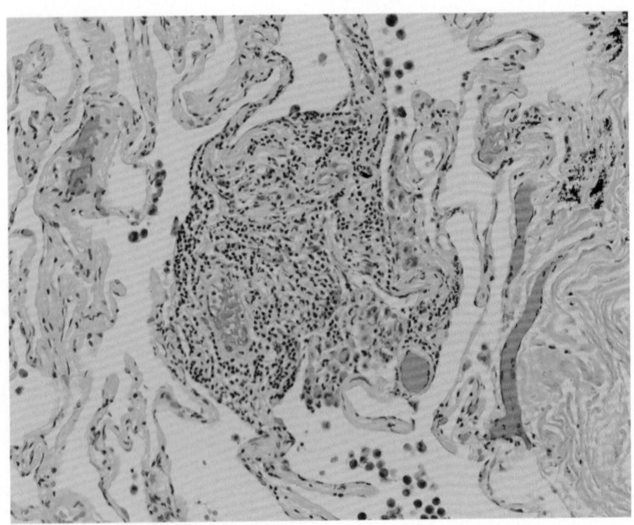

Figure 101.2 A centrilobular aggregate of mixed inflammatory infiltrates can be seen involving the terminal airway structure. Lymphocytes predominate; however, macrophages and eosinophils are also visible. Pigmented smoker's macrophages are visible in the surrounding airspaces.

Respiratory Bronchiolitis-Interstitial Lung Disease/ Desquamative Interstitial Pneumonia

102

▶ Lynette M. Sholl

The pathologic definition of respiratory bronchiolitis-interstitial lung disease is an area of controversy among pulmonary pathologists. Reports of respiratory bronchiolitis-interstitial lung disease describe the presence of respiratory bronchiolitis with the extension of fibrosis and inflammation into the alveolar structures. Patients are heavy smokers with restrictive pulmonary function tests or interstitial markings on standard chest X-ray. In contrast to respiratory bronchiolitis, these patients are symptomatic, with complaints of cough and shortness of breath; the symptoms, however, tend to be nonprogressive, in contrast to other defined forms of interstitial lung disease.

Although many studies have used the presence of alveolar wall fibrosis to distinguish between respiratory bronchiolitis and respiratory bronchiolitis-interstitial lung disease, this distinction has been challenged by studies that demonstrate peribronchiolar alveolar wall fibrosis in a large minority of (asymptomatic) smokers. Thus, it is not clear that histologic characteristics can distinguish between respiratory bronchiolitis and respiratory bronchiolitis-interstitial lung disease. Similarly, the findings on high-resolution computed tomography—including centrilobular nodularity and ground glass opacities—overlap in the two groups; however, the presence of reticular changes has only been described in the context of respiratory bronchiolitis-interstitial lung disease.

Desquamative interstitial pneumonia is considered to be on a spectrum with respiratory bronchiolitis-interstitial lung disease. Although desquamative interstitial pneumonia pattern can be seen in a variety of contexts—including connective tissue diseases, drug reactions, and as an idiopathic process (see also Chapters 97 and 135)—it is most highly associated with smoking. On computed tomography scanning, desquamative interstitial pneumonia appears as lower lobe–predominant ground glass opacities admixed with normal-appearing lung. Microscopically, desquamative interstitial pneumonia in smokers is characterized by large clusters and sheets of pigmented macrophages and giant cells within the airspaces. Interstitial fibrosis and inflammation should be present in a pattern that resembles nonspecific interstitial pneumonia; indeed some radiology studies have suggested that desquamative interstitial pneumonia can progress to nonspecific interstitial pneumonia. Progressive disease is reported in a minority of patients, but most patients stabilize or improve with smoking cessation and corticosteroid therapy.

HISTOLOGIC FEATURES

- Airspace macrophages containing fine yellow to tan pigment are visible.
- Alveolar septa show patchy chronic inflammation and fibrosis radiating from the respiratory bronchioles.
- In desquamative interstitial pneumonia, the pigmented macrophages form clusters and sheets with filling of the alveolar spaces, with associated inflammation and fibrosis of the alveolar septa.

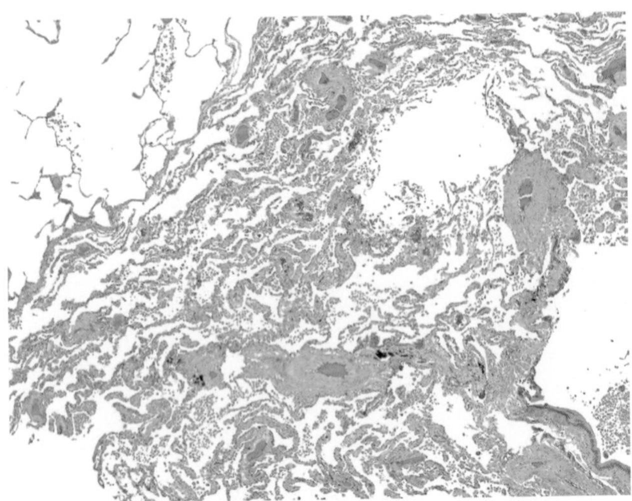

Figure 102.1 Patchy interstitial fibrosis is evident, with the most pronounced fibrosis emanating from the respiratory bronchiole *(lower midfield)*. Relatively spared emphysematous lung is visible in the *top left*. Pigmented "smoker's" macrophages are prominent within the airspaces.

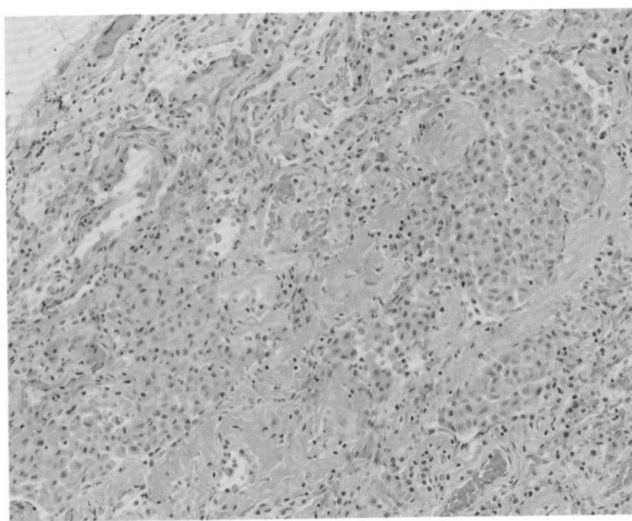

Figure 102.2 Clusters and sheets of macrophages containing yellow to tan finely granular pigment filling airspaces in a patient with desquamative interstitial pneumonia.

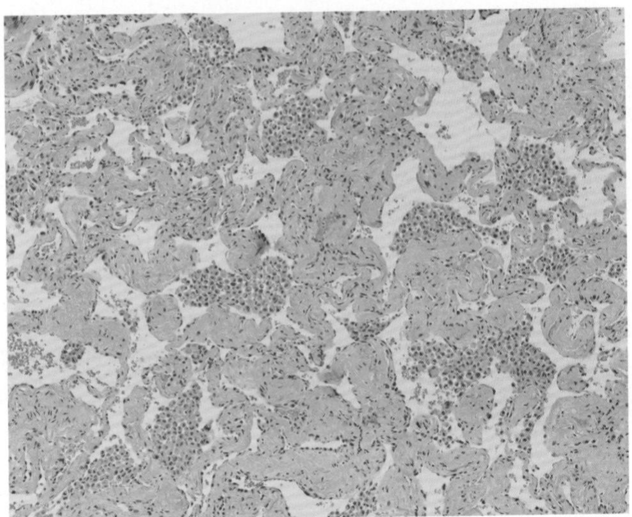

Figure 102.3 Clusters of airspace macrophages and interstitial fibrosis in a case of desquamative interstitial pneumonia in a smoker. Pulmonary Langerhans cell histiocytosis was identified in other areas of this patient's lung and was the indication for a surgical lung biopsy.

Part 1

Pulmonary Langerhans Cell Histiocytosis

▸ Lynette M. Sholl

Cigarette smoking leads to a proinflammatory chemokine milieu that triggers the differentiation and activation of Langerhans cells; consequently, smokers demonstrate an increased number of Langerhans cells in the lung. A small subset will go on to develop pulmonary Langerhans cell histiocytosis, a process that is now generally recognized as a clonal proliferation of these specialized histiocytes driven by activating mutations in mitogen-activated protein kinase pathway genes including *BRAF* and *MAP2K1*.

Patients may present with cough and dyspnea, or spontaneous pneumothorax, or they may have lung nodules detected incidentally on imaging studies. Computed tomography studies show small nodules and cysts; the latter become more pronounced with disease progression. Smoking cessation is the first line of therapy and will lead to disease remission in many patients. Immunosuppression is indicated in patients with progressive disease (see also Chapter 47).

HISTOLOGIC FEATURES

- Granulomatous inflammation centered on the bronchioles; the bronchiolar epithelium is typically denuded and the bronchiolar wall may appear dilated.
- The granulomatous inflammation contains Langerhans cells with characteristic folded nuclei, eosinophils, and pigment similar to that of smoker's macrophages in the airspaces.
- "Burned-out" Langerhans cell histiocytosis appears as stellate scars; the characteristic inflammatory cell components may not be evident in this setting.
- In smokers, pulmonary Langerhans cell histiocytosis will be seen on a background of respiratory bronchiolitis.

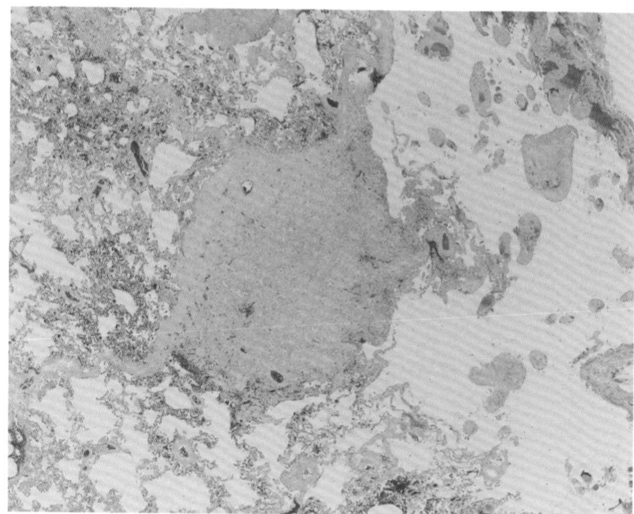

Figure 102.4 Pulmonary Langerhans cell histiocytosis manifests as a bronchiolocentric nodule comprised of admixed granulomatous inflammation and scar tissue *(center)*. Severe emphysematous change is evident in the distal, subpleural lung tissue *(right side of image)*.

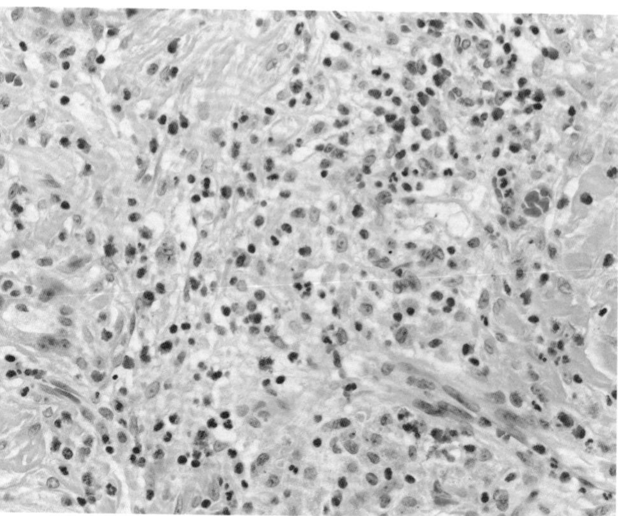

Figure 102.5 High-power examination of the granuloma shows numerous eosinophils, scattered neutrophils, fine to coarse tan, granular pigment, and abundant Langerhans cells with vesicular, folded nuclei and pale, indistinct cytoplasm.

103

Smoking-Related Interstitial Fibrosis

Lynette M. Sholl

Katzenstein et al. coined the term *smoking-related interstitial fibrosis* in 2010 following the observation that a subset of smokers display severe interstitial fibrosis on pathologic review despite lacking clinical features of interstitial lung disease. Histologically, smoking-related interstitial fibrosis was described as alveolar septal thickening by dense acellular collagen invariably accompanied by respiratory bronchiolitis and emphysematous changes. The severity of the fibrosis varies throughout the involved lung, with accentuation in the subpleural and peribronchiolar compartments.

These changes are observed in both current and former smokers, including those who quit several decades prior. In the original description, all patients had undergone lobectomy for a local neoplastic process, mostly commonly non–small cell lung carcinoma, and the cohort was biased toward upper lobe resections. The majority of patients with smoking-related interstitial fibrosis did have mild to moderate obstructive defects on pulmonary function testing and the minority showed reduced diffusion capacity; a subset of these showed reduced diffusion capacity despite normal spirometry. The radiographic correlates in the original description of smoking-related interstitial fibrosis were nonspecific, described as areas of fibrosis or scarring; the minority showed emphysema. Clinically, smokers with combined fibrosis and emphysema on high-resolution computed tomography scans can have unexpectedly normal spirometry findings despite reduced total lung capacity, and some authors have speculated that smoking-related interstitial fibrosis may be the pathologic correlate of this mixed physiologic disturbance.

The differential diagnosis of smoking-related interstitial fibrosis includes usual interstitial pneumonia (which can be distinguished based on its temporal variability and the presence of numerous fibroblast foci), asbestosis, and pulmonary Langerhans cell histiocytosis. The clinical and radiographic correlates of smoking-related interstitial fibrosis are not fully defined, and it has been proposed that this entity overlaps with or is possibly the same as respiratory bronchiolitis-interstitial lung disease or "airspace enlargement with fibrosis," a pathologic pattern described by Kawabata et al. in lung specimens resected for cancer in a cohort of Japanese smokers.

HISTOLOGIC FEATURES

- Uniform, acellular collagen deposition leads to thickening of the alveolar septae. Interstitial inflammation is minimal to absent.
- The interstitial thickening may show accentuation in the subpleural and peribronchiolar compartments of the lung. Peribronchiolar metaplasia and focal honeycomb change may be present.
- Respiratory bronchiolitis is invariably present; a desquamative interstitial pneumonia pattern of abundant airspace macrophages may be seen.
- Emphysematous changes are inevitably present.
- Fibroblast foci, when present, should be rare.

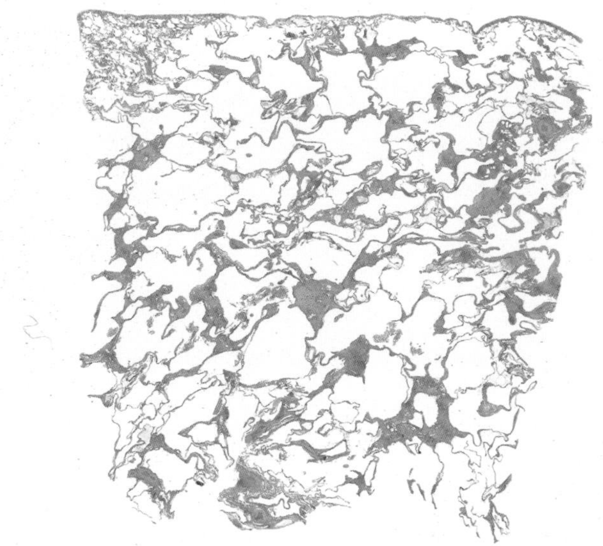

Figure 103.1 Scanning view of airspace enlargement by emphysema with concomitant alveolar septal thickening including nodular scarring in a peribronchiolar-predominant distribution.

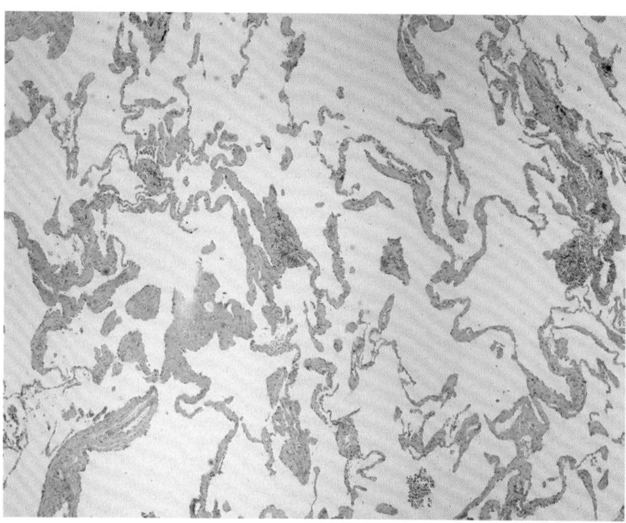

Figure 103.2 Bland, uniform interstitial thickening of the alveolar septae by hyalinized collagen. Inflammatory cells are sparse and are enriched in the respiratory bronchioles consistent with the association with respiratory bronchiolitis. Pigmented airspace "smoker's" macrophages are visible as a small cluster at the bottom of the field.

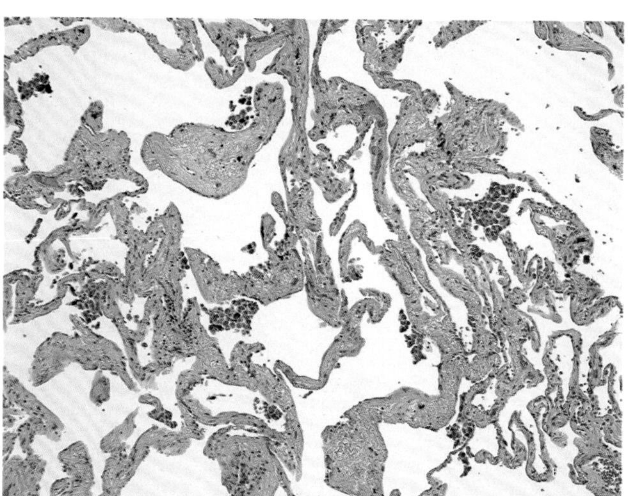

Figure 103.3 High-power image of alveolar septal collagenous fibrosis with sparse lymphocytic infiltrates, numerous intra-alveolar pigmented macrophages, and emphysematous change.

Section **15**

Diffuse Interstitial Lung Diseases

Maxwell L. Smith

Hypersensitivity Pneumonitis

104

Maxwell L. Smith
Stacey A. Kim

Hypersensitivity pneumonitis is a diffuse lung disease caused by inhalational exposure to organic antigens. Other names for the disease include extrinsic allergic alveolitis, farmer's lung, and bird fancier's lung. The former term, extrinsic allergic alveolitis, underscores the importance of the diffuse cellular interstitial infiltrate in this disease. In general, females are more commonly affected than males. Interestingly, smoking seems to provide a protective benefit, as smokers are less likely to suffer from hypersensitivity pneumonitis. Hypersensitivity pneumonitis presents as acute, subacute, and chronic forms. In the acute and subacute forms, patients often present with shortness of breath, cough, and occasionally systemic symptoms, such as malaise and fever. The chronic form develops over a longer period, with progressive dyspnea, cough, weight loss, and end-stage fibrotic lung disease. The classic imaging findings are described as upper lobe predominant, ill-defined ground glass nodules, with a centrilobular distribution and immediate subpleural sparing. In chronic forms, there may still be some vague centrilobular nodules, but increased reticulation, fibrosis, and even radiographic cysts of honeycombing may be identified.

HISTOLOGIC FEATURES

Acute Hypersensitivity Pneumonitis

- Acute and organizing lung injury with fibrin, diffuse alveolar damage, granulomatous pneumonitis, and organizing pneumonia.

Subacute Hypersensitivity Pneumonitis

- Diffuse cellular interstitial infiltrates, which may show a centrilobular distribution.
- Centrilobular poorly formed interstitial granulomas, consisting of loose aggregates of histiocytes with or without multinucleated giant cells in a background of lymphoplasmacytic inflammation.
- Patchy organizing pneumonia with or without fibrin.
- Granulomas should be difficult to identify; if granulomas are numerous, show necrosis, or are obvious from scanning magnification, an alternative diagnosis should be considered.

Chronic Hypersensitivity Pneumonitis

- Fibrotic nonspecific interstitial pneumonia pattern of fibrosis or airway-centered pattern of fibrosis.
- Chronic hypersensitivity pneumonitis may be advanced with microscopic honeycomb remodeling and fibroblast foci, mimicking the usual interstitial pneumonia pattern of pulmonary fibrosis.
- Extensive chronic small airways remodeling in the form of peribronchiolar metaplasia, mucostasis, and chronic bronchiolitis.
- Scattered interstitial poorly formed granulomas with or without multinucleated giant cells.

- Airspace giant cells are of questionable significance.
- Lack of peripheral and subpleural predominant fibrosis of usual interstitial pneumonia of idiopathic pulmonary fibrosis.
- Bridging fibrosis joining adjacent centrilobular regions.

DIFFERENTIAL DIAGNOSIS

Various entities in the differential diagnosis depend on the phase of presentation: acute, subacute, or chronic. In the acute form, the differential diagnosis is similar to that of acute and organizing lung injury and includes infection, adverse drug reaction, connective tissue disease, widespread aspiration, and idiopathic (acute respiratory distress syndrome). The presence of airway centricity with vague granulomas or multinucleated giant cells can help support a diagnosis of acute hypersensitivity pneumonitis. In the subacute phase, the differential diagnosis is similar to that of a cellular interstitial pneumonia, such as cellular nonspecific interstitial pneumonia, and includes connective tissue disease, adverse drug reaction, aspiration, and infection. Because the granulomas are typically small, poorly formed, and difficult to identify, other granulomatous diseases (such as granulomatosis with polyangiitis, necrotizing granulomas of infection, and sarcoidosis) rarely enter into the differential diagnosis. The accentuation of changes within the centrilobular regions strongly supports a diagnosis of hypersensitivity pneumonitis, as does the presence of background chronic small airways remodeling. In chronic hypersensitivity pneumonitis, the main differential diagnosis includes fibrotic nonspecific interstitial pneumonia and usual interstitial pneumonia patterns of pulmonary fibrosis. In cases of otherwise typical usual interstitial pneumonia, close scrutiny of the interstitium for poorly formed granulomas and multinucleated giant cells, along with the presence of chronic small airways remodeling, can help support chronic hypersensitivity pneumonitis as an etiology for the advanced pulmonary fibrosis. Histologic features that have been shown to be more often found in the setting of chronic hypersensitivity pneumonitis as opposed to usual interstitial pneumonia include the presence of granulomas, giant cells, organizing pneumonia, bridging fibrosis, cellular nonspecific interstitial pneumonia areas, lymphoid follicles, centrilobular fibrosis, and chronic bronchiolitis.

The prognosis for hypersensitivity pneumonitis is variable. In the subacute phase, treatment with steroids can improve outcome; however, removal of the offending antigen is the best predictor of a favorable outcome. Once the disease has reached the chronic phase with advanced fibrosis, steroid treatment may or may not be beneficial. Histologic patterns of fibrotic nonspecific interstitial pneumonia or usual interstitial pneumonia, older age, and longer/more intense exposure are associated with worse prognosis.

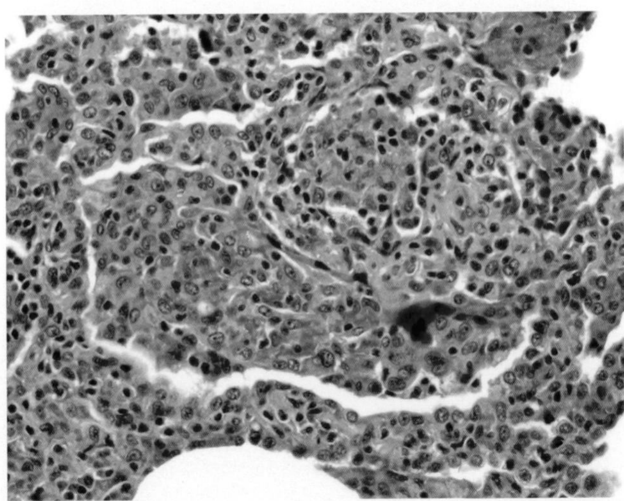

Figure 104.1 In acute hypersensitivity pneumonitis, it is common to find fibrin within airspaces with associated lymphoplasmacytic inflammation.

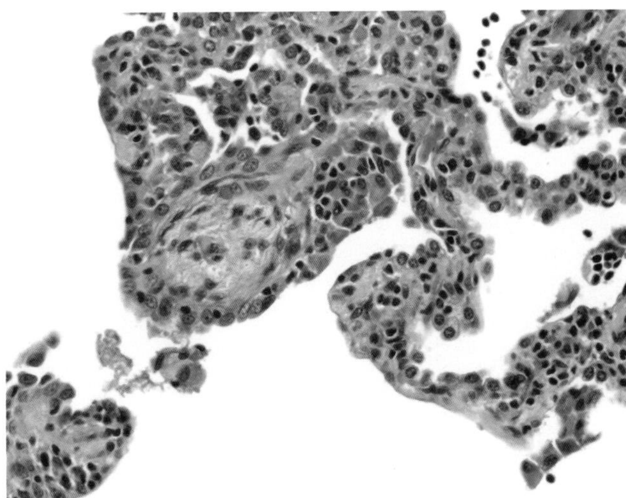

Figure 104.2 Polyps of organizing pneumonia may be prominent in the acute phase.

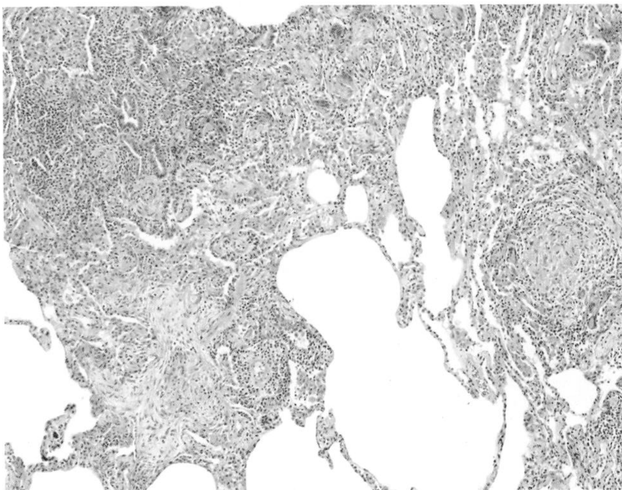

Figure 104.3 Other cases of acute hypersensitivity pneumonitis may show a granulomatous pneumonitis reaction pattern with multiple granulomas, multinucleated giant cells, and large polyps of organizing pneumonia.

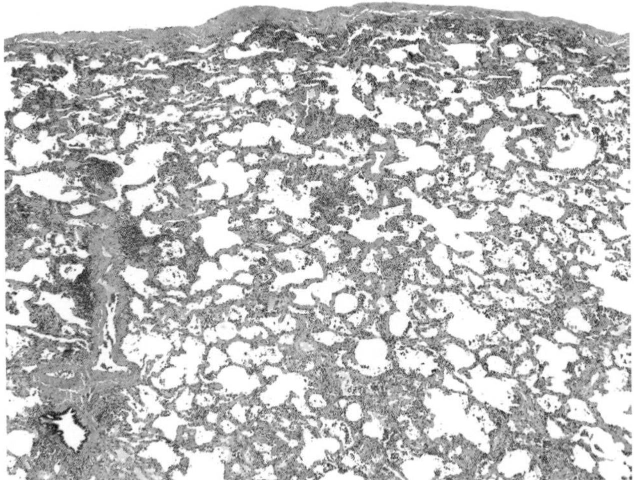

Figure 104.4 Subacute hypersensitivity pneumonitis classically shows a diffuse cellular interstitial infiltrate, reminiscent of cellular nonspecific interstitial pneumonia.

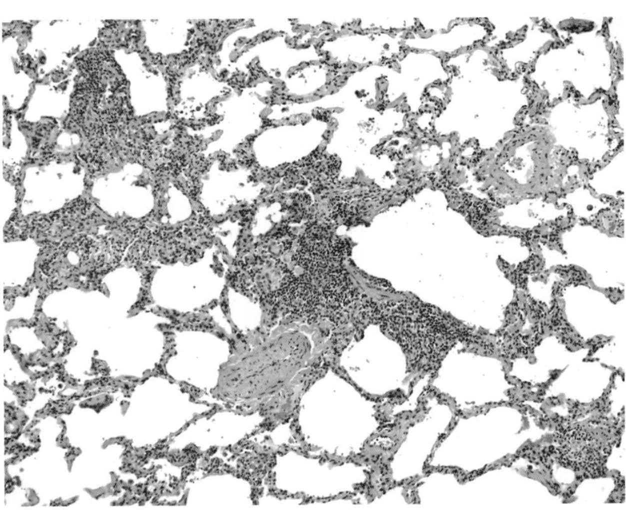

Figure 104.5 The histologic hallmark of subacute hypersensitivity pneumonitis is the collection of loose aggregates of histiocytes and multinucleated giant cells within the interstitium in a centrilobular distribution.

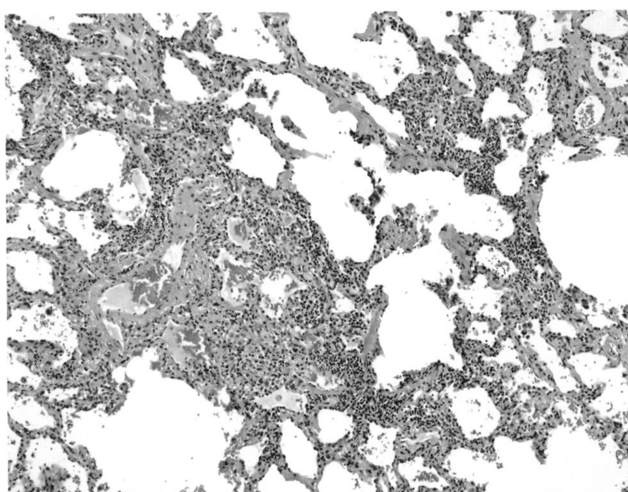

Figure 104.6 Some cases consist only of loose aggregates of histiocytes within the interstitium.

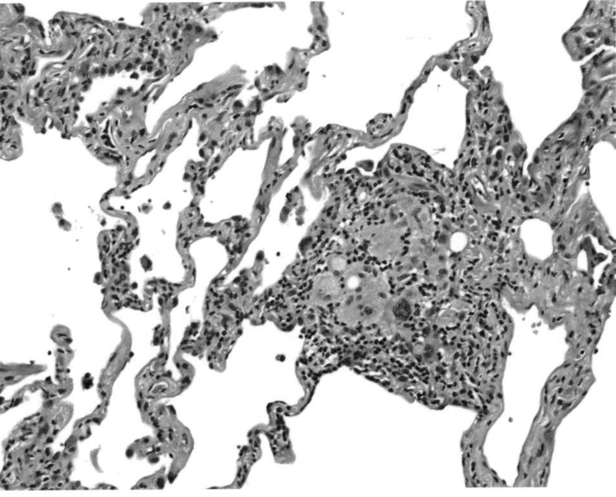

Figure 104.7 A classic poorly formed loose granuloma of subacute hypersensitivity pneumonitis.

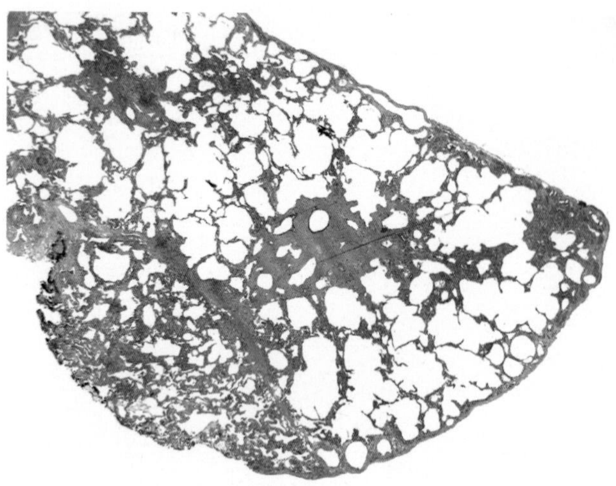

Figure 104.8 In chronic hypersensitivity pneumonitis, the most common histologic feature is the presence of centrilobular stellate scars. Some cases may show more of a fibrotic nonspecific interstitial pneumonia pattern of injury. Note the bridging of fibrosis from the centrilobular region to the interlobular septa. Scattered poorly formed interstitial granulomas were present in this case, supporting hypersensitivity pneumonitis as an etiology for the advanced fibrosis.

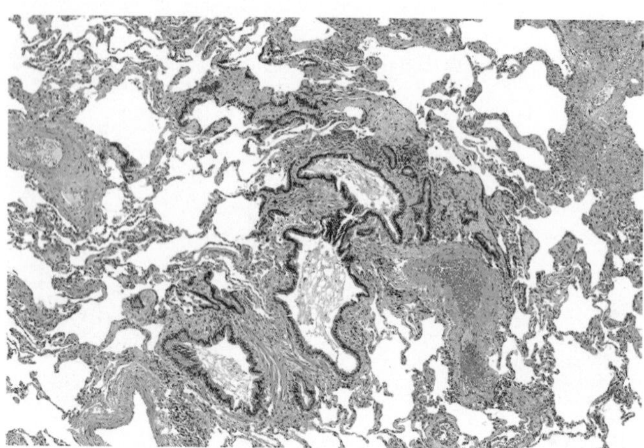

Figure 104.9 Chronic hypersensitivity pneumonitis often shows prominent small airways remodeling in the form of mucostasis, peribronchiolar fibrosis, and peribronchiolar metaplasia.

105

Hot Tub Lung

Maxwell L. Smith
Fang Zhou

Nontuberculous mycobacterial infection of the lung manifests as a wide spectrum of pathologic patterns, including cavitary disease, nodules with bronchiectasis, and diffuse interstitial infiltrates. Hot tub lung is the clinicopathologic manifestation of nontuberculous mycobacterial involvement secondary to the inhalation of aerosolized *Mycobacterium avium* complex, often in the setting of contaminated hot tubs or other water sources. This typically occurs in immunocompetent patients with a wide age range and equal distribution between males and females. Patients typically present with cough, hypoxia, dyspnea, and fever. Imaging studies show bilateral diffuse infiltrates, occasionally with finely nodular interstitial infiltrates. Oftentimes, the imaging studies are mistaken for hypersensitivity pneumonitis.

HISTOLOGIC FEATURES

- The predominant histopathologic feature is the presence of nonnecrotizing granulomas. Rare cases may show occasional necrosis. The granulomas typically show loose clustering of epithelioid histiocytes with occasional multinucleated giant cells. They are predominantly located within air spaces and bronchiolar lumens. Occasional involvement of the interstitium is present.
- There is often mild cuffing with a lymphoplasmacytic inflammatory infiltrate.
- Granulomas may be random or show a centrilobular distribution. There is rare to nonexistent involvement of the intralobular septa and pleura.
- Cases show a variable cellular interstitial infiltrate.
- Polyps of organizing pneumonia are frequently seen in the airspaces and terminal airways.
- The demonstration of acid-fast bacilli is exceedingly rare, even in classic cases.
- Confirmation by culture studies is the preferred method of confirming the diagnosis.

Despite the presence of *M. avium* complex as the pathophysiologic mechanism of injury, oral corticosteroids are often used in the treatment of hot tub lung. Antimycobacterial therapy may also be used. Patients tend to have a good prognosis, particularly if the exposure is removed or the water is decontaminated.

DIFFERENTIAL DIAGNOSIS

The differential diagnosis for the presence of nonnecrotizing granulomas includes hypersensitivity pneumonitis, sarcoidosis, and diffuse granulomatous infections due to other organisms. Hypersensitivity pneumonitis typically shows a far more robust cellular interstitial infiltrate that overshadows the presence of granulomatous inflammation. Furthermore, the granulomas of hypersensitivity pneumonitis are typically located within the interstitium in a centrilobular distribution and should only rarely show granulomas in the airspaces.

Polyps of organizing pneumonia can be seen in both entities. Obviously, the demonstration of acid-fast bacilli on acid-fast staining would support a diagnosis of hot tub lung.

The granulomas of sarcoidosis typically show less surrounding inflammation compared with the granulomas of hot tub lung. In addition, they have a tendency to coalesce together with background hyaline sclerosis, a feature not seen in the setting of hot tub lung. Furthermore, the granulomas of sarcoidosis show a distinct lymphangitic distribution, involving the bronchovascular bundle, intralobular septa, and pleura, whereas the granulomas of hot tub lung are limited to the airspaces.

The distinction between hot tub lung and infectious granulomatous pneumonitis due to other organisms can be challenging. The presence of necrotizing granulomas would favor a different infectious etiology over *M. avium* complex. In addition, patients with diffuse lung disease secondary to other organisms are typically far more ill than patients presenting with hot tub lung.

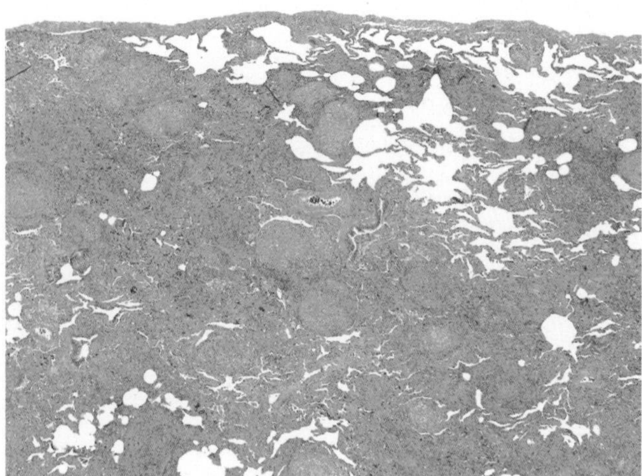

Figure 105.1 Low-power examination of a hot tub lung biopsy showing numerous nonnecrotizing granulomas randomly distributed throughout the biopsy.

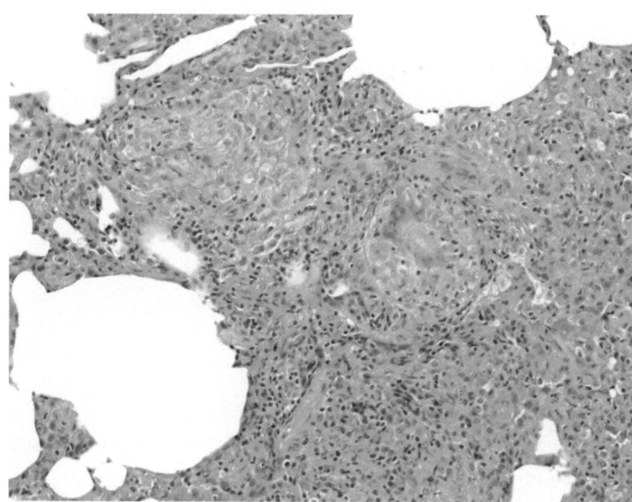

Figure 105.2 Loose clusters of epithelioid histiocytes with rare multinucleated giant cells are characteristic of the granulomas in hot tub lung.

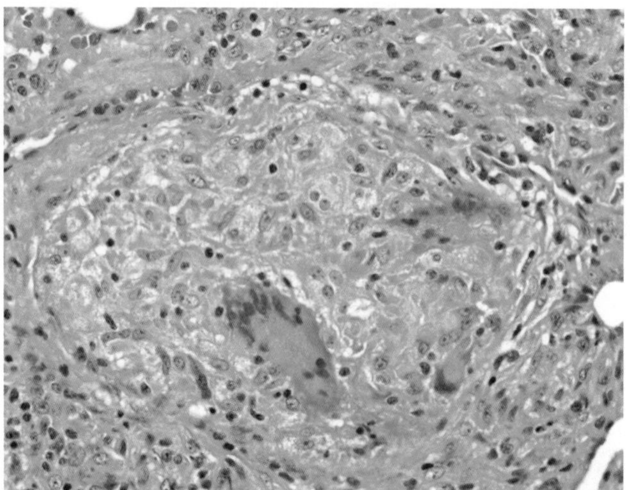

Figure 105.3 Granulomas are seen with or without multinucleated giant cells.

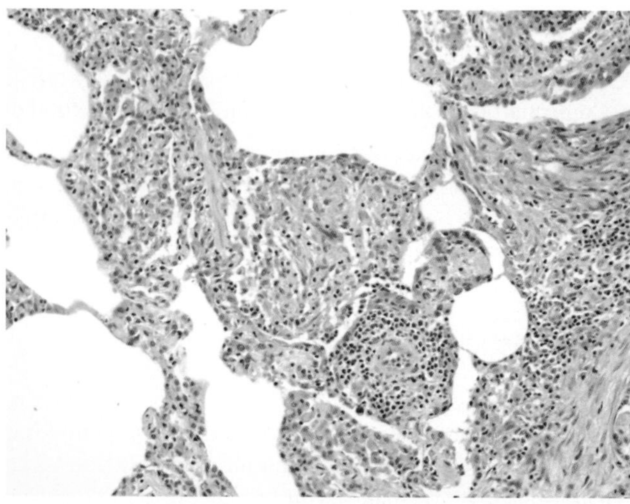

Figure 105.4 The loose aggregates of histiocytes and granulomas are predominantly located within airspaces. Rare interstitial involvement may be seen. Oftentimes, because of the robust number of granulomas, it is difficult to discern airspace versus interstitial involvement.

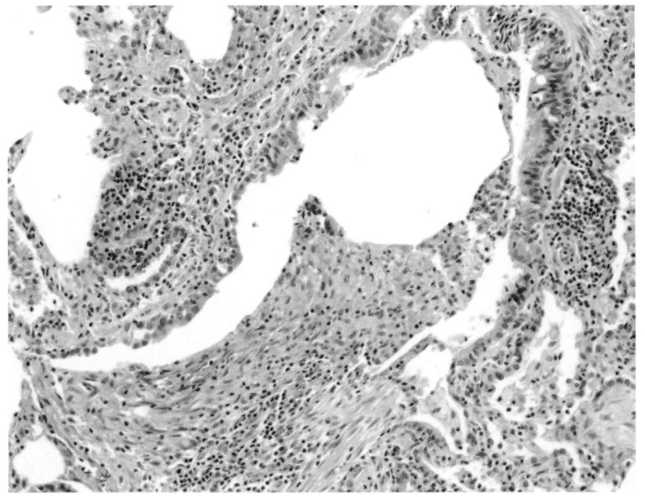

Figure 105.5 Many granulomas involve the terminal bronchiolar lumens.

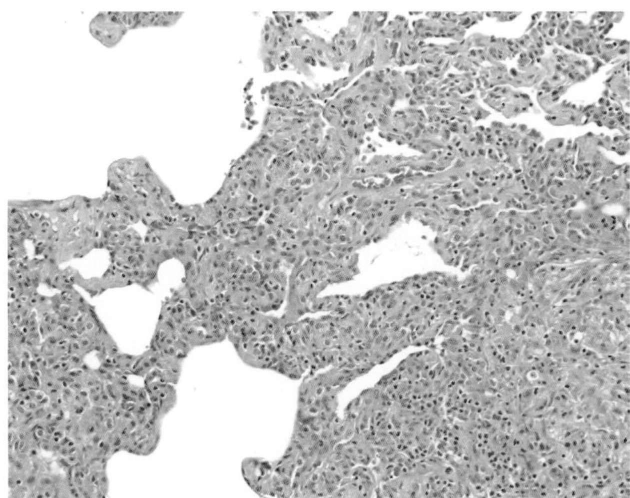

Figure 105.6 Cases of hot tub lung show a variable cellular interstitial infiltrate consisting mostly of lymphocytes and plasma cells. Scattered granulomas may be seen.

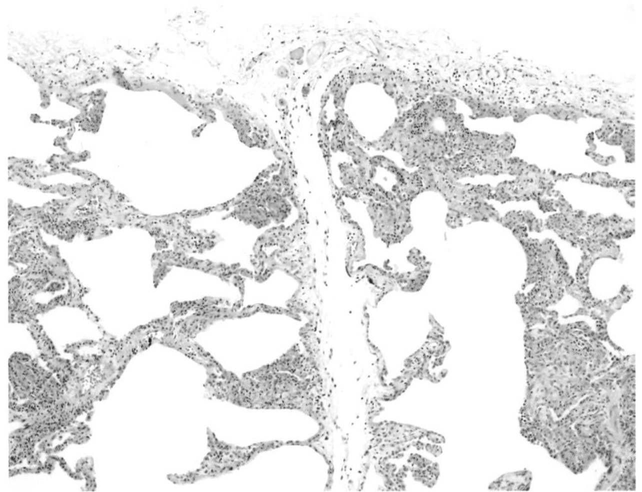

Figure 105.7 Note the absence of involvement of the pleura and interlobular septa. This is a useful feature in the differential diagnosis from sarcoidosis.

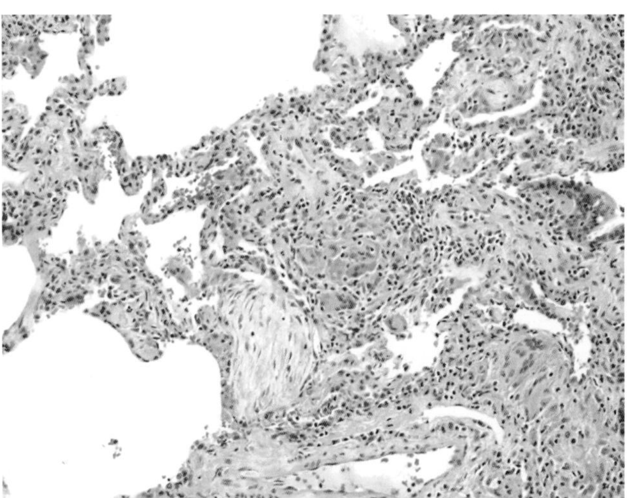

Figure 105.8 Rare polyps of organizing pneumonia may be seen in association with the airspace granulomas.

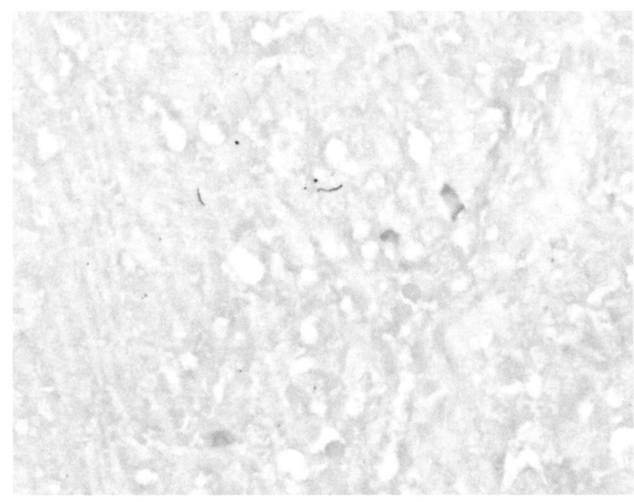

Figure 105.9 The demonstration of acid-fast bacilli is exceedingly rare in cases of hot tub lung. However, if they are identified, it can be useful in making a definitive diagnosis.

106

Flock Lung

Maxwell L. Smith
Fang Zhou

Flock lung is a rare interstitial lung disease associated with the inhalation of flock, which is a pulverized synthetic or natural fiber of small diameter that is used to create a soft, velvet-like coating when applied to fabrics. The primary risk factor is working in a flock factory; multiple outbreaks of interstitial pneumonia have been identified among nylon flock workers. There is no male or female predilection. Patients usually present with chronic dyspnea and cough. Pulmonary function testing typically reveals a restrictive pattern and a reduced diffusing capacity. Imaging studies, most often on high-resolution CT scanning, show peripheral ground-glass opacities without significant hilar adenopathy.

HISTOLOGIC FEATURES

- Chronic lymphocytic bronchiolitis.
- Peribronchiolitis with lymphoid hyperplasia, often as nodular aggregates of lymphocytes. Secondary follicles are rare.
- Giant cells nearly always absent.
- Associated diffuse alveolar damage or organizing pneumonia may be present.
- Rare cases show a desquamative interstitial pneumonia pattern of injury.
- Fibrosis is minimal to absent.
- Granulomas are absent.

Because of the rarity of the disease, treatment strategies are not well characterized. Treatment most often includes corticosteroids, and removal from further flock exposure is probably the best measure to prevent progression of disease.

DIFFERENTIAL DIAGNOSIS

The differential diagnosis for the characteristic histologic changes in flock lung is broad. Other considerations for chronic bronchiolitis include common variable immunodeficiency disease (CVID), IgG4-related disease, chronic aspiration bronchiolitis, hypersensitivity pneumonitis, hot tub lung, and lung disease associated with inflammatory bowel disease. Several of the differential diagnostic possibilities commonly show granulomas (CVID-associated lung disease, chronic aspiration bronchiolitis, hypersensitivity pneumonitis, hot tub lung, and lung disease associated with inflammatory bowel disease), which should help exclude them as possibilities. IgG4-related pulmonary disease usually has a component of fibrosis, which is more extensive than what is seen in flock lung. In addition, immunohistochemistry for IgG4 and IgG can help exclude this possibility. As is the case with many interstitial lung diseases, clinical correlation is most helpful to make a definitive diagnosis of flock worker's lung.

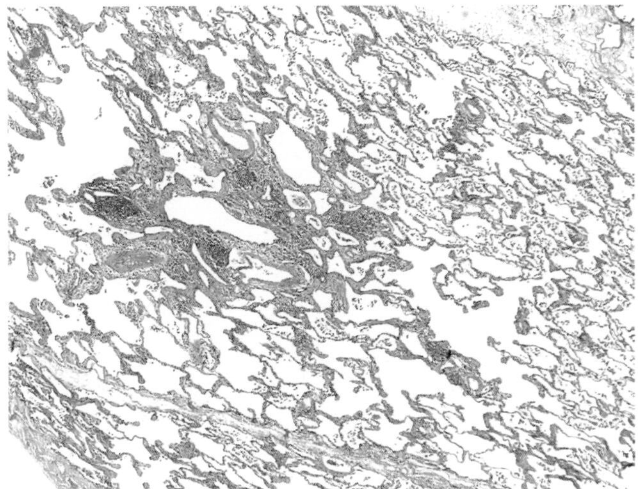

Figure 106.1 Cases of flock lung typically show prominent chronic lymphocytic bronchiolitis.

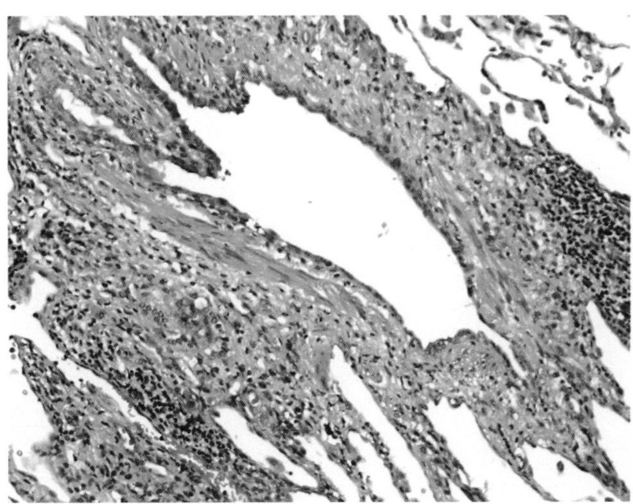

Figure 106.2 Chronic bronchiolitis characterized by lymphocytes within the respiratory epithelium and reactive epithelial changes. Note the peribronchiolar chronic inflammatory cell infiltrate consisting mostly of lymphocytes.

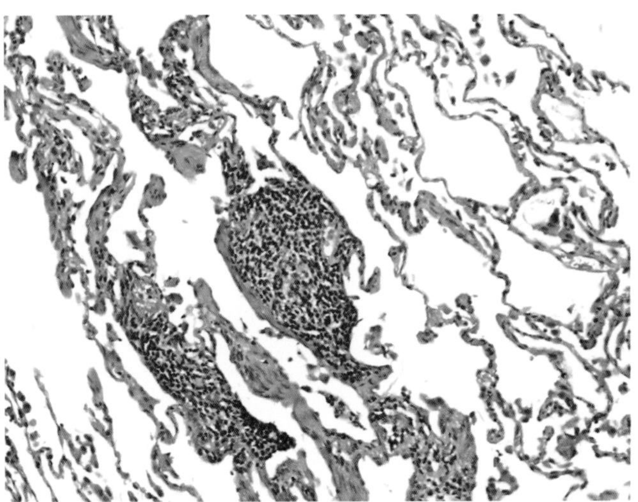

Figure 106.3 Some cases may show nodular aggregates of lymphocytes in the interstitium, but secondary follicles are rare.

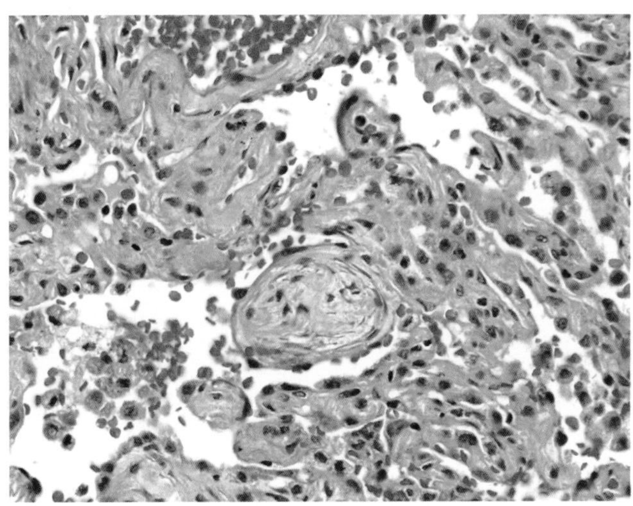

Figure 106.4 Polyps of organizing pneumonia may be seen within the airspaces.

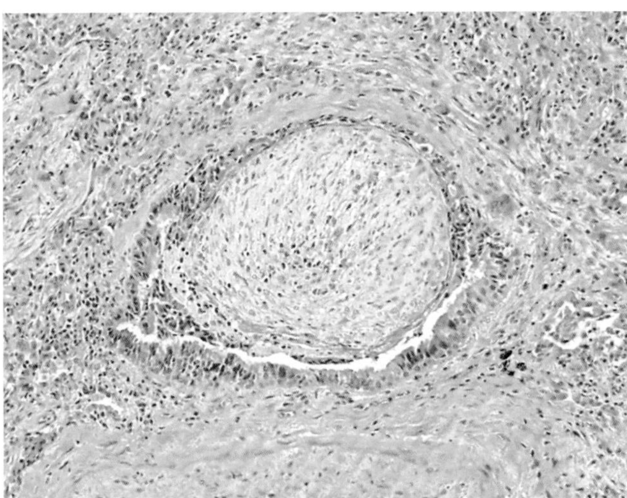

Figure 106.5 Bronchiolitis obliterans organizing pneumonia is a rare feature.

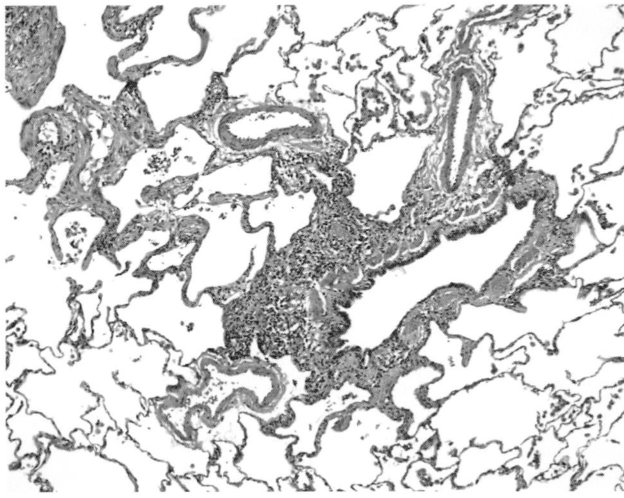

Figure 106.6 Although cases show chronic lymphocytic bronchiolitis, the peribronchiolar fibrosis is relatively minimal.

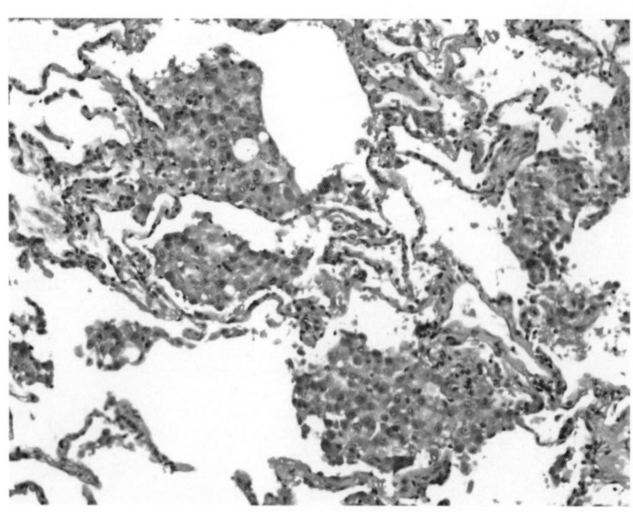

Figure 106.7 Rare cases may show a desquamative interstitial pneumonia pattern of injury with collections of macrophages within the airspaces.

Airway-Centered Fibrosis

107

▸ Maxwell L. Smith
▸ Raghavendra Pillappa

Over the past 15 years, there has been increased recognition of a potential idiopathic interstitial lung disease that is centered around airways and shows variable fibroinflammatory changes. Because of this increased recognition, the 2013 update on idiopathic interstitial pneumonias from the American Thoracic Society and European Respiratory Society included the term *bronchiolocentric patterns of interstitial pneumonia* under the section of rare histologic patterns. Airway-centered fibrosis is one of the main patterns of injury seen in his setting. Additional study will be required to determine if this represents a true idiopathic interstitial pneumonia or is secondary to another form of chronic centrilobular injury, perhaps inhalational. Patients with airway-centered fibrosis typically present with chronic cough and slowly progressive dyspnea. There is often a female predominance. The disease typically affects older adults between the ages of 40 and 65 years. Patients showed a predominantly restrictive pattern with decreased forced vital capacity on pulmonary function testing. Imaging studies often show centrilobular changes with traction bronchiectasis, interstitial thickening, and fibrosis. Variable honeycombing and bronchiolectasia are identified radiographically.

HISTOLOGIC FEATURES

- At scanning magnification, one can appreciate "stellate" appearing scars beginning in the centrilobular regions.
- In more advanced cases, the entire pulmonary lobule can be destroyed, making it difficult to distinguish from a usual interstitial pneumonia pattern of fibrosis.
- There is often extensive chronic small airways remodeling in the background including peribronchiolar metaplasia with extension of respiratory epithelium into adjacent alveoli (bronchiolization) and mucostasis.
- Occasional bridges of fibrosis from one centrilobular region to the next may be observed (Figure 107.4). There typically is distinct sparing of the periphery of the pulmonary lobules.
- Interstitial inflammation is variable.
- The presence of foreign material is suggestive of aspiration predominantly chronic aspiration of gastric contents.
- The presence of scattered interstitial granulomas and multinucleated giant cells is suggestive of chronic hypersensitivity pneumonitis.
- Fibroblast foci may be present in a minority of cases.

Because of insufficient studies of these patients and lack of adequate clinical follow-up, it has been difficult to suggest a treatment strategy.

Airway-centered fibrosis must be distinguished from fibrotic nonspecific interstitial pneumonia and from the usual interstitial pneumonia pattern of pulmonary fibrosis. This is best done at low magnification noting the "stellate" centrilobular scars of airway-centered fibrosis, which are in contrast to the peripheral and subpleural predominant scars as seen in the usual interstitial pneumonia pattern of fibrosis. Fibrotic nonspecific interstitial pneumonia typically involves all alveolar walls, at least to some extent. Once the general pattern of airway-centered fibrosis is identified, close inspection of the specimen for features to suggest a specific etiology is required. Should any foreign material be seen, consideration should be given to a chronic aspiration syndrome. It should be noted that aspiration may be subclinical in many cases. Furthermore, the identification of foreign material can be quite difficult.

In cases with more significant cellular interstitial infiltrates and poorly formed interstitial granulomas, or giant cells entrapped within the fibrosis, strong consideration should be given to the possibility of hypersensitivity pneumonitis. In addition, the patient's history should be closely evaluated for the presence of any chronic inhalational exposures including fumes and toxins.

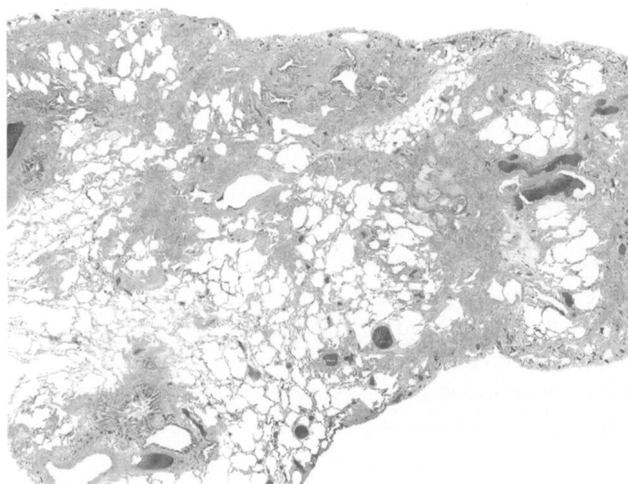

Figure 107.1 From scanning magnification one can appreciate central lobular predominance fibrosis often producing "stellate" scars centered around the bronchovascular bundle.

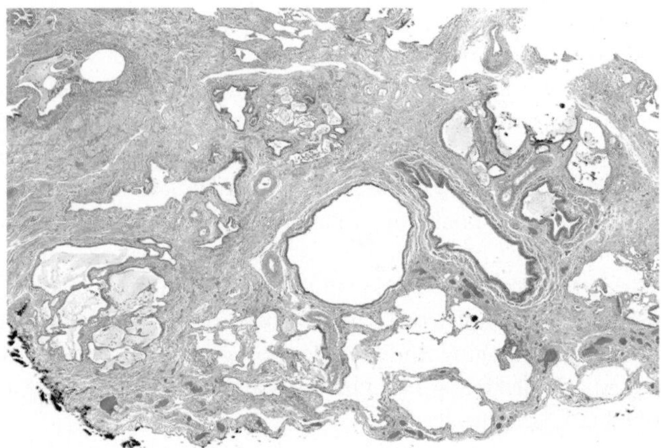

Figure 107.2 In cases with advanced fibrosis, the distinction between airway-centered fibrosis and the usual interstitial pneumonia pattern of fibrosis can be quite challenging. This case shows microscopic honeycomb remodeling and advanced fibrosis. However, other sections from this case showed a distinct airway-centered distribution.

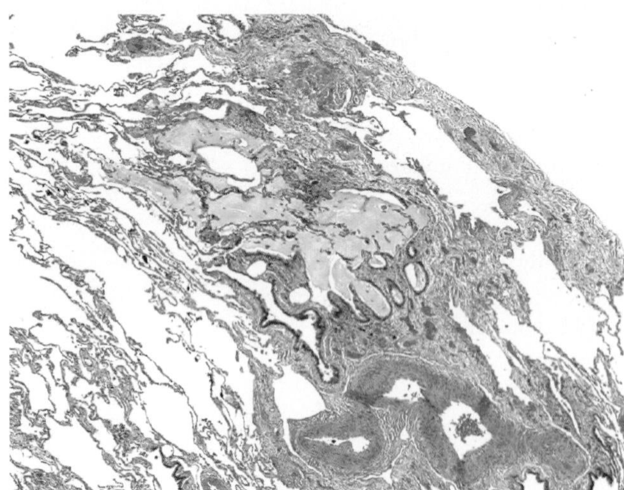

Figure 107.3 The presence of chronic small airways remodeling is a relatively constant finding, characterized by mucostasis and peribronchiolar metaplasia with focal bronchiolization.

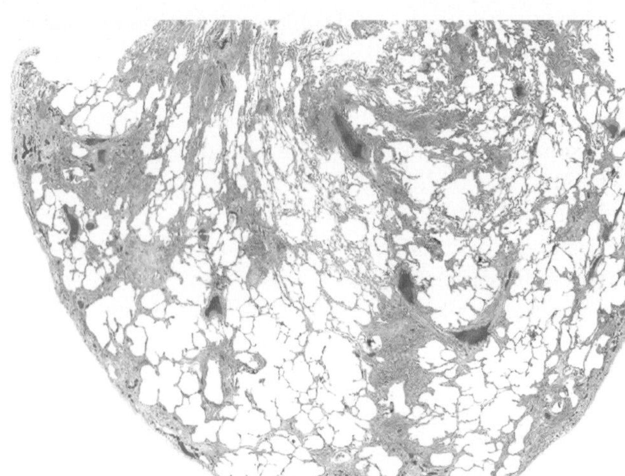

Figure 107.4 In some cases the demonstration of bridging fibrosis from one bronchovascular bundle to an adjacent bronchovascular bundle can be observed, as seen on the *left side* of this image.

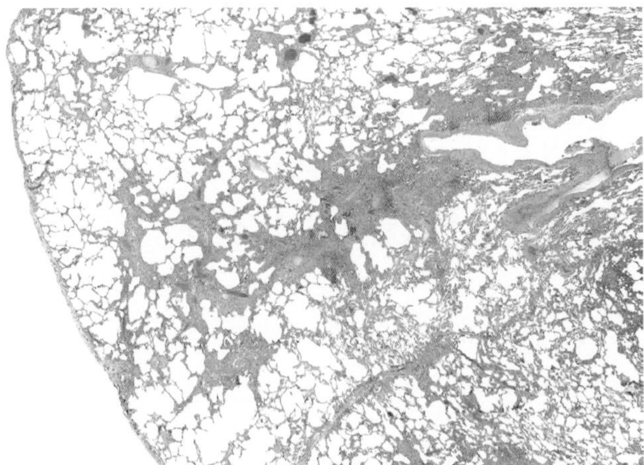

Figure 107.5 The degree of cellular interstitial inflammation is variable in cases of airway-centered fibrosis. However, the more significant the associated cellular interstitial infiltrates, the more suspicious one should become for more definitive diagnoses such as hypersensitivity pneumonitis or interstitial lung disease associated with connective tissue disease.

108 Diffuse Alveolar Septal Amyloidosis

Maxwell L. Smith
Melanie C. Bois

Pulmonary amyloidosis presents in three main patterns: nodular, tracheobronchial, or diffuse alveolar septal. Each of these may be further dichotomized into primary (isolated pulmonary) or systemic amyloidosis, with the former being the most common in the nodular and tracheobronchial presentations. In contrast, diffuse alveolar septal amyloidosis is most commonly found in the setting of systemic disease and is usually secondary to a plasma cell dyscrasia. In such situations diffuse alveolar septal amyloidosis is almost invariably associated with concurrent cardiac amyloidosis. While generally associated with systemic disease, primary (isolated-pulmonary) diffuse alveolar septal amyloidosis can occur but is an exceedingly rare phenomenon.

Men of advanced age are preferentially affected by this disease. It is generally clinically silent, with patients presenting to medical attention due to end-organ damage (and symptoms therein) from their systemic amyloidosis, including kidney failure, restrictive cardiomyopathy, and peripheral neuropathy. Despite this, cases with pulmonary symptoms have been reported and are commonly, although not always, associated with cardiac dysfunction.

Imaging features of parenchymal disease are variable and may mimic interstitial lung disease. Specifically, high-resolution computed tomography often shows diffuse septal thickening with air space opacities in bilateral lungs, subtle nodule formation, and lack of significant honeycomb change. Such radiographic presentation is often misinterpreted as an interstitial lung disease, with amyloidosis discovered on subsequent biopsy.

In keeping with its association with plasma cell dyscrasia, diffuse alveolar septal amyloidosis is commonly composed of immunoglobulin light chains (AL amyloidosis). Rare presentations of parenchymal involvement by systemic serum amyloid A and transthyretin amyloidosis have been reported.

As diffuse alveolar septal amyloidosis is generally associated with systemic amyloidosis, cardiac involvement, and underlying hematologic malignancy, it carries a less favorable prognosis than the other (lung-limited) pulmonary amyloidosis subtypes. The prognosis for diffuse alveolar septal amyloidosis is therefore poor and frequently complicated by the underlying systemic amyloidosis and/or the primary disease process.

Once recognized, congophilic material can be sent for mass spectroscopy and definitive amyloid subtyping. If AL-type amyloid is identified, a thorough hematologic workup for identification of a plasma cell dyscrasia is necessary to help treat and minimize the progression of amyloidosis.

HISTOLOGIC FEATURES

- Diffuse deposition of amorphous eosinophilic material within bronchovascular bundles and interstitium, which may often resemble fibrotic nonspecific interstitial pneumonia at first glance.
- Coalescing of amorphous eosinophilic material into vague nodules, often appreciated at lower power.
- Occasional multinucleated giant-cell reaction.
- Minimal cellular interstitial infiltrate.

- Early cases may be quite subtle and only appreciated at high power.
- The amyloid material is often accentuated around pulmonary vessels.
- Trichrome staining shows a "steel blue" appearance to the material, in stark contrast to the bright blue staining expected for mature collagen.
- Congo red staining shows characteristic salmon pink reactivity under normal-phase microscopy.
- Cross-polarized light microscopy of Congo red stain shows characteristic apple-green birefringence.
- Crystal violet staining may also be used to highlight the amyloid material.

DIFFERENTIAL DIAGNOSIS

From scanning magnification, cases of diffuse alveolar septal amyloidosis may be mistaken for fibrotic interstitial processes. Fibrotic nonspecific interstitial pneumonia (NSIP) commonly mimics this disease because of the diffuse involvement of the interstitium. Close inspection of alveolar septa to identify the amorphous eosinophilic material characteristic of amyloid helps differentiate diffuse alveolar septal amyloidosis from fibrotic NSIP. Likewise, smoking-related interstitial fibrosis (SRIF) may also come into the differential diagnosis because of fibrotic and paucicellular interstitial thickening. However, SRIF differs from diffuse alveolar septal amyloidosis by dense collagenous fibrosis, often with individual fibroblasts within the interstitium.

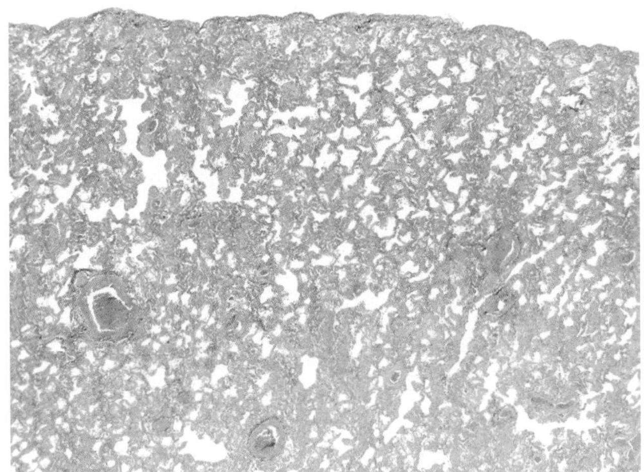

Figure 108.1 Diffuse interstitial thickening by paucicellular material is a common presentation in diffuse alveolar septal amyloidosis. This pattern may mimic fibrosing interstitial processes such as nonspecific interstitial pneumonia.

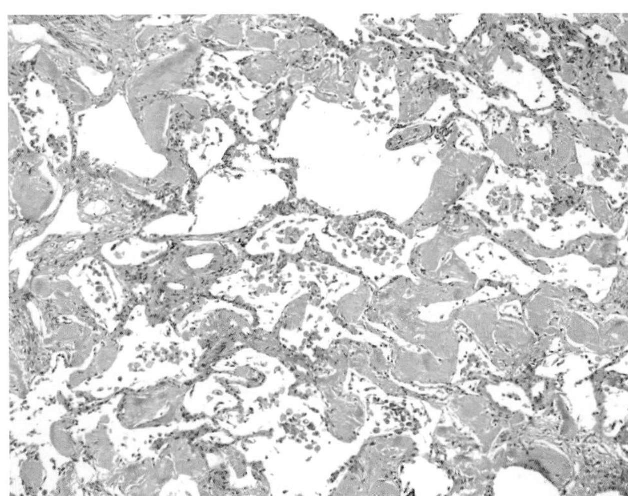

Figure 108.2 Amyloidosis may show mild, homogenous interstitial involvement or vaguely nodular deposition (as shown) in more advanced disease.

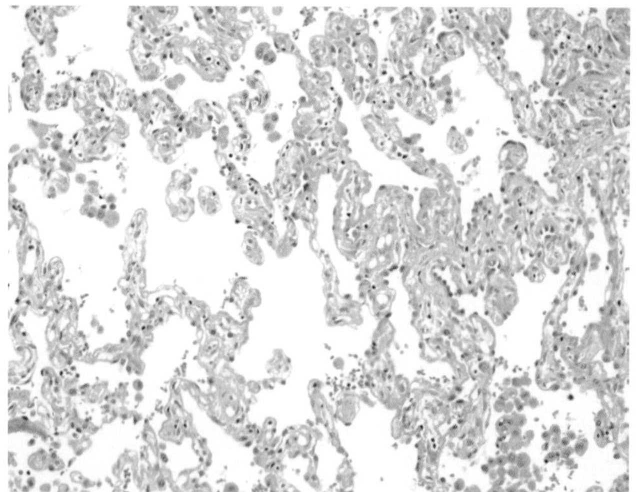

Figure 108.3 Early cases of diffuse alveolar septal amyloidosis may be easily overlooked because of the subtle deposition of interstitial.

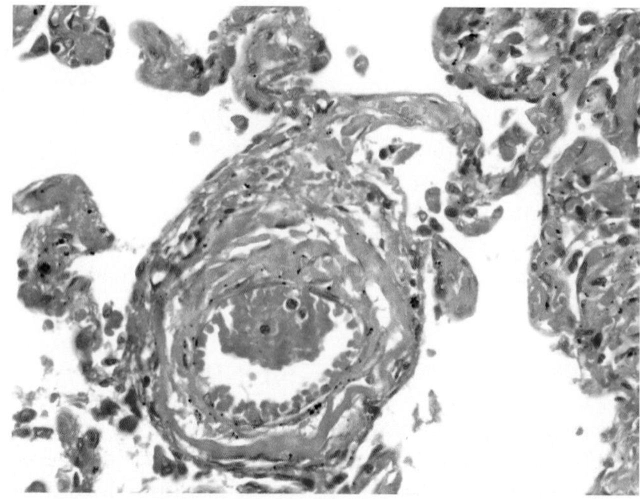

Figure 108.4 Pulmonary vasculature is frequently involved in diffuse alveolar septal amyloidosis, demonstrating amorphous eosinophilic deposits in the vessel wall.

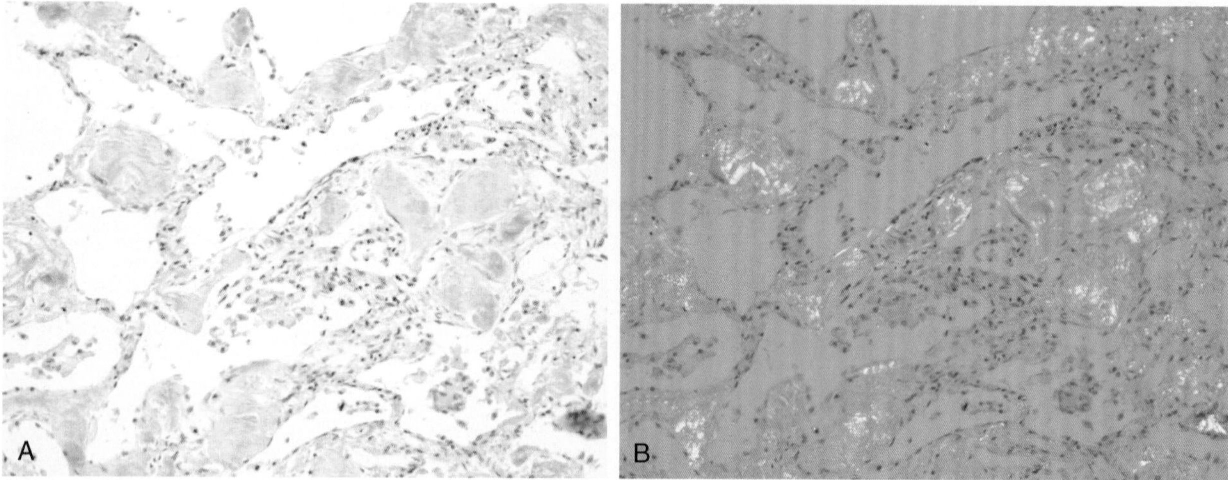

Figure 108.5 Amyloid deposits are congophilic under light microscopy (**A**), with characteristic apple-green birefringence under cross-polarized light (**B**).

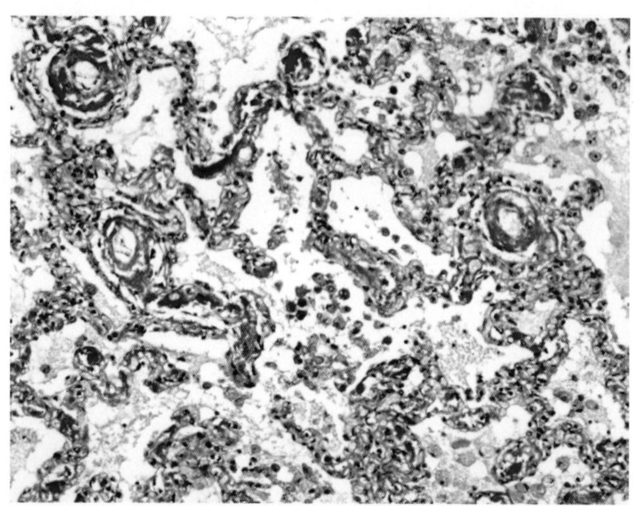

Figure 108.6 Metachromatic stains, including crystal violet, accentuate amyloid deposits without the need for cross-polarized light.

Honeycomb Lung

▶ Maxwell L. Smith
▶ Maria Cecilia Mengoli

Honeycomb lung represents the late, end stage, of various lung diseases. Honeycombing is classically associated with idiopathic pulmonary fibrosis (IPF) but may be seen in any advanced fibrosing disease. The term *honeycombing* per se is uniquely a pathologic and radiologic sign of terminally damaged lung and is not a specific diagnosis. When the honeycombing involves most of the parenchyma, the definition *honeycomb lung* is applied. Innumerable chronic and progressive lung disease other than usual interstitial pneumonia (UIP) of IPF may led to honeycomb lung, including chronic hypersensitivity pneumonitis (HP), chronic connective tissue disease, chronic sarcoidosis, fibrotic nonspecific pneumonia, iatrogenic reactions to drugs, toxic inhalations, or chronic aspirations. In addition, any severe acute lung injury may evolve into honeycomb scars, such as old healed bronchopneumonia. Rarely some neoplastic lesions may mimic honeycomb lung, or honeycomb changes can be detected in the parenchyma proximal to primary lung cancers.

Radiologically, honeycombing appears as clusters of cystic air spaces typically of comparable dimensions on the order of 3 to 10 mm, rarely as large as 2.5 cm, with well-defined walls resembling a honeycomb, and is considered a computed tomography finding of established pulmonary fibrosis. Honeycomb cysts are typically located beneath the visceral pleura, stacking on one another sharing their walls, and are often associated with traction bronchiectasis and fibrotic architectural distortion. Microscopic honeycomb cysts (recognized by pathologists) are much smaller than their radiology counterparts. Thoracic surgeons trend to avoid areas with radiographic honeycombing, as biopsies from these areas increase the risk of postoperative air leaks. The distribution of the honeycomb changes largely depends on the primary etiology with typical basal and posterior predilection in patients with IPF, frequent upper lung and midlung predominance in chronic HP, and upper prevalence in chronic aspiration and sarcoidosis. Clinical presentation, age of onset, and sex are dependent on the primary disease. Patients with IPF are mostly men, smokers, older than 60 years with progressive cough and shortness of breath. On the contrary, patients with chronic HP are frequently younger, nonsmoker, and exposed to inhaled antigens. Lung diseases in the context of connective tissue disease mostly affect young people with systemic symptoms and serologic abnormalities of the autoimmune system. Chronic aspiration affects older patients, and frequently predisposing factors such as obesity, gastroesophageal reflux, hiatal hernia, habitual use of chronic pain medication are detected. Rarely well-differentiated mucinous or nonmucinous adenocarcinoma may arise in a honeycomb lung or closely mimic it.

HISTOLOGIC FEATURES

Microscopic honeycomb remodeling is characterized by the following:

- Replacement of parenchyma by enlarged, distorted, cystic airspaces surrounded by thick fibrous walls with complete loss of acinar architecture.
- Residual intact bronchioles frequently detected within honeycomb lung and recognized by the surrounding smooth muscle layer.
- Varying amounts of mucin and admixed inflammatory cells, including neutrophils, macrophages, and lymphocytes in the cystic air spaces.
- A ciliated metaplastic bronchiolar epithelium lining the cysts.

DIFFERENTIAL DIAGNOSIS

Honeycomb lung is an unspecific pattern of injury detected in many end-stage lung diseases. Although honeycombing is characteristic of the UIP pattern, it is not pathognomonic of IPF and can be encountered in other forms of fibrotic lung disease because of chronic and/or old severe injury. As pathologists, we can only describe the pattern of injury of end-stage lung disease. The rarely encountered pitfall of an adenocarcinoma arising in the context of honeycomb lung should induce careful inspection of the epithelium for the presence of cilia that are absent in adenocarcinoma and preserved in the metaplastic bronchiolar epithelium lining of the honeycomb cysts. Caution is suggested when using the term *honeycombing*, as many clinicians equate this term with the clinical syndrome of IPF.

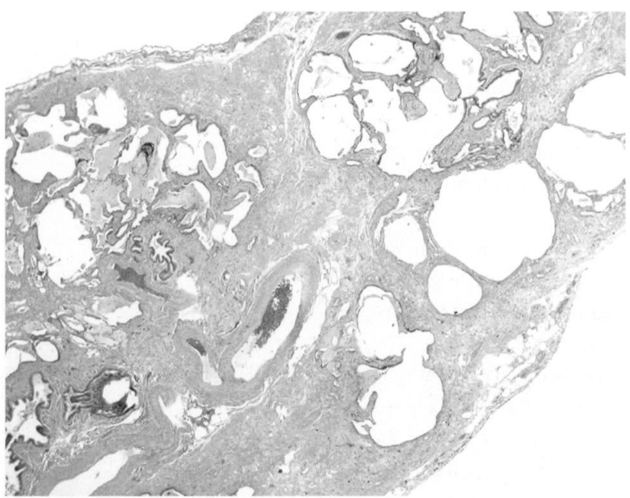

Figure 109.1 Complete destruction of the lung architecture by a severe fibrosing process, leaving residual cystic spaces separated by broad bands of mature scar.

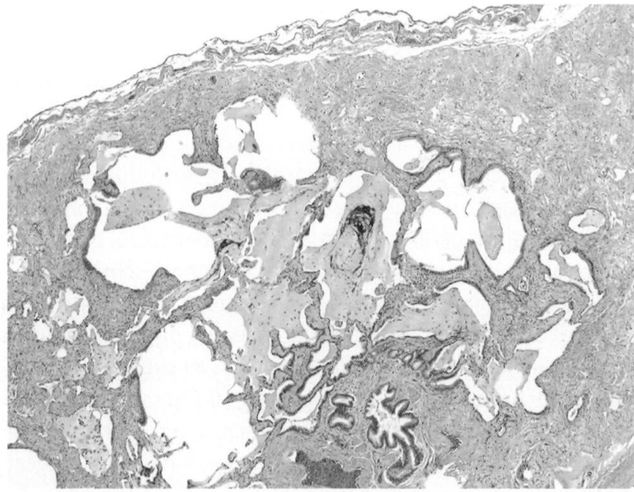

Figure 109.2 Honeycomb remodeling with dilated terminal airways lined by respiratory epithelium and filled with blue mucus.

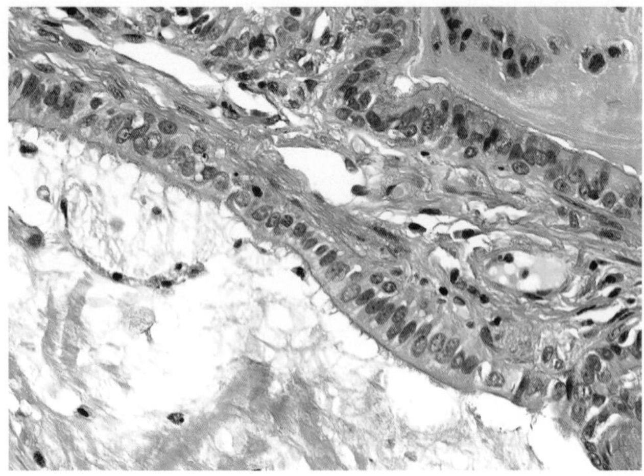

Figure 109.3 Metaplastic ciliated respiratory bronchiolar epithelium lines some cysts.

Lung Disease in Inflammatory Bowel Disease

110

▶ Maxwell L. Smith
▶ Maria Cecilia Mengoli

The term *inflammatory bowel disease (IBD)* is used to describe two distinct diseases, namely ulcerative colitis (UC) and Crohn's disease (CD). Approximately 6% to 47% of patients develop extraintestinal manifestation during the course of IBD. The true prevalence of lung involvement is unknown, as it is estimated that 40% to 60% of patients have some degree of subclinical lung involvement. Pulmonary involvement is more common in UC than CD, and in most patients (72% to 84%), pulmonary involvement follows the onset of IBD with variable time interval ranging from weeks to decades. Severe bronchopulmonary involvement has been reported following colectomy, as the inflammatory process shifts from the bowel to the lung. In rare instances (13%), respiratory symptoms predate intestinal manifestation. The bronchopulmonary involvement in IBD is seen most often in female, nonsmoking patients. Patients with small airway involvement usually present with productive or nonproductive cough and shortness of breath. Upper airway involvement manifests as purulent expectoration, bronchorrhea, or wheezing frequently misdiagnosed and treated as asthma. The pleural involvement may present pleuritic chest pain, dyspnea, and fever. Patients with IBD are also at increased risk of pulmonary embolism; therefore thromboembolism should always be considered in cases of acute pulmonary symptoms.

Imaging features are protean and variable, including bronchial wall thickening, bronchiectasis with air trapping, thickening of the wall of the trachea, and main bronchi with/without bronchial stenosis, diffuse bilateral infiltrates or ground-glass opacities, and bilateral nodules with possible internal cavitation and pleural effusion.

Bronchoscopy may reveal tracheal or bronchial edema, hyperemia, suppurative bronchitis, or strictures. In tracheobronchial involvement, bronchoalveolar lavage may be dominated by neutrophils, thus requiring a careful exclusion of a possible infectious agent.

A subset of patients with UC demonstrates antineutrophilic cytoplasmic (ANCA) antibodies, most often MPO antigen (p-ANCA).

Because the respiratory involvement in IBD is inflammatory in nature, it is usually responsive to steroids, and inhaled beclomethasone and budesonide are the first line of therapy of IBD-related interstitial lung disease (ILD).

HISTOLOGIC FEATURES

Ulcerative Colitis

- Upper and large airway disease: glottis/subglottic stenosis; tracheal inflammation and stenosis; chronic bronchitis with dense peribronchiolar lymphoplasmacytic infiltrate possibly extending into submucosal bronchial glands often lacking germinal centers; chronic bronchial suppuration with pools of luminal neutrophils; bronchiectasis with mucus stasis.
- Small airway disease: chronic bronchiolitis with dense peribronchiolar lymphoplasmacytic infiltrates and frequent absence of germinal centers; necrotizing bronchiolitis with erosion and squamous metaplasia of the overlying mucosa and luminal exudate rich in neutrophils; diffuse panbronchiolitis-like pattern characterized by acute and chronic

bronchiolitis with lymphoid hyperplasia and distinctive clusters of interstitial foamy macrophages; chronic constrictive bronchiolitis with fibrosis and luminal narrowing of bronchioles with relatively little inflammatory infiltrate (rare).

- ILD: organizing pneumonia (OP) pattern often associated with a distinctive marked edematous septal thickening and infiltration by chronic inflammatory cells including eosinophils and plasma cells; cellular, fibrotic, or mixed nonspecific interstitial pneumonia (NSIP) pattern or eosinophilic pneumonia.
- Necrobiotic sterile parenchymal nodules, histologically reminiscent of pyoderma gangrenosum of the skin ("pyoderma lung") with central necrosis composed of neutrophils, fibrin, and neutrophil debris and cavitation and a rim of fibrous tissue and histiocytes; absence of granulomas and/or giant cells; no microorganisms on methenamine silver stain, Gram stain, or acid-fast bacilli stain; possible secondary vascular injury, but absence of true vasculitis and capillaritis.
- Serositis (pleural effusion with huge number of neutrophils, pleuropericarditis).

Crohn's Disease

Pulmonary manifestations of CD are similar to UC-related lung disease with the only exception of necrobiotic parenchymal nodules, which have only been reported in patients with UC. Other findings in CD include the following:

- Bronchiolitis with nonnecrotizing granulomas and giant cells, some containing cholesterol clefts and calcium oxalate crystals.
- NSIP pattern with rare giant cells or scattered nonnecrotizing granulomas.

DIFFERENTIAL DIAGNOSIS

The main differential diagnosis includes infection and drug reaction, as these patients are often immunosuppressed and on biologic agents. Special stains for infectious organisms and culture studies should be performed. Chronic medications required for the management of IBD, particularly sulphasalazine, mesalamine (5-aminosalicylic acid), methotrexate, and anti–tumor necrosis factor, can cause drug-induced lung diseases. The patterns of lung injuries related to the abovementioned drugs are variable and similar to those seen in IBD-related ILD, including eosinophilic pneumonia with peripheral eosinophilia, OP, NSIP, acute lung injury patterns, eosinophilic pleural effusion, and granulomatous reaction. Granulomatosis with polyangiitis looks similar to the "pyoderma lung" and consequently enters the differential diagnosis; however, this possibility is excluded by the negativity for c-ANCA and the lack of hyperchromatic giant cells and vasculitis at morphologic evaluation. IBD-associated NSIP pattern with/without granulomatous features may be identical to hypersensitivity pneumonitis and only a positive exposure history with/without serologic evaluation can discriminate the two entities. Sometimes differentiating CD affecting lung from sarcoidosis, based on the presence of nonnecrotizing granulomas, is difficult. As a rule, the presence of a lymphangitic distribution of pink, coalescing, naked granulomas, associated with minimal interstitial inflammation or chronic bronchiolitis, strongly favors a diagnosis of sarcoidosis.

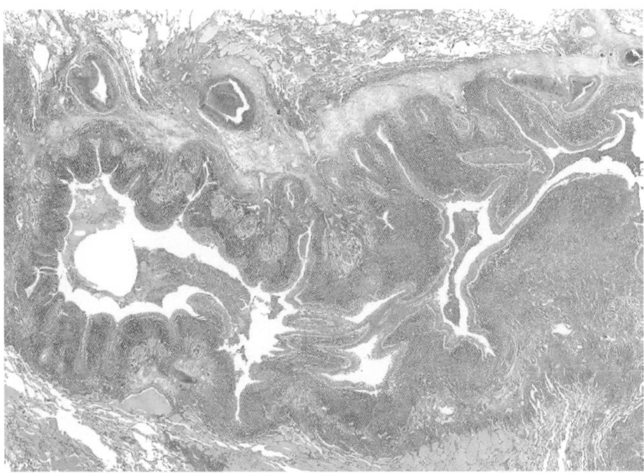

Figure 110.1 Bronchiole with marked bronchioloectasia and mucostasis and prominent peribronchiolar lymphoplasmacytic infiltrate in a case of UC.

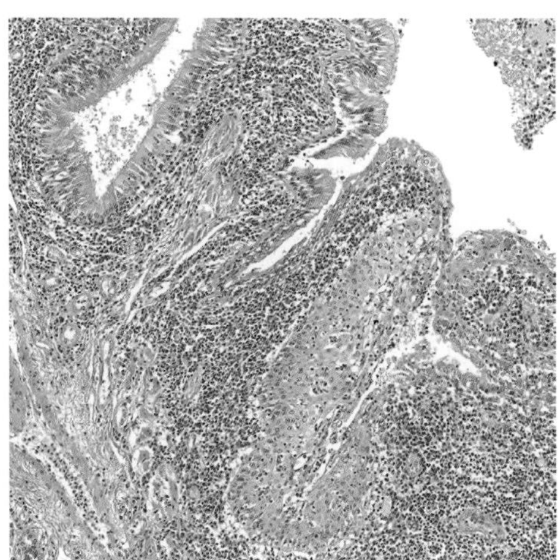

Figure 110.2 High-power magnification of acute and chronic bronchiolitis with squamous metaplasia of the respiratory epithelium, which is infiltrated by neutrophils.

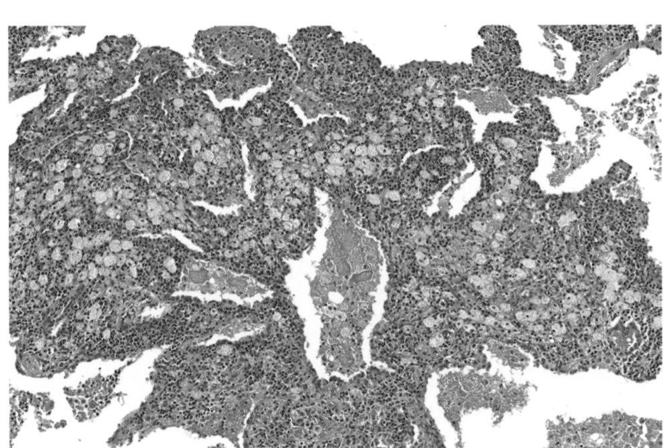

Figure 110.3 Diffuse panbronchiolitis-like pattern with prominent widening of the alveolar walls because of collection of distinctive clusters of interstitial foamy macrophages and lymphocytes.

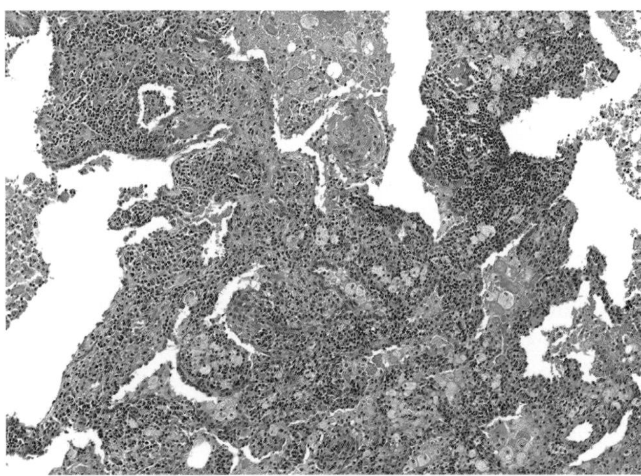

Figure 110.4 Nonspecific interstitial pneumonia pattern with interstitial widening by a chronic inflammatory infiltrate with clusters of foamy macrophages and foci of organizing pneumonia with polyps of fibromyxoid inflammatory tissue protruding into a central alveolar space.

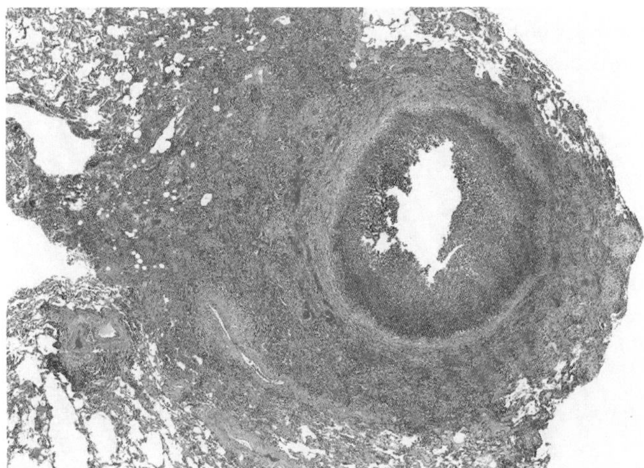

Figure 110.5 Necrobiotic sterile parenchymal nodule (so-called pyoderma lung) with a central cavitated area of necrosis and a peripheral rim of fibrous tissue.

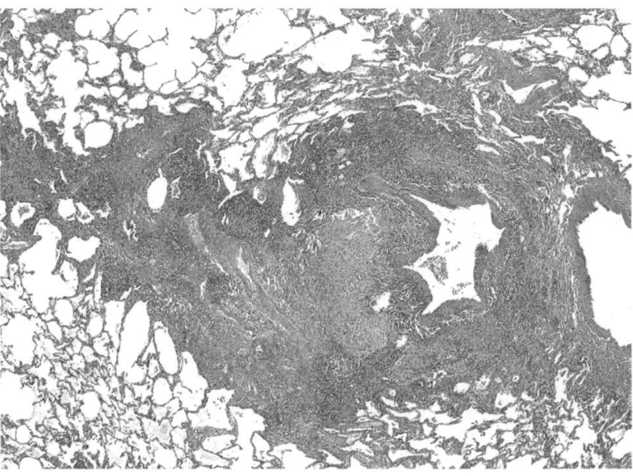

Figure 110.6 Chronic bronchiolitis with constrictive fibrosis and several lymphoid follicles lacking germinal centers.

Common Variable Immunodeficiency Disorders/ Granulomatous–Lymphocytic Interstitial Lung Disease (CVID/ GLILD)–Associated Lung Disease

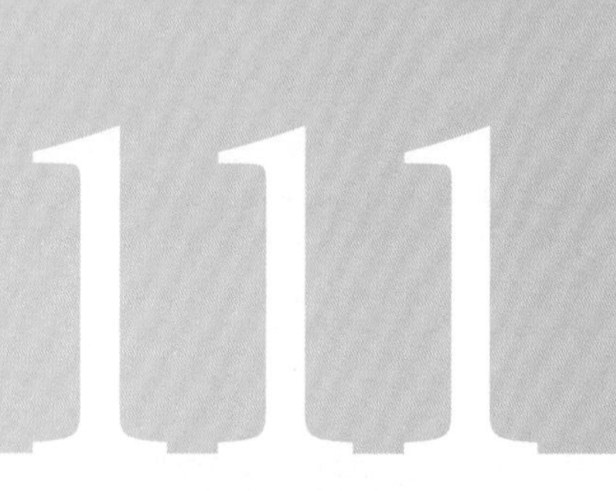

▶ Ying-Han (Roger) Hsu
▶ Maxwell L. Smith

Common variable immunodeficiency (CVID) is a clinical syndrome that comprises a heterogeneous group of primary immunodeficiency disorders characterized by low serum IgG and the inability to generate specific antibodies in response to antigens. The prevalence of CVID ranges from 1:25,000 to 1:50,000. Patients with CVID present at a variable age but often between the second and fourth decades. These patients are not only predisposed to systemic infections but also at particularly increased risk for recurrent respiratory tract infections from encapsulated and atypical bacterial species. As a result, multifocal infection with bronchiectasis is a common infectious complication. Infections are covered elsewhere in this atlas and, in the setting of CVID, do not show any specific histopathologic features.

Approximately 10% to 30% of patients with CVID develop noninfectious diffuse lung disease complications collectively termed *granulomatous–lymphocytic interstitial lung disease (GLILD)*, which seems to portend a worse prognosis compared with patients with CVID alone. GLILD is a clinical term encompassing a spectrum of histopathologic changes seen in CVID patients, who also have clinical and radiographic manifestations of a diffuse parenchymal lung disease. There is often a history of autoimmune cytopenias and splenomegaly in these patients.

HISTOLOGIC FEATURES

- Diffuse cellular interstitial infiltrates expanding the interstitium and consisting predominantly of lymphocytes and plasma cells. This pattern of infiltration is reminiscent of cellular nonspecific interstitial pneumonia (NSIP) and lymphoid interstitial pneumonia (LIP).
- Follicular bronchiolitis characterized by dense airway-centered lymphoid follicles with germinal centers.
- Acute and chronic bronchiolitis is a common associated finding, along with polyps of organizing pneumonia in the airspaces.

- Nonnecrotizing granulomas consisting of loose aggregates of epithelioid histiocytes and multinucleated giant cells, often with dense lymphoid hyperplasia in the background.
- It is not uncommon to have polyps of organizing pneumonia associated with the chronic inflammatory cell infiltrates.
- Plasma cells may be a significant component of the infiltrate.
- As the disease progresses, a component of interstitial fibrosis with remodeling of the lobular architecture of the lung may occur.
- Many cases show advanced fibrosis with microscopic honeycomb change and traction bronchiectasis.
- Areas resembling usual interstitial pneumonia (UIP) or fibrotic NSIP pattern of fibrosis can be present.

DIFFERENTIAL DIAGNOSIS

Because of the spectrum of histopathologic findings in GLILD, it is not surprising that a broad differential diagnosis must be considered, depending on the predominant patterns. If the predominant changes are those of a diffuse cellular interstitial infiltrate with only rare poorly formed granulomas, subacute hypersensitivity pneumonitis (HP) may be at the top of the differential diagnosis. Without a clinical history of CVID, the distinction between GLILD and subacute HP can be quite difficult, if not impossible. In addition to CVID, all other possible causes for a histopathologic pattern of LIP including HP, connective tissue diseases (CTDs, particularly Sjogren syndrome), other primary or acquired immunodeficiency disorders, and low-grade B-cell lymphomas should be excluded with appropriate workup. Idiopathic NSIP is also a consideration, albeit less likely when granulomas are also observed. The presence of more significant interstitial fibrosis warrants consideration of fibrotic NSIP and UIP. If the fibrosis is airway-centered and secondary to long-term bronchiolitis, one might entertain the possibility of airway-centered fibrosis of various etiologies, such as chronic HP, CTDs, and chronic aspiration.

Sarcoidosis is often included in the differential diagnosis of robust granulomatous diseases; however, the granulomas of sarcoidosis are typically set in a densely hyalinized background and consist of tight aggregates of histiocytes and multinucleated giant cells. This is in contrast to the loose aggregates of epithelioid histiocytes in GLILD.

The differential diagnosis for follicular bronchiolitis, including CTDs (in particular, rheumatoid arthritis, systemic lupus erythematosus, and Sjogren syndrome), other primary or acquired immunodeficiency disorders (e.g., human immunodeficiency virus infection/acquired immunodeficiency syndrome), and low-grade B-cell lymphomas of mucosa-associated lymphoid tissue, should all be explored and appropriately excluded. Finally, if the predominant pattern of injury is airway-centered, consideration should be given to chronic or diffuse aspiration pneumonia, as well as inflammatory bowel disease–associated interstitial lung disease.

Owing to the diverse histopathologic findings in GLILD, it is rare to make an outright diagnosis unless the patient is known to have CVID. However, it must remain an important consideration in the differential diagnosis for otherwise unexplained lymphocytic and/or granulomatous infiltrates with or without fibrosis.

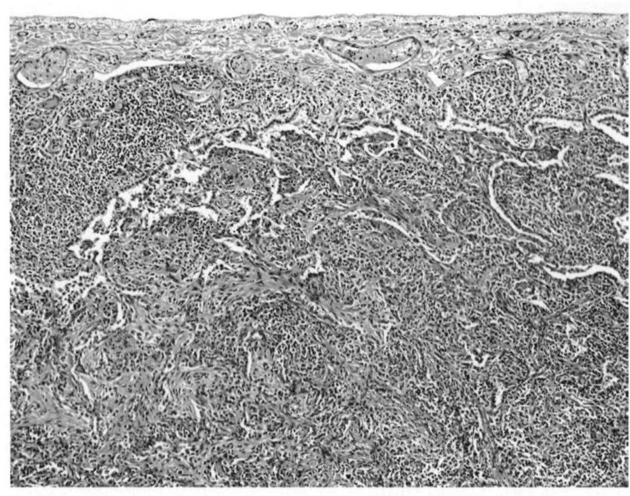

Figure 111.1 Diffuse cellular interstitial infiltrate. The alveolar interstitium is markedly expanded by a dense collection of mature lymphocytes and plasma cells. Polyps of organizing pneumonia are often present. These histopathologic findings may overlap with those of cellular NSIP, LIP, or low-grade B-cell lymphomas; immunohistochemical studies, which typically demonstrate a predominantly CD3+/CD4+ T-cell infiltrate in GLILD, would be helpful in excluding the latter.

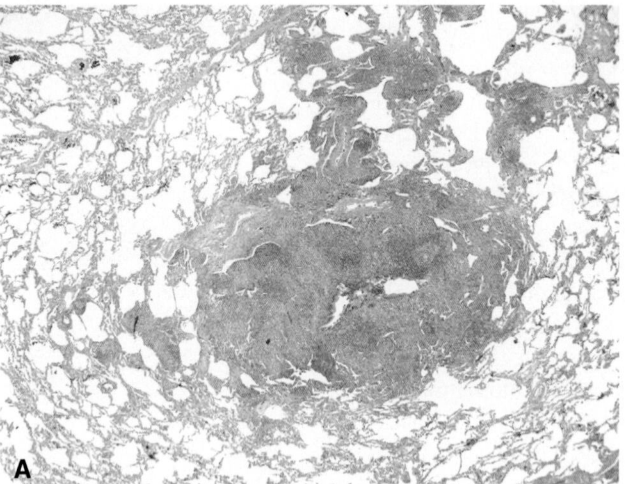

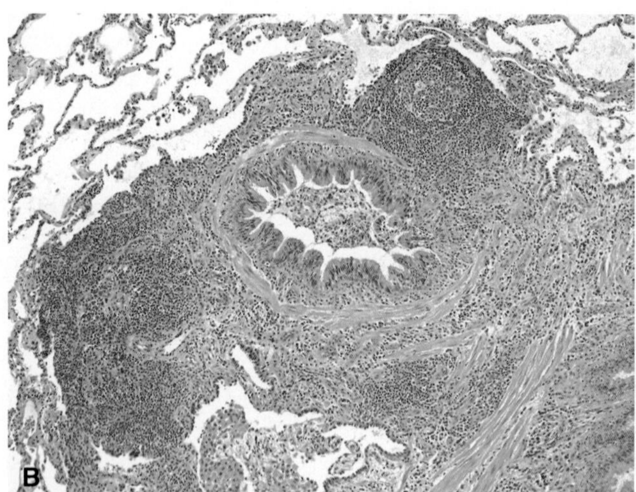

Figure 111.2 Follicular bronchiolitis. Dense airway-centered lymphoid hyperplasia with several small nodular lymphoid aggregates (**A**). On higher magnification, there is chronic bronchiolitis accompanied by submucosal lymphoplasmacytic infiltrate and a well-developed lymphoid follicle with germinal center (**B**).

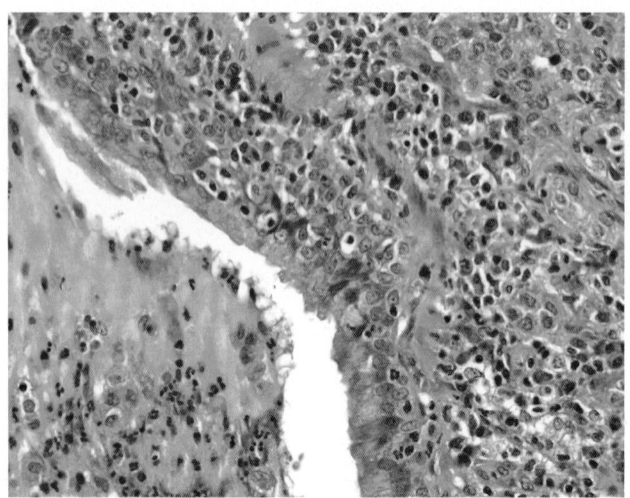

Figure 111.3 Acute and chronic bronchiolitis. This bronchiolar wall is infiltrated by a mixture of acute and chronic inflammatory cells, including epithelial and intraluminal collections of neutrophils. A superimposed infection should be excluded.

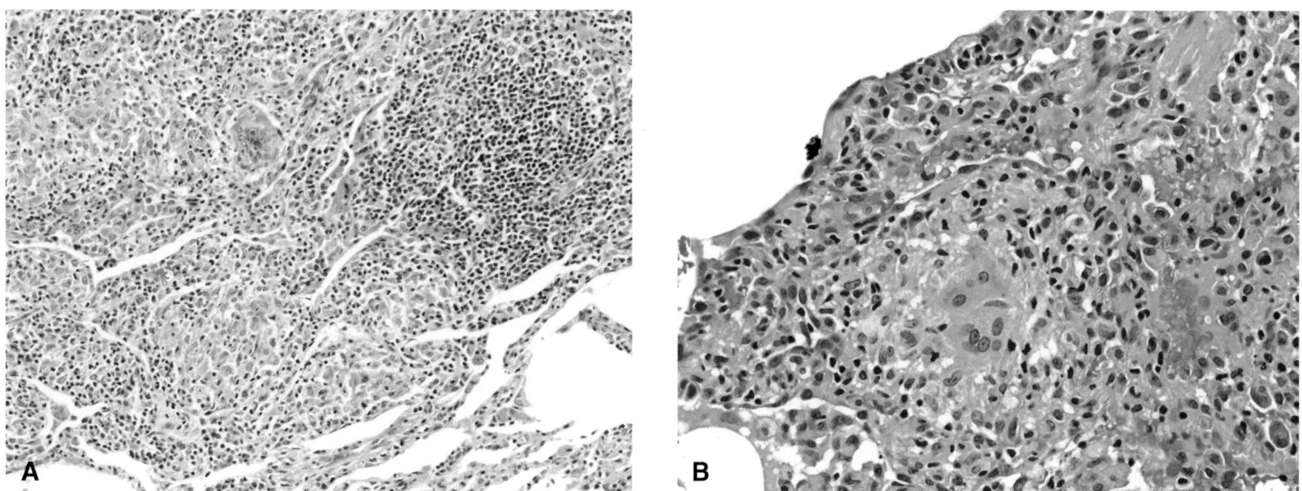

Figure 111.4 Nonnecrotizing granulomatous inflammation. Scattered loose aggregates of epithelioid histiocytes (**A**) and multinucleated giant cells (**B**), often found within the dense peribronchiolar and interstitial lymphoid background, are characteristic features of GLILD. These findings can sometimes be difficult to distinguish from those of HP or granulomatous infections. Special stains and microbiological studies for *Mycobacterial* and fungal microorganisms should be obtained.

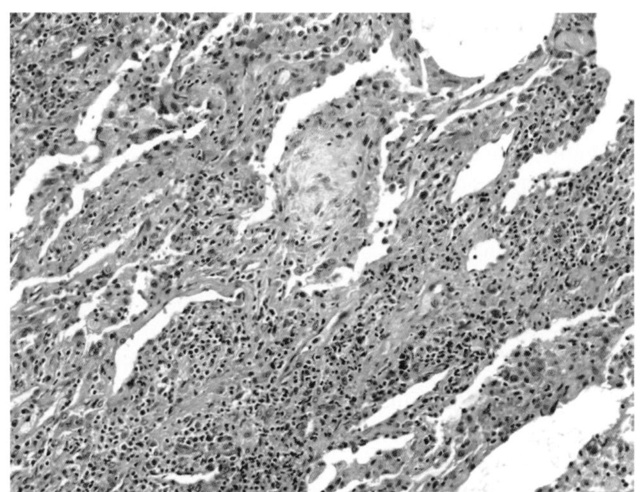

Figure 111.5 Organizing pneumonia. Intraluminal plugs of fibroblastic proliferation representing organizing pneumonia are a common and sometimes prominent feature in GLILD and may potentially lead to misinterpretation as cryptogenic organizing pneumonia if other causes including GLILD have not been considered.

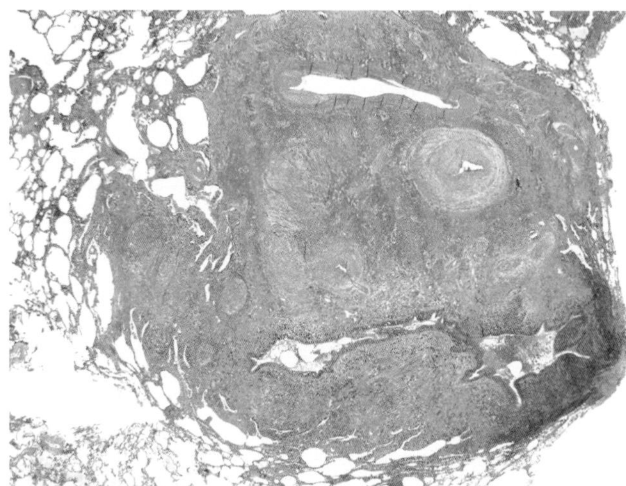

Figure 111.6 Fibrosis associated with lymphoid hyperplasia. There is remodeling of the bronchovascular architecture by lymphoid proliferation and abundant collagen deposition with thickened pulmonary vessels. GLILD may progress to significant airway and interstitial fibrosis, which may become challenging to differentiate from other etiologies, such as chronic HP, CTDs, drug toxicity, and chronic infection.

112

Chronic Aspiration Bronchiolitis

▶ Maxwell L. Smith
▶ Paul Wawryko

Aspiration of oral contents can create a variety of clinical pulmonary syndromes with distinct pathologic features. Aspiration pneumonitis occurs following large volume inhalation of gastric contents and shows acute and organizing diffuse alveolar damage on biopsy. Aspiration pneumonia is infection following aspiration of oropharyngeal microorganisms into the lung. Pathologically, this appears as a typical lobar bronchopneumonia. There is increasing evidence that aspiration can cause interstitial lung disease and is recognized as a risk factor for progression in the clinical syndrome idiopathic pulmonary fibrosis. Diffuse aspiration bronchiolitis is one of the more common aspiration-associated diseases to cross the surgical pathologist's desk. The disease onset is usually subacute to chronic with nonspecific complaints, including cough, sputum production, and shortness of breath. Risk factors for aspiration include altered level of consciousness (e.g., alcohol, drugs, and seizures), abnormalities of the stomach or esophagus, gastroesophageal reflux disease, recurrent vomiting, and dysphagia. Interestingly, aspiration is uncommonly suspected by the clinical services. Imaging findings are nonspecific but may show lobar or diffuse centrilobular nodules with variable tree-in-bud opacities. Some patients have traction bronchiectasis.

HISTOLOGIC FEATURES

- Scanning magnification typically shows airway-centered disease in the form of chronic bronchiolitis and/or fibrosis.
- The histologic hallmark is the identification of foreign material within the terminal airways or lung parenchyma. The foreign material can take on a variety of appearances depending on its origin (e.g., meat, vegetable material, and so forth).
- There is often a vague granulomatous response surrounding the foreign material. Multinucleated giant cells are common.
- A number of other nonspecific histologic findings can be seen in the setting of diffuse aspiration bronchiolitis, including organizing pneumonia, fibrotic organizing pneumonia, airway-centered "fibroblast foci," acute and chronic bronchiolitis, vasculopathic changes, neutrophilic infiltrates in the airspace similar to acute bronchopneumonia, and vague interstitial granulomas.
- The degree of foreign material may not correlate with the degree of histologic changes.
- Aspiration of saliva alone leads to a number of nonspecific histologic changes but may not show foreign material.

DIFFERENTIAL DIAGNOSIS

If the pathologic features include a prominent granulomatous component in addition to acute and chronic bronchiolitis, a long list of differential diagnostic considerations must be entertained, including infection (especially nontuberculous mycobacterial infection), antineutrophilic cytoplasmic–associated diseases, sarcoidosis, connective tissue disease, hypersensitivity pneumonitis, inflammatory bowel disease–associated interstitial lung disease, and adverse drug reaction. If no definitive foreign material is identified, cases are often left with a differential diagnosis. The differential diagnosis for airway-centered fibrosis with associated chronic bronchiolitis includes chronic hypersensitivity pneumonitis, connective tissue disease–associated interstitial lung disease, smoking or other inhalational disease, recurrent infection, and potentially an idiopathic disease (idiopathic airway-centered fibrosis). Again, the identification of foreign material can help clench the diagnosis. Some authors believe that polyps of organizing pneumonia with a prominent central core of plasma cell aggregates (the "jelly doughnut" sign) are suggestive of aspiration as an etiology (Figure 112.6). Anytime the pathologic features are suggestive of airway-centered disease, whether it is subacute or chronic, regardless of the presence of foreign material, aspiration should be considered as a potential etiology.

The prognosis for chronic aspiration bronchiolitis is variable. If the risk factors for aspiration can be addressed and corrected, disease progression is minimal. However, many of the risk factors for aspiration are difficult to modulate and therefore progressive disease with increased scarring and functional deficit is the more common course.

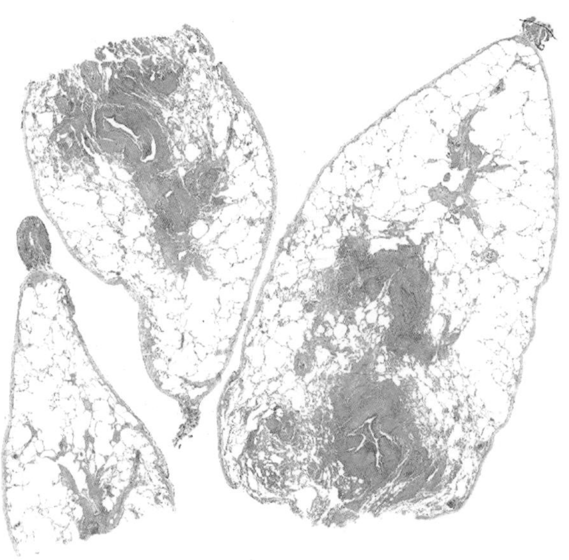

Figure 112.1 In chronic aspiration bronchiolitis, low-power magnification often shows evidence of airway-centered disease. Note the peribronchiolar fibrosis and chronic small airways remodeling in this example.

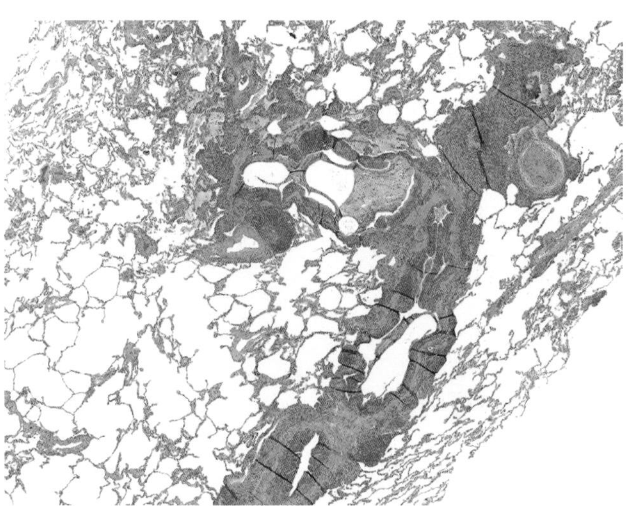

Figure 112.2 A number of nonspecific airway-centered changes may be seen in the setting of chronic aspiration bronchiolitis, including chronic bronchiolitis, mucostasis, nodular peribronchiolar lymphoid hyperplasia, and peribronchiolar metaplasia.

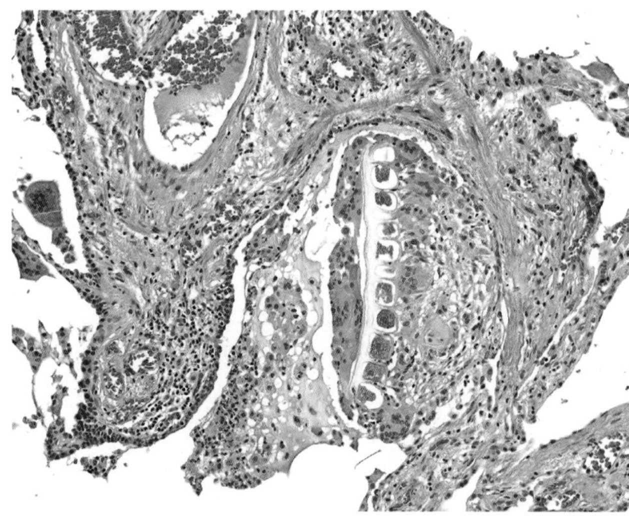

Figure 112.3 The histologic hallmark of chronic aspiration bronchiolitis is the identification of foreign food material within airspaces. This is an example of vegetable material with a surrounding multinucleated giant-cell foreign-body response, chronic inflammation, and fibrosis. Despite the dramatic airway-centered changes throughout the biopsy, this was the only piece of foreign material identified.

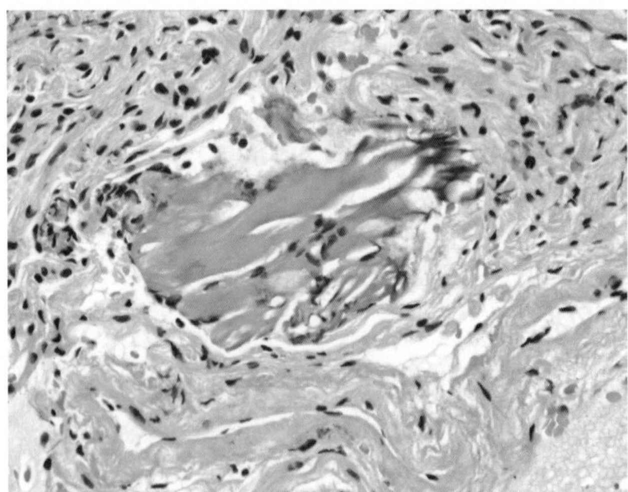

Figure 112.4 An example of aspirated skeletal muscle with surrounding fibrosis.

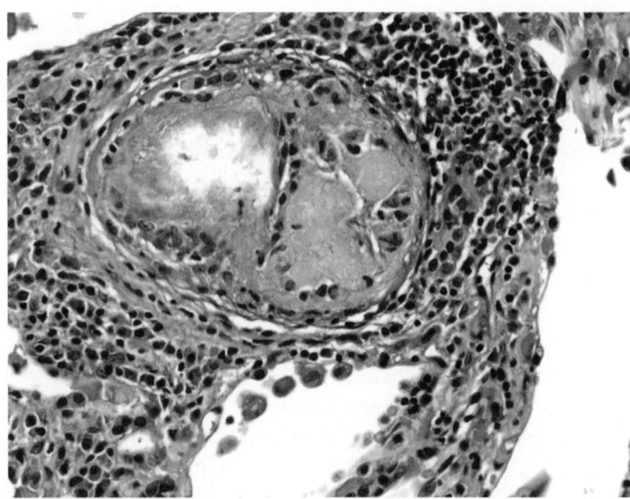

Figure 112.5 Eosinophilic amorphous debris with surrounding granulomatous infiltrate commonly seen in aspiration.

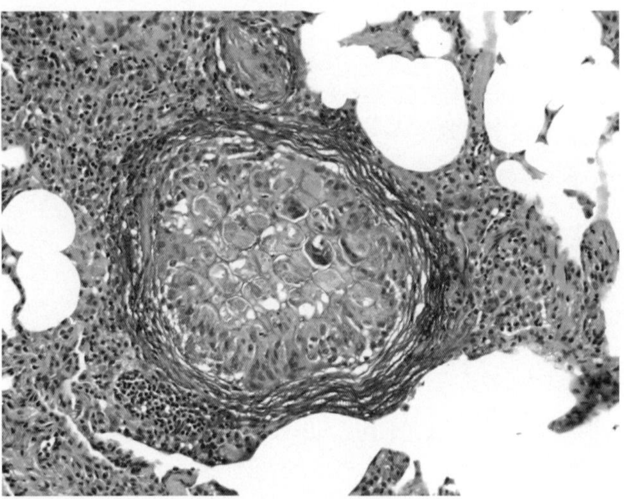

Figure 112.6 Another example of vegetable material with a granulomatous reaction.

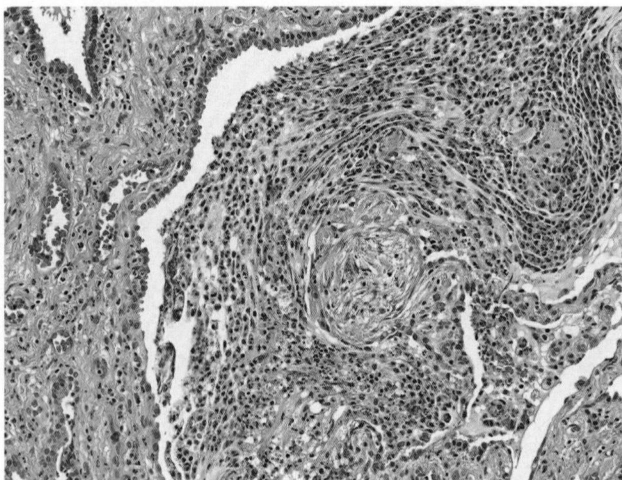

Figure 112.7 Nonspecific changes including mucostasis, polyps of organizing pneumonia, and prominent neutrophilic inflammation are often seen in the setting of chronic aspiration bronchiolitis.

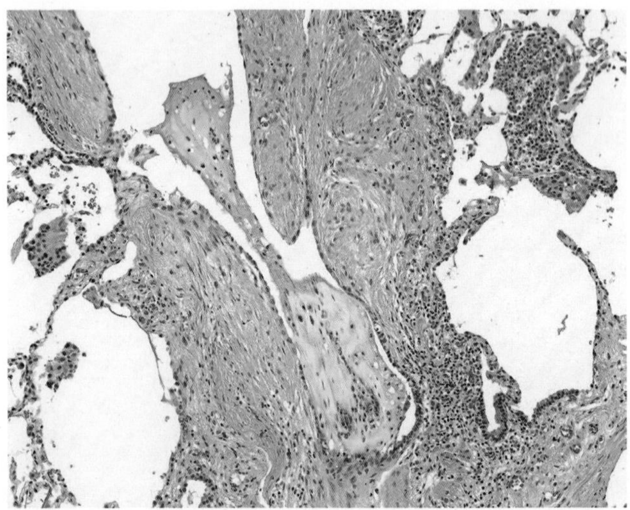

Figure 112.8 "Fibroblast foci" seen in the terminal bronchial respiratory epithelium should raise the possibility of chronic aspiration bronchiolitis. In this distribution, fibroblast foci are not suggestive of the usual interstitial pneumonia pattern of idiopathic pulmonary fibrosis.

IgG4-Related Pulmonary Disease

113

▸ Maxwell L. Smith
▸ Maria Cecilia Mengoli

IgG4-related disease is a fibroinflammatory condition of unknown origin, characterized by tumefactive lesions, involving virtually every organ system, dense lymphoplasmacytic infiltrates rich in IgG4+ plasma cells, storiform fibrosis, obliterative phlebitis, and frequent elevated serum concentration of IgG4. The majority of affected patients are men (62% to 83%), older than 50 years. Pulmonary involvement occurs in 12% to 54% of patients with IgG4-related disease. Thoracic IgG4-related disease may present subacutely with mild nonspecific clinical symptoms, such as cough, shortness of breath, exertional dyspnea, chest pain, and pleural effusion. However, greater than 75% of cases are identified incidentally via imaging studies. Many patients with IgG4-related disease (up to 40%) manifest allergic features, such as atopy, eczema, asthma, and peripheral blood eosinophilia. Intrathoracic disease could manifest as mediastinal lesions (such as mediastinal lymphadenopathy and sclerosing mediastinitis) or parenchymal lung disease and is usually associated with involvement of at least one extrathoracic organ. At imaging, IgG4-related lung disease is categorized into four major subtypes: (1) solid nodular lesions, (2) round-shaped ground-glass opacities, (3) alveolar interstitial lesions showing honeycombing, bronchiectasis, and diffuse ground-glass opacities, and (4) bronchovascular type showing thickening of bronchovascular bundles and interlobular septa with possible involvement of the pleura. Glucocorticoids are typically the first line of treatment and are effective in most patients. The major determinant of treatment responsiveness is the degree of fibrosis, as long-standing lesions with prominent sclerosis are unlikely to respond.

HISTOLOGIC FEATURES

The three major histopathologic features of IgG4-related lung disease are as follows:

- Dense lymphoplasmacytic inflammatory infiltrate (composed predominantly of T cells) rich in IgG4-positive plasma cells with lymphangitic distribution, involving visceral pleura, interlobular septa, and bronchovascular bundles.
- Dense fibrosis arranged at least focally in a storiform pattern with hyaline/keloid-like features.
- Obliterative phlebitis without necrosis.

Other morphologic features possibly associated with IgG4-related lung disease are as follows:

- Phlebitis without obliteration of the lumen and nonnecrotizing lymphoplasmacytic arteritis.
- Mild to moderate number of eosinophils.
- Concentric bronchiolar chronic inflammatory infiltration associated with lymphoid hyperplasia with germinal centers.
- Pleuritis possibly associated with pleural effusion.
- Features consistent with postcapillary pulmonary hypertension (i.e., dilated lymphatics, widened of interlobular septa, congested capillaries, and pulmonary edema) secondary to pulmonary venous obstruction in patients with sclerosing IgG4-related mediastinitis and/or obliterative phlebitis.

IgG4 and IgG immunohistochemical staining is required for the pathologic assessment of IgG4-related disease, especially in patients without elevation of serum IgG4. Because the IgG4 cell distribution may be patchy, the consensus statement recommends to count the three 40× microscopic fields with the highest number of IgG4+ plasma cells (so called hot spots) and calculate the average number. The same three fields should be counted for IgG+ cells to calculate the IgG4/IgG ratio.

- In surgical lung biopsies, cases of IgG4-related disease should show greater than 50 IgG4-positive plasma cells per high-power field with a ratio of IgG4 to IgG of greater than 40%.
- In nonsurgical lung biopsies (transbronchial or cryobiopsies), cases of IgG4-related disease should show greater than 20 IgG4-positive plasma cells per high-power field with a ratio of IgG4 to IgG of greater than 40%.
- In pleural specimens, cases of IgG4-related disease should show greater than 50 IgG4-positive plasma cells per high-power field with a ratio of IgG4 to IgG of greater than 40%.

DIFFERENTIAL DIAGNOSIS

A number of both neoplastic and nonneoplastic conditions enter the differential diagnosis for IgG4-related disease. IgG4 disease is one of many fibroinflammatory diseases of the lung, including inflammatory pseudotumor, inflammatory myofibroblastic tumor (IMT), plasma cell granuloma, and hyalinizing granuloma. IMT is distinguished from the others by overexpression of the ALK-1 protein. Many cases designated inflammatory pseudotumor, plasma cell granuloma, and hyalinizing granuloma in the past likely were related to IgG4 disease.

Many cases will require at least a limited set of additional studies (kappa and lambda clonality studies, CD3, CD20, and Epstein–Barr virus [EBV] in situ hybridization) to evaluate for lymphoproliferative disorders. Low-grade B-cell lymphomas will have a CD20-dominant infiltrate compared with the CD3-dominant infiltrate characteristic of IgG4-related disease. The EBV-positive large B cells characteristic of lymphomatoid granulomatosis and its angiodestructive pathognomonic feature are lacking in IgG4-related disease. The distinction between Castleman disease and IgG4-related disease is important because they differ in their responsiveness to steroids. Castleman disease does not typically show the degree of fibrosis seen in IgG4-related disease and lacks the increased numbers of IgG4-positive plasma cells. Serum levels of IgA are reported to be elevated in Castleman disease and may be helpful in the evaluation of the patient.

Connective tissue diseases involving lung and pleura are best excluded with appropriate clinical and serologic correlation.

Rosai–Dorfman disease and IgG4-related disease largely overlap, both in terms of morphologic features and in the presence of increased IgG4-positive plasma cells. The prevalence of an S100-positive histiocytic infiltrate showing prominent lymphatic dilation with emperipolesis favors the former diagnosis.

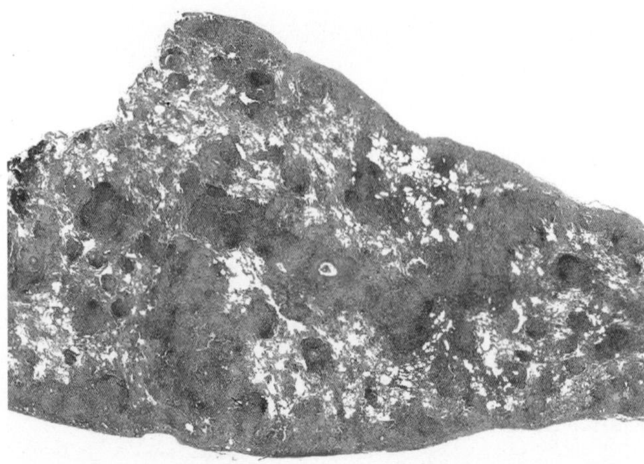

Figure 113.1 Lymphangitic distribution of a dense lymphoplasmacytic reactive infiltrate, involving visceral pleura, interlobular septa, and bronchovascular bundles.

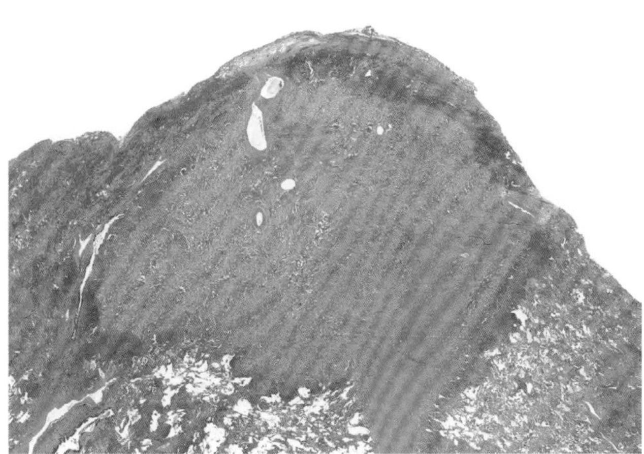

Figure 113.2 Dense hyaline fibrosis with storiform arrangement.

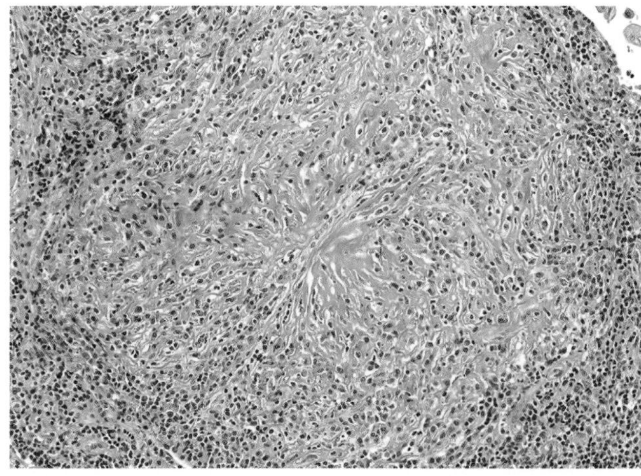

Figure 113.3 Venous channel completely obliterated by a dense lymphoplasmacytic infiltrate.

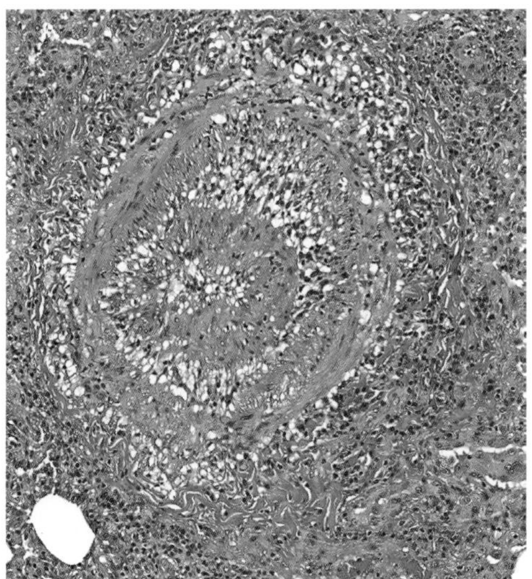

Figure 113.4 Nonnecrotizing lymphoplasmacytic arteritis, a fairly common feature of IgG4-related disease involving lung parenchyma.

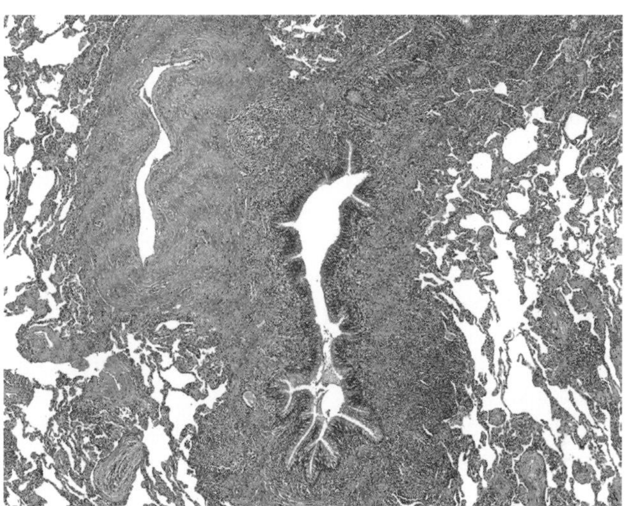

Figure 113.5 Concentric chronic bronchiolitis displaying lymphoid follicles, a nonspecific morphologic feature frequently encountered in IgG4-related disease.

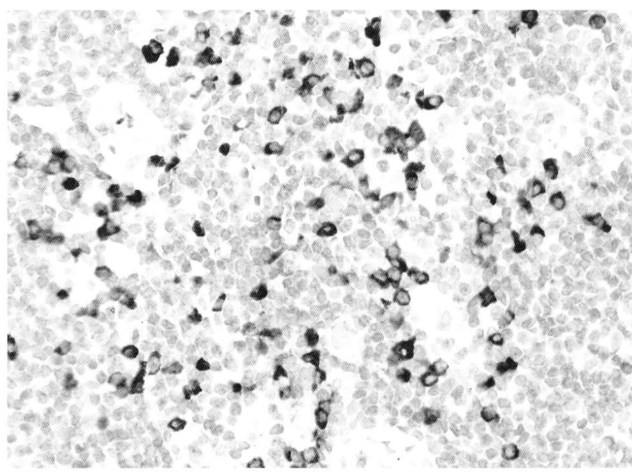

Figure 113.6 Immunohistochemistry revealing numerous IgG4+ plasma cells (>50 cells per high-power field).

114 Diffuse Meningotheliomatosis

▶ Maria Cecilia Mengoli
▶ Maxwell L. Smith

Diffuse pulmonary meningotheliomatosis (DPM) is a rare condition characterized by the presence of multiple bilateral meningothelial nodules. Patients show clinical symptoms of restrictive pulmonary disease and radiologic evidence of diffuse reticulonodular pulmonary infiltrates. DPM must be distinguished from incidental meningothelial nodules (previously known as *pulmonary chemodectomas*) that are of no clinical significance. Most incidental meningothelial nodules occurred in adults older than 40 years. Meningothelial nodules take their name by their striking similarities, on morphologic, immunohistochemical, and ultrastructural grounds, with meningiomas. Rarely, meningothelial nodules are so numerous (range from 30 to >100 per lung) to cause clinical and radiographic abnormalities in patients without other identifiable underlining lung disease. This is the condition of DPM. Most patients with DPM are females in their sixth and seventh decades of life with restrictive physiology and diffuse reticulonodular bilateral infiltrates on imaging studies.

HISTOLOGIC FEATURES

- Patients with DPM show multiple interstitial nodules ranging in size from a few cells to multiple centimeters.
- Nodules may be in the bronchovascular bundle or the peripheral/subpleural regions of the lobules.
- Nodules are composed of oval to spindle-shaped cells with abundant pink cytoplasm, indistinct cellular borders, and uniform bland oval nuclei with finely dispersed chromatin reminiscent of meningothelial cells.
- Many nodules will have cells with clear pseudonuclear inclusions, nuclear grooves/indentation, and prominent hyalinization of the vessel walls.
- No necrosis or increased mitotic figures are seen.
- The meningothelial cells are positive for EMA (weak but diffuse), vimentin, progesterone receptor, and CD56.
- The meningothelial cells are negative for cytokeratin, TTF-1, smooth muscle actin, muscle-specific actin, type IV collagen, desmin, S-100, CD1a, chromogranin A, synaptophysin, vascular markers (such as CD31, CD34, and D2-40), CD68, HER2/neu, E-cadherin, HMB45, and estrogen receptor.

DIFFERENTIAL DIAGNOSIS

The major differential diagnosis is with primary or metastatic neoplasms. The distribution of multiple bilateral pulmonary nodules is highly suspicious for metastatic neoplasm and recognition of the characteristic cytologic features and confirmatory immunohistochemical stains (EMA, vimentin, and progesterone receptor) can help confirm the diagnosis of DPM. Because of the exceedingly low frequency of intraspinal meningioma metastases, this is rarely considered. Primary pulmonary meningioma is an uncommon primary tumor of the lung that is typically a single isolated lesion. The possibility should be considered if a limited biopsy shows meningothelial cells. The differential diagnosis with neuroendocrine proliferations of the lung, namely tumorlets and carcinoids, is based on the expression of cytokeratin, chromogranin A, and synaptophysin in neuroendocrine lesions. Morphologically, meningothelial nodules may look similar to paraganglioma. Paraganglioma distinguishes itself by the positivity for neuroendocrine markers coupled with negativity for cytokeratin and presence of intermingled stellate S100+ spindle cells.

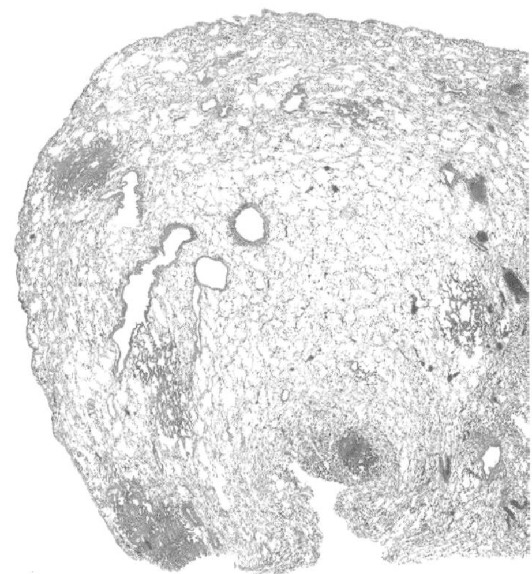

Figure 114.1 Multiple interstitial, subpleural, and peribronchovascular meningothelial-like nodules in diffuse meningotheliomatosis.

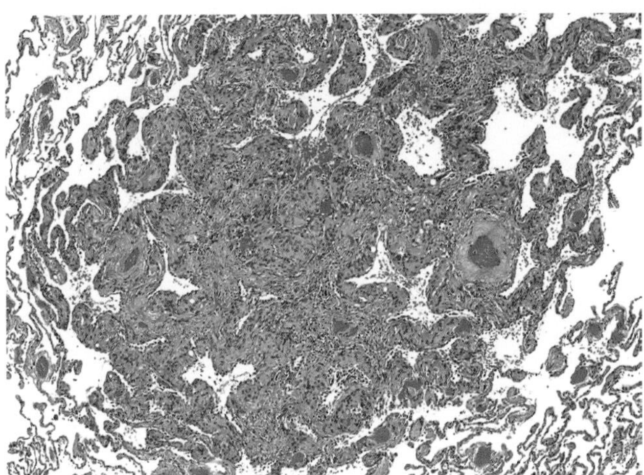

Figure 114.2 Meningothelial-like nodule with prominent hyalinization of the intermingled vessel walls.

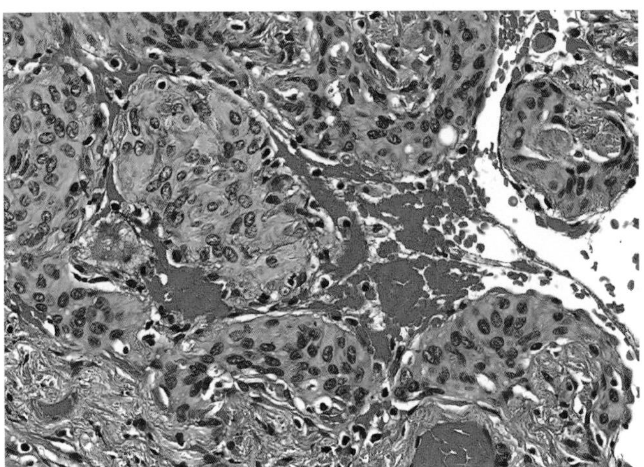

Figure 114.3 Oval to spindle-shaped cells with abundant pink glassy cytoplasm reminiscent of meningothelial cells with interstitial pattern of growth define meningothelial-like nodules.

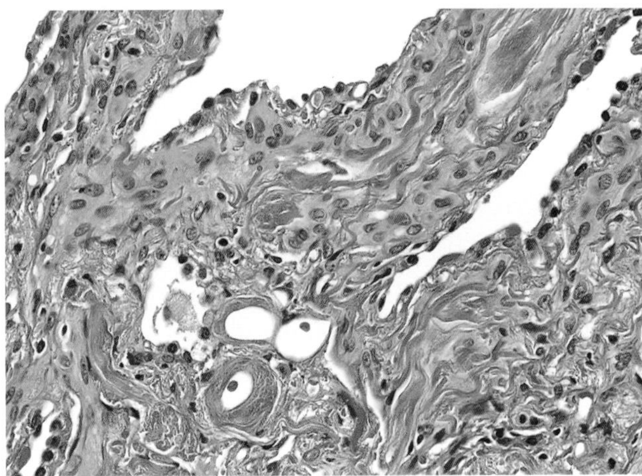

Figure 114.4 Nuclei are bland with finely dispersed chromatin and occasional pseudoinclusion.

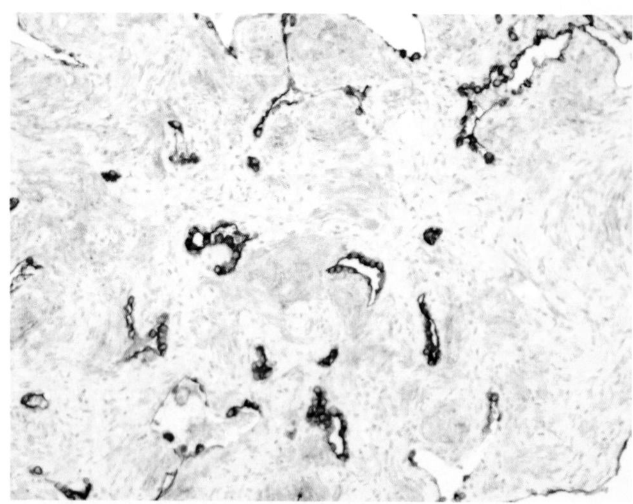

Figure 114.5 Diffuse cytoplasmic immunostaining with EMA in meningothelial-like nodules, weaker in comparison to the adjacent alveoli.

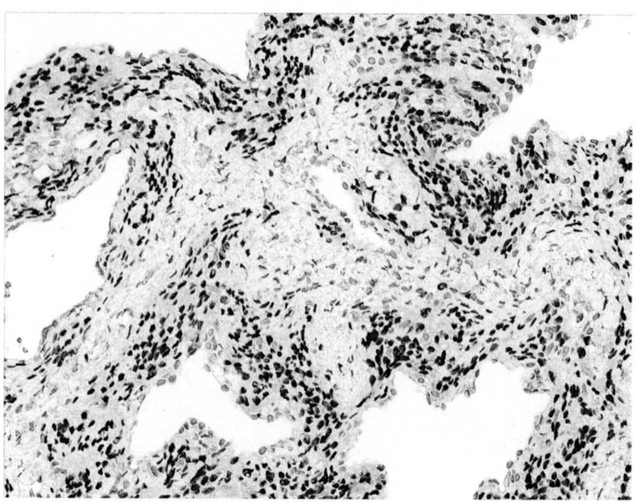

Figure 114.6 Diffuse nuclear positivity for progesterone receptor.

Section 16

Idiopathic Interstitial Pneumonias

▸ Kirtee Raparia

115

Acute Interstitial Pneumonia

▸ Kirtee Raparia

Acute interstitial pneumonia (AIP) is the pathologic correlate of Hamman–Rich syndrome, a rapidly progressive idiopathic interstitial pneumonia. The onset of shortness of breath is typically preceded by a prodrome of viral-like illness with cough and fever and respiratory failure within days or weeks. AIP can show pathologic features of early exudative phase and later organizing phase of diffuse alveolar damage. There is no known precipitating factor for AIP, although it is important to rule out infections (such as bacteria, viruses, mycoplasma, rickettsia, atypical mycobacteria, and pneumocystis), drug reactions, collagen vascular diseases, vasculitis, aspiration, and inhalational injuries in these patients. High-resolution computed tomography findings are usually not specific for the pathologic findings in patients with AIP. Mortality is high in these patients, up to 60%. Patients with sepsis, advanced age, and multiorgan failure have a worse prognosis.

HISTOLOGIC FEATURES

- The early exudative phases show necrosis of pneumocytes, endothelial cells, intra-alveolar fibrinous exudates, and formation of hyaline membranes.
- Diffuse interstitial fibroblastic proliferation associated with edematous myxomatous stroma and collapse of alveolar parenchyma is seen.
- Organizing phase shows organization of hyaline membranes with formation of airway space granulation tissue.
- Pulmonary vessels may have organizing and recent thrombi.
- In such cases, it is important to perform immunostains for viral antigens and special stains to rule out other infectious organisms.

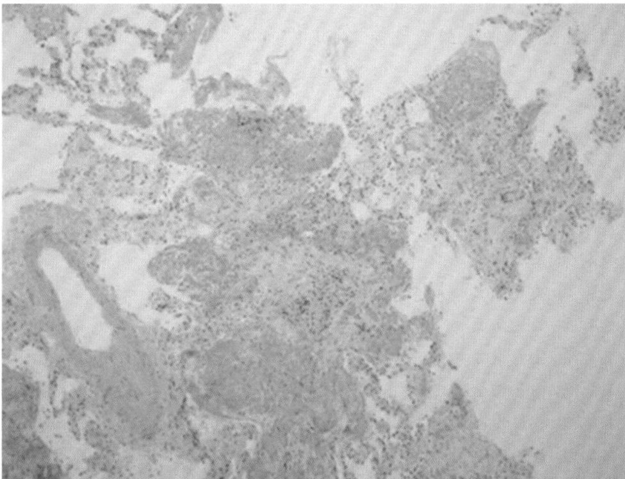

Figure 115.1 Early exudative phase shows intra-alveolar fibrinous exudates with formation of hyaline membranes and mild expansion of interstitium with myxomatous edematous stroma.

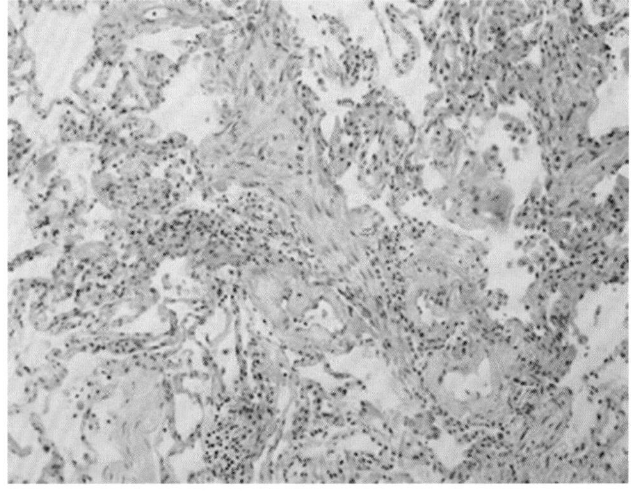

Figure 115.2 Organizing phase shows organization of hyaline membranes with formation of airway space granulation tissue, mimicking organizing pneumonia.

116 Usual Interstitial Pneumonia

Kirtee Raparia

Idiopathic cases of usual interstitial pneumonia (UIP) pattern on pathology are clinically referred to as *idiopathic pulmonary fibrosis* (IPF). The 2011 American Thoracic Society/European Respiratory Society statement on the diagnosis and management of IPF requires the exclusion of other known causes of interstitial lung diseases (e.g., domestic and occupational environmental exposures, connective tissue disease, and drug toxicity); presence of a UIP pattern on high-resolution computed tomography (HRCT) in patients not subjected to surgical lung biopsy; and specific combinations of HRCT and surgical lung biopsy pattern in patients subjected to surgical lung biopsy. Patients with IPF are characterized clinically by the insidious onset of dyspnea with a chronic and progressive downhill course. The great majority of patients with IPF are smokers, which may play a causative role apart from other environmental and genetic factors. Pulmonary function tests demonstrate restrictive defects in these patients. UIP is characterized histologically and radiologically by progressive chronic fibrosis of the parenchyma that is more prominent in the periphery of the lungs and in the lower lobes. UIP is the most common idiopathic interstitial pneumonia, comprising more than 60% of cases previously included under the category of IPF. Most patients are between the ages of 50 and 70 years, with an average age of onset in the sixth decade. Occasional cases have been reported in younger individuals. Men are affected about twice as often as women. UIP affects the lower lobes and the periphery of the lung first, eventually extending to the other areas of the lung. UIP in collagen vascular disease is typically seen in patients with slightly younger age and with less number of fibroblastic foci in their biopsies. These patients carry a slightly better prognosis than patients with IPF. Other diseases that may produce UIP pattern include drug reactions (e.g., amiodarone, nitrofurantoin, and some chemotherapeutic agents), chronic hypersensitivity pneumonitis, some cases of pneumoconiosis such as asbestosis, and rare cases of familial/genetic UIP. HRCT in classic cases show bilateral interstitial reticular markings that are most prominent at the bases and periphery of the lungs. Traction bronchiectasis and honeycomb changes can also be seen in similar distribution. These radiographic findings in an appropriate clinical setting may be diagnostic of UIP without the need for a surgical lung biopsy. However, often in 50% of cases, there may be other nonspecific findings, such as ground-glass opacities, upper lobe distribution, and absence of honeycomb changes, thus necessitating the need for a surgical lung biopsy. Appropriately controlled and blinded studies have shown that the traditionally used combination of corticosteroids and cytotoxic agent (azathioprine) to treat IPF actually resulted in worse outcomes in the treated group compared with the untreated group. Two novel agents pirfenidone and nintedanib have been shown to slow the rate of progression of pulmonary fibrosis in patients with IPF. The disease is usually progressive and ultimately fatal in most patients. These patients are at increased risk for lung cancer, pulmonary hypertension/cor pulmonale, respiratory failure secondary to progressive fibrosis, and increased pulmonary infections. Acute lung injury superimposed on UIP (acute exacerbation of UIP) is a cause of death in approximately 50% of patients with UIP. Median survival rates vary in the average range of 2 to 3 years in large series but approaching 4 to 6 years in few. The presence of underlying collagen vascular disease is associated with longer survival.

HISTOLOGIC FEATURES

- Heterogenous, patchwork pattern of lung fibrosis whereby scarred areas of lung are present adjacent to normal lung parenchyma resulting in spatial variability is a characteristic feature.
- Clear evidence of chronic scarring and architectural destruction in the form of microscopic honeycombing and traction bronchiectasis.
- The patchy pattern of interstitial fibrosis also results in temporal heterogeneity demonstrated by the presence of active fibroblastic foci representing "younger" foci of active ongoing disease compared with the more abundant "older" mature scarring areas.
- Fibroblastic foci consisting of proliferating fibroblasts and myofibroblasts in a myxoid or edematous stroma, typically at the interface between fibrotic and normal lung, representing sites of acute lung injury and comprising type III and type VI collagen.
- Fibrosis has a typical peripheral/subpleural accentuation and paraseptal distribution.
- End-stage honeycomb changes are characterized by enlarged airspaces with thickened fibrotic walls, lined by bronchiolar epithelium and inspissated mucus in the lumen of these spaces.
- Squamous metaplasia of the epithelial lining and hyperplasia of the smooth muscle are also common associated findings.
- Although UIP is primarily a fibrosing process, there is minimal to mild associated inflammation composed of lymphocytes and plasma cells and associated with hyperplasia of type II pneumocytes and bronchiolar epithelium.
- Lymphoid follicles with germinal centers in the fibrotic lung and pleura tend to be prominent in cases associated with collagen vascular diseases such as rheumatoid arthritis.
- Vascular changes are also common in the scarred areas, including intimal proliferation and medial thickening of muscular pulmonary arteries.
- Some patients may show areas of increased intra-alveolar macrophages in the alveolar spaces (desquamative interstitial pneumonia–like reactions) or areas of eosinophilic pneumonia.
- Sometimes, acute lung injury in the form of diffuse alveolar damage is superimposed in patients with UIP and is referred to as *acute exacerbation of UIP*.
- An isolated or occasional granuloma and/or a mild component of organizing pneumonia pattern may rarely be seen in biopsies with UIP pattern.

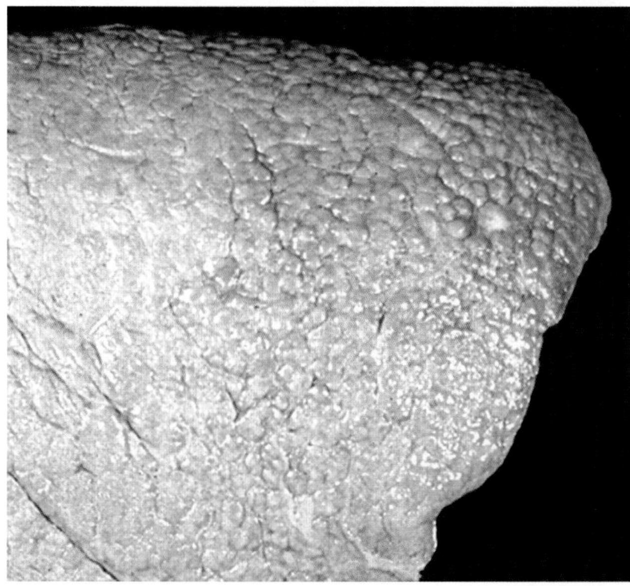

Figure 116.1 "Cobblestoning" of the pleural surface in UIP caused by retraction of interlobular septa due to subpleural fibrosis.

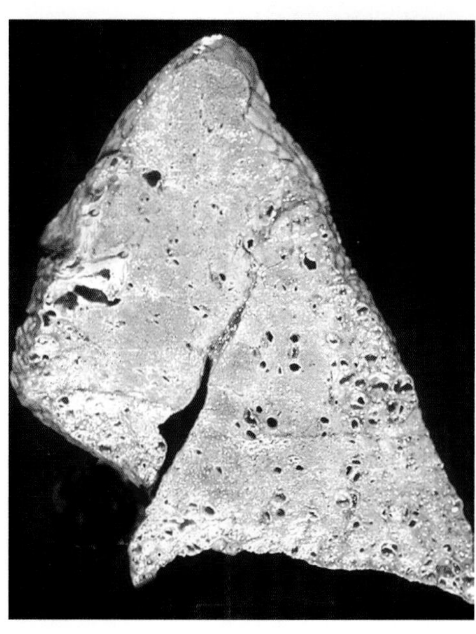

Figure 116.2 Cut surface shows more severe fibrosis subpleurally and in the lower lung zones.

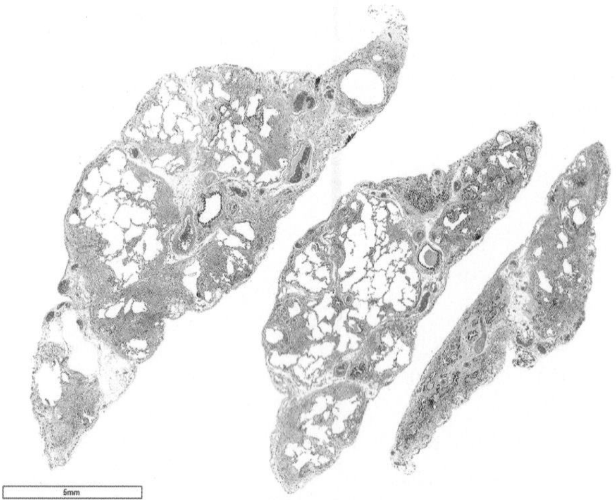

Figure 116.3 Low-power scanning image of patient with UIP pattern with architectural distortion and advanced fibrosis in a predominantly subpleural/paraseptal distribution.

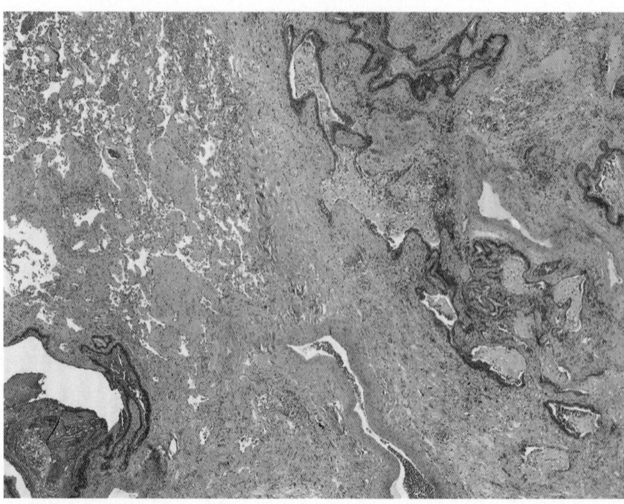

Figure 116.4 Spatial heterogeneity with areas of advanced fibrosis and honeycomb lung, next to less-affected lung parenchyma, can be seen.

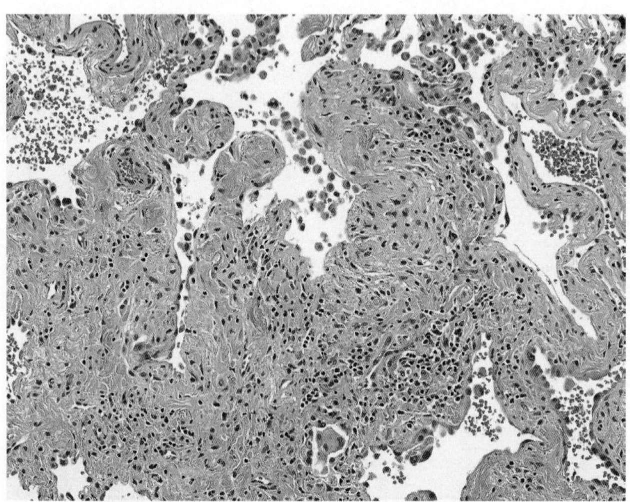

Figure 116.5 Fibroblastic foci are typically seen at the interface of normal and fibrotic lung and are composed of fibroblasts and myofibroblasts in a myxoid stroma.

117 Nonspecific Interstitial Pneumonia

Kirtee Raparia

Nonspecific interstitial pneumonia (NSIP) is defined as temporally and geographically homogeneous chronic interstitial pneumonia with variable degrees of inflammation and fibrosis. Biopsies of several specific entities, such as hypersensitivity pneumonitis, drug reactions (methotrexate and anti-TNF agents), and collagen vascular diseases (e.g., scleroderma), can show features that meet criteria of NSIP. Less often, NSIP pattern on a small biopsy might reflect a nonrepresentative biopsy of another disease or process. NSIP occurs often in middle-aged adults with female predominance and usually presents as shortness of breath, cough, and often constitutional symptoms including fever and fatigue. Most patients with NSIP pattern are nonsmokers. Physical examination features mild hypoxemia and inspiratory rales. Pulmonary function tests demonstrate restriction and a low diffusing capacity for carbon monoxide. High-resolution computed tomography abnormalities include predominantly lower lobe subpleural reticular changes, traction bronchiectasis, and ground-glass opacities; honeycombing is rarely seen. An evaluation of the underlying pathology is necessary for a firm diagnosis. Idiopathic NSIP is a diagnosis of exclusion and the 2013 update of the International Multidisciplinary Classification of the Idiopathic Interstitial Pneumonias accepts idiopathic NSIP as a specific clinicopathologic entity. Studies have shown that the clinical progression in patients with NSIP is highly heterogeneous and prognosis depends on the absence or presence of fibrosis. The cellular pattern of NSIP responds better to steroids compared to the fibrotic form.

HISTOLOGIC FEATURES

- NSIP is divided into cellular and fibrotic forms. Most cases of NSIP show cellular interstitial infiltrates composed of lymphocytes and plasma cells in a homogeneous pattern with preservation of underlying lung architecture.
- The fibrotic form of NSIP shows homogenous fibrosis, which widens the alveolar septa, producing architectural distortion in severe cases.
- Fibroblastic foci are rarely seen in NSIP but have been reported in the fibrotic form.

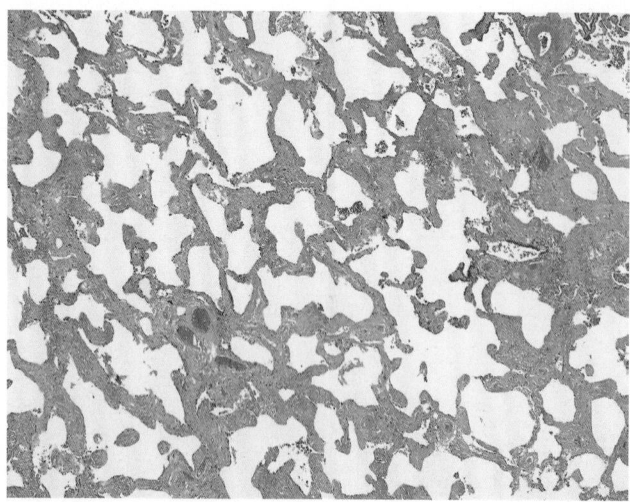

Figure 117.1 Diffuse alveolar wall expansion by increased lymphoplasmacytic infiltrate and preservation of underlying alveolar architecture (cellular NSIP).

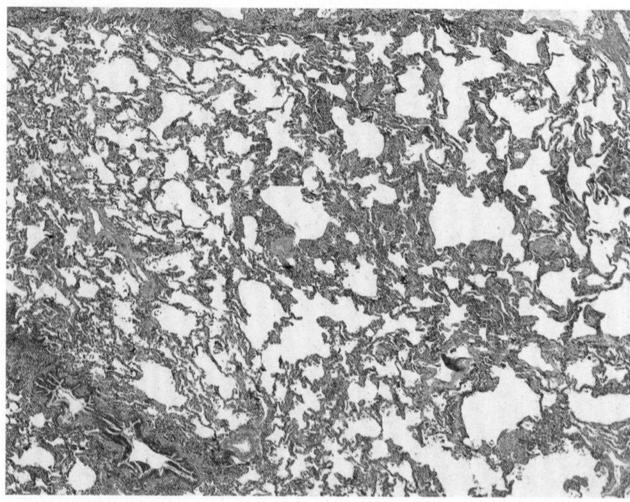

Figure 117.2 Diffuse alveolar wall thickening by uniform fibrosis with preservation of the alveolar architecture and no honeycombing or fibroblastic foci are seen (fibrotic NSIP).

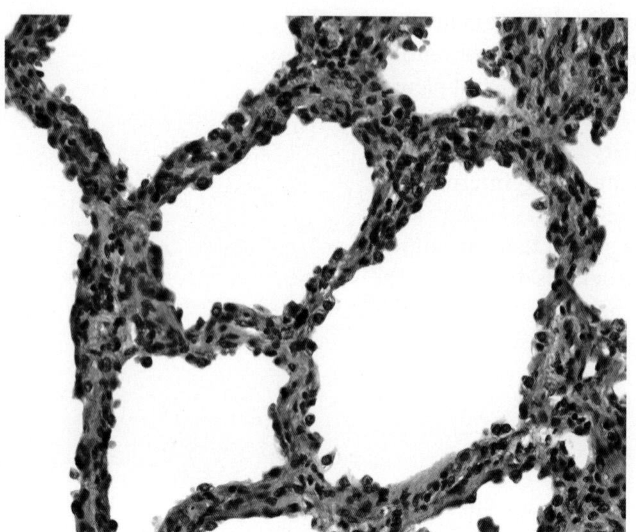

Figure 117.3 Higher power view shows homogeneous "linear" pattern of lymphoplasmacytic infiltrates in alveolar septa in cellular NSIP.

118 Cryptogenic Organizing Pneumonia

Kirtee Raparia

Organizing pneumonia, formerly referred to as *bronchiolitis obliterans organizing pneumonia*, consists of proliferation of granulation tissue within small airways, alveolar ducts, and alveoli with a typical branching appearance. It is commonly seen in middle-aged to older adults and is often preceded by a flu-like illness. Persistent nonproductive cough and shortness of breath are the usual presenting symptoms. It is a common histopathologic pattern seen in patients with subacute lung injury, which can be seen secondary to infections (bacterial or fungal), aspiration pneumonia, and drug reactions and can be seen as a minor component of many other diseases, such as hypersensitivity pneumonitis, collagen vascular disease, and Wegener granulomatosis. The idiopathic cases of organizing pneumonia are referred to as *cryptogenic organizing pneumonia*. Most, but not all, patients respond rapidly to steroids, and in most cases, prognosis is excellent. Relapses are commonly seen in patients when steroids are tapered. Prognosis of patients with secondary organizing pneumonia depends on the underlying condition.

HISTOLOGIC FEATURES

- Nodules of granulation tissue (fibroblasts in an edematous or myxoid stroma) in and around small airways with typical branching appearance.
- Mild to moderate interstitial inflammation composed of lymphocytes and plasma cells is typically seen.
- Areas of bronchiolitis and intra-alveolar foamy macrophages can be seen.
- No significant architectural destruction, neutrophils, eosinophils, vasculitis, or granulomas are seen.

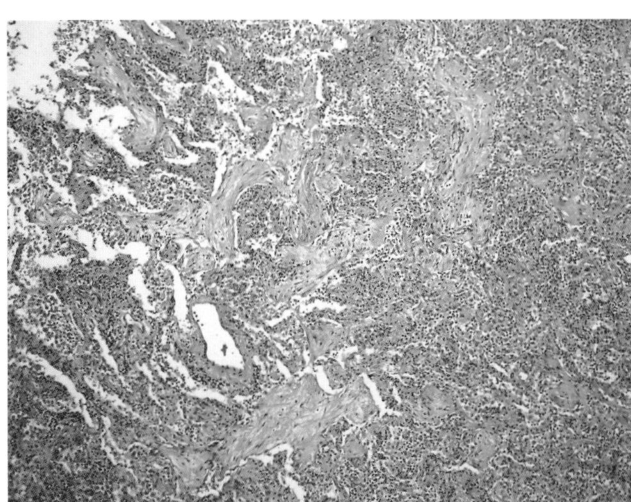

Figure 118.1 Plugs of granulation tissue with typical branching appearance and moderate interstitial inflammation can be seen in organizing pneumonia.

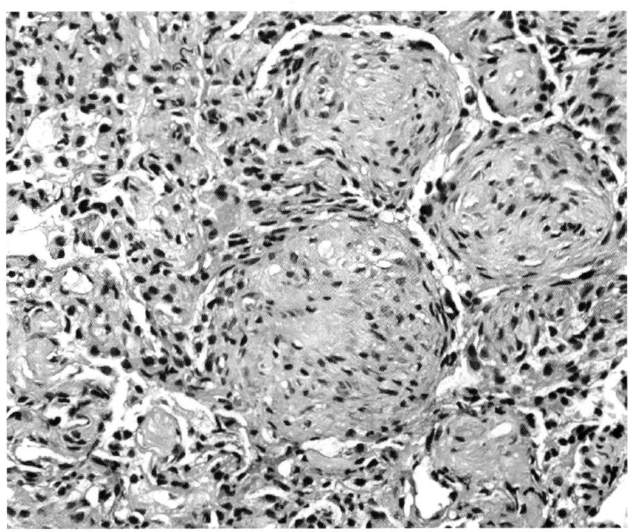

Figure 118.2 Higher power view of rounded Masson bodies shows that they are composed of fibroblasts in an edematous or myxoid stroma.

Idiopathic Pleuroparenchymal Fibroelastosis

119

▸ Kirtee Raparia
▸ John C. English

Idiopathic pleuroparenchymal fibroelastosis (PPFE) is a rare condition that consists of fibrosis involving the pleura and subpleural lung parenchyma, predominately in the upper lobes. PPFE is now a defined clinicopathologic entity in the updated 2013 American Thoracic Society (ATS)/European Respiratory Society (ERS) classification of idiopathic interstitial pneumonias. The fibrosis seen in PPFE is characterized by the deposition of collagen and elastic tissue, with the presence of intra-alveolar fibrosis. Localized PPFE is a common finding on surgical lung biopsies, which includes the apical region of the lung. Initial reports, originated in Japanese literature, were referred to as *idiopathic pulmonary upper lobe fibrosis*, also termed *Amitani disease*. Most cases are considered idiopathic, although a variety of associated conditions have been described, including posttreatment carcinoma with chemotherapy and/or radiotherapy, hematopoietic malignancies treated with chemotherapy and bone marrow transplantation, inhalation exposures, infections, gastrointestinal reflux disease, postlung transplantation, and in coexistence with usual interstitial pneumonia (UIP). This disease presents in adults with a median age of 57 years with no sex predilection. Most patients are nonsmokers. Approximately half of the patients experience recurrent infections or may have an autoimmune condition, whereas few may have familial interstitial lung disease and nonspecific autoantibodies. Most patients present with dyspnea on exertion and dry cough and have restrictive lung function tests. A small number of patients are asymptomatic despite abnormalities on imaging. High-resolution computed tomography show subpleural reticular/nodular opacities, initially favoring the upper zones followed by pleural fibrosis and linear or wedge-shaped extension down secondary lobular septa. The middle and lower zones may not be affected initially, but progressive envelopment of these regions occurs with time. In more advanced cases, volume loss and traction bronchiectasis may be prominent features. An increased incidence of pneumothorax is noted in these patients. Clinical outcome in PPFE is variable with a significant number of patients demonstrating progressive decline and death, particularly those with lung or bone marrow transplants. Survival characteristics depend on the stage of the disease at presentation because some patients are diagnosed in a relatively asymptomatic phase. Aside from lung transplantation, there is no demonstrated effective treatment.

HISTOLOGICAL FEATURES

- Gross specimen description in the literature is limited, likely reflecting the paucity of recognized cases at autopsy or the rare cases of transplantation.
- Microscopic examination shows dense collagenous fibrosis with or without concomitant elastosis of the visceral pleura; encasement of the lung begins in the apical region, with progressive extension into the inferior zones.
- Dense subpleural bands of parenchymal fibroelastosis follow this same distribution. The pattern is histologically distinctive in that vague outlines of alveoli are preserved or even accentuated by elastotic proliferation, presumably within the alveolar septa.

- The enclosed airspaces are filled with collagenous fibrosis of variable density. At the (typically sharp) interface with normal parenchyma, the intra-alveolar fibrosis may assume the features of fibroblastic foci.
- The inflammatory component within the fibrous regions is typically sparse and lymphocytic, occasionally with lymphoid follicles.
- Patients diagnosed with PPFE may also show concurrent histologic patterns, including UIP, nonspecific interstitial pneumonitis, and hypersensitivity pneumonitis in the underlying lung parenchyma.

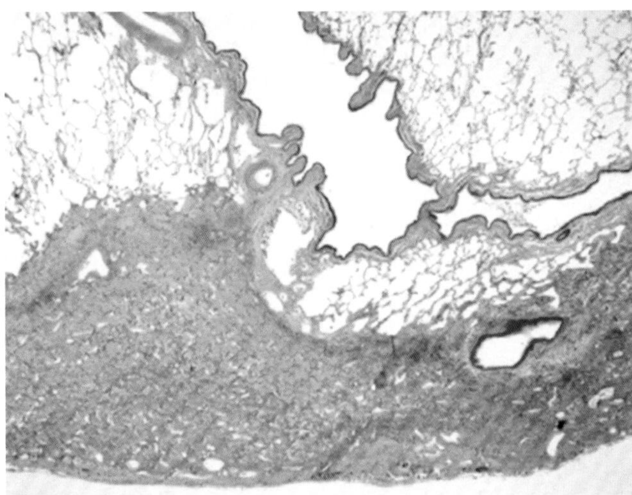

Figure 119.1 Low-power image shows subpleural fibroelastosis, which focally extends into lung parenchyma, but shows an abrupt interface with the uninvolved lung.

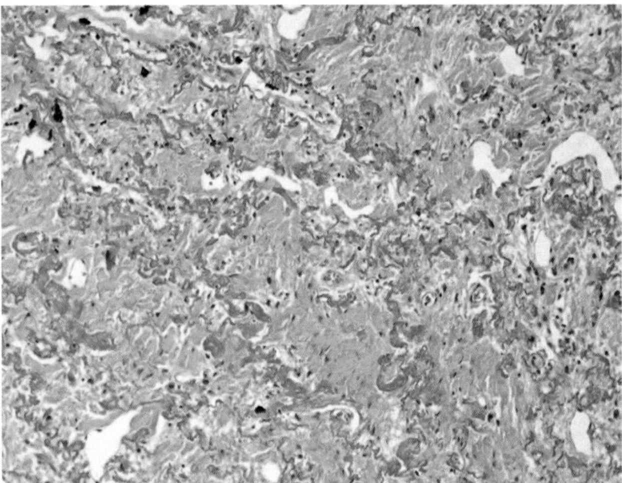

Figure 119.2 Higher power image shows characteristic intra-alveolar fibrosis.

Section 17

Specific Infectious Agents

▶ Alain Borczuk

Viruses

120

Many pulmonary viral infections are diagnosed based on laboratory testing, such as culture, serologies, viral load, or molecular testing. In these settings, pulmonary histology may reflect general lung injury patterns, such as bronchiolitis or diffuse alveolar damage. However, some viruses cause characteristic cytopathic changes, including multinucleation, cytomegaly, and inclusions (nuclear and/or cytoplasmic). These findings can be supported using immunohistochemistry in some instances.

Part 1

Cytomegalovirus

▸ Alain Borczuk

Cytomegalovirus (CMV) is a herpes virus that causes pneumonia in patients with compromised immune systems. CMV can be transmitted by infected body fluids. Patients can present with fever and a mononucleosis-like illness. It rarely causes pneumonia in immunocompetent individuals. In the immunocompromised host, CMV pneumonia can be severe and life-threatening.

HISTOLOGIC FEATURES

- Cellular enlargement.
- Dense single nuclear inclusion that follows the contour of the nucleus, with a clear halo around it (Cowdry type A, "owl's eye" appearance). The nuclear inclusions can be seen in other herpes virus family infections.
- Cytoplasmic inclusions, usually basophilic, but occasionally may be more eosinophilic. These cytoplasmic inclusions are characteristic of CMV infection.
- Inclusions are seen in pneumocytes and endothelial cells; however, mesenchymal cells such as smooth muscle cells can also be involved.
- The interstitial pneumonitis is mild and lymphocytic, but severe lung injury with diffuse alveolar damage can also occur.

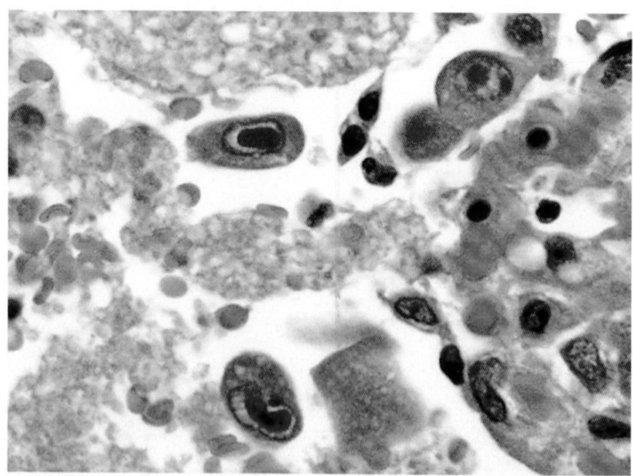

Figure 120.1 CMV infection causes basophilic, "owl's eye" nuclear inclusions with a clear halo.

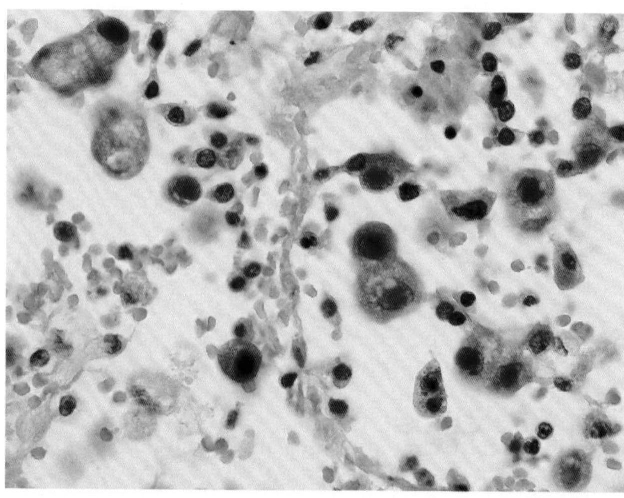

Figure 120.2 Cytoplasmic inclusion imparts a basophilic appearance to the cytoplasm, with peripheral distribution in this cell.

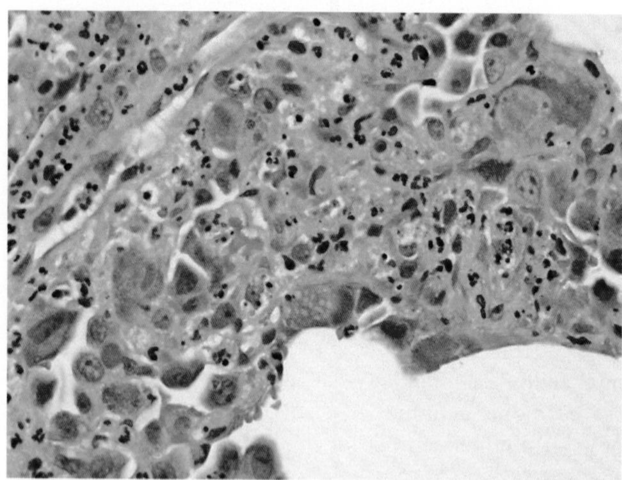

Figure 120.3 In some cases, inclusion in the cytoplasm can appear more eosinophilic.

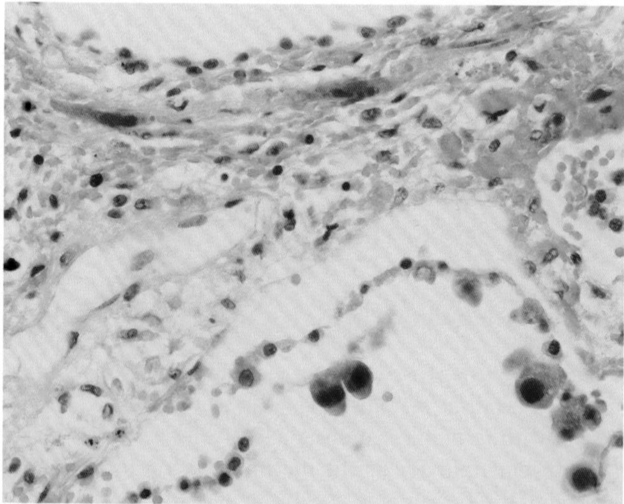

Figure 120.4 Both pneumocytes and mesenchymal cells (endothelial and smooth muscle) can show cytomegalic changes.

Part 2

Herpes Simplex Virus

▶ Alain Borczuk

Herpes simplex virus (HSV) infections cause a necrotizing pneumonia or tracheobronchitis, usually in immunocompromised individuals. The degree of acute inflammation may be severe, and as a result HSV pneumonia may show morphologic overlap with bacterial bronchopneumonia. Nuclear enlargement and multinucleation are characteristic, but nuclear inclusions, while present, can be harder to identify. Immunohistochemistry can be very useful in confirming the diagnosis in suspicious cases.

HISTOLOGIC FEATURES

- Multinucleated and enlarged cells.
- Nuclear inclusions are more eosinophilic than the basophilic, dense inclusions of CMV; these inclusions can be glassy, filling the majority of the nucleus or a single eosinophilic inclusion with a surrounding halo.
- Cytoplasmic inclusions are not seen.

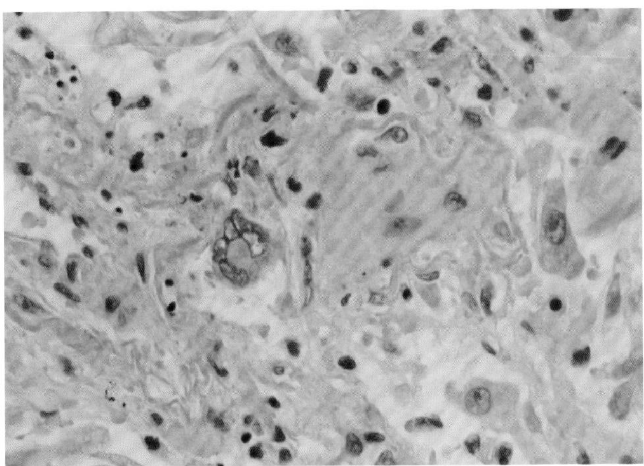

Figure 120.5 Herpes pneumonia results in multinucleated cells, here with intranuclear inclusions that are eosinophilic with a clear halo.

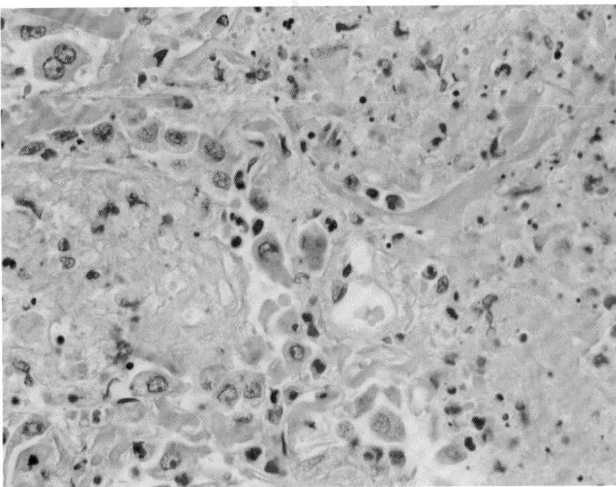

Figure 120.6 Some nuclear inclusions have a more glassy appearance. Pneumonia can be necrotizing with neutrophils.

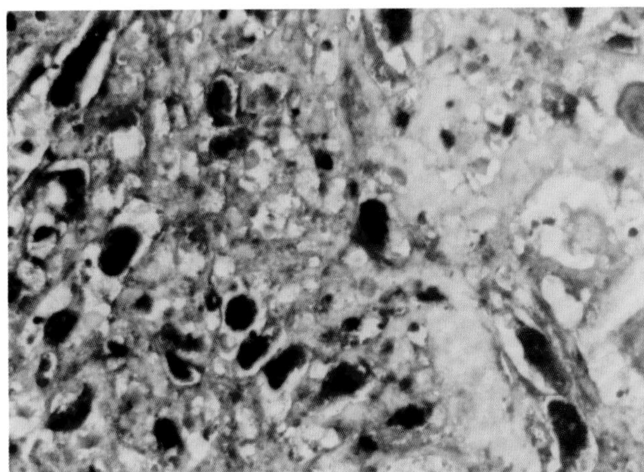

Figure 120.7 Immunohistochemistry can highlight numerous infected cells, some of which do not have visible inclusions on hematoxylin and eosin (H&E) stains.

Part 3

Varicella Zoster Virus

Alain Borczuk

Varicella zoster virus (VZV) is a herpes virus that causes chicken pox and shingles (herpes zoster). Adults and immunocompromised patients may develop VZV pneumonia. Although VZV pneumonia can manifest with diffuse lung injury, in later stages the pneumonia consists of small nodules that can resolve or calcify.

HISTOLOGIC FEATURES

- Cytopathic features are similar to those of HSV.
- Nodules can have central necrosis but are not granulomatous; they can become fibrotic and hyalinized or can calcify.

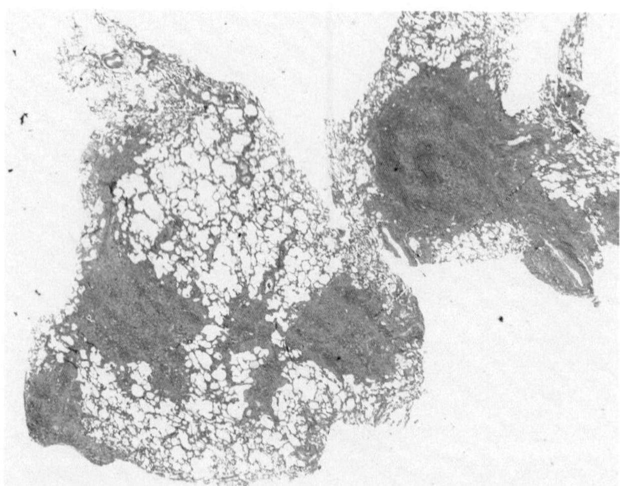

Figure 120.8 Varicella can cause multiple nodules that can resemble military infection; these eventually hyalinize.

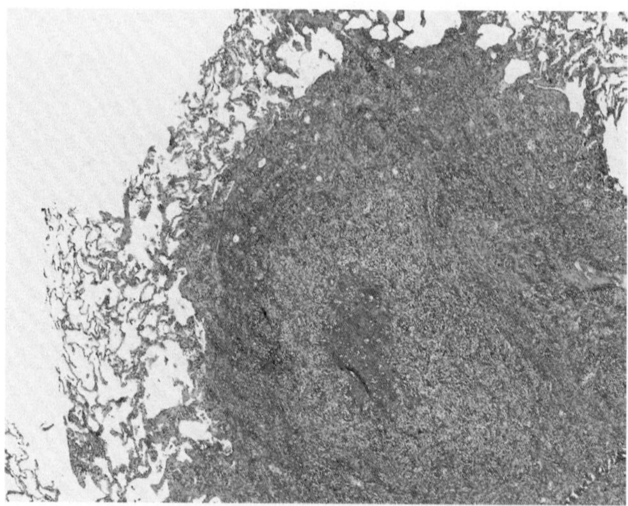

Figure 120.9 These nodules can show central necrosis (and calcification, not shown) but are not surrounded by a histiocytic rim.

Part 4

Adenovirus

▸ Alain Borczuk

Adenovirus is a DNA virus that can cause pneumonia in immunocompetent and immunocompromised hosts. It can result in upper respiratory infection, pneumonia with bronchiolitis, and conjunctivitis. Necrosis in small airways can be seen. More serious infections can result in diffuse alveolar damage.

HISTOLOGIC FEATURES

- Intranuclear inclusions can resemble Cowdry type A inclusions as seen in CMV, but more characteristic are smudge cells with basophilic blurring of nuclear chromatin.
- The inclusions are dark and basophilic on H&E stain.
- Cytomegaly, multinucleation, and cytoplasmic inclusions are not seen, in contrast to VZV, HSV, and CMV.
- Immunohistochemistry can be helpful in establishing the diagnosis.

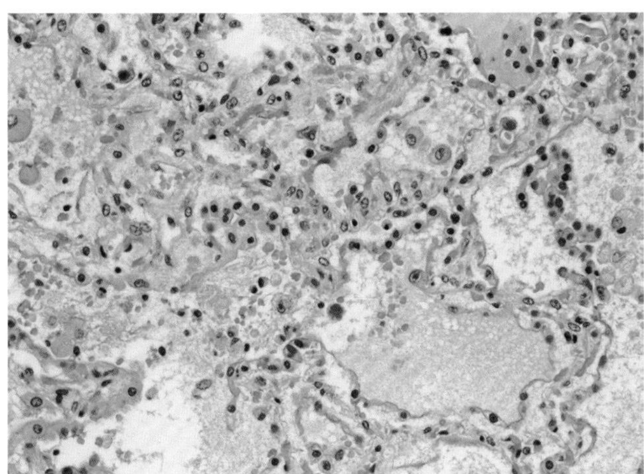

Figure 120.10 Adenoviral pneumonia leads to acute respiratory distress syndrome with type II pneumocyte hyperplasia.

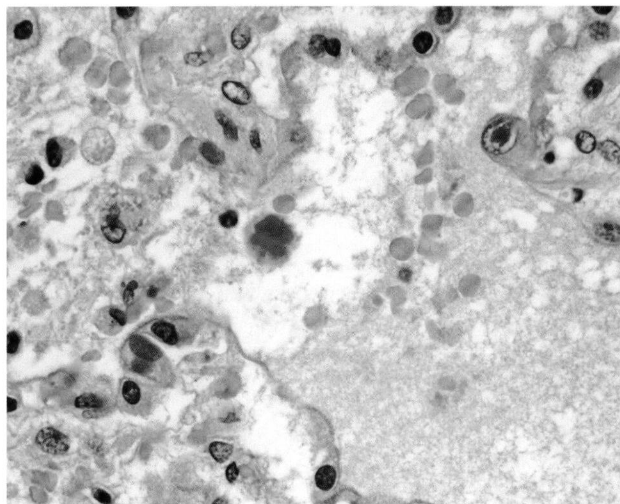

Figure 120.11 Pneumocytes can show two patterns of cytopathic change with smudge cells *(center)* and Cowdry type A inclusions *(right)*.

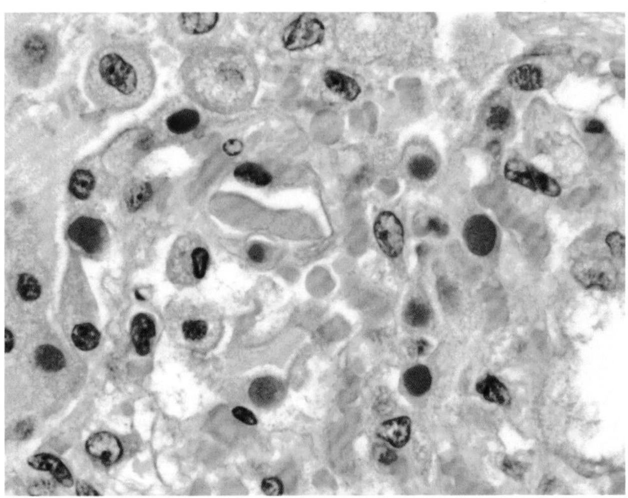

Figure 120.12 Smudge cells with basophilic homogeneous chromatin.

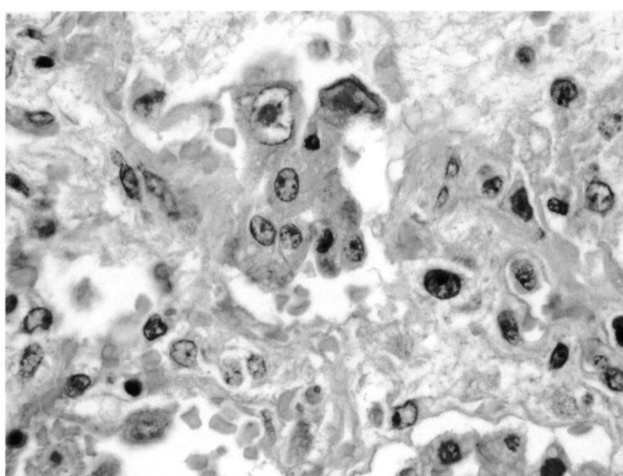

Figure 120.13 Cowdry type A–like inclusions can be seen in adenoviral infection.

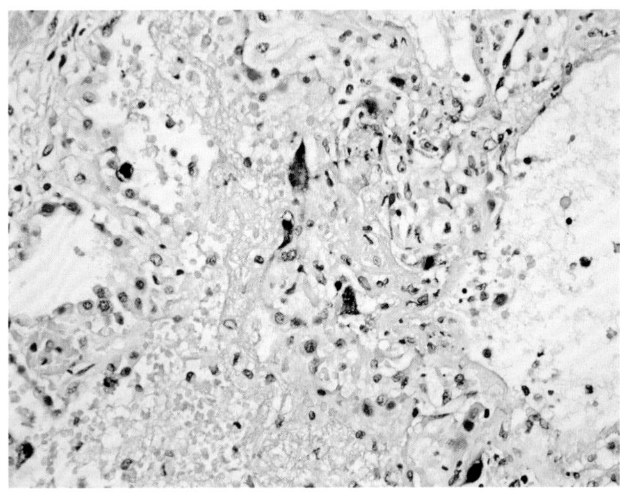

Figure 120.14 Immunohistochemistry for adenovirus can confirm the diagnosis.

Part 5

Influenza

▶ Alain Borczuk

Influenza viruses are RNA viruses that can infect respiratory epithelial cells. Influenza viruses have two types, A and B, and cause seasonal outbreaks. It can cause mild and severe symptoms and can lead to pneumonia.

HISTOLOGIC FEATURES

- Diffuse alveolar damage with hyaline membranes is a feature of severe influenza virus infection.
- No characteristic cytopathic changes are associated with influenza infection.

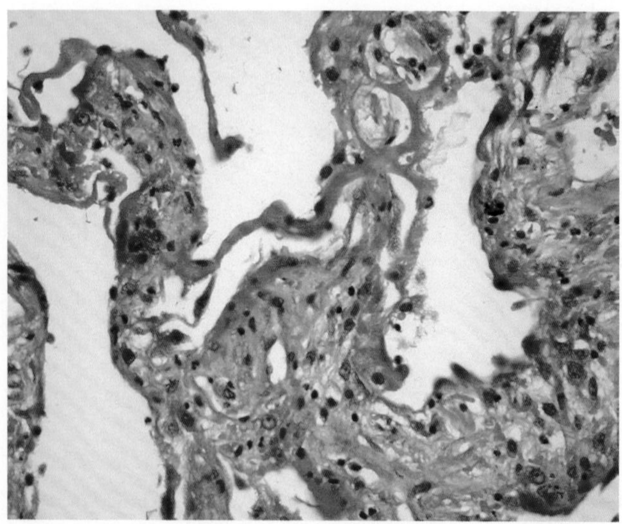

Figure 120.15 Influenza pneumonia causes histologic changes of acute respiratory distress syndrome with hyaline membranes.

Part 6

Parainfluenza

▶ Alain Borczuk

Human parainfluenza virus infections can cause upper and lower respiratory infections in children and adults. Croup and bronchiolitis can be seen in children and immunocompromised adults. Pneumonia can be seen due to parainfluenza virus 3. Immunohistochemistry can be supportive of the diagnosis.

HISTOLOGIC FEATURES

- Parainfluenza pneumonia causes syncytial giant cells. Giant cell pneumonia with multinucleation can be seen in measles and respiratory syncytial virus as well as parainfluenza virus.

- Nuclear inclusions are not seen, but cytoplasmic inclusions can be present.
- Bronchiolitis with epithelial infection can lead to epithelial injury and squamous metaplasia.

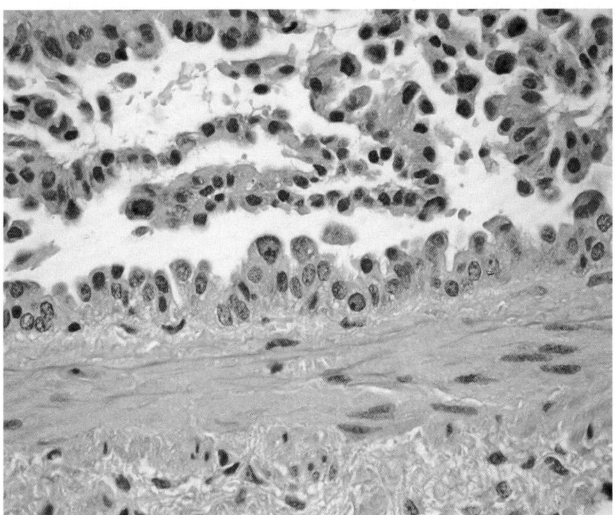

Figure 120.16 Bronchiolar lining cells show regenerative changes and some nuclear atypia.

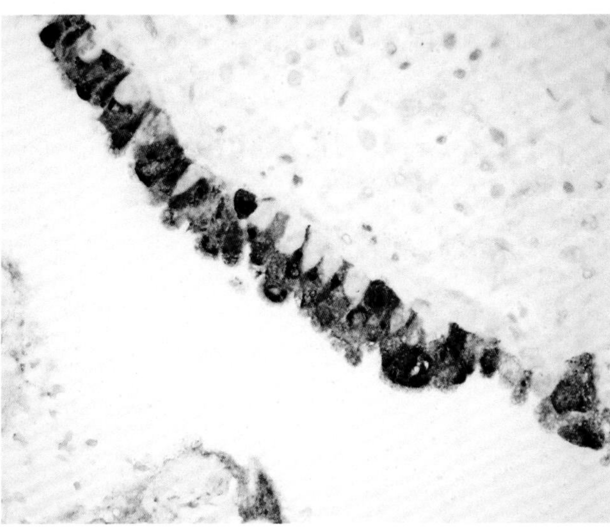

Figure 120.17 Immunohistochemistry for parainfluenza virus strongly stains these atypical bronchiolar cells.

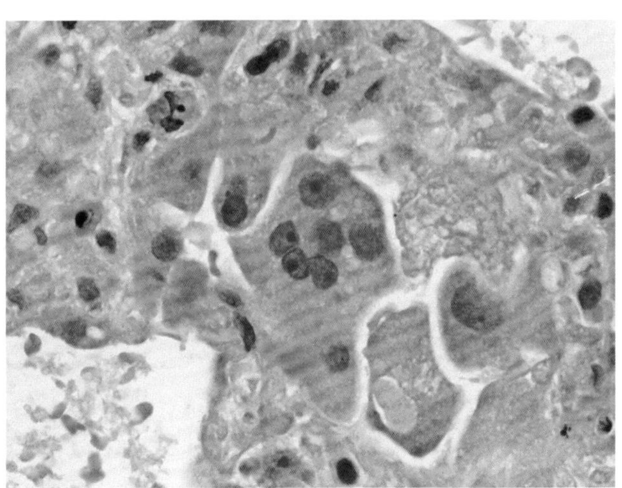

Figure 120.18 Multinucleation is a feature of parainfluenza infection, as are eosinophilic cytoplasmic inclusions.

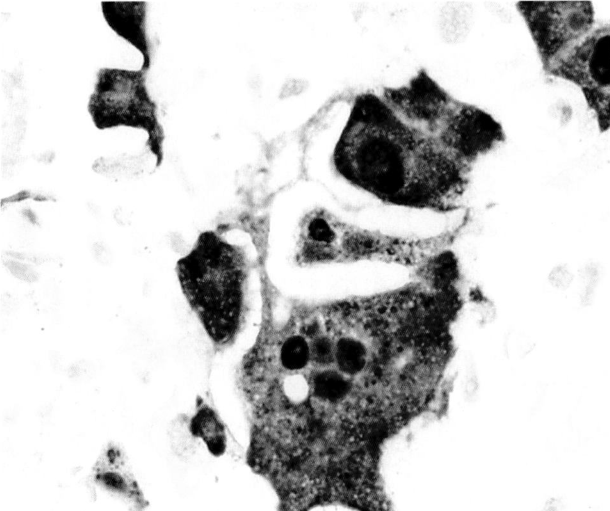

Figure 120.19 Immunohistochemistry for parainfluenza virus stains the multinucleated cell cytoplasm and the cytoplasmic inclusions.

Part 7

Measles

▶ Alain Borczuk

Measles is an RNA virus of the paramyxovirus family. It is highly contagious and causes fever, cough, runny nose, sore throat, and white spots inside the mouth. These symptoms are followed by skin rash and upper respiratory symptoms. In young children and adults, measles can result in pneumonia and encephalitis, with potentially life-threatening consequences. Outbreaks can occur in unvaccinated populations and in immunosuppressed individuals.

- The Warthin–Finkeldey giant cell is a syncytial giant cell with numerous nuclei.
- Measles causes intranuclear eosinophilic inclusions with a pale halo around them.
- In addition, eosinophilic cytoplasmic inclusions are seen.

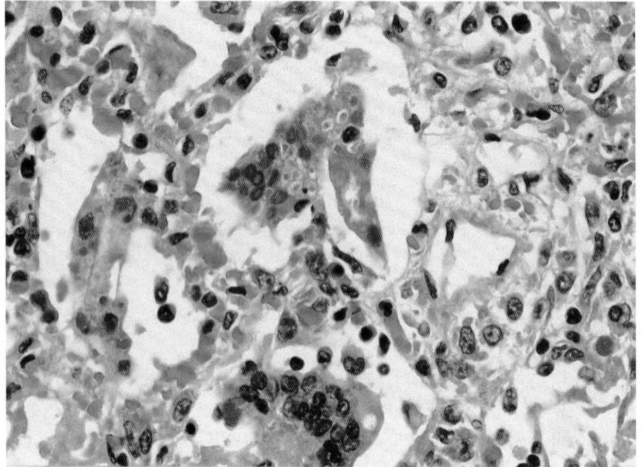

Figure 120.20 These multinucleated syncytial cells show eosinophilic cytoplasmic inclusions, and the lower cell shows visible nuclear inclusions.

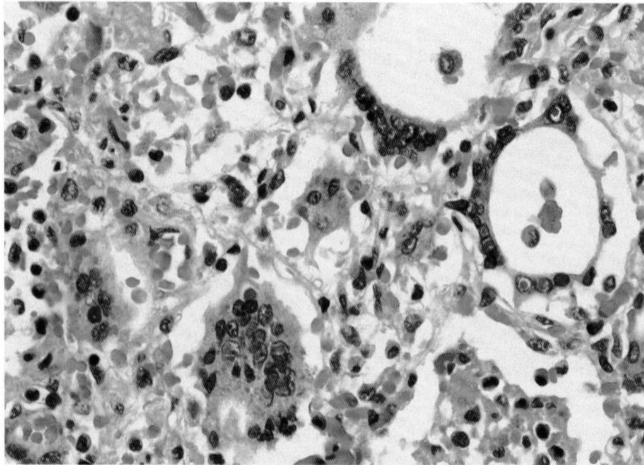

Figure 120.21 Eosinophilic nuclear inclusions with a clear halo around them are better visualized in the giant cell on the *lower left*.

Part 8

Respiratory Syncytial Virus

▸ Alain Borczuk and Debra Beneck

Respiratory syncytial virus (RSV) is an RNA virus of the paramyxovirus family that also consists of measles and mumps. It is a common respiratory virus that results in common cold–like symptoms, most often in infants and children, and causes bronchiolitis when it involves the lung. Lung involvement in children occurs in up to 40% of cases. Disease can be especially severe in premature infants and in the immunocompromised individuals. Patients with heart and lung disease can also be susceptible.

HISTOLOGIC FEATURES

- Conducting airways show evidence of epithelial injury and regeneration, with basal layer hyperplasia that can eventually result in squamous metaplasia.
- It represents a giant-cell pneumonia with multinucleated syncytial giant cells.
- Eosinophilic cytoplasmic inclusion of variable size can be identified.
- No nuclear inclusions.
- Inflammation, mostly lymphocytic, is seen in the lung tissue.

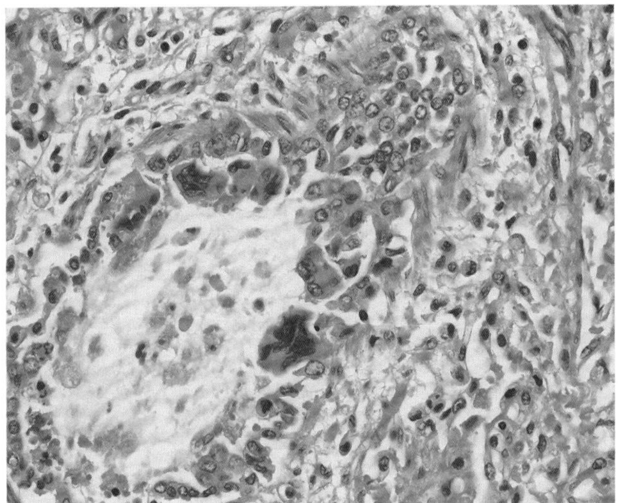

Figure 120.22 This small airway shows regenerative epithelium and numerous syncytial giant cells of RSV infection.

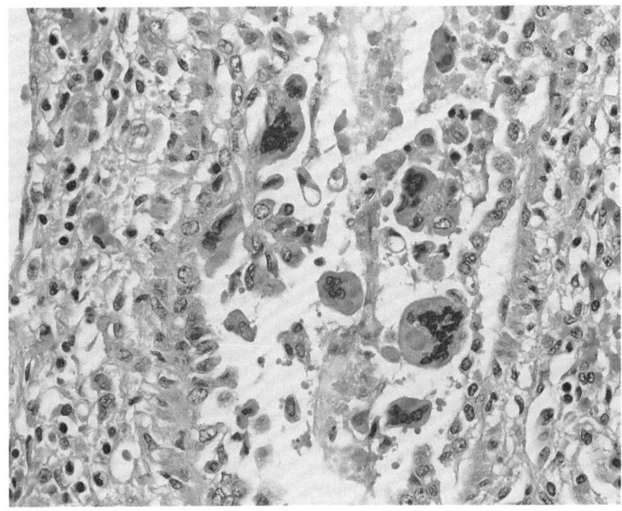

Figure 120.23 These syncytial giant cells show dark nuclei without inclusions. Eosinophilic cytoplasmic inclusions are seen.

Part 9

Hantavirus

Alain Borczuk

Hantavirus pulmonary syndrome is a severe respiratory illness that is caused by exposure to rodents. Person-to-person transmission has not been reported. This infection causes progressive pulmonary edema and acute respiratory distress syndrome and can occur in otherwise healthy individuals. Muscle aches are characteristic in early phases, especially of large muscles.

HISTOLOGIC FEATURES

- A mild mononuclear interstitial inflammation is seen along with edema.
- This progresses to diffuse alveolar damage with hyaline membranes and type 2 pneumocyte hyperplasia.

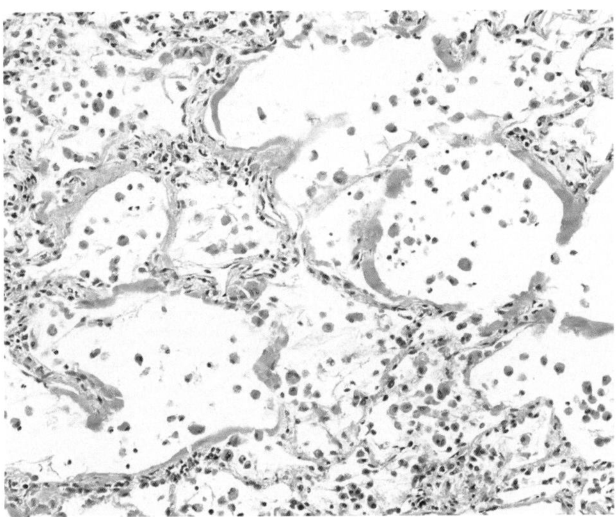

Figure 120.24 A diffuse mild mononuclear cell infiltrate is seen along with interstitial widening and hyaline membranes.

Bacteria

121

Part 1

Streptococcus

▸ Alain Borczuk

Streptococcal pneumonia, mostly frequently caused by *Streptococcus pneumoniae*, is the most common cause of community-acquired bacterial pneumonia internationally (earning its name "pneumococcus"). In addition to pneumonia, it can cause meningitis and otitis media. Pneumococcal pneumonia can be complicated by bacteremia, pericarditis, and empyema. Although young children and elderly individuals are more susceptible to pneumonia and prone to complications, pneumococcal pneumonia remains a significant cause of pneumonia in otherwise healthy adults. Even in the antibiotic era, the fatality rate remains significant. Pneumococcal vaccine can prevent infection and is offered to patients older than 65 years, as well as to those with immunocompromised states, hemoglobinopathies, and asplenia.

HISTOLOGIC FEATURES

- Classic descriptions of pneumococcal pneumonia included "lobar pneumonia," a fast-spreading infection involving a lobe of lung, all at the same age of development.
- Acute infection consists of intra-alveolar accumulation of neutrophils; with time, organization includes an influx of macrophages.
- The organism is a gram-positive diplococcus.

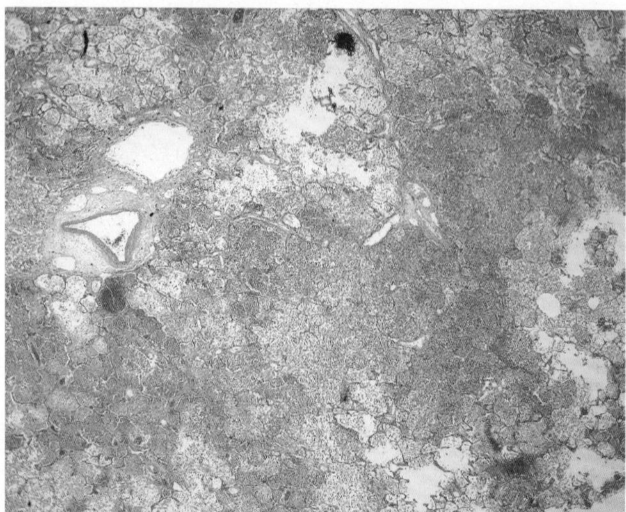

Figure 121.1 Low-power view of pneumococcal pneumonia showing a relatively uniform diffuse alveolar filling process.

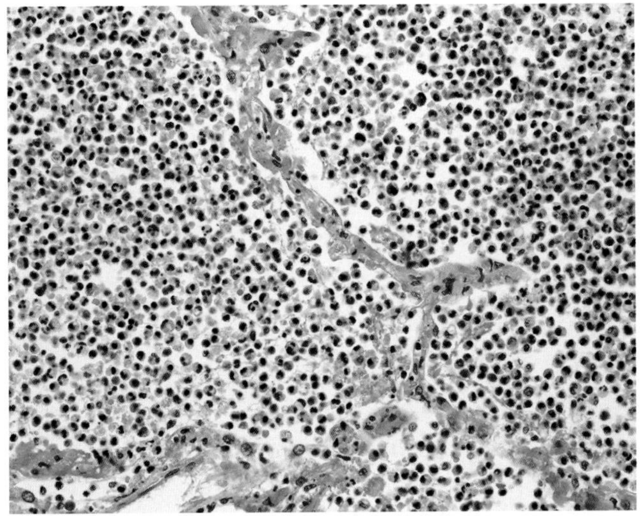

Figure 121.2 The alveolar filling process, in the acute phase, represents a robust accumulation of neutrophils.

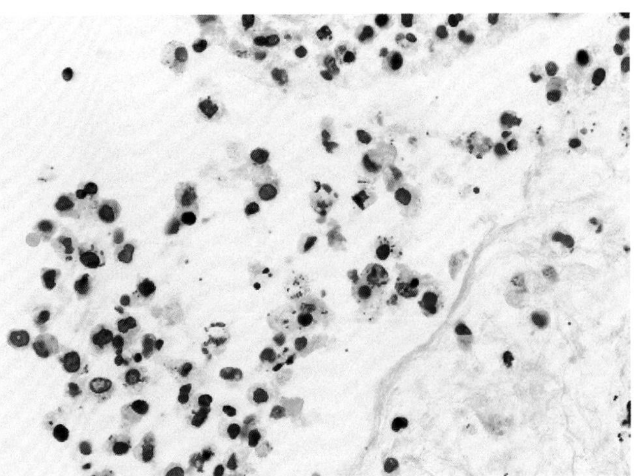

Figure 121.3 *Streptococcus* organisms are gram-positive diplococci (Gram stain).

Part 2

Staphylococcus

Alain Borczuk

Staphylococcus aureus is a gram-positive coccus that is carried in the nasal cavity in a subset of the population. Pneumonia can result when a large inoculum of organisms reaches the lower airway. This can occur via aspiration, via mechanical ventilation, and in situations where normal airway function is compromised (such as postviral airway metaplasia). In addition, *Staphylococcus* can reach the lung via the bloodstream, for example, in patients with bacterial endocarditis. The tendency of this organism to cause necrotizing pneumonia leads to abscess formation and can result in pleural extensions, resulting in empyema.

HISTOLOGIC FEATURES

- Staphylococcal pneumonia is necrotizing and can result in abscess formation.
- Cases of tracheobronchitis can result in membrane formation.
- The organism is a gram-positive coccus, and abundant organisms can be seen in sheets and clusters.

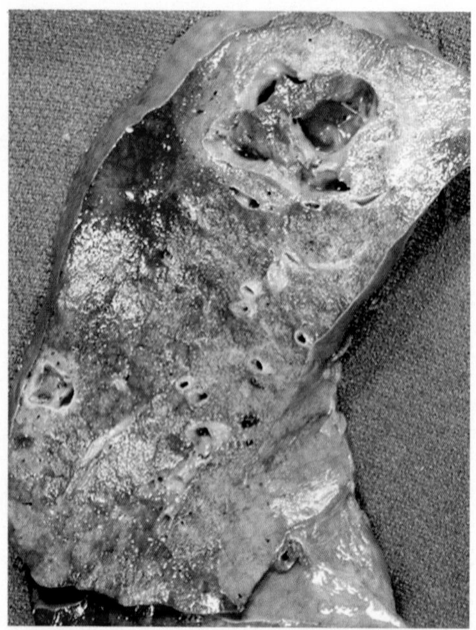

Figure 121.4 Staphylococcal pneumonia resulting in abscess formation.

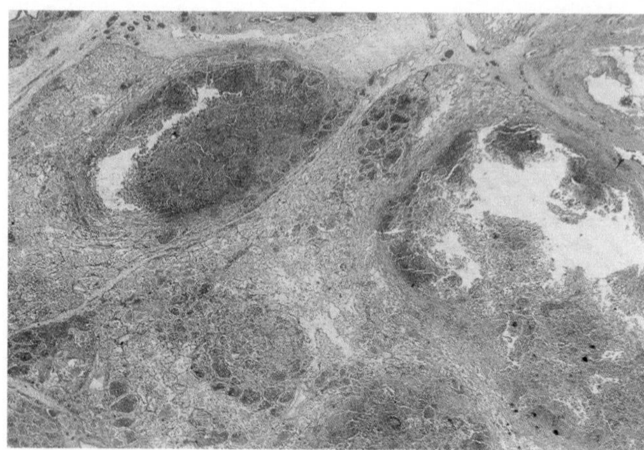

Figure 121.5 Regions of suppuration lead to tissue destruction and abscess formation.

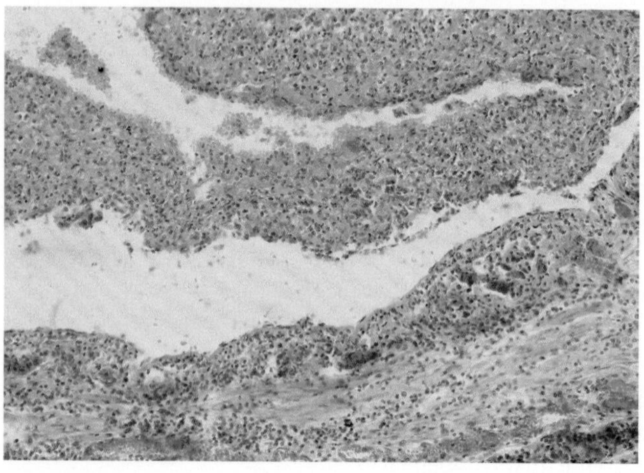

Figure 121.6 Rare cases of *Staphylococcus* cause a necrotizing bronchitis with membrane formation, mimicking diphtheria infection.

Part 3

Klebsiella

Alain Borczuk

While *Klebsiella pneumoniae* is a rare cause of community-acquired pneumonia (restricted to certain endemic areas), when it occurs, it has a risk factor association with alcoholism. In addition, it continues to be a wider health problem, as it has increased as a cause of hospital-acquired pneumonia. It is spread through contact and can affect individuals on ventilators and with intravenous catheters. Antibiotic-resistant strains have emerged as a significant health risk. Risk of spread to healthy adults is low.

HISTOLOGIC FEATURES

- As in other acute pneumonias, stages go from neutrophil influx to increasing numbers of macrophages, with resolution, organization, or scarring.
- The organism is a gram-negative bacillus.

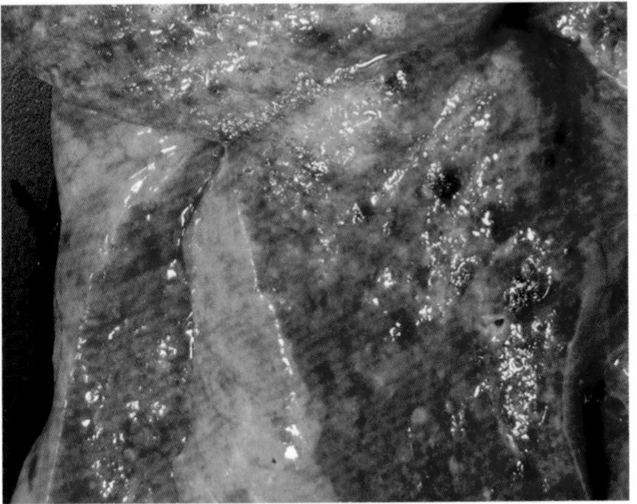

Figure 121.7 Bronchopneumonia with patchy pneumonia at different stages of development as manifested by differences in color.

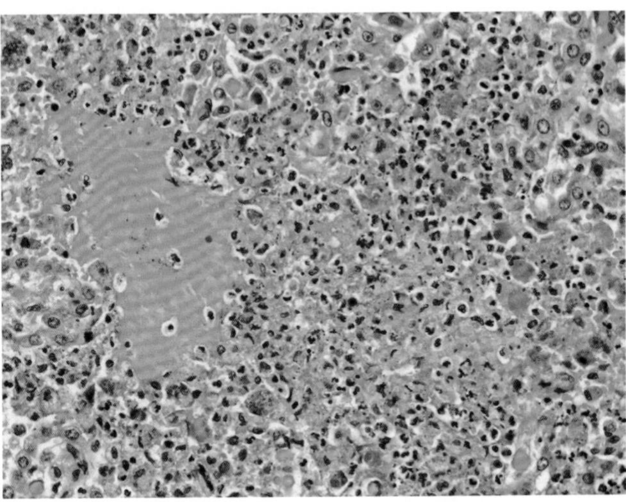

Figure 121.8 Necrotizing pneumonia with neutrophils.

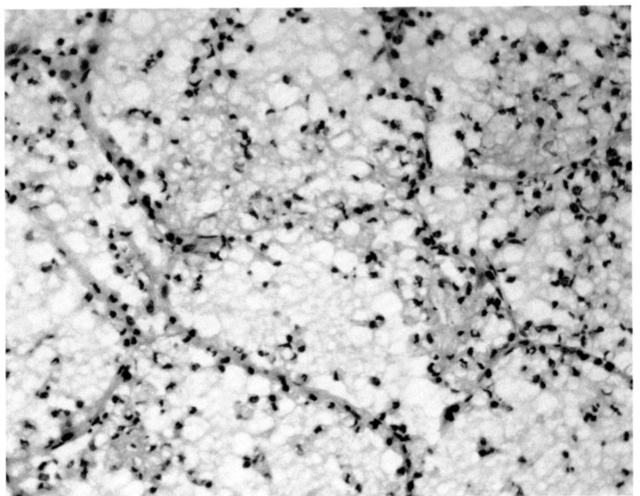

Figure 121.9 More sparse neutrophils and a mucoid background.

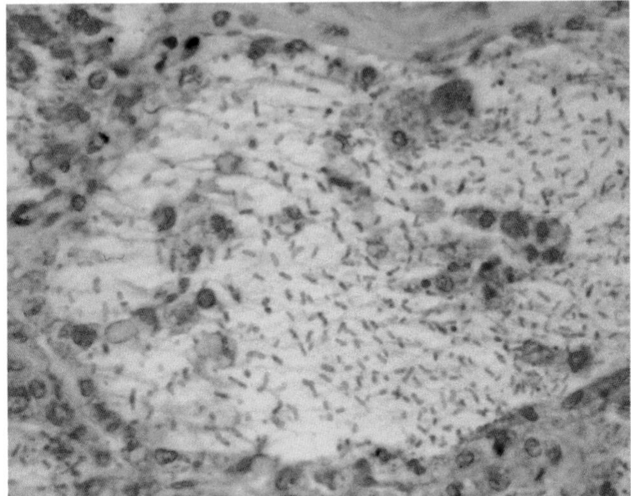

Figure 121.10 Gram-negative rods of *K. pneumoniae*.

Part 4

Pseudomonas

Alain Borczuk

Pseudomonas pneumonia is usually a hospital-acquired infection. However, patients with cystic fibrosis are susceptible to infection with *Pseudomonas*, as well as with *Burkholderia cepacia* and *Stenotrophomonas maltophilia* (formerly *Pseudomonas cepacia* and *Pseudomonas maltophilia*). Bronchopneumonia extending from colonized intrabronchial secretion can occur, as can hematogenous infection. The organism can cause an infectious vasculitis with resultant hemorrhage and infarction.

HISTOLOGIC FEATURES

- Necrosis, abscess, and infarct-like areas with hemorrhage.
- Infectious vasculitis can be seen.
- In cystic fibrosis, bronchiectatic airways filled with neutrophils.
- Gram-negative bacillus.

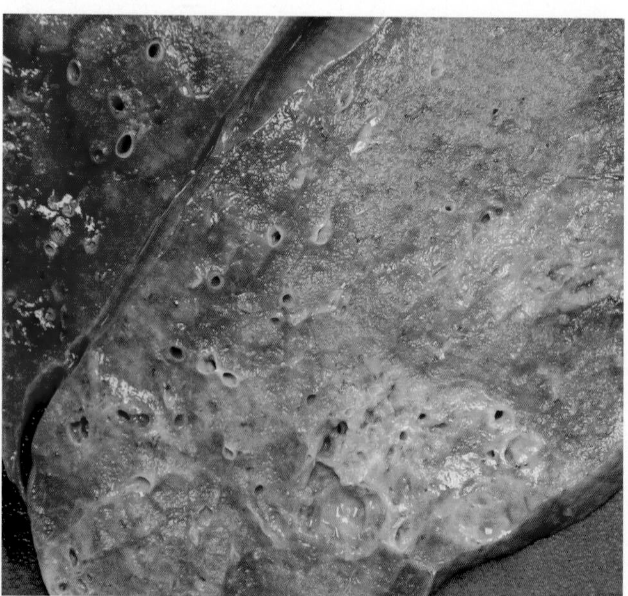

Figure 121.11 Pseudomonas pneumonia with tissue destruction and abscess formation.

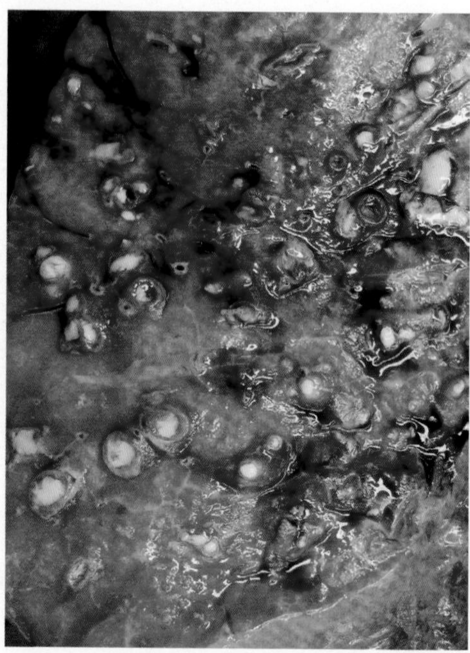

Figure 121.12 Cystic fibrosis lungs with yellow–green purulent intrabronchial secretions.

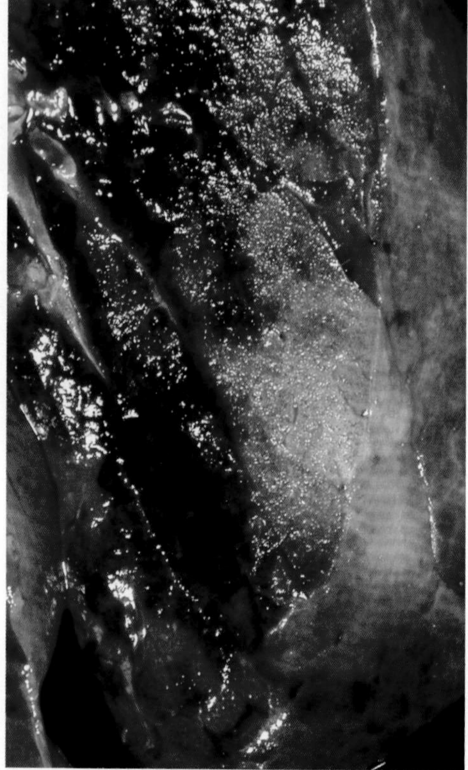

Figure 121.13 Hemorrhagic pneumonia with areas of bland infarction.

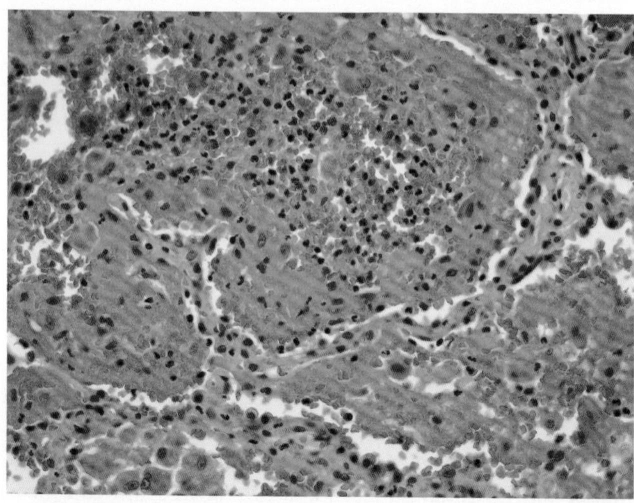

Figure 121.14 Hemorrhagic pneumonia with neutrophils.

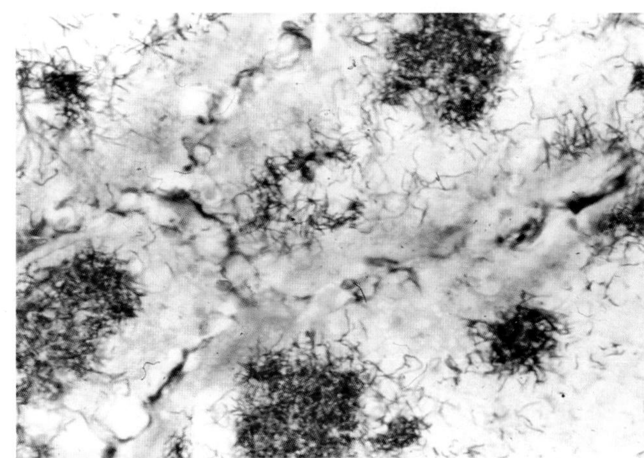

Figure 121.15 A Warthin–Starry stain highlights numerous slender rod-shaped organisms.

Part 5

Legionella

Alain Borczuk

Legionnaire's disease was named after a serious outbreak of pneumonia that occurred during an American Legion convention in 1976. Pontiac fever, a less severe manifestation of the disease also caused by *Legionella*, does not result in pneumonia. It is thought that the infection is derived from contaminated freshwater, and outbreaks are often linked to contaminated man-made water sources, such as plumbing or cooling towers. Although exposed individuals do not always develop the disease, people older than 50 years or with preexisting lung disease are at risk for developing pneumonia.

The most common cause of Legionnaire's disease is *Legionella pneumophila*. It can result in a severe pneumonia with progression to diffuse alveolar damage. The organism is a gram-negative bacillus with a wide range of lengths from short (2 μm) to long (20 μm) organisms. It grows within alveolar macrophages. Although described as gram-negative, it can be difficult to detect without silver stains such as Warthin–Starry, Steiner, or Dieterle stains.

HISTOLOGIC FEATURES

- Diffuse alveolar damage, characterized by interstitial neutrophils and karyorrhexis ("dirty diffuse alveolar damage").
- Intra-alveolar macrophages, although this varies based on the timing of tissue sampling.
- Short rods on Warthin–Starry stains.
- Pitfalls—species such as *Legionella micdadei* are positive on acid-fast bacilli stain, but shorter than *Mycobacteria*.

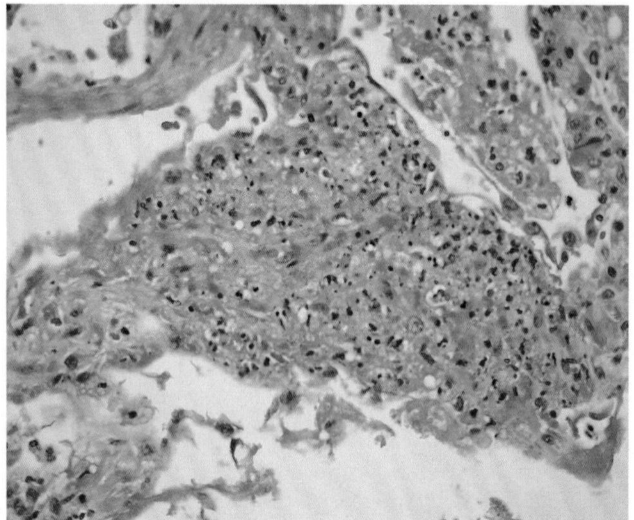

Figure 121.16 Diffuse alveolar damage with neutrophils and karyorrhexis.

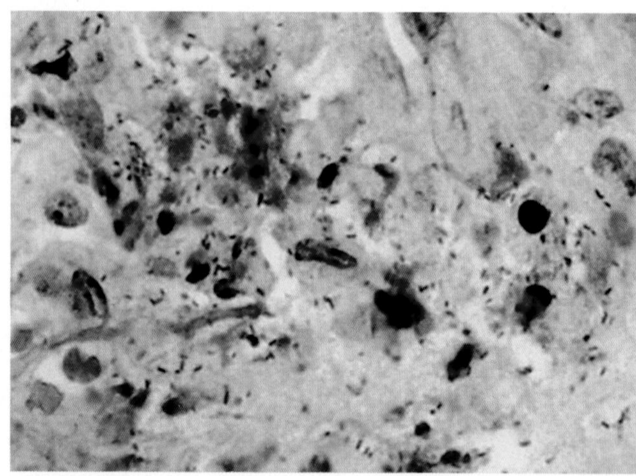

Figure 121.17 Short rods best identified with silver impregnation stains (Warthin–Starry) are shown.

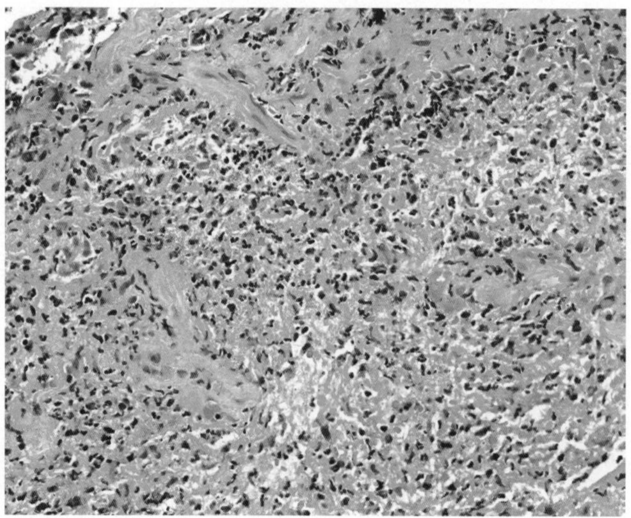

Figure 121.18 An acute pneumonia/abscess without granulomatous inflammation caused by *L. micdadei*.

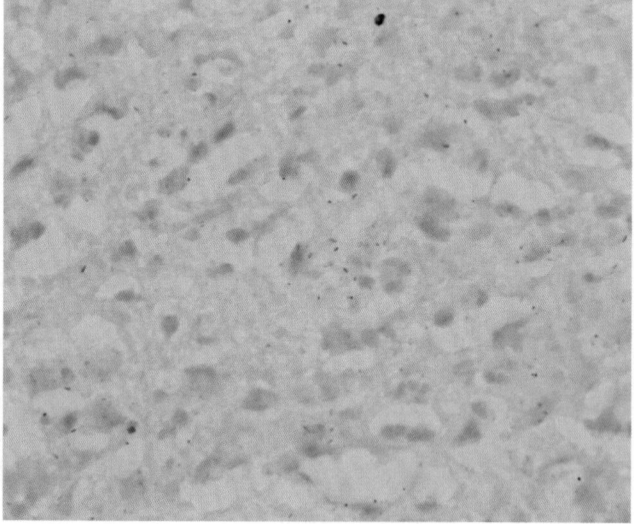

Figure 121.19 An acid-fast stain showing short acid-fast rods in this abscess caused by *L. micdadei*.

Part 6

Actinomyces

Alain Borczuk

Actinomyces are filamentous anaerobic gram-positive bacteria that are commonly encountered in the oropharynx. Pulmonary infection derives from aspiration of oropharyngeal contents, and presentation is often with a mass lesion that can show cavitation.

HISTOLOGIC FEATURES

- Abscess formation.
- Sulfur granules within the abscess—aggregates of the filamentous bacteria surrounded by a proteinaceous material that may help resist phagocytosis (Splendore–Hoeppli phenomenon).
- Organisms are gram-positive filamentous bacteria that also stain on silver stains such as Gomori methenamine silver (GMS).

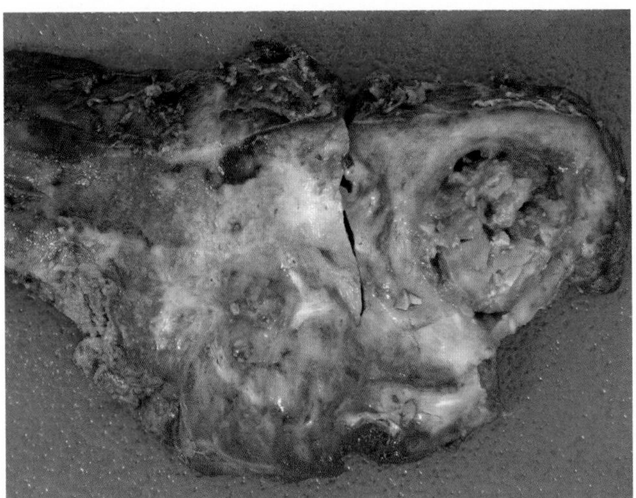

Figure 121.20 Cavitary mass due to *Actinomyces* infection.

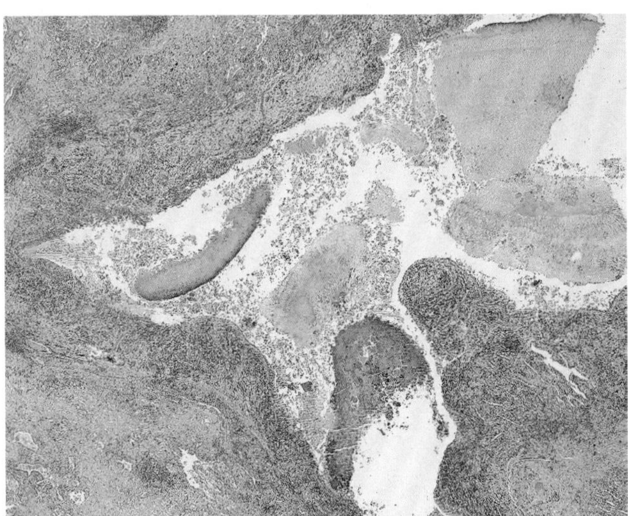

Figure 121.21 Bronchiolectasia filled with neutrophils and amorphous basophilic aggregates of organisms.

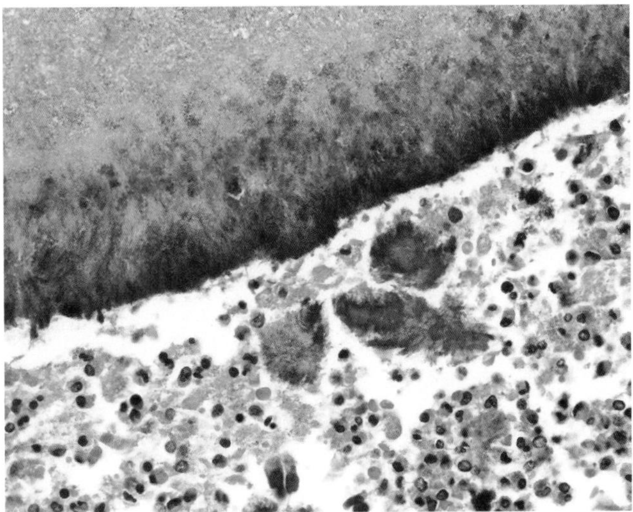

Figure 121.22 Aggregates of bacteria for the sulfur granule surrounded by neutrophils and eosinophilic proteinaceous material.

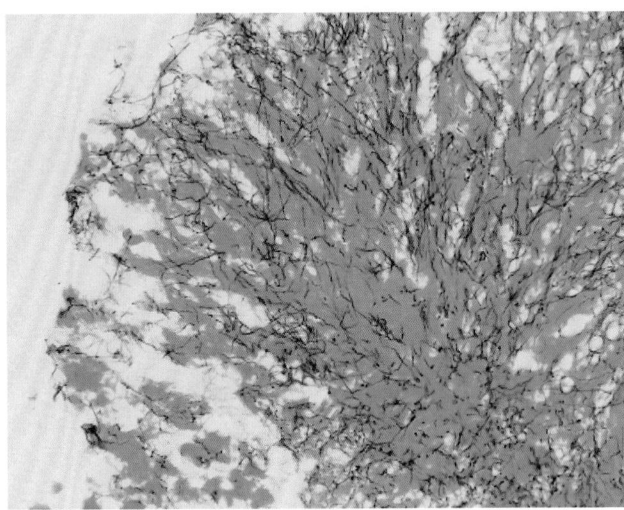

Figure 121.23 GMS stain shows the long slender branching filamentous bacteria.

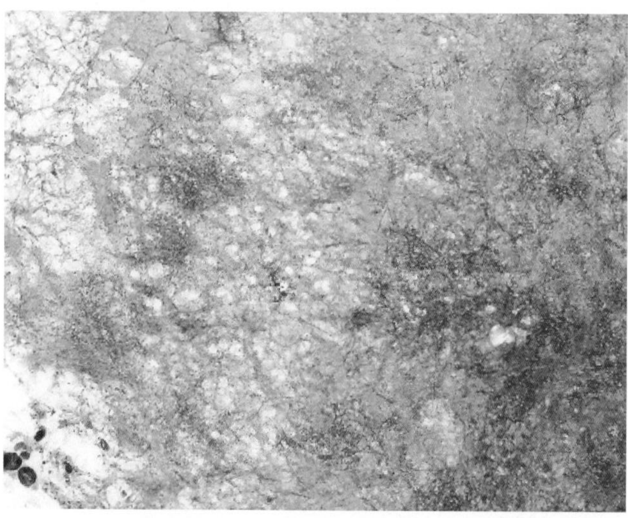

Figure 121.24 These bacteria are also gram-positive.

Part 7

Nocardia

▶ Alain Borczuk

Nocardia are filamentous bacteria that cause pneumonia after inhalation of contaminated soil. Immunocompetent hosts can develop a necrotizing pneumonia with abscess formation, and immunocompromised patients can have a more severe acute pneumonia with dissemination. *Nocardia asteroides* and *Nocardia brasiliensis* are the most common causes.

HISTOLOGIC FEATURES

- Necrotizing pneumonia with abscess.
- Organisms are filamentous bacteria with right-angle branching.
- Organisms are gram-positive, GMS-positive, and weakly acid fast.

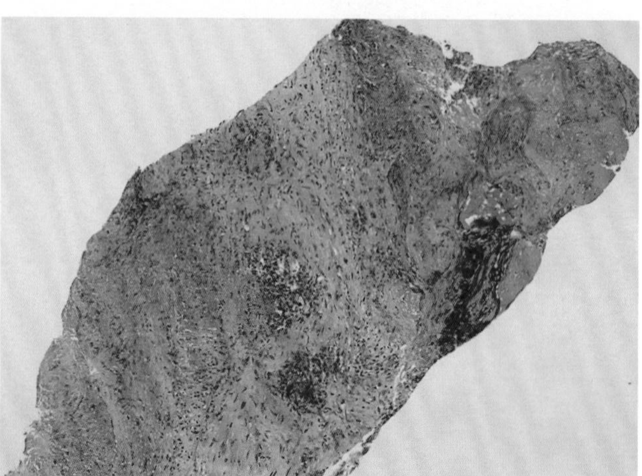

Figure 121.25 Tissue biopsy shows suppuration with surrounding fibrous tissue.

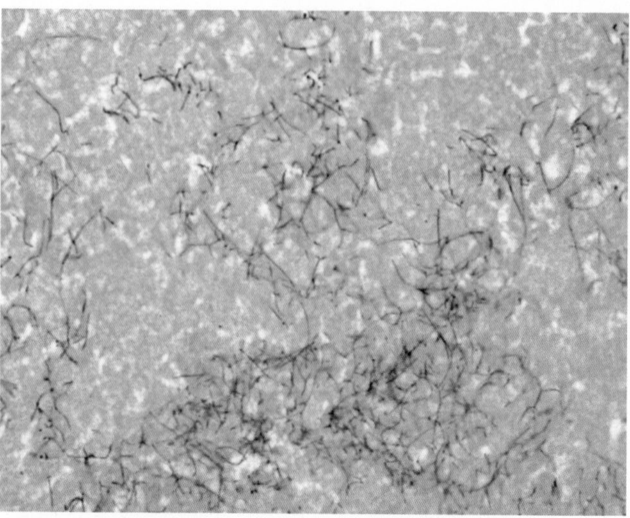

Figure 121.26 On GMS stain, filamentous bacteria are long and slender with right-angle branching.

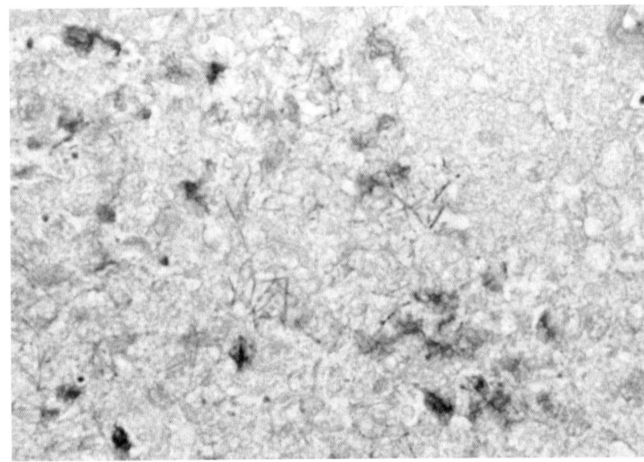

Figure 121.27 Nocardia is weakly acid fast.

Part 8

Mycoplasma

Alain Borczuk

Mycoplasma pneumoniae causes upper respiratory infection and pneumonia. It is often referred to as *walking pneumonia*, as *Mycoplasma* infection may be less severe than classical pneumococcal pneumonia. It is a common cause of community-acquired pneumonia, although its incidence may be underestimated. It was referred to as *atypical pneumonia* in which patients did not respond to the antibiotics used for pneumococcal pneumonia. The organism is smaller than most bacilli and is the smallest self-replicating organism. As a result, conventional and special stains used for morphologic evaluation do not identify the organism. They attach to the surface of respiratory epithelial cells.

HISTOLOGIC FEATURES

- Organizing pneumonia and bronchiolitis are typical features of infection but are not specific.

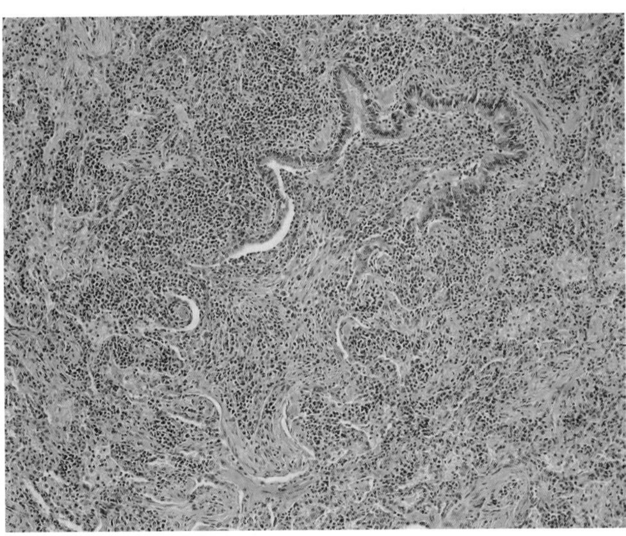

Figure 121.28 Organizing pneumonia and chronic bronchiolitis are characteristic of *Mycoplasma* pneumonia.

Part 9

Coxiella burneti

▸ Alain Borczuk

Coxiella burneti is the cause of Q fever. This bacterium is found in livestock and can be transmitted via body fluids such as milk, urine, blood, and feces. As the organism can survive after desiccation, spread can occur via contaminated dust. Increased risk is associated with working near livestock, in places such as ranches or slaughterhouses.

Q fever presents with chills, fatigue, headache, and fever. Severe cases result in hepatitis and pneumonia, and chronic forms can also occur.

HISTOLOGIC FEATURES

- Lung tissue shows patchy chronic inflammation with poorly formed granulomas.
- In the liver and bone marrow, a characteristic histologic feature is a ring granuloma, a poorly formed granuloma with a prominent central vacuole.

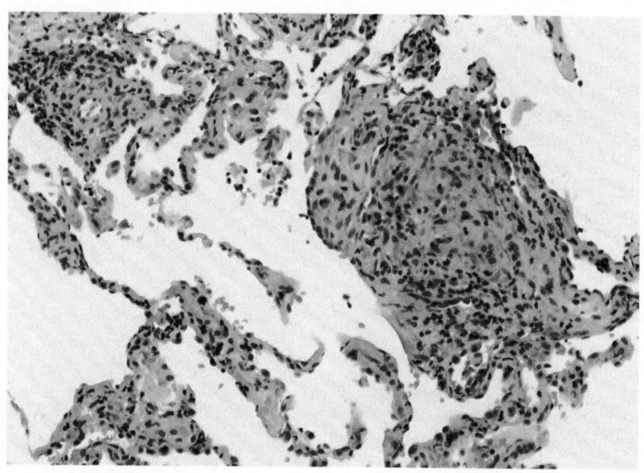

Figure 121.29 Q fever pneumonia with mild lymphocytic inflammation and poorly formed granuloma.

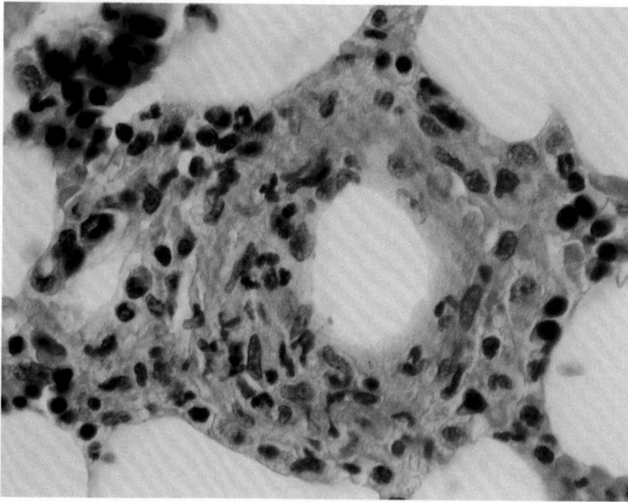

Figure 121.30 Bone marrow biopsy with poorly formed granuloma with central vacuole described as ring or "doughnut" granuloma.

Part 10

Rhodococcus

▸ Alain Borczuk

Rhodococcus equi is a coccobacillus that causes lung consolidation in immunocompromised individuals. It results in a massive histiocytic accumulation of pulmonary malakoplakia. It is covered in the chapter on granulomatous diseases of the lung (Chapter 68, Part 2).

HISTOLOGIC FEATURES

- Organisms are gram-positive and weakly acid fast.

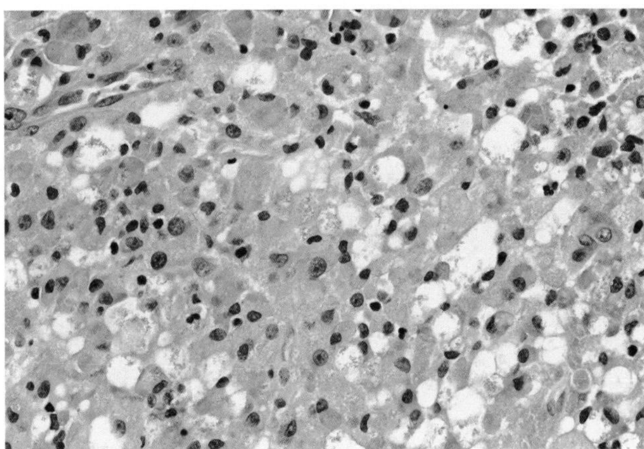

Figure 121.31 Histiocytic accumulation showing intracytoplasmic granular material that represents aggregates of *Rhodococcus*.

122 Mycobacteria

Alain Borczuk

Mycobacterial infections include tuberculosis that is caused by *Mycobacterium tuberculosis*. In some individuals, tuberculous mycobacteria cause sickness when the organisms actively multiply. In others, tuberculosis can infect without overt disease and is contained by the immune system. This represents latent tuberculosis. These individuals can reactivate disease later in life if they develop a weakened immune system.

Atypical mycobacterial infections are caused by a diverse set of nontuberculous mycobacteria. These organisms are found in the environment, including drinking water. These organisms can infect the lungs, especially in patients with chronic lung disease such as chronic obstructive pulmonary disease.

TUBERCULOSIS

Pulmonary tuberculosis causes granulomatous lung disease, with necrosis in classic examples. Initial infection can lead to containment of the organism, with a granuloma in lung and lymph node, which can calcify, called a Ghon complex. Reactivation of tuberculosis can take the form of an expanding nodule with necrosis (fibrocaseous tuberculosis), pneumonia, or miliary spread that is lymphohematogenous.

Histologic and Pathologic Features

- Gross pathology can include a cavity and white cheesy material, which has been described as caseating necrosis.
- Miliary tuberculosis has innumerable small nodules of 2 to 3 mm.
- Granulomas are histiocytic collections often with multinucleated giant cells. Necrosis, corresponding to gross caseation, is typical of tuberculous infection.
- *M. tuberculosis* is a long beaded rod-shaped organism that is red on Ziehl–Nielsen stain, described as acid fast. These organisms can also stain on Gomori methenamine silver (GMS).
- Nodules can become fibrotic and calcified.

ATYPICAL MYCOBACTERIA

Mycobacterium avium, *Mycobacterium intracellulare*, *Mycobacterium kansasii*, *Mycobacterium xenopi*, *Mycobacterium fortuitum*, *Mycobacterium abscesses*, and *Mycobacterium marinum* represent species of mycobacteria that are considered to be atypical mycobacteria. Pulmonary infection is associated with abnormal lungs and in immunocompromised hosts such as patients with acquired immunodeficiency syndrome (AIDS).

Histologic Features

- Necrotizing granulomas are seen in patients with atypical mycobacteria, as are nonnecrotizing granulomas.
- In immunocompromised patients, granulomas may not be seen but rather sheets of histiocytic cells filled with organisms.

- Organisms are acid-fast bacilli on Ziehl–Nielsen stain and can also stain on GMS.
- Mass-forming lesions can be composed of spindle cells, known as mycobacterial spindle-cell pseudotumor.

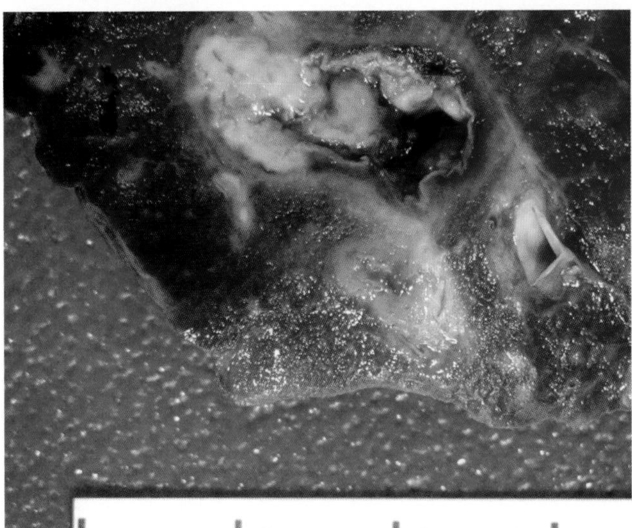

Figure 122.1 A gross nodule with cavitation and caseating necrosis of tuberculosis.

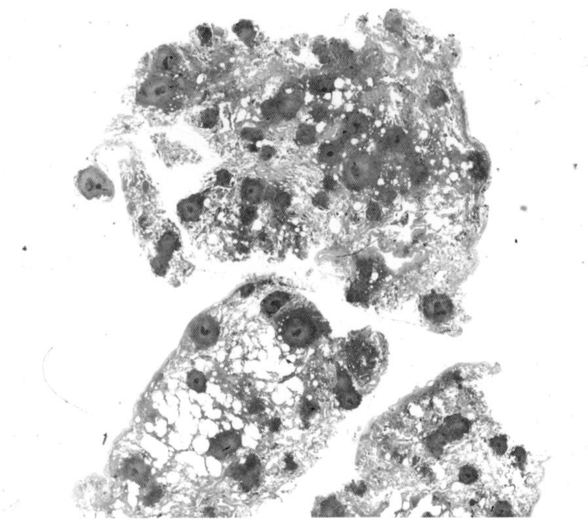

Figure 122.2 Whole mount lung tissue from a patient with miliary tuberculosis showing numerous 1 to 2 mm nodules.

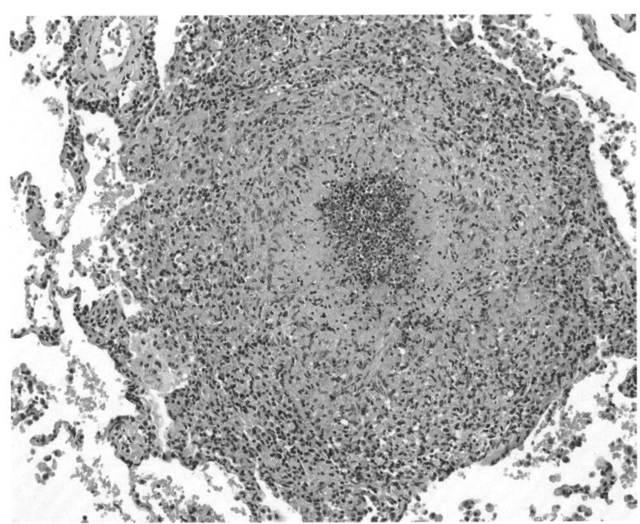

Figure 122.3 Each nodule represents a necrotizing granuloma.

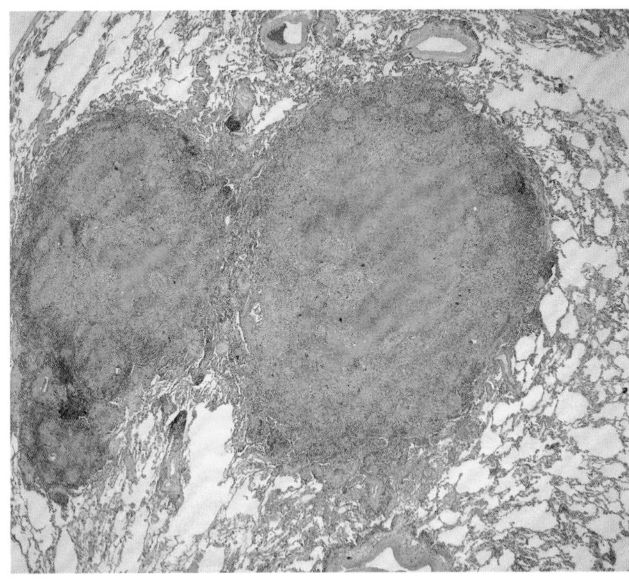

Figure 122.4 A fibrocaseous nodule with central necrosis, a histiocytic rim, fibrosis, and chronic inflammation.

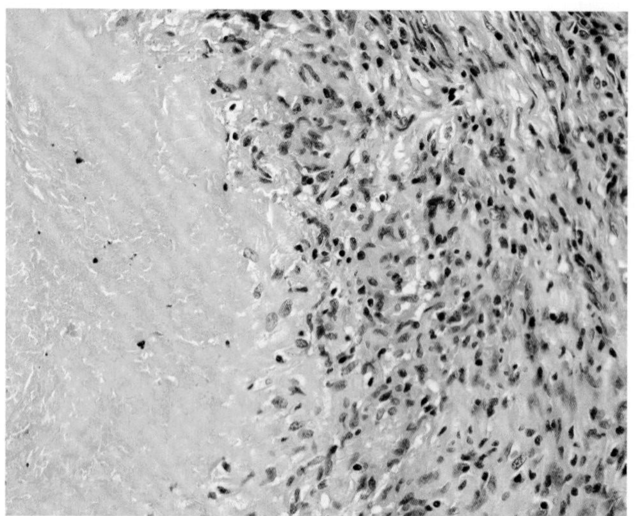

Figure 122.5 Necrotizing granuloma with necrosis, histiocytic rim, and multinucleated giant cells.

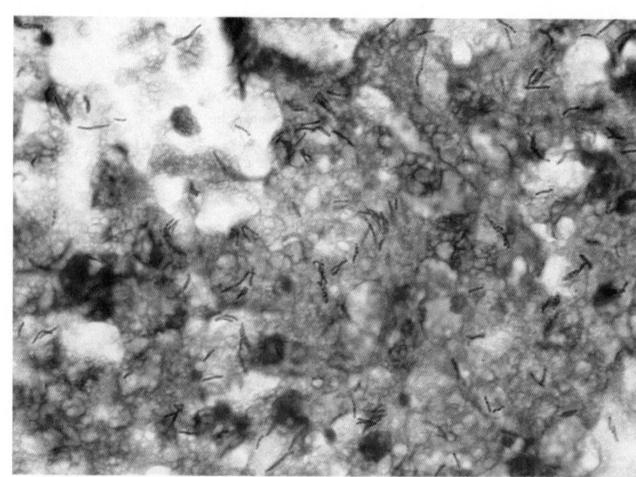

Figure 122.6 A Ziehl–Nielsen stain shows red acid-fast bacilli.

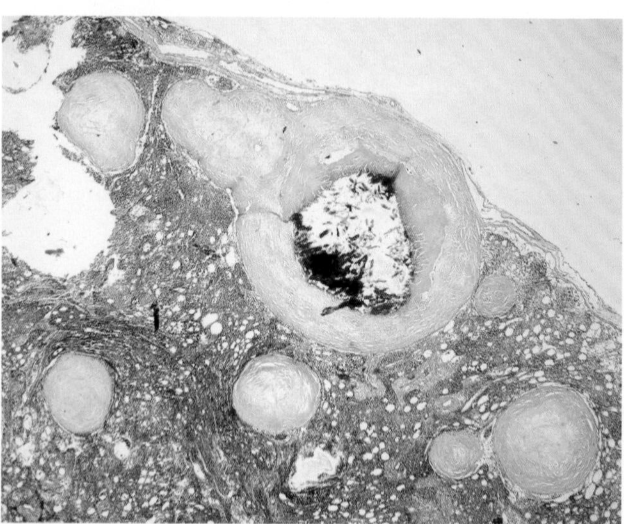

Figure 122.7 Prior tuberculous infection with calcified fibrous nodule in a lymph node, part of a Ghon complex.

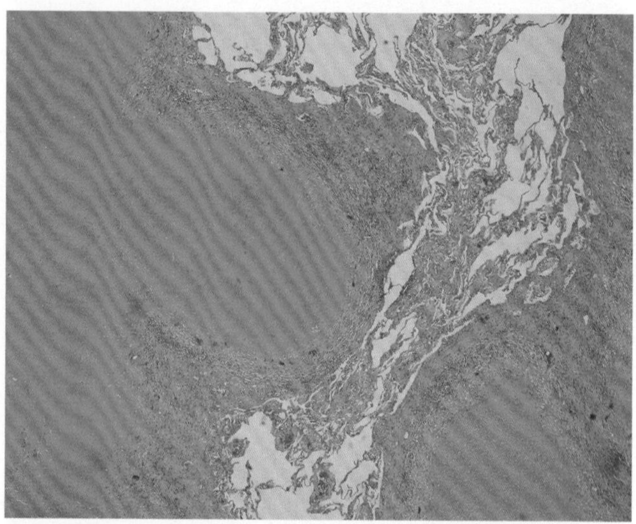

Figure 122.8 Extensive confluent granulomas with central necrosis.

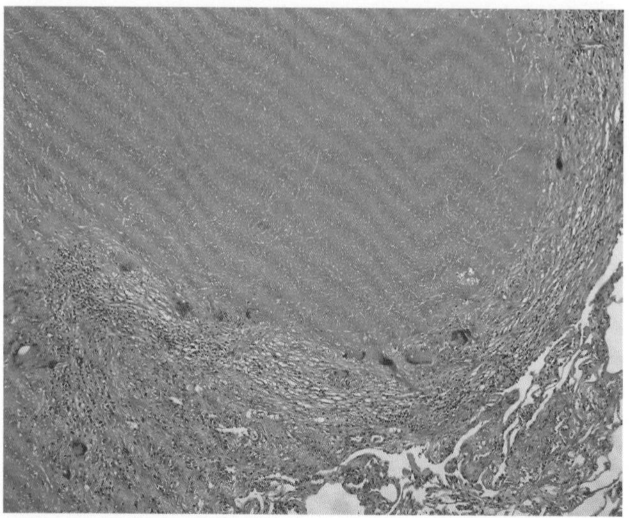

Figure 122.9 Necrotizing granuloma with a fibrous and histiocytic rim with multinucleated giant cells.

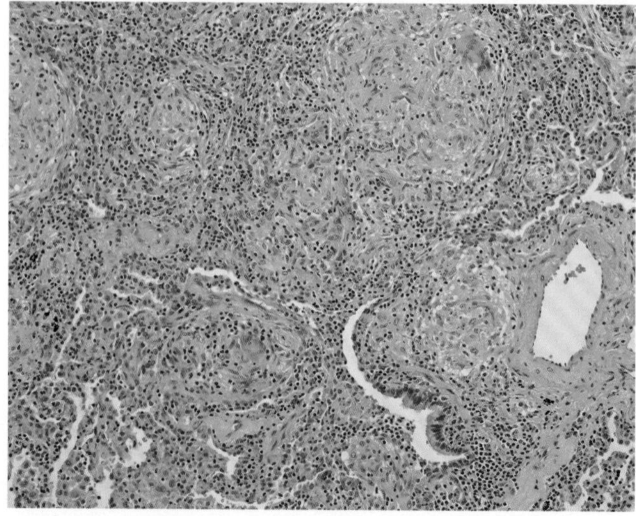

Figure 122.10 Poorly formed confluent nonnecrotizing granulomas surrounding a small airway in a case of atypical mycobacterial infection.

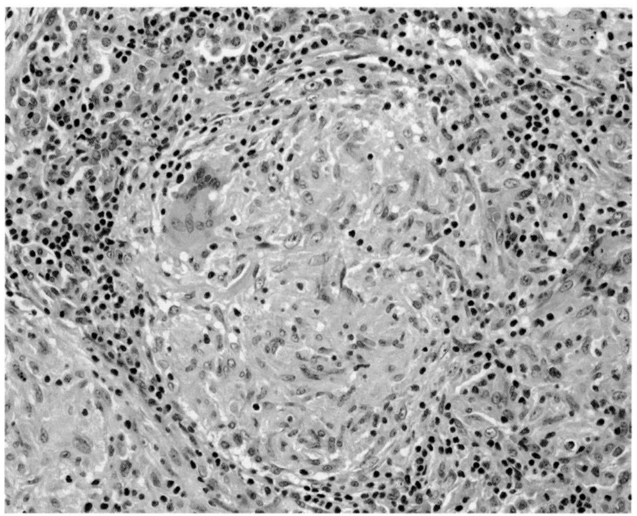

Figure 122.11 Mycobacterial granulomas, nonnecrotizing, with multinucleated giant cell.

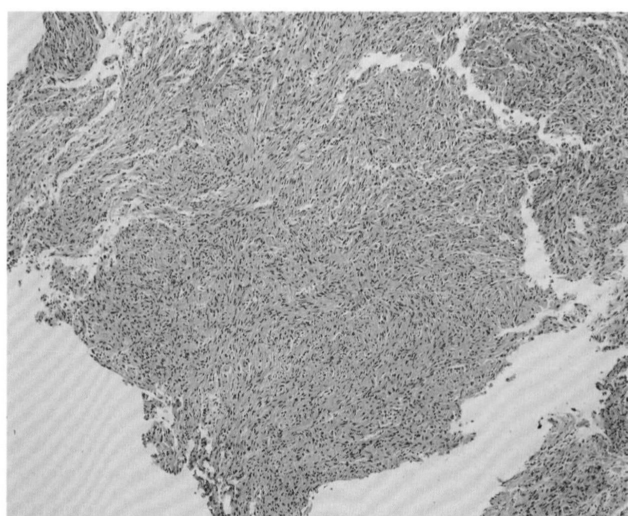

Figure 122.12 Mycobacterial spindle-cell pseudotumor in an immunocompromised patient.

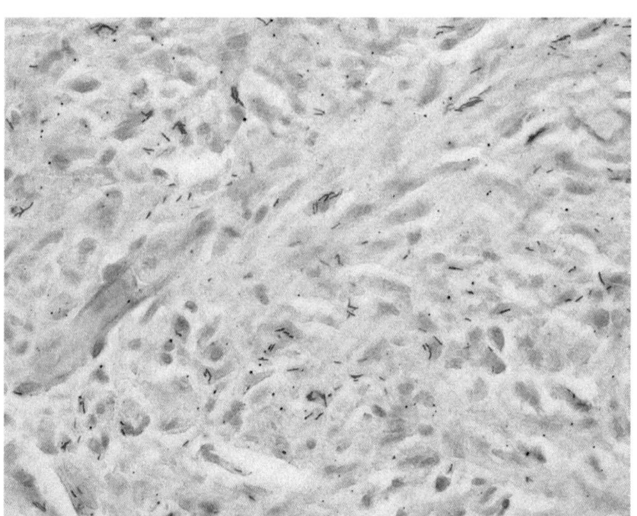

Figure 122.13 Numerous acid-fast bacilli in a mycobacterial spindle-cell pseudotumor.

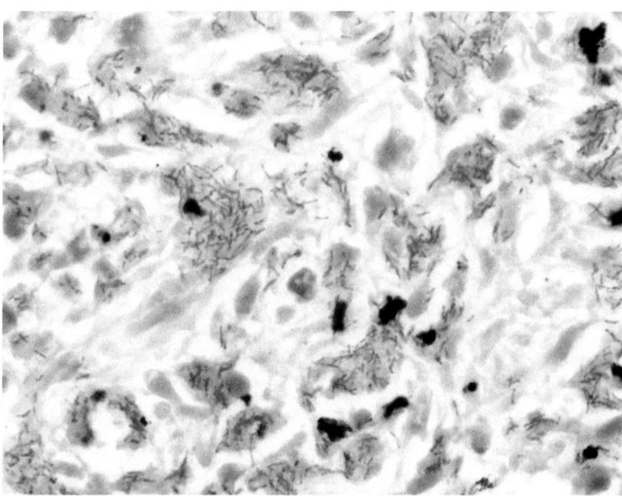

Figure 122.14 Atypical mycobacteria in a patient with AIDS showing numerous acid-fast bacilli in histiocytes. These are long slender beaded rods.

123 Fungi

Pulmonary fungal infections can occur in immunocompetent hosts but are more frequently encountered in immunosuppressed hosts where they represent opportunistic infections. Granulomatous reaction is typical of coccidioidomycosis, blastomycosis, and paracoccidioidomycosis, as well as infections with *Histoplasma* and *Cryptococcus*, whereas it is less frequently encountered in *Candida*, *Aspergillus*, or Mucorales infections, which are more often suppurative or invasive. However, exceptions to these typical tissue reactions can occur depending on factors such as host immunity and treatment effects.

Although organisms can be identified on hematoxylin and eosin (H&E) stains, special stains such as Gomori methenamine silver (GMS) and periodic acid–Schiff (PAS) can help document the presence of fungi and can also help assess morphology and extent of invasion.

Part 1

Aspergillus

Alain Borczuk

Aspergillosis is caused by a common mold that is encountered in both indoor and outdoor environments. It can affect people with compromised immune systems.

Aspergillus infection has several manifestations in lung pathology. Allergic bronchopulmonary aspergillosis represents an allergic response to fungus within mucin. A localized mass of *Aspergillus* that grows within a dilated airway or preexisting mass is an aspergilloma. Chronic disease can occur in which there are tissue reaction and minimal invasion, and frankly invasive aspergillosis with tissue destruction and vascular invasion.

HISTOLOGIC FEATURES

- Hyphae are septated and show acute-angle branching; their contours are distinct and parallel.
- They are often visible on H&E stain and stain intensely on GMS stain.
- Invasive aspergillosis is vasculoinvasive and can cause infarcts.
- Fruiting bodies are occasionally encountered.
- Some species are associated with pigments and polarizable oxalate crystals.

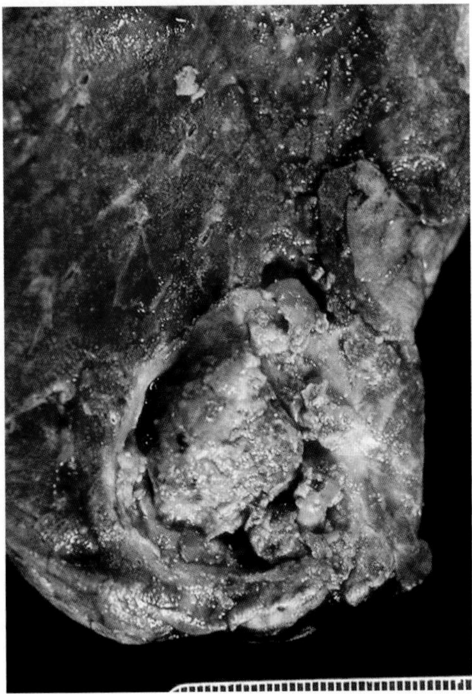

Figure 123.1 Brown necrotic material is seen within a thin-walled cavity in this aspergilloma.

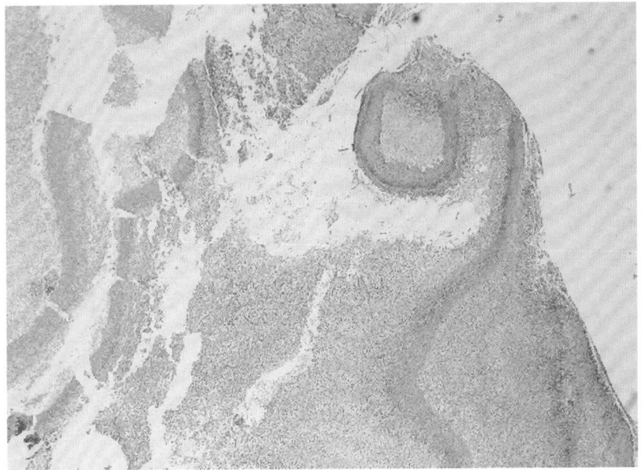

Figure 123.2 Aspergilloma contents show a higher density of fungal organisms and often appear in concentric rows.

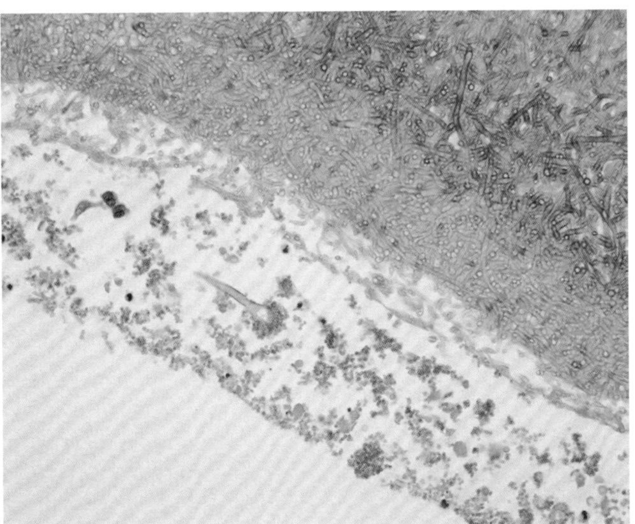

Figure 123.3 Dense accumulation of fungal hyphae associated with a fruiting body (conidial head).

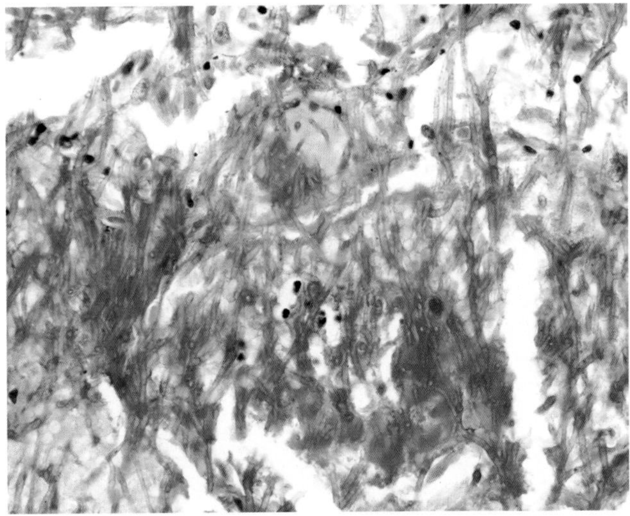

Figure 123.4 Invasive disease involves vessels with a large number of fungal hyphae that appear to overrun the tissue (PAS stain).

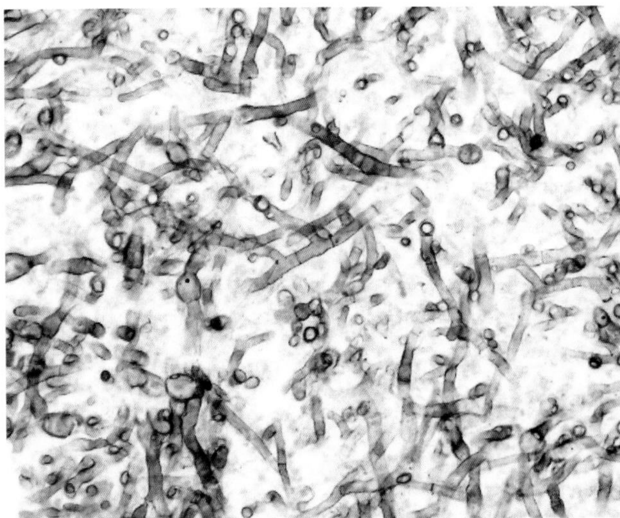

Figure 123.5 A GMS stain highlights the parallel contour, septation, and acute-angle branching.

Part 2

Mucorales

Alain Borczuk

Several different fungi are members of the suborder Mucorales, including *Rhizopus*, *Lichtheimia*, and *Mucor*. It is an uncommon infection seen in immunocompromised patients, as well as patients with diabetes. Pulmonary infection occurs in patients with neutropenia from a variety of causes including treatment of hematologic malignancy. The organism is ubiquitous, and spores are inhaled from the environment as a cause of pneumonia.

HISTOLOGIC FEATURES

- Organisms are associated with necrosis and vascular invasion.
- The fungi have broad hyphae without septation.
- Branching is wide angled rather than acute angled.
- They are weakly GMS-positive, so that often they are best seen on H&E stain.
- Infections are usually suppurative, but occasionally granulomas to fungal fragments can be seen in chronic infections.
- Organism fragments can sometimes look wrinkled or twisted.

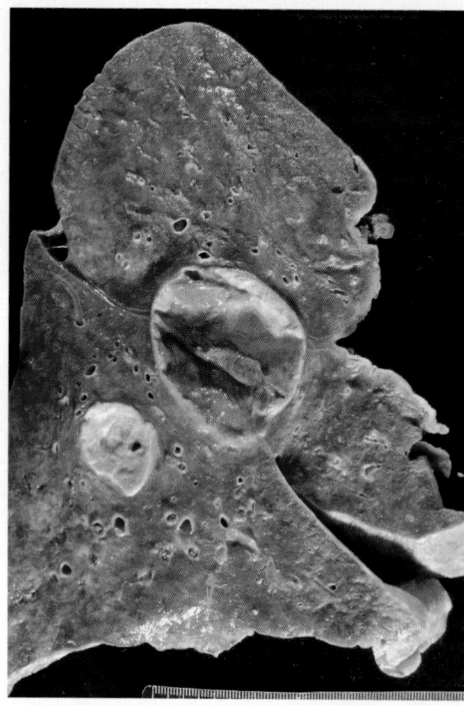

Figure 123.6 Lung with multiple areas of necrosis and invasive growth across the fissure.

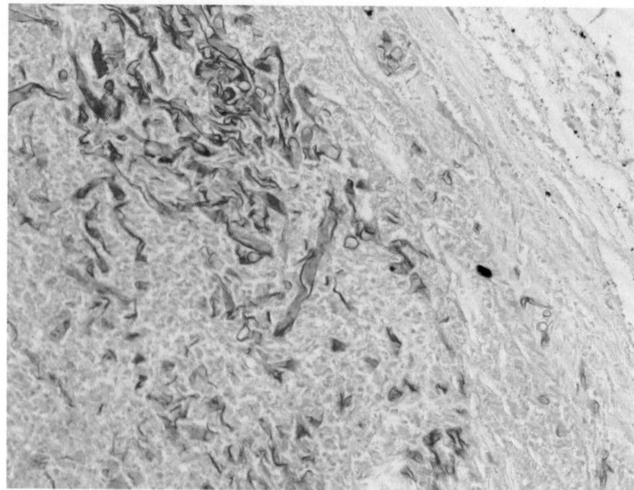

Figure 123.7 Organisms are quite visible on H&E stain and have irregular twisted contours.

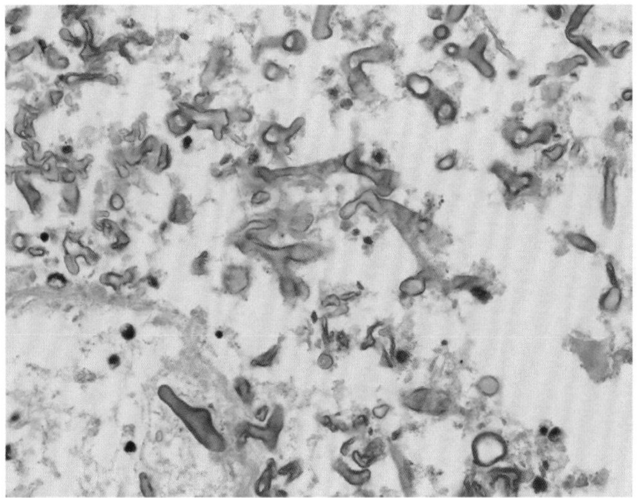

Figure 123.8 Hyphae are broad, show no septation, and demonstrate wide-angle branching.

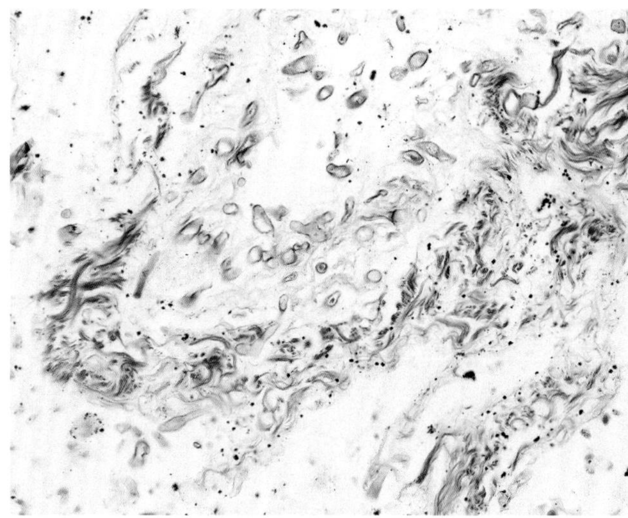

Figure 123.9 Mucorales are only weakly GMS-positive, and these broad empty-appearing structures can be mistaken for an artifact.

Part 3

Pneumocystis

Alain Borczuk

Pneumocystis pneumonia (PCP) is caused by *Pneumocystis jiroveci* (formerly *Pneumocystis carinii*). It is an opportunistic pathogen that was originally described in infants and pediatric patients with occasional hospital outbreaks. It was originally considered to be a protozoan but was reclassified as fungal. This infection is seen in patients with immunosuppression such as HIV/AIDS or malignancies such as lymphoma. Importantly, this infection can occur after steroid therapy, so PCP prophylaxis is administered in conjunction with long-term steroid therapy.

The terminology to describe these organisms remains to be cysts, sporozoites, and trophozoites. Cysts are demonstrated by GMS stain.

HISTOLOGIC FEATURES

- The hallmark of PCP is foamy intra-alveolar exudate, which is eosinophilic on H&E stain but can be observed in Papanicolaou (PAP) and Diff-Quik stains as well.
- GMS stain shows the cysts that are 4 to 7 μm and appear cup-shaped and round. When a round profile is seen, a dense black "dot" is seen within the organism.
- Lung tissue can show chronic inflammation but can also show diffuse alveolar damage.
- Some cases will show granulomatous inflammation with little foamy exudate.

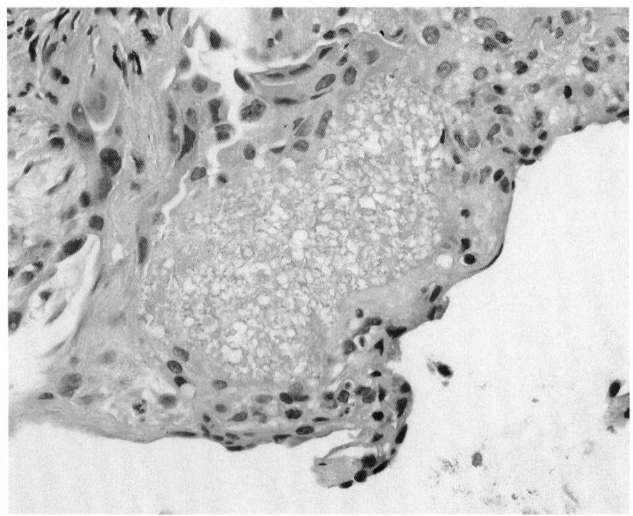

Figure 123.10 Typical foamy eosinophilic exudate is seen within alveolar spaces. Foamy appearance represents the negative images of the organisms.

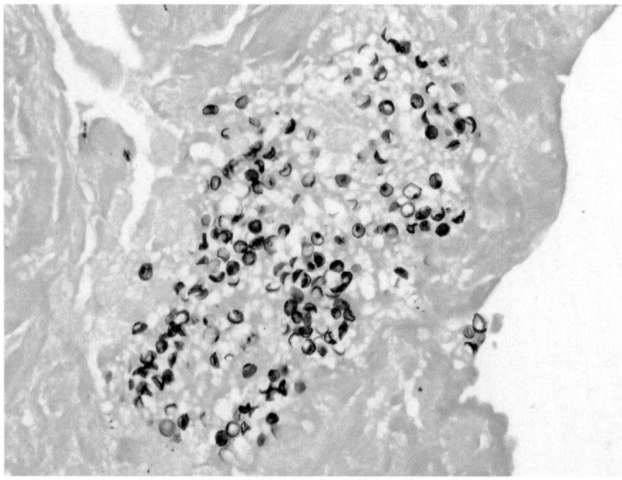

Figure 123.11 GMS stain shows cup-shaped and round profile of organisms without budding. Organisms seen "en face" show an eccentrically placed black density.

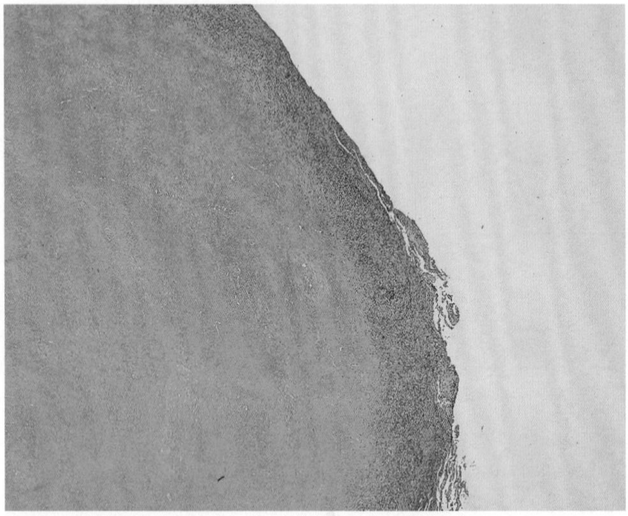

Figure 123.12 Some cases will show a granulomatous reaction, which can present as small nodules.

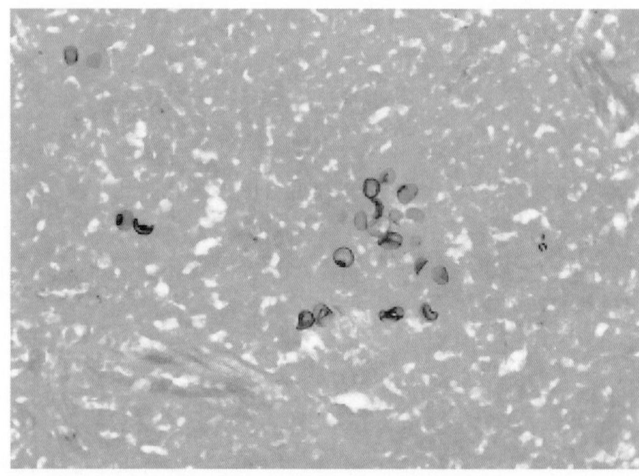

Figure 123.13 Organisms within the granuloma will have the same appearance as in the foamy exudate. In these cases, the differential diagnosis might include yeasts such as *Histoplasma*. However, *Pneumocystis* does not show budding and is rounder and PAS-negative.

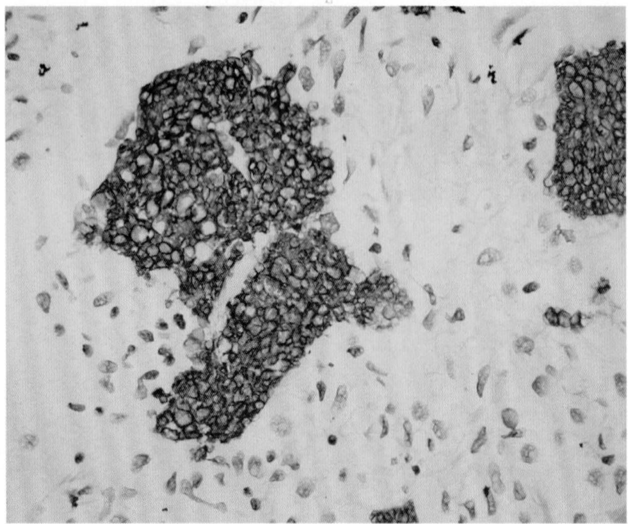

Figure 123.14 Immunohistochemistry for *Pneumocystis* can be helpful in difficult cases.

Part 4

Histoplasma

Histoplasma capsulatum is a dimorphic fungus that lives in soil. It is found in bat and bird droppings. In the United States, it is endemic to the Ohio and Mississippi River valleys. Human infection is through inhalation of fungus. It can result in an asymptomatic infection that gets contained within granulomatous inflammation, which eventually calcifies. However, chronic infection can be symptomatic and severe, especially in immunocompromised individuals. Lung disease and lymph node disease can be nodular; dissemination can occur. Disease can include pericarditis and mediastinal disease, including sclerosing mediastinitis.

HISTOLOGIC FEATURES

- *Histoplasma* infection typically results in granulomatous disease with or without necrosis.
- The organism is ovoid and small (2 to 5 μm) with narrow-based asymmetrical budding.
- Both GMS and PAS stains demonstrate organisms within necrosis and within macrophages.
- The differential diagnosis includes other yeasts such as *Cryptococcus*, *Torulopsis*, and *Penicillium*.

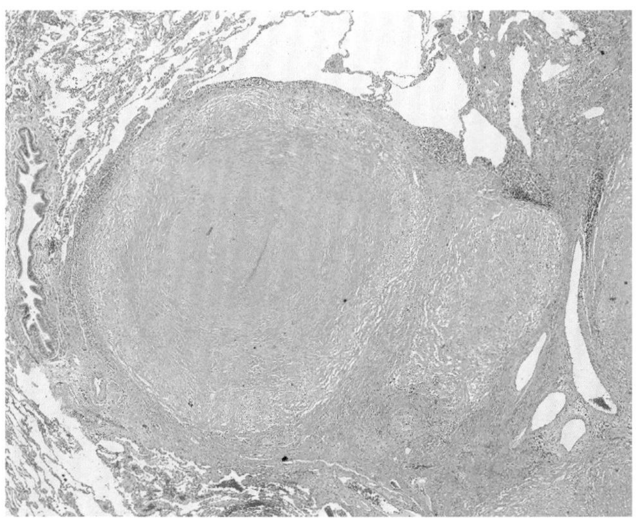

Figure 123.15 Necrotizing granuloma in lung parenchyma.

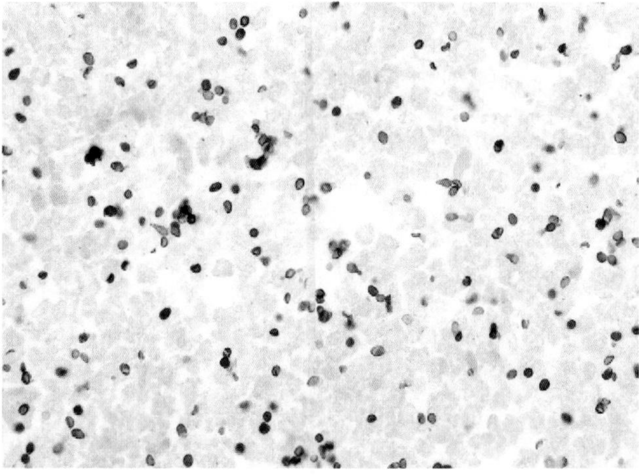

Figure 123.16 Necrotic center of granuloma shows numerous yeasts on GMS stain. Organisms are ovoid with dense capsule and narrow-based asymmetrical budding.

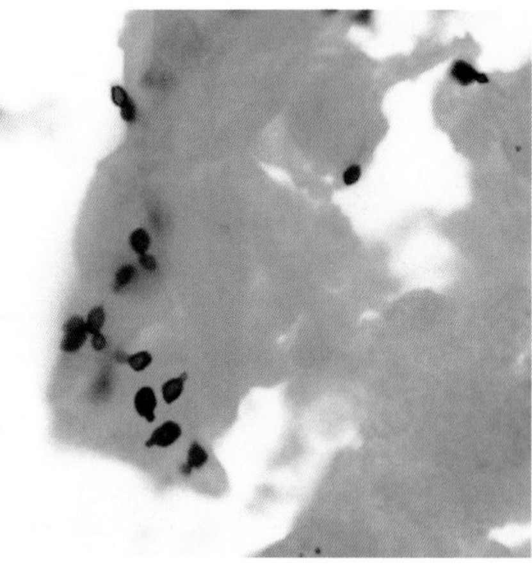

Figure 123.17 Higher magnification of GMS stain highlights narrow-based asymmetrical budding ("mother–daughter" budding).

Part 5

Cryptococcus

Alain Borczuk

Cryptococcal infection in the lung is most often due to *Cryptococcus neoformans*, although recent cases have been described it to be due to *Cryptococcus gattii*. It is a fungus that is observed in the environment and is associated with bird droppings. Cryptococcal granuloma can be a cause of a solitary lung nodule. However, significant infection is usually but not always associated with immunosuppression. Pneumonia is the most common manifestation of infection, but meningitis can occur as a significant life-threatening complication.

HISTOLOGIC FEATURES

- Organisms are usually larger than *Histoplasma*, with a wider size range (2 to 20 μm). They are round to ovoid.
- Organisms show narrow-based asymmetrical budding.
- The thick capsule of the organisms can be seen on H&E stain and is refractile in appearance, causing a space ("soap-bubble" appearance).
- Granulomatous inflammation is frequent, although severely immunosuppressed individuals can have numerous organisms with little inflammatory response.
- Special stains can help identify the organism. In addition to GMS stain, the capsule of *Cryptococcus* can be strongly positive on mucicarmine stain.
- In immunocompromised individuals, the mucicarmine capsule of *Cryptococcus* can be lost or not produced. Fontana stain continues to stain a melanin-like substance in the organism wall.

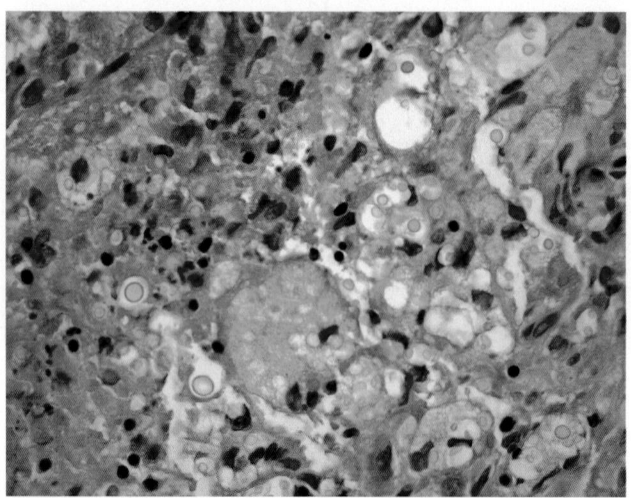

Figure 123.18 Variably sized yeast forms are seen on H&E stain with a clear zone around the organisms ("soap-bubble" appearance).

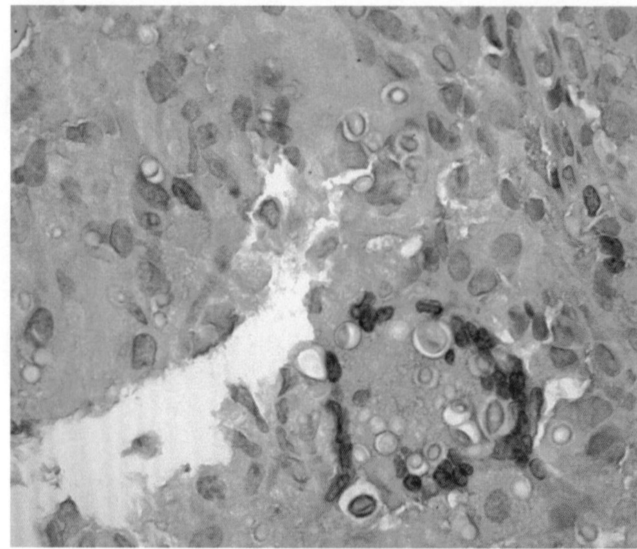

Figure 123.19 Mucicarmine stain shows round to ovoid organisms.

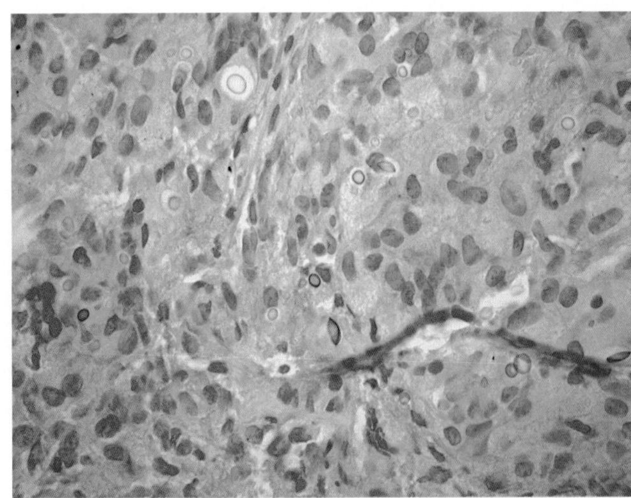

Figure 123.20 Organisms are also highlighted by Fontana stain.

Part 6

Coccidioides

Alain Borczuk

Coccidioides immitis is a fungus endemic to the southwest United States, although cases have been described in Mexico, Central America, and South America. Dry periods lead to aerosolization of fungus from soil, and subsequent inhalation can result in valley fever in exposed individuals. Infection can be acute with fever and cough but self-limited. Some patients will develop chronic infection; dissemination can also occur but is uncommon.

HISTOLOGIC FEATURES

- Granulomatous reaction is the typical tissue reaction encountered in lung samples.
- Organisms form large cystic spherules (up to 100 μm) filled with endospores. These are visible on H&E stain.
- Spherules are GMS-positive, but endospores are only variably so.
- Empty spherules can be seen on GMS stain.
- Rarely, hyphae can be seen in tissue. While rare, this should not be confused with a second fungal infection.

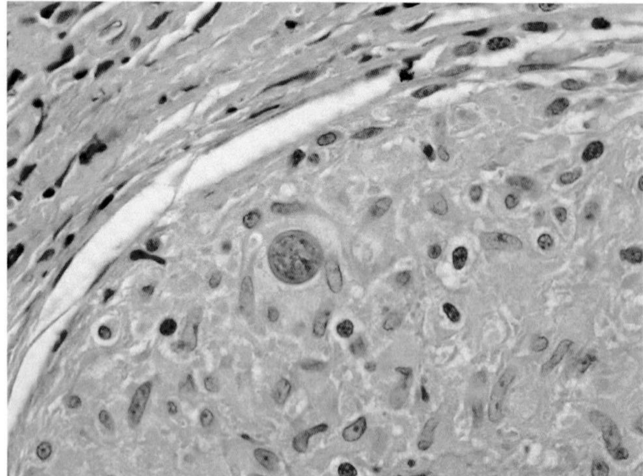

Figure 123.21 Granuloma showing a spherule of *Coccidioides*.

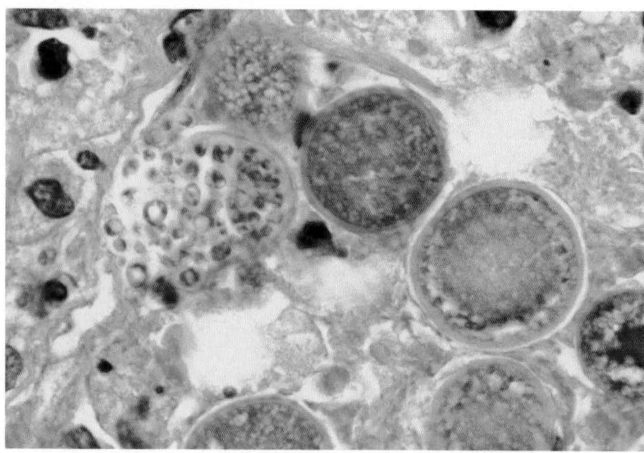

Figure 123.22 High-magnification view shows spherules with endospores, one showing rupture.

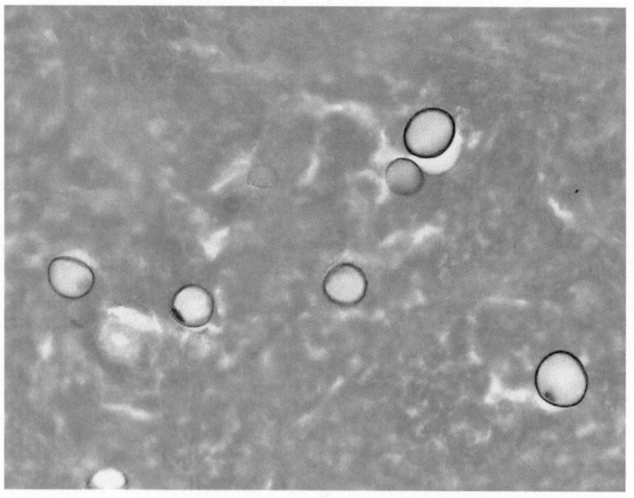

Figure 123.23 GMS stain highlights spherules, but endospores are less evident.

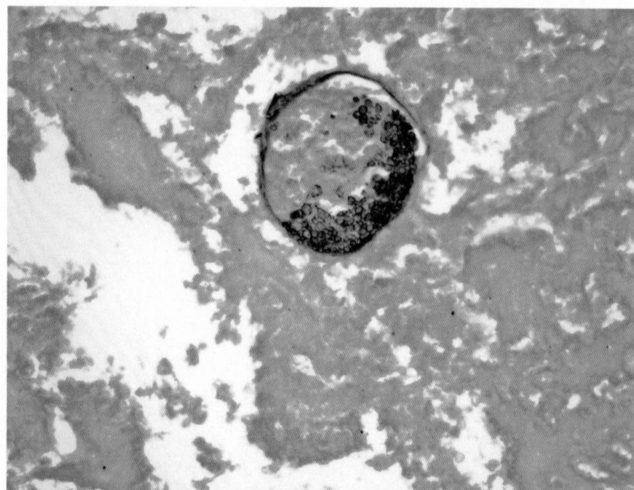

Figure 123.24 A large spherule filled with endospores on GMS stain.

Part 7

Paracoccidioides

Alain Borczuk, Marcelo L. Balancin, and Vera Capelozzi

Paracoccidioides brasiliensis is endemic to South and Central America and can cause a granulomatous infection of the skin and lungs.

HISTOLOGIC FEATURES

- Granulomatous disease containing fungal organisms.
- Organisms are up to 30 μm in diameter, with thick refractile wall.
- Budding can occur and shows a radial pattern characteristic of the organism.

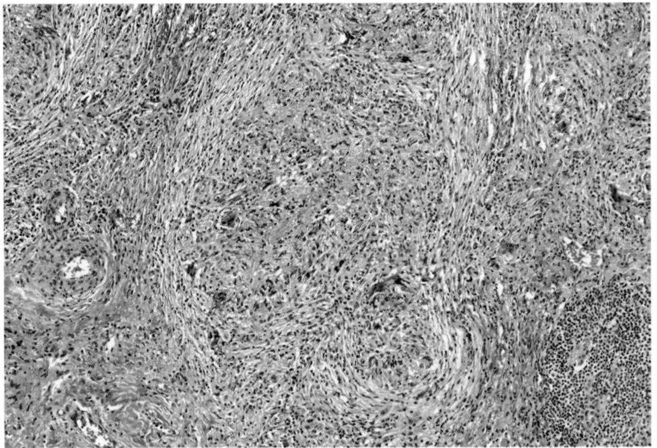

Figure 123.25 Granulomatous inflammation from a case of cutaneous *Paracoccidioides* infection.

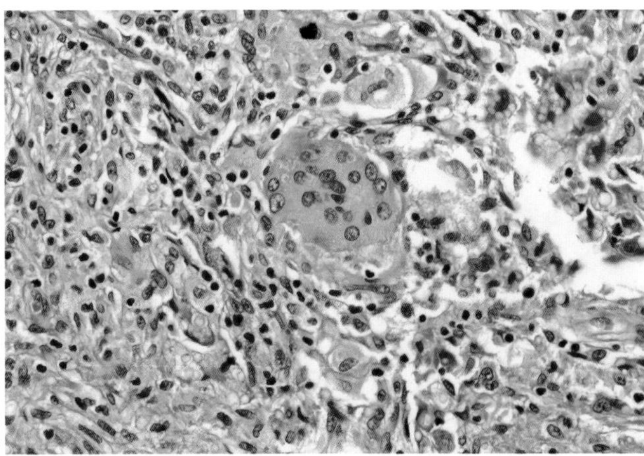

Figure 123.26 Organisms are visible within the granuloma as pale-staining structures.

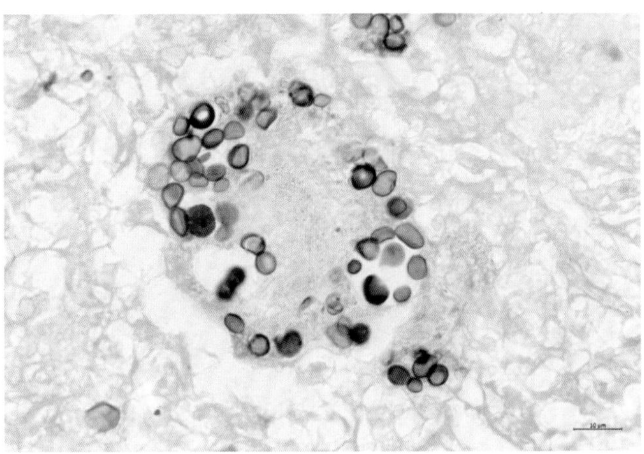

Figure 123.27 GMS stain highlights the yeast forms within a giant cell.

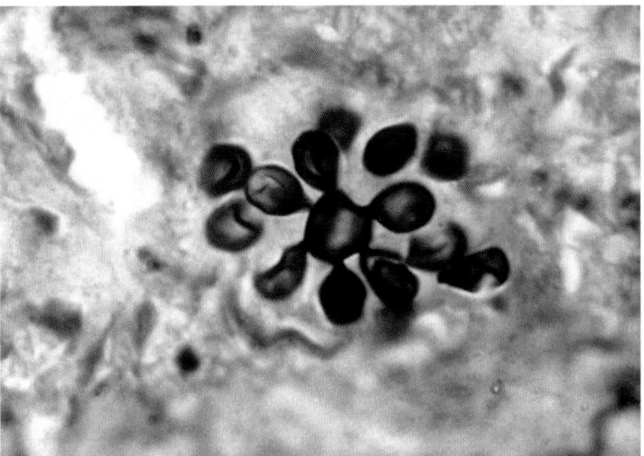

Figure 123.28 GMS stain shows the radially arranged budding of the organism. (Image from Public Health Image Library, CDC.)

Part 8

Blastomycosis

Alain Borczuk

Blastomyces dermatitidis is a dimorphic fungus that is endemic to the Ohio and Mississippi River valleys in the United States. It is inhaled from aerosolized fungus of soil origin. Infection results in fever and cough, as well as other constitutional symptoms. Infection can lead to extrapulmonary involvement in a subset of patients, and severe pulmonary infection can lead to diffuse alveolar damage.

HISTOLOGIC FEATURES

- Pulmonary infection is in the form of granulomas.
- Organisms are yeasts with thick walls and broad budding, with more symmetrical division. They are 8 to 15 μm.

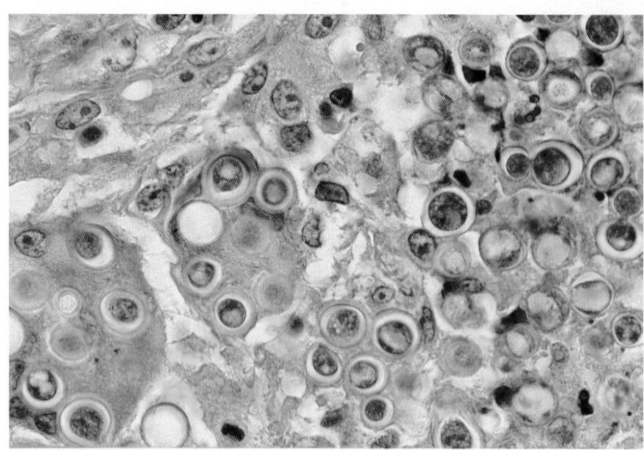

Figure 123.29 Granulomatous reaction with numerous yeast forms of *Blastomyces*.

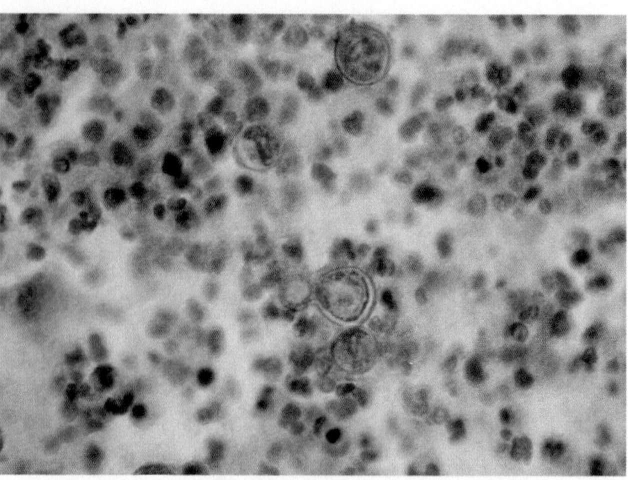

Figure 123.30 A PAP-stained smear shows *Blastomyces* with broad-based budding with more symmetrical division.

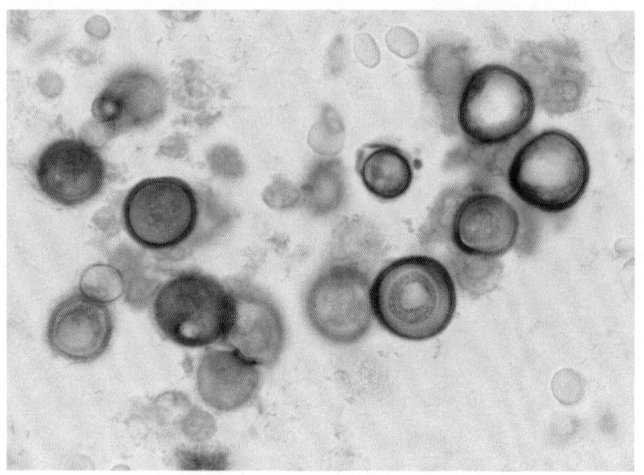

Figure 123.31 *Blastomyces* on GMS stain highlights the thick wall of the organism, somewhat larger than *Histoplasma* or *Cryptococcus*.

Part 9

Candida

Alain Borczuk

Candidal pneumonia is a suppurative process that occurs in immunocompromised individuals. It results in an acute necrotizing pneumonia.

HISTOLOGIC FEATURES

- Suppurative necrotizing process that is not usually granulomatous.
- Organisms are dimorphic in tissue with yeast forms and pseudohyphae.

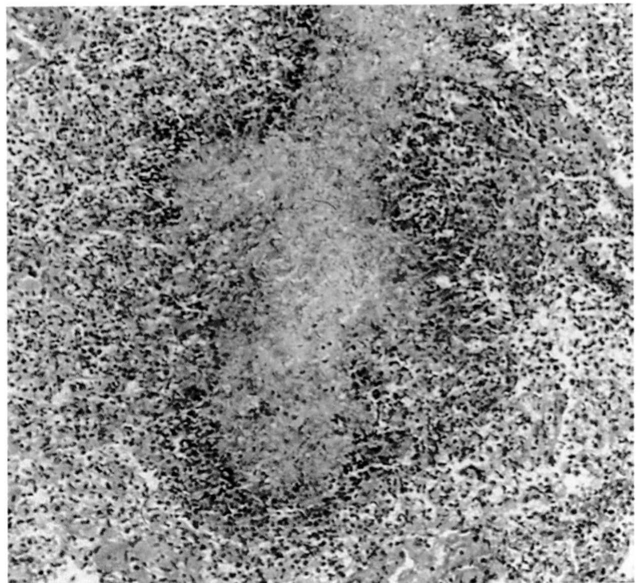

Figure 123.32 A patch of necrosis with surrounding acute inflammation.

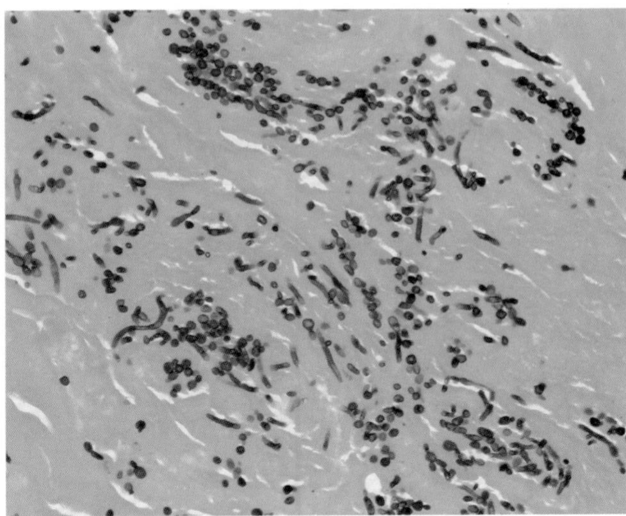

Figure 123.33 On GMS, both yeast forms and pseudohyphae are seen, the so-called spaghetti and meatballs appearance.

Part 10

Phaeohyphomycosis

Alain Borczuk and Jeannette Guarner

This is a heterogeneous group of fungal infections caused by dematiaceous fungi found in soil and decomposing organic matter. Infection occurs in immunocompromised individuals. Pneumonia can occur; systemic and central nervous system infections are also described.

HISTOLOGIC FEATURES

- Inflammation can be granulomatous with necrosis.
- Organisms show septated and branched hyphae with brown pigment. Brown pigment can be seen on H&E stain or enhanced by Fontana stains.
- Budding yeast forms can also be seen.

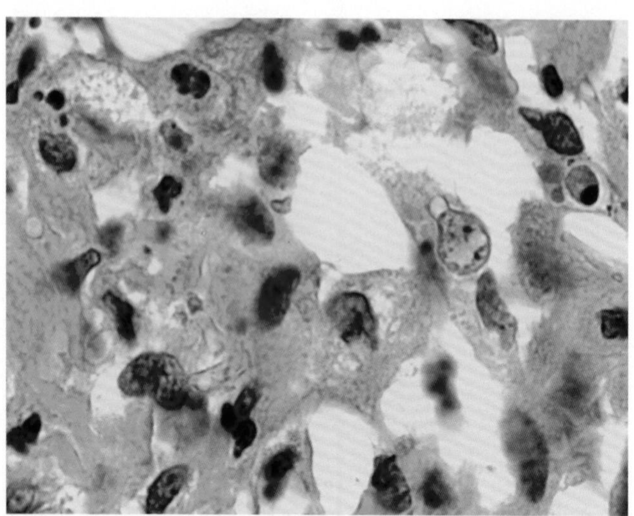

Figure 123.34 Pigmented budding yeast forms are present in the lung tissue.

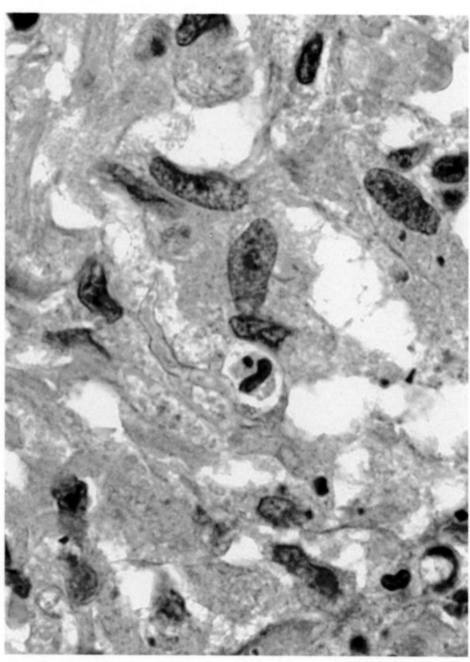

Figure 123.35 A branching pigmented hyphal form is seen amidst granulomatous inflammation.

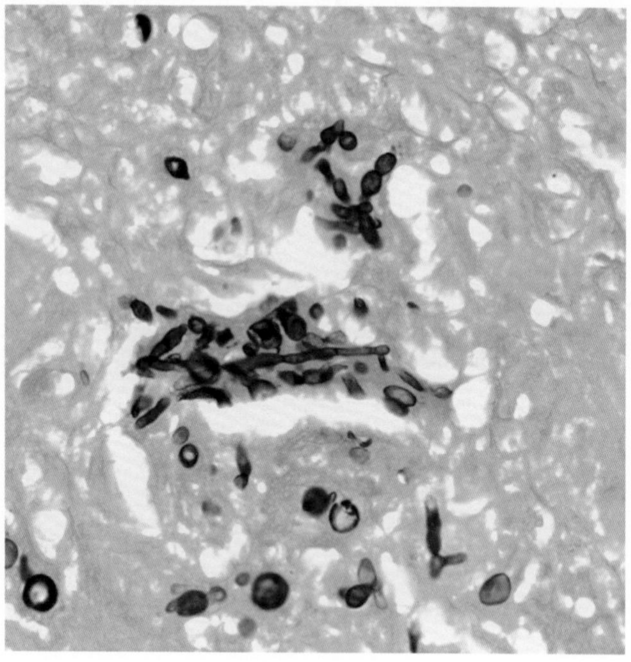

Figure 123.36 GMS stain shows yeast and hyphal forms with budding.

124 Parasites

Parasitic infections frequently involve the lung as part of the life cycle of the organism. However, disseminated disease from a variety of parasites can involve the lung. In some instances, the lung is the primary site of infestation.

Part 1

Strongyloides

Alain Borczuk

Strongyloidiasis is caused by a nematode, most commonly *Strongyloides stercoralis.* It is a soil pathogen that enters through exposed skin. During its life cycle, it not only passes through the lungs but also can enter the intestine where eggs hatch into larvae. These larvae can reenter the circulation as part of autoinfection. These states can be latent for many years. In immunocompromised patients, this can result in a hyperinfection state.

HISTOLOGIC FEATURES

- Lungs can show inflammation, hemorrhage, and necrosis, although some cases show little tissue reaction.
- Granulomatous inflammation and eosinophilia can be seen in chronic infection.
- Most common form seen in the lungs is the filariform larvae, although with hyperinfection other forms can be seen.

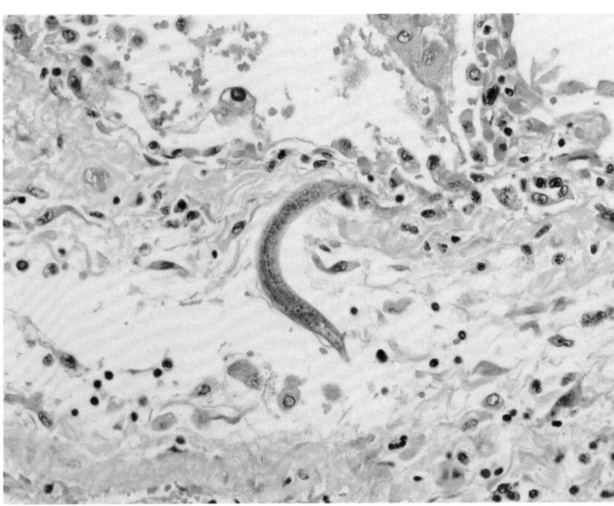

Figure 124.1 An autopsy case with hyperinfection showed numerous larvae in the lung.

Part 2

Dirofilaria

Alain Borczuk

Dirofilaria immitis is the dog heartworm that can infect humans, despite the fact that humans are not the definitive host. As a result, the worms travel to the heart, where they die. The fragments of worm can embolize into the lung where they cause pulmonary nodules. These nodules include vessels with plugging by worm fragments, causing infarction. *Dirofilaria repens* has a similar life cycle and is seen in Europe rather than in North America.

HISTOLOGIC FEATURES

- The coin lesions represent an area of necrosis with an involved pulmonary artery branch.
- Pulmonary artery is plugged with fragments of embolized worm.
- Cross sections of worm show thick cuticle and muscular walls.
- The entire lesion resembles an infarct, and multiple level sections should be performed for parasite fragments.

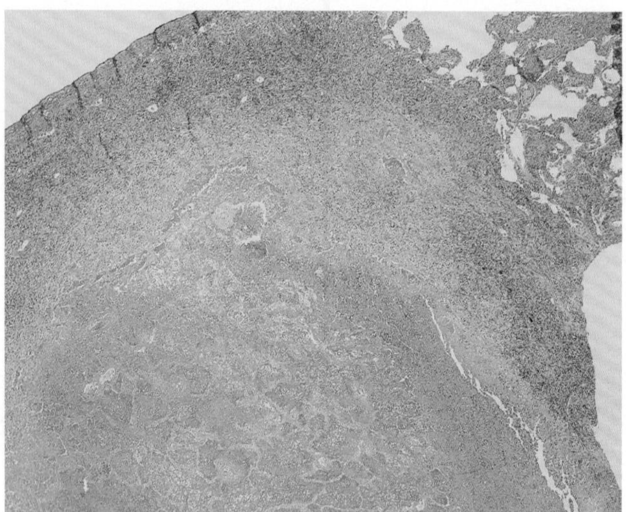

Figure 124.2 A coin lesion with fibrous reaction surrounding an area of necrosis.

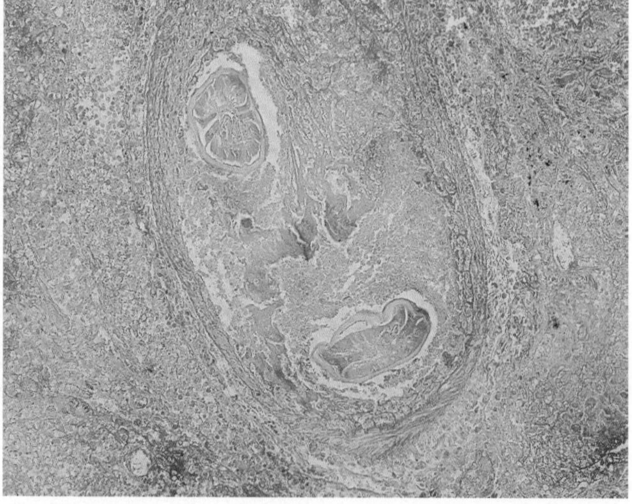

Figure 124.3 Pulmonary artery with thrombus and fragments of dead parasite are seen.

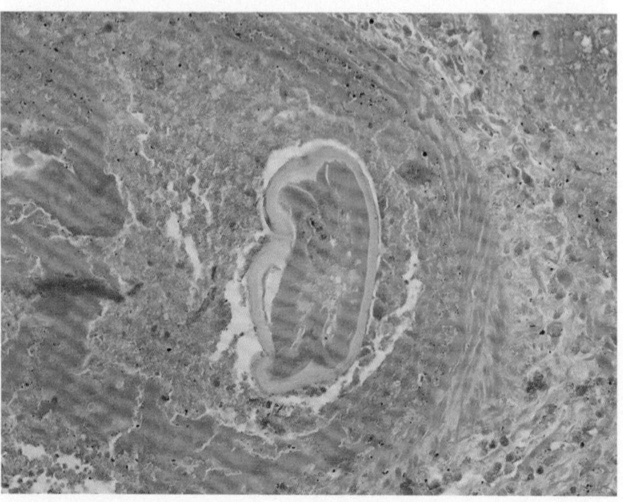

Figure 124.4 High magnification shows the thick cuticle and muscular wall of the *Dirofilaria* worm inside a pulmonary artery.

Part 3

Toxoplasma

Alain Borczuk

Toxoplasma gondii is an intracellular parasitic protozoan. It infects humans not only via undercooked meat but also through handling of cat litter/feces. Although most people who are infected are asymptomatic, it can be a significant problem in pregnant women in the form of stillbirth or the development of ocular and central nervous system (CNS) problems in their children. However, infected individuals can develop a flu-like syndrome with lymphadenopathy. Immunocompromised patients can reactivate prior infections, and this can include pneumonia.

HISTOLOGIC FEATURES

- Interstitial chronic inflammation.
- Pneumocytes and macrophages can show accumulation of tachyzoites in their cytoplasm.
- Tachyzoites accumulate within a defined intracytoplasmic parasitophorous vacuole.

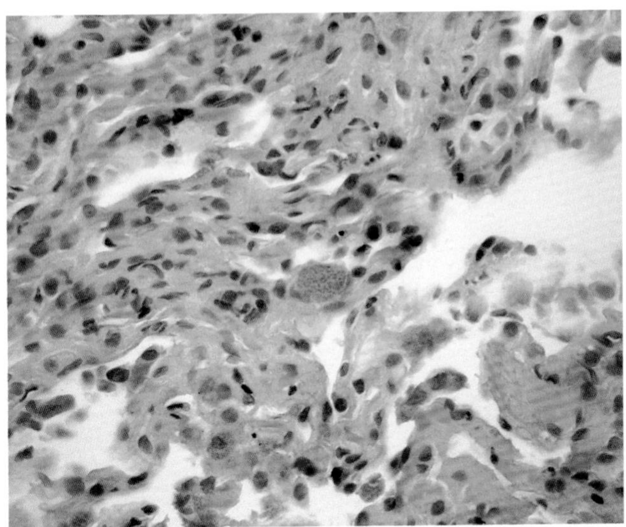

Figure 124.5 Pneumocyte with accumulation of tachyzoites in the cytoplasm with interstitial chronic inflammation.

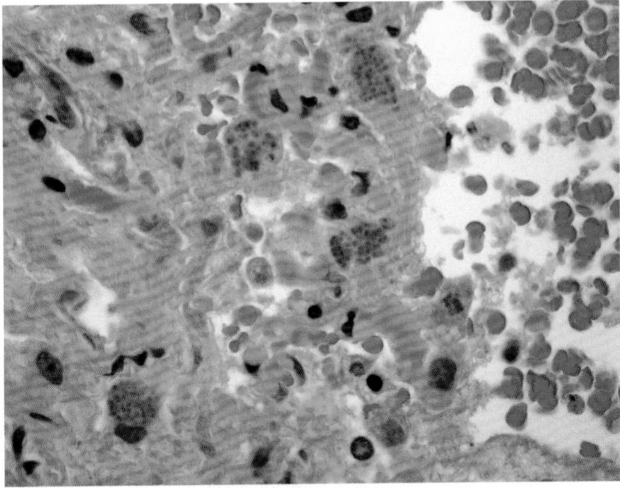

Figure 124.6 Numerous cells show multiple pneumocytes with tachyzoites as part of an active infection.

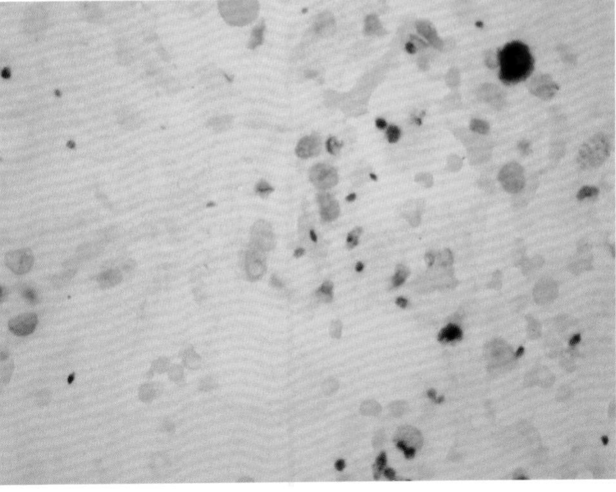

Figure 124.7 Immunohistochemistry highlights both intracellular tachyzoites and free tachyzoites of *Toxoplasma*.

Part 4

Acanthamoeba

▶ Alain Borczuk

Acanthamoeba is among a group of amebic organisms that are found living in freshwater and soil. Although exposure is frequent, disease is rare and can include keratitis, and CNS and cutaneous infection. In addition, more disseminated infection can occur to include lungs and other organs. *Balamuthia mandrillaris* and *Naegleria fowleri* can also cause serious and often fatal disease. *Naegleria* has not been reported to result in disseminated disease in contrast to the other two organisms.

HISTOLOGIC FEATURES

- Cysts and trophozoites are seen in *Acanthamoeba* and *Balamuthia*, whereas only trophozoites are seen in *Naegleria*.
- Cysts have a thick wall and a crinkled external wall.
- Trophozoites resemble macrophages, with granular cytoplasm and a round nucleus.
- Trophozoite nuclei are round and targetoid, with an eosinophilic hue.

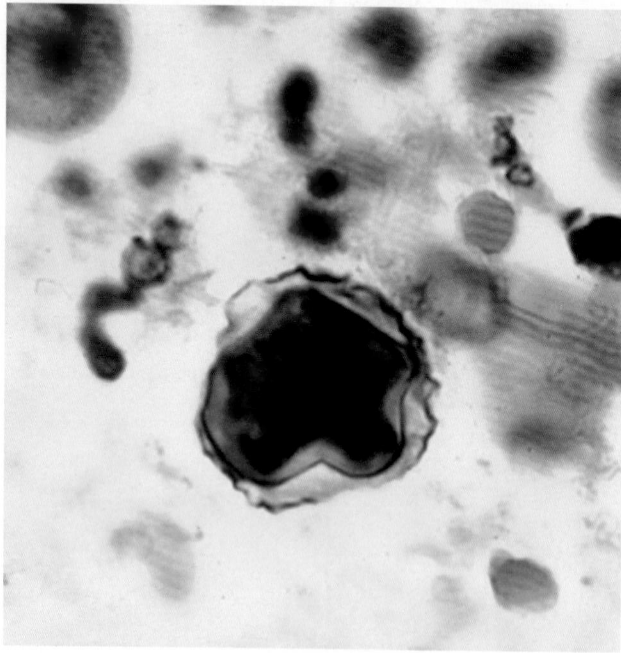

Figure 124.8 Cyst of *Acanthamoeba*. (Image from www.cdc.gov/dpdx/freeLivingAmebic/index.html, a publically available resource.)

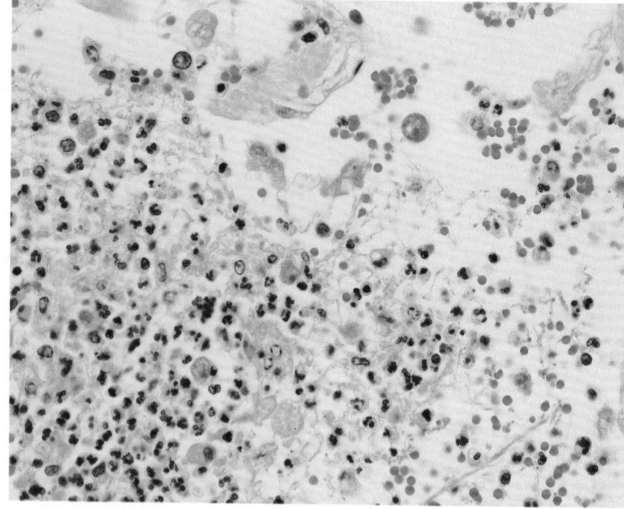

Figure 124.9 *Acanthamoeba* pneumonia with intra-alveolar inflammation including neutrophils and macrophages. (Courtesy of Dr. Thomas V. Colby.)

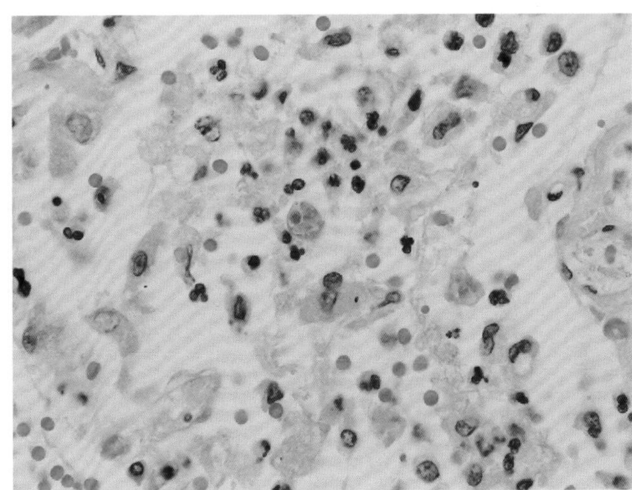

Figure 124.10 An *Acanthamoeba* trophozoite with a round nucleus and granular cytoplasm. (Courtesy of Dr. Thomas V. Colby.)

Part 5

Paragonimus

Alain Borczuk

Paragonimus infection is the result of infection by a trematode that humans ingest when eating raw freshwater crabs or crayfish. Larvae can penetrate the small intestine, travel through the diaphragm, and enter the pleural space or lung parenchyma. Worms lay eggs in the thoracic space or lung with resultant inflammatory reaction.

The most common organism causing infection in humans is *Paragonimus westermani*. This organism is endemic to Asia, in countries such as China, Japan, Vietnam, South Korea, Taiwan, Thailand, and the Philippines. Other species cause disease in Africa (*Paragonimus africanus*), Central and South America (*Paragonimus mexicanus*), and North America (*Paragonimus kellicotti*). Aspects of the organism's life cycle may influence the frequency of human disease.

Acute infection can be symptomatic, with fever, abdominal pain, cough, and chest discomfort. Chronic infection can lead to hemoptysis and pleural effusion.

HISTOLOGIC FEATURES

- *Paragonimus* eggs can elicit an inflammatory response—granulomatous and eosinophilic.
- Eggs in tissue.

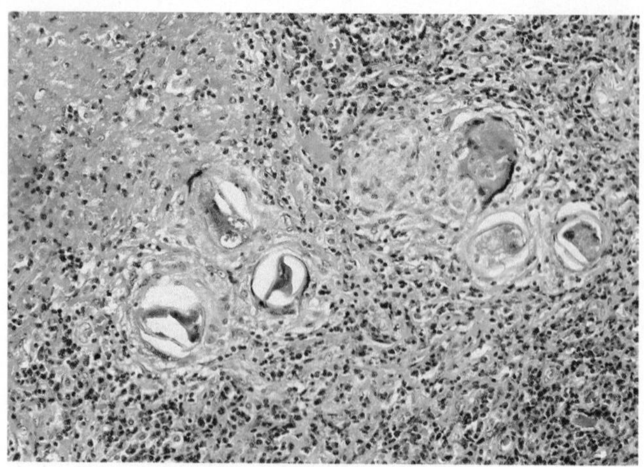

Figure 124.11 A granulomatous and mixed inflammatory reaction with eosinophils surrounding *Paragonimus* eggs in this lung biopsy.

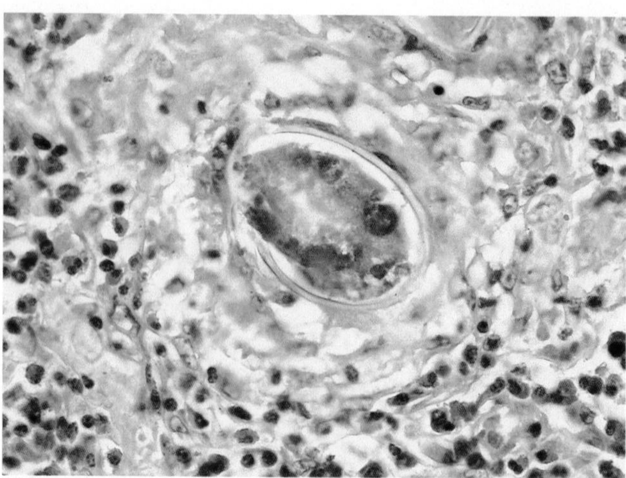

Figure 124.12 Higher magnification of a *Paragonimus* egg shows a thick refractile shell and internal nuclei. More precise identification is better obtained in fresh samples such as those obtained from sputum or lavage.

Part 6

Schistosoma

Alain Borczuk

Schistosoma infection is caused by a trematode (fluke). It is acquired from freshwater swimming in contaminated waters. Contamination comes from freshwater snails that harbor the parasite and facilitate its life cycle.

Schistosome infection can involve the lungs as an acute and chronic disease. In the acute setting, fever can occur, and this is an allergic reaction: type III hypersensitivity reaction. In the chronic setting, eggs can travel to the lung via the vasculature, resulting in a granulomatous reaction. This can result in pulmonary hypertension.

HISTOLOGIC FEATURES

- Eggs cause a granulomatous and fibrous reaction.
- These can be seen in pulmonary circulation, causing a granulomatous reaction.
- Eggs are about 100 μm, with variation by species. They have a lateral spine (*Schistosoma mansoni*), a terminal spine (*Schistosoma haematobium*), or an absent or indistinct lateral spine (*Schistosoma japonicum*).

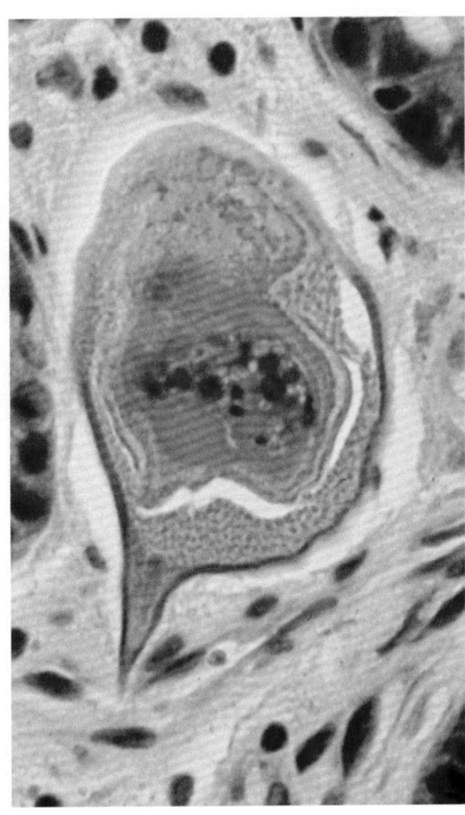

Figure 124.13 High magnification of a schistosome egg showing a lateral spike and internal nuclei.

Part 7

Leishmania

Alain Borczuk

Visceral leishmaniasis is caused by *Leishmania donovani* and is spread by the bite of the sand fly. It is found in Africa, Asia, South America, and southern Europe. Skin is a common site of infection, but in visceral leishmaniasis, solid organs are affected. Hepatosplenomegaly, anemia, leukopenia, and thrombocytopenia can result. Diagnosis can be made on bone marrow biopsy. In lungs, organisms can be found within macrophages.

HISTOLOGIC FEATURES

- Granulomatous inflammation.
- Amastigotes have a nucleus and a kinetoplast, which imparts a clothespin appearance to the organism.

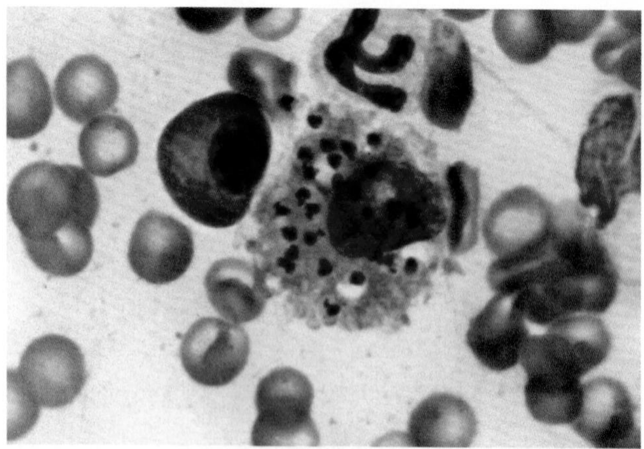

Figure 124.14 Histiocytic cell containing *Leishmania* amastigotes. (From the CDC Public Health Image Library, image by Dr. Francis W. Chandler, 1979.)

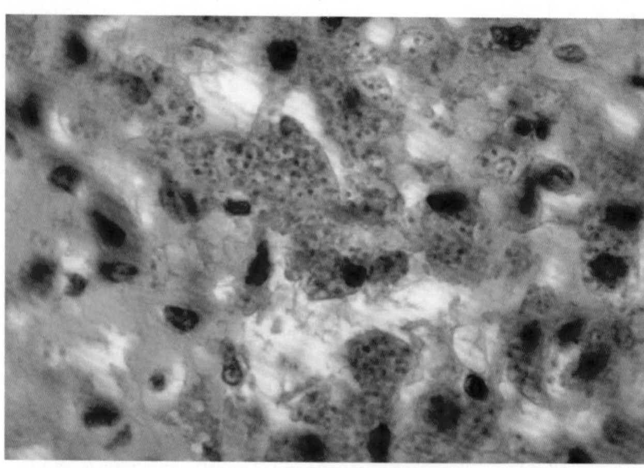

Figure 124.15 Skin infection showing macrophages with *Leishmania* amastigotes. (From the CDC Public Health Image Library, image by Dr. Martin D. Hicklin, 1964.)

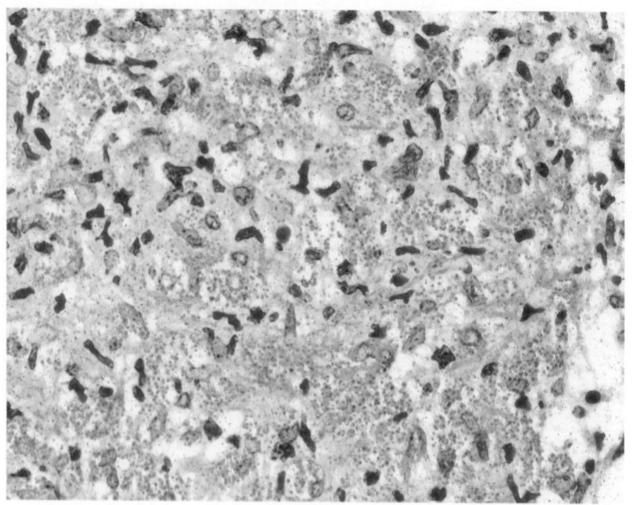

Figure 124.16 Numerous macrophages expand in the interstitium, filled with *Leishmania* amastigotes, stained on Warthin–Starry stain.

Part 8

Echinococcus

Alain Borczuk

Echinococcal infection is usually caused by the tapeworm *Echinococcus granulosus*. Infection is acquired from fecal contamination often from an infected dog. Dogs can become infected through ingestion of contaminated organs of sheep, cattle, goats, or pigs; livestock get infected from fecal contamination in soil.

Most human cases are hepatic, which is called hydatid cysts. However, lungs can be involved, and this can include cyst formation and reaction to cyst fragments. Humans are not a definitive host, so there is no human-to-human transmission.

HISTOLOGIC FEATURES

- Cysts have a characteristic multilamellated structure that is strongly positive on periodic acid–Schiff stain.
- Scolices contain hooklets and have a distinctive microscopic appearance.

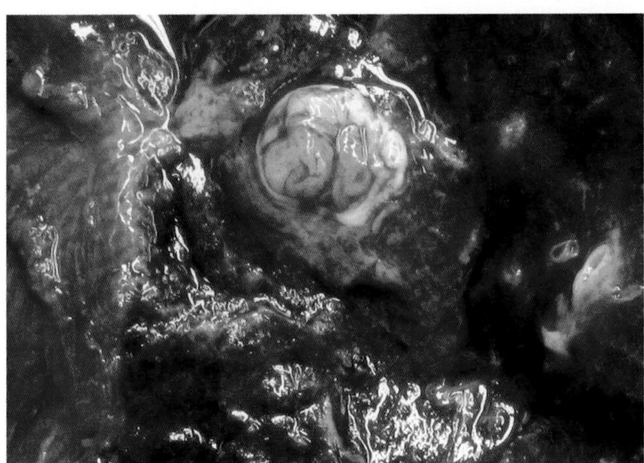

Figure 124.17 Gross image of an echinococcal cyst.

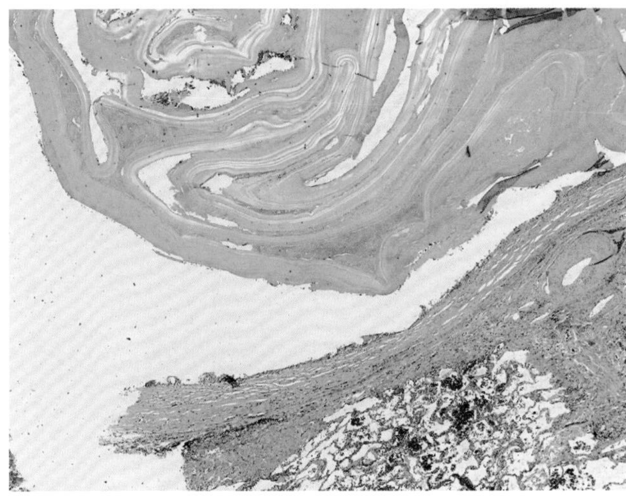

Figure 124.18 Lower power histology showing eosinophilic cyst wall with infolding.

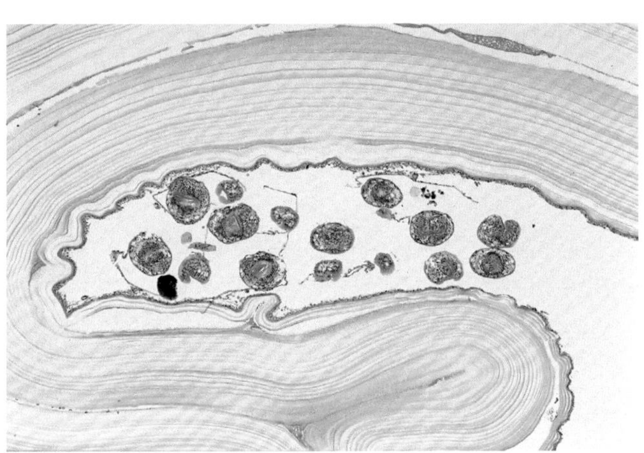

Figure 124.19 Multilamellated cyst wall containing scolices.

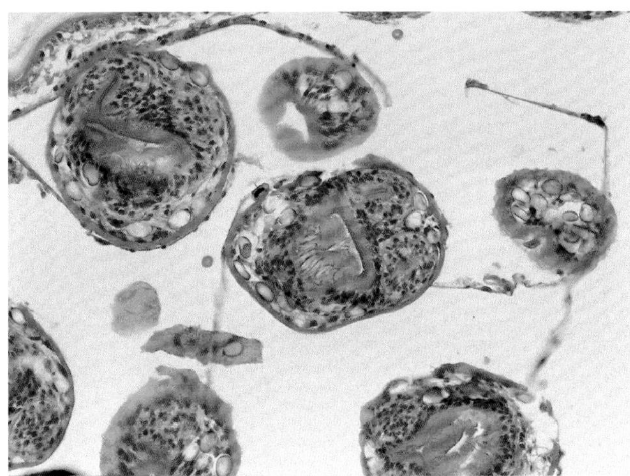

Figure 124.20 High magnification of echinococcal scolices with refractile hooklets.

Section **18**

Transplant-Related Pathology

Aliya N. Husain

125 Acute Lung Transplant Rejection

Aliya N. Husain

The term *acute* does not imply a time course; rather, acute rejection is a cell-mediated process with progressive infiltration of the graft by a characteristic mixture of immune cells. Although acute cellular rejection can develop as early as 3 days to many years posttransplant, patients experience rejection commonly around 3 months, with most episodes occurring between 2 and 9 months. Of total posttransplant patients, 34% develop at least one episode of rejection during the first year. Noncompliance with immunosuppressive medications is a significant cause of late episodes of acute rejection. Patients often present with a low-grade fever, cough, and dyspnea, and some are hypoxemic with greater than 10% decrease in pulmonary function tests. Aspiration and infection may precipitate episodes of acute rejection. The intensity and distribution of the immune infiltrate form the basis of the International Society for Heart and Lung Transplantation (ISHLT) grading system. The main differential diagnosis is infection caused by bacteria, viruses, or fungi. The clinical and radiologic features are similar to those of rejection. Microbiologic cultures and transbronchial biopsies are most useful. Special stains, including immunohistochemistry for cytomegalovirus, Gomori methenamine silver stain for fungus and *Pneumocystis jiroveci*, and Ziehl–Neelsen stain for acid-fast bacteria, should be performed as indicated.

The term *acute cellular rejection* implies a perivascular infiltrate, which is graded from none (0) to severe (4), while airway inflammation (bronchiolitis) has been considered to be difficult to differentiate from infection. Once infection has been ruled out clinically, and the biopsy does not show the classic features of infection, i.e., predominance of neutrophils, especially intraepithelial neutrophils, the airway inflammation most likely represents acute airway rejection. In the 2007 ISHLT grading system, airway inflammation is divided into low and high grades (B1R–B2R). Although a two-tier grading is more reproducible, the problem is that in many transplant centers the decision to treat lies between minimal and mild (B1 and B2) airway rejection according to the 1996 grading scheme. In the current classification, these two grades are lumped into B1R. Because severe airway rejection is extremely rare, the grade B2R is essentially equivalent to B3. Thus, it may be prudent to use the 1996 classification with the revised 2007 grade in parentheses. Whatever the cause of airway inflammation (e.g., ischemia, acute rejection, and infection), it appears to significantly increase the risk of chronic lung allograft dysfunction and bronchiolitis obliterans syndrome (discussed later).

HISTOLOGIC FEATURES

- Minimal acute rejection (grade A1): perivascular infiltrates infrequent; blood vessels, particularly venules, cuffed by small, round, plasmacytoid, and transformed lymphocytes forming 2- to 3-cell-thick layer.
- Mild acute rejection (grade A2): perivascular infiltrates more frequent; greater than three layers of lymphocytes, with eosinophils around venules and arterioles. Grade A2 or higher grade acute rejection is often accompanied by lymphocytic airway inflammation.
- Moderate acute rejection (grade A3): characterized by an extension of the perivascular inflammation into alveolar septa.

- Severe acute rejection (grade A4): diffuse perivascular, interstitial, and airspace infiltrates associated with pneumocyte damage, macrophages, hyaline membranes, hemorrhage, and neutrophils or epithelial ulceration with fibrinopurulent exudates are seen.
- Acute airway rejection (lymphocytic bronchiolitis): the inflammatory infiltrate is the same as seen in perivascular rejection with the predominant cell being the activated lymphocyte, with smaller numbers of eosinophils and neutrophils.
- Low-grade lymphocytic bronchiolitis (B1R): mononuclear cells, with occasional eosinophils, are present in submucosa of the bronchioli as either scattered cells or a circumferential band, without infiltration or necrosis of the epithelium. Minimal airway rejection (B1) has only a few inflammatory infiltrates, whereas mild airway rejection (B2) has a band-like infiltrate in the submucosa.
- High-grade lymphocytic bronchiolitis (B2R): dense bronchiolar inflammatory cell infiltrates with epithelial cell dropout, lymphocytic infiltration of the epithelium, and sometimes ulceration. Moderate airway rejection (B3) has extension of the inflammation into the epithelium, whereas severe airway rejection, with extensive inflammation and ulceration of mucosa, is rarely seen.
- Airway infection: the submucosal inflammation has predominance of neutrophils, which extend into the epithelium.

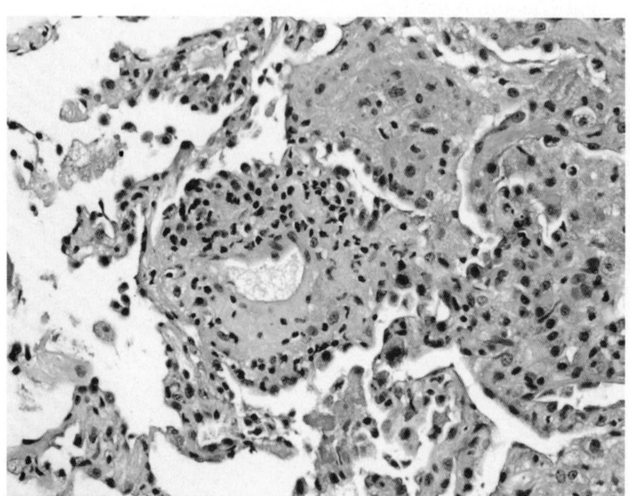

Figure 125.1 Minimal acute rejection (grade A1): perivascular infiltrate forming an incomplete cuff, which is 2- to 3-cell-thick layer.

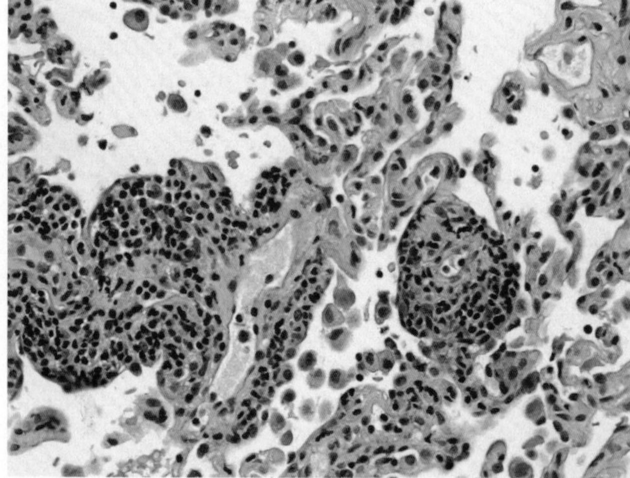

Figure 125.2 Mild acute rejection (grade A2): prominent perivascular infiltrate with more than three layers of lymphocytes and rare eosinophils.

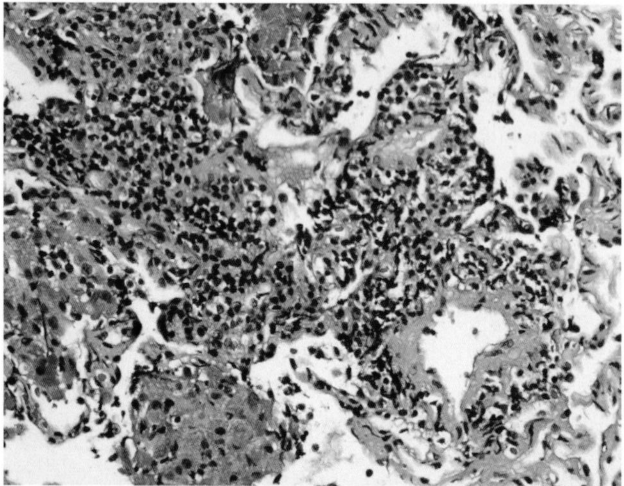

Figure 125.3 Moderate acute rejection (grade A3): the perivascular inflammation extends into alveolar septa.

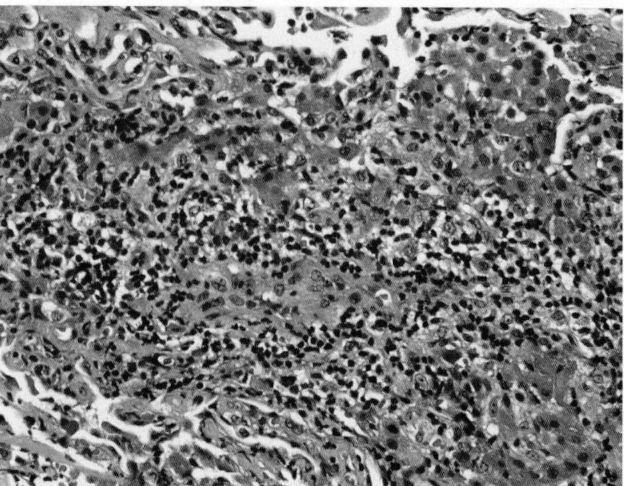

Figure 125.4 Severe acute rejection (grade A4): extensive perivascular, interstitial, and airspace infiltrates associated with pneumocyte damage and macrophages.

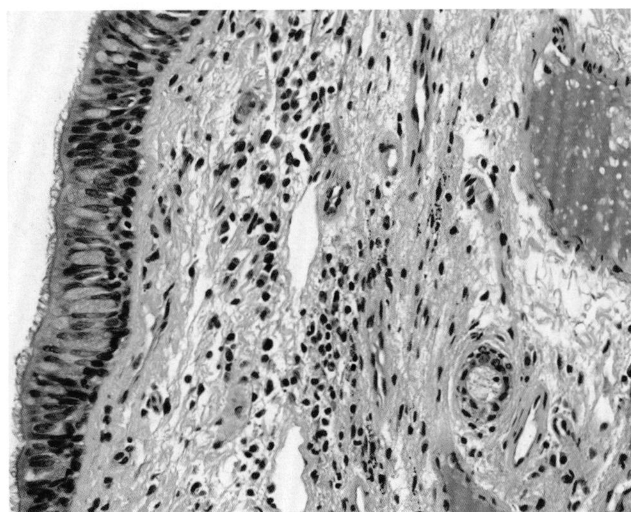

Figure 125.5 Minimal airway rejection (B1): only a few inflammatory cells (lymphocytes and plasma cells) are present in the submucosa.

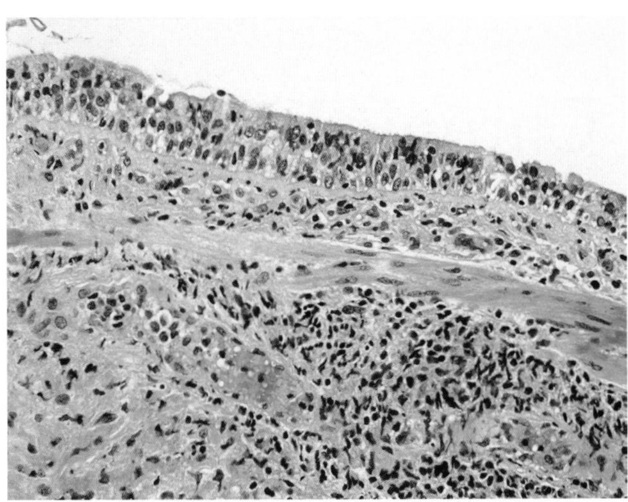

Figure 125.6 Mild airway rejection (B2): there is a band-like inflammatory infiltrate (lymphocytes and few eosinophils) in the submucosa.

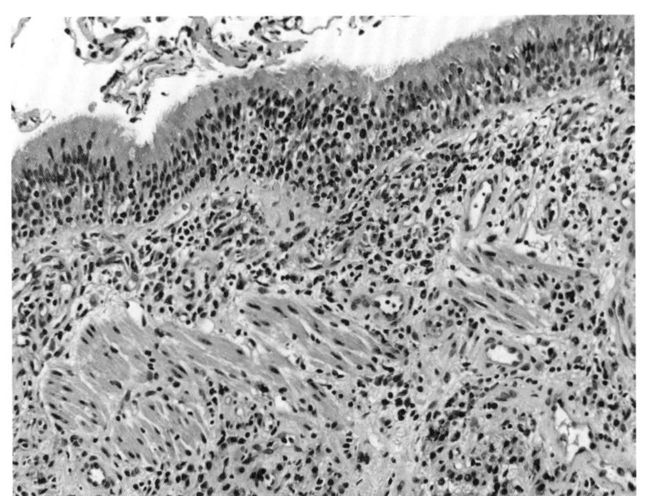

Figure 125.7 Moderate airway rejection (B3): there is extension of the submucosal inflammation (lymphocytes, eosinophils, and plasma cells) into the epithelium.

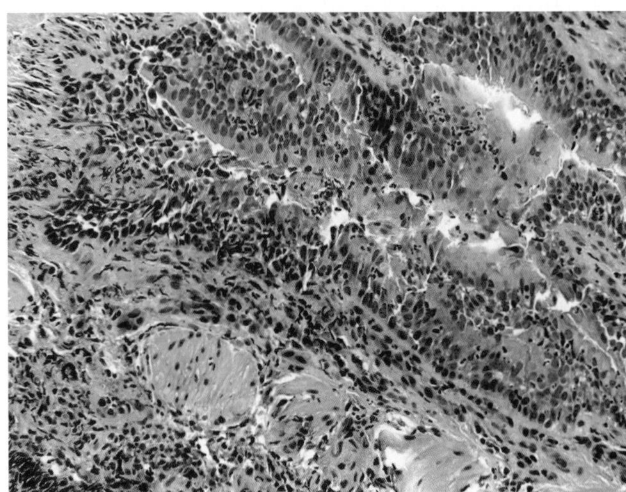

Figure 125.8 Airway infection: the submucosal inflammation has neutrophils (and lymphocytes), which extend into the epithelium, a characteristic feature of infection.

126

Chronic Lung Allograft Dysfunction

Aliya N. Husain

Compared with other solid organ transplants, survival after lung transplantation is shorter due to 50% of patients developing chronic lung allograft dysfunction (CLAD) within 5 years after transplant. CLAD is clinically defined and graded by the degree of permanent decrease in lung function tests and is divided into obstructive, bronchiolitis obliterans syndrome (BOS) and restrictive allograft syndrome (RAS). Although the term *chronic* implies a late temporal process, bronchiolitis obliterans (BO) can be seen as early as 3 to 6 weeks after transplantation, but primarily occurs one or more years later. BOS histologically manifests as obstructive bronchiolitis (BO), which is a fibroinflammatory process that affects mainly bronchioles and also bronchi. It develops as a result of injury and inflammation involving epithelial and subepithelial cells, leading to extensive fibroproliferation. Both alloimmune and nonalloimmune mechanisms are involved in the development of BOS; however, several studies have shown strongest correlation with acute cellular rejection and lymphocytic bronchiolitis (acute airway rejection). Other contributing factors include infections (cytomegalovirus [CMV] and non-CMV), HLA mismatching, primary graft dysfunction, and gastroesophageal reflux. When the clinical diagnosis is not clear, a wedge biopsy is often needed, as BO is a patchy process and diagnostic yield of transbronchial biopsy is low. Development of pleuroparenchymal fibrosis in RAS is commonly preceded by acute lung injury (diffuse alveolar damage). Chronic vascular rejection may be present with either BO or RAS but is mostly not clinically significant.

HISTOLOGIC FINDINGS

Bronchiolitis Obliterans

- Patchy submucosal fibrosis resulting in partial or complete occlusion of bronchiolar lumen, with or without inflammatory infiltrates.
- Submucosal fibrosis either bulges asymmetrically into the lumen and causes partial obstruction or is concentric and causes total obstruction.
- The histologic grading of BO is based only on the presence or absence of the lesion and does not classify them further based on inflammation.
- Secondary changes often seen include mucostasis, postobstructive endogenous lipoid pneumonia, and foci of acute inflammation.
- The main histologic differential diagnosis is organizing pneumonia, which is a healing response to various forms of lung injury and manifests as loose fibromyxoid plugs of connective tissue within alveoli and bronchioles.

Restrictive Allograft Syndrome

- Pleuroparenchymal fibrosis, with or without BO, is predominantly a subpleural process of the upper lobes, with occasional paraseptal and centrilobular fibrosis.

Chronic Vascular Rejection

- Intimal fibrosis and thickening of small blood vessels.

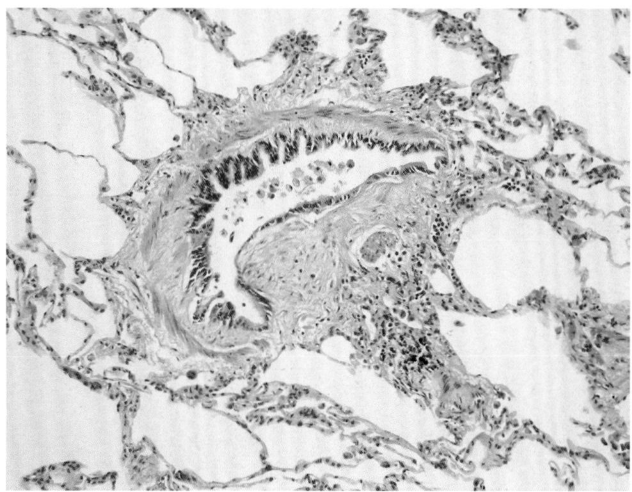

Figure 126.1 BO: the airway lumen is partially occluded by asymmetric submucosal fibrosis.

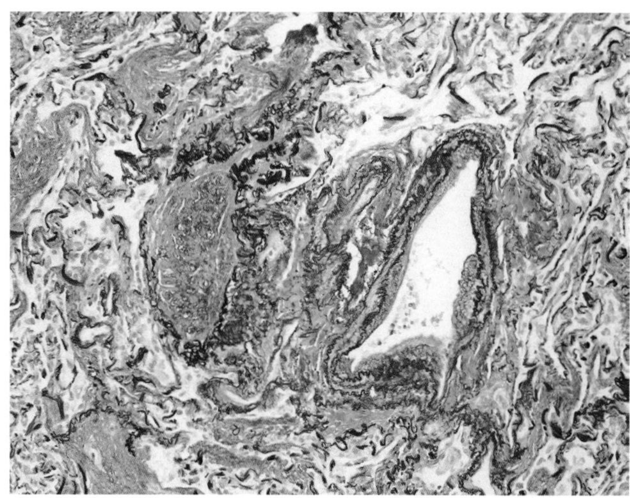

Figure 126.2 Elastic stain highlights the obliterated bronchiole on the *left*. Note relatively normal accompanying pulmonary artery branch on the *right*.

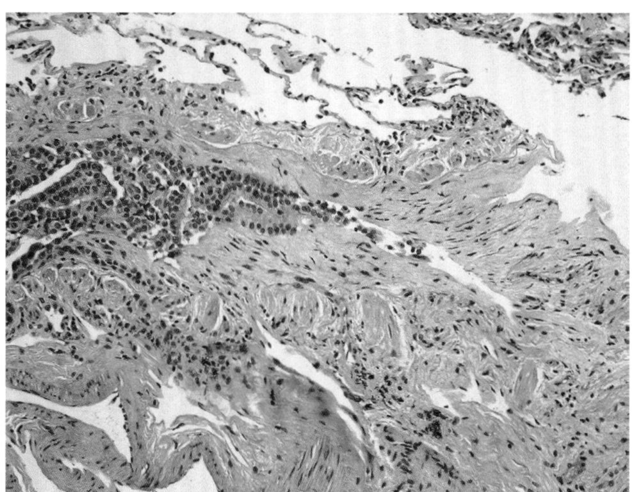

Figure 126.3 The lumen of this distorted bronchiole is partially obliterated by fibrosis; however, the residual smooth muscle outlines the original airway.

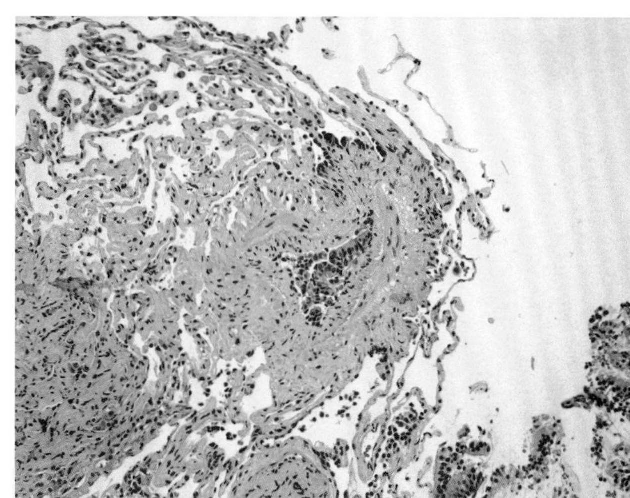

Figure 126.4 Circumferential submucosal fibrosis is present in this case of BO.

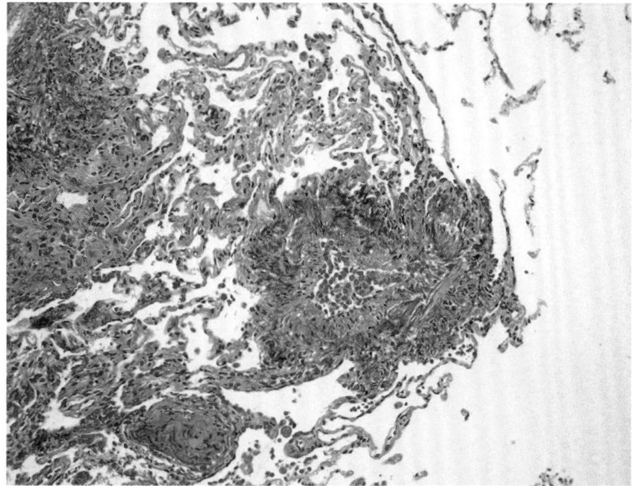

Figure 126.5 Trichrome stain highlights the fibrosis seen in Figure 126.4.

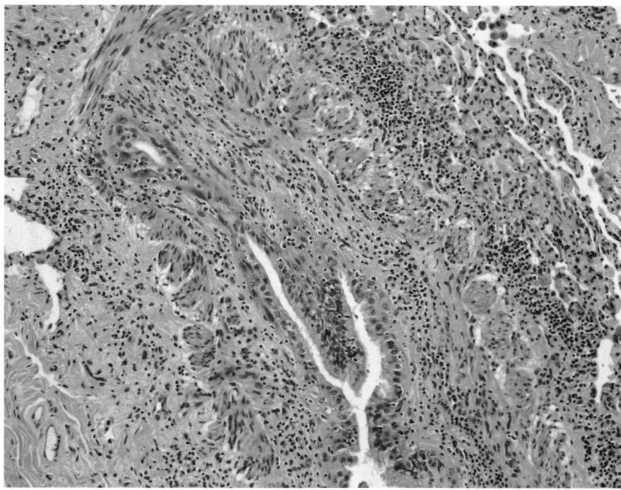

Figure 126.6 The submucosal fibrosis in this case of BO contains inflammatory infiltrates (mainly lymphocytes).

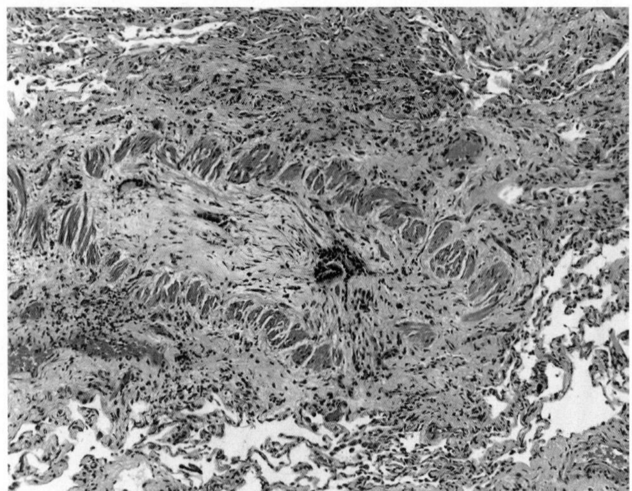

Figure 126.7 Near complete obliteration of the lumen is present in this case of BO.

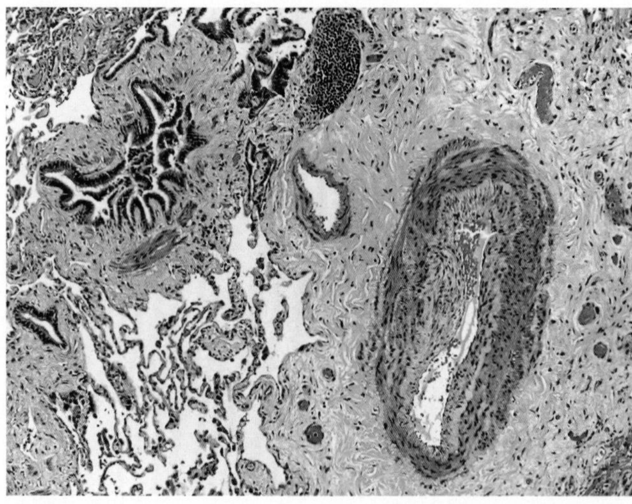

Figure 126.8 Chronic vascular rejection (intimal fibrosis) is also present in the case illustrated in Figure 126.7.

Antibody-Mediated Lung Transplant Rejection

127

Aliya N. Husain

In the lung, antibody-mediated rejection (AMR) is a diagnostic challenge because of the lack of widely accepted diagnostic criteria. AMR is caused by binding of preformed or de novo donor-specific human leukocyte antigen (HLA) antibodies to the antigen on the capillary endothelial cells. Interaction between antibody and antigen leads to allograft injury through activation of complement and complement cascade and leukocyte recruitment. Incidence of AMR is not known. Currently, diagnosis of AMR is based on clinical evidence of allograft dysfunction, presence of circulating donor-specific antibodies (DSAs) and pathologic findings. Small number of patients with preformed DSAs may develop hyperacute rejection during or immediately after the transplant, leading to respiratory failure. Most patients develop DSAs during first posttransplant year and present with breathlessness, hypoxia, and radiographic finding of diffuse pulmonary infiltrates. Hyperacute rejection is usually fatal. Most of the patients with AMR initially improve but are at a higher risk of developing chronic lung allograft dysfunction. Treatment includes removal of the circulating antibodies by plasmapheresis, intravenous immunoglobulins, and B cell–mediated therapy.

HISTOLOGIC FEATURES

- Histologic findings in AMR are nonspecific and overlap with those of acute cellular rejection, ischemia–reperfusion injury, infection, and drug reaction.
- In hyperacute rejection there is evidence of pulmonary infarction associated with vascular thrombosis, vascular fibrinoid necrosis, vasculitis, and neutrophil margination.
- Histologic patterns described in patients with graft dysfunction and de novo DSAs include capillary inflammation, acute lung injury, and endothelialitis.
- Immunostain for complement fragment 4d (C4d) deposition can be seen in various pulmonary structures; however, only staining of the vascular endothelium of the interstitial alveolar capillaries is considered significant. C4d is positive when >50% of interstitial capillaries stain strongly. However, this is seen only rarely, which limits its usefulness.

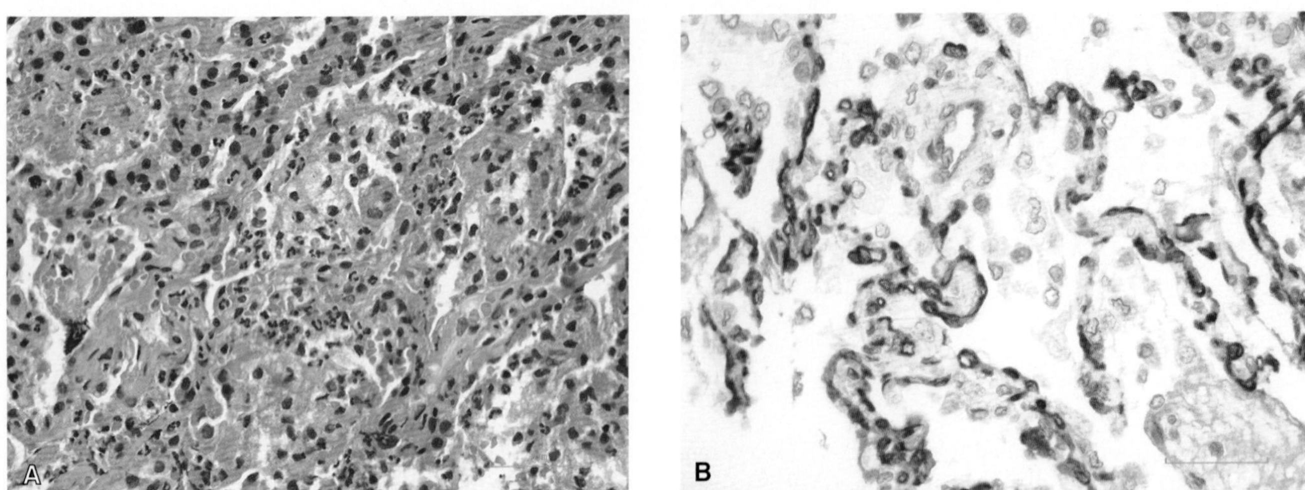

Figure 127.1 This transbronchial biopsy shows capillaritis, focal hemorrhage, and intra-alveolar macrophages (**A**). Immunohistochemical stain for C4d shows strong diffuse endothelial staining of alveolar capillaries (**B**). (Figures courtesy of M. Angeles Montero MD, PhD, London, England.)

128 Anastomotic Complications

Aliya N. Husain

Anastomotic complications have become much less common in the current transplant era because of better surgical techniques and patient management. They may occur in the airway or vascular anastomosis due to ischemia or infection. Necrosis at the airway anastomotic site is common 1 to 5 weeks after transplantation and is part of the normal healing process. In 7% to 24% of patients, excessive granulation tissue is formed at the site of anastomosis causing airway obstruction, which may be removed bronchoscopically. In rare instances, extensive necrosis and ischemia lead to dehiscence of the anastomosis. Bronchial stenosis most commonly develops 2 to 9 months after transplantation and is the most common complication, occurring in 1.6% to 32% of transplanted patients. Management depends on the type of airway complication and on its severity. Vascular complications are very rare.

HISTOLOGIC FEATURES

- Most common specimen received in surgical pathology is granulation tissue with only mild acute and chronic inflammation.
- When ischemic changes are more extensive, the anastomotic site is debrided, which often shows necrotic cartilage.
- If superimposed infection is present, bacterial colonies or invasive fungal hyphae may be seen for which a silver stain is very helpful.

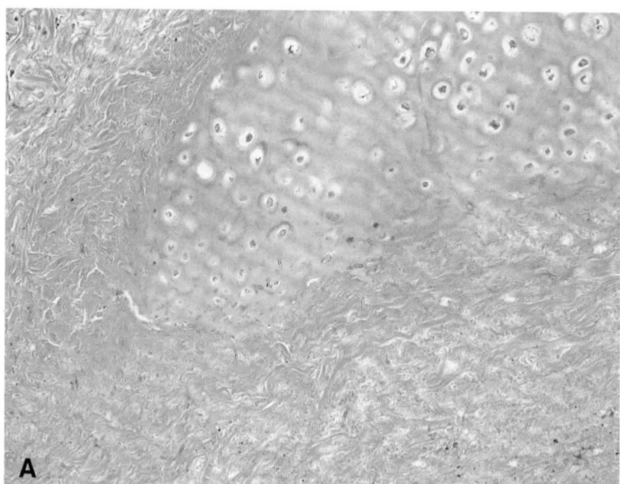

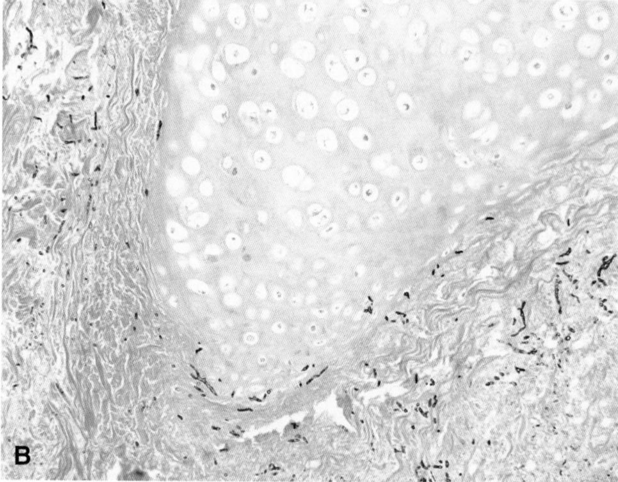

Figure 128.1 Airway anastomotic site showing necrosis of soft tissue and cartilage with invasive fungus (**A**). GMS stain highlights the invasive fungal hyphae (**B**).

129 Transplant-Related Infections

Aliya N. Husain

Lung transplant recipients are at high risk of developing infections due to exposure to the environment, immunosuppression, loss of cough reflex, compromised lymphatic drainage, and ischemia of bronchial anastomosis. Both community-acquired and opportunistic infections are seen, including bacterial, viral, and fungal infections. Patients present with one or more of the following: fever, cough, sputum production, dyspnea, hypoxemia, and decline in spirometry. Most bacterial infections occur in the first posttransplant month and are commonly caused by health care–associated organisms. Viral and fungal infections are more commonly seen 3 to 6 months after transplantation. Cytomegalovirus (CMV) infections are the most common viral infections in transplanted patients and are a contributing factor in the development of chronic lung allograft dysfunction (CLAD). Incidence of fungal infection ranges from 15% to 35% with *Aspergillus* and *Candida* species being the most common organisms. *Aspergillus* commonly colonizes airways and also causes infection of the anastomotic site and invasive pneumonia. Patients with CLAD are particularly vulnerable to development of late-onset pneumonia, which may be fatal.

HISTOLOGIC FEATURES

- These depend on the etiology of the infection and the host response, which may be minimal.
- Neutrophilic inflammation is often seen in bacterial infections. Occasionally, there is only bacterial growth with no inflammation.
- The most common viral infection is caused by CMV, which infects endothelial cells and pneumocytes, and is diagnosed by the presence of classical single intranuclear inclusion and multiple small cytoplasmic inclusions. Treated CMV infection is difficult to identify because it results in fragmented or smudged, eosinophilic inclusions. Immunohistochemistry (IHC) stain is helpful in identifying early infection without cytopathic effect. Rejection may be seen in the same biopsy as infection.
- Fungal infection manifests as infiltrating hyphae in necrotic tissue, which can be highlighted by periodic acid–Schiff or Gomori methenamine silver stain. There may be minimal inflammation.

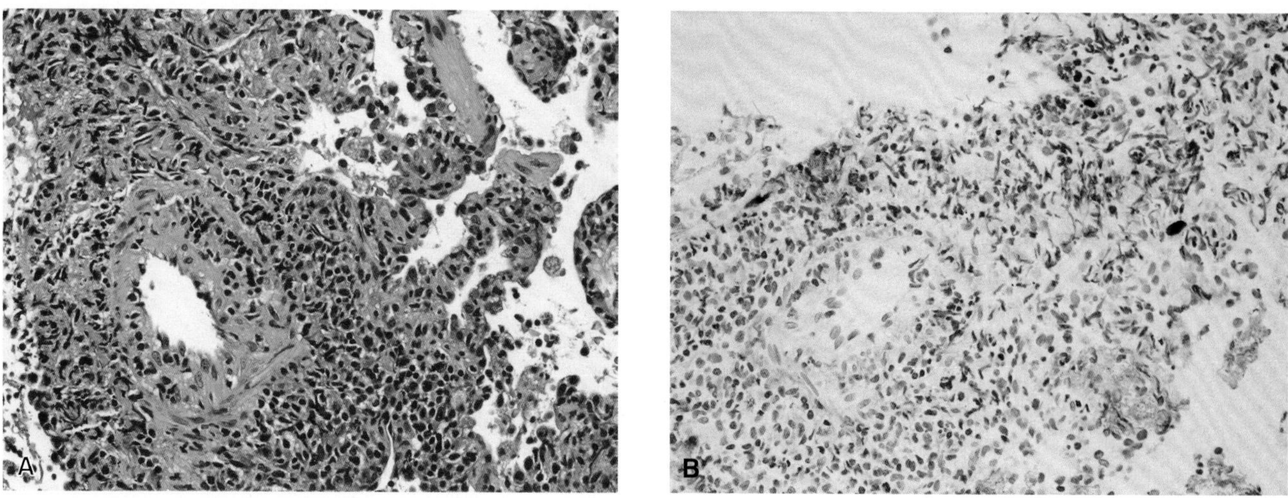

Figure 129.1 Infection can precipitate acute cellular rejection, as seen in this case with perivascular inflammatory cuff (**A**), and CMV pneumonitis demonstrated by IHC stain (**B**).

130 Primary Graft Dysfunction

Aliya N. Husain

Primary graft dysfunction (PGD), a form of acute lung injury occurring within 72 hours of lung transplantation, is characterized by hypoxemia and alveolar infiltrates in the allograft. PGD is the end result of multiple deleterious mechanisms, including donor brain death, mechanical ventilation, procurement, storage, and ischemia–reperfusion injury (IRI). IRI refers to sterile inflammation that occurs after substrate supply is restored following a period of absent blood flow. As a result, there is innate immune activation, epithelial cell injury, endothelial cell dysfunction, and cytokine release. Mechanisms leading to acute lung injury with diffuse alveolar damage include ischemia-induced endothelial and epithelial injury, abnormalities in coagulation and fibrinolysis, alterations in cell adhesion, and chemotaxis. Absence of perivascular and airway mononuclear cell infiltrates helps distinguish PGD from acute rejection. Severe PGD occurs in approximately 30% of patients and is associated with increased risk of mortality (both early and late) and increased incidence of chronic lung allograft dysfunction/bronchiolitis obliterans syndrome.

HISTOLOGIC FEATURES

- The transplanted lung is only rarely biopsied for PGD.
- Pathologic findings depend on the duration and severity of symptoms.
- Early changes include edema, reactive pneumocytes, and, if severe, hyaline membranes.
- In the recovery phase, organizing diffuse alveolar damage is seen.

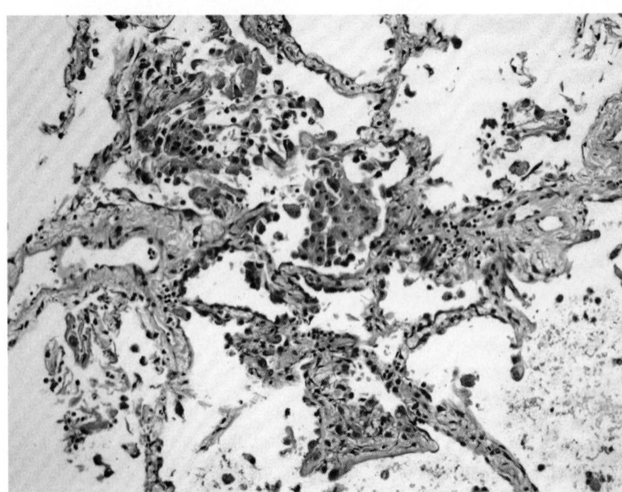

Figure 130.1 This early posttransplant lung biopsy shows intra-alveolar edema, scattered macrophages, and reactive pneumocytes.

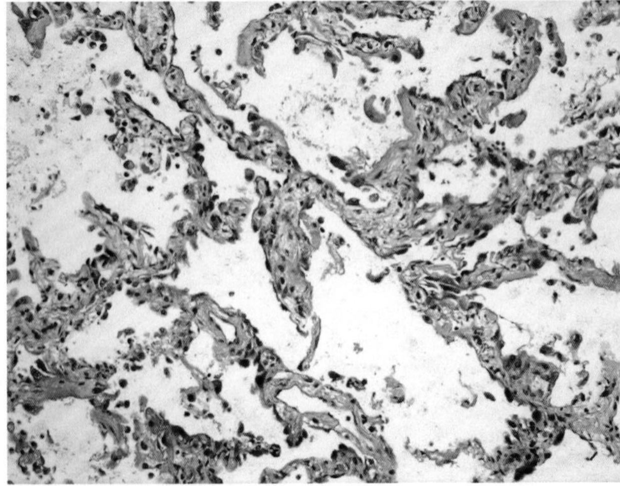

Figure 130.2 This transbronchial lung biopsy shows organizing hyaline membranes and reactive pneumocytes.

Organizing Pneumonia in the Transplanted Lung

131

Aliya N. Husain

Organizing pneumonia (formerly known as *bronchiolitis obliterans organizing pneumonia* or *BOOP*), is a healing response to various forms of lung injury and manifests as loose fibromyxoid plugs of connective tissue within alveoli and bronchioles. It may be seen in patients recovering from acute rejection, infection, or any other damage to the transplanted lung. The main differential diagnosis is from bronchiolitis obliterans, which is dense scar tissue (mature collagen) in the submucosa of small airways.

HISTOLOGIC FEATURES

- Organizing pneumonia in the transplanted lung is similar to that seen in the nontransplant setting.
- There are intra-alveolar plugs of loose myxoid fibrous tissue (Masson bodies), which may have few inflammatory cells, such as macrophages, lymphocytes, and plasma cells. Hemosiderin may also be present.

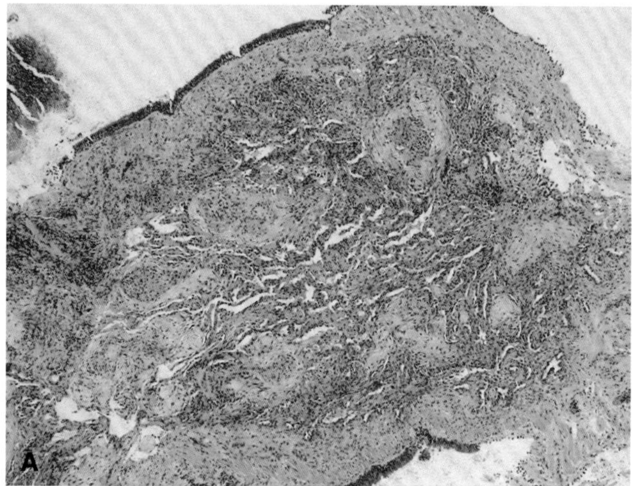

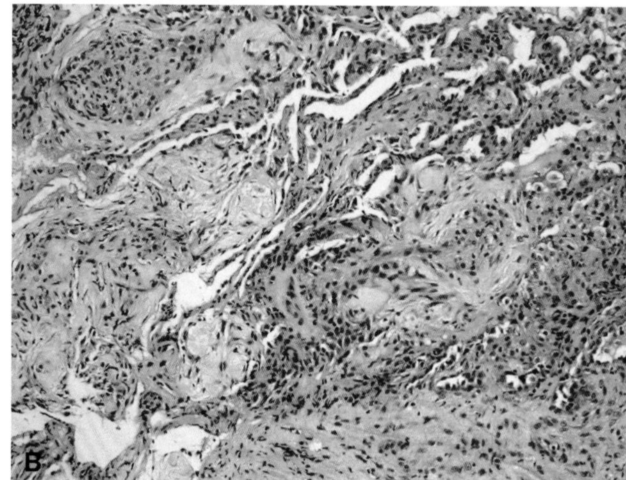

Figure 131.1 This transbronchial biopsy specimen from a transplant patient shows intra-alveolar Masson bodies at low (**A**) and high (**B**) powers. Note the presence of hemosiderin and reactive type II pneumocytes.

Other Lung Transplant–Related Pathology

132

Aliya N. Husain

Most posttransplant lung biopsies are performed either as rejection surveillance or to evaluate symptoms suggestive of infection or rejection. Several other pathologies may be present, which need to be considered in the differential diagnosis.

HISTOLOGIC FEATURES

- Bronchus-associated lymphoid tissue (BALT) is often hyperplastic in posttransplant patients. It is a localized collection of mature small lymphocytes, often with several capillaries, and may have anthracotic pigment or hemosiderin in it. Central CD21-positive network of dendritic cells can be demonstrated in lesions that are larger.
- Microaspiration is common and may trigger acute rejection. Small poorly formed granulomas with multinucleated giant cells or intra-alveolar foreign body–type giant cells are highly suggestive. Foreign material is only occasionally seen.
- Acute inflammation often signifies infection. Neutrophils can be present in alveoli or within bronchial and bronchiolar epithelium, with or without other inflammatory cells.
- Nonspecific changes may be seen in any biopsy, such as intra-alveolar fibrin, reactive type II pneumocytes, and interstitial fibrosis.
- Hemosiderin, a very common finding, can be present in the interstitium or in intra-alveolar macrophages.
- Lipoid pneumonia may be seen in aspiration (exogenous, with large intracytoplasmic vacuoles) or postobstruction (endogenous, small intracytoplasmic vacuoles).
- Kaposi sarcoma is characterized by a spindle-cell proliferation with extravasated red blood cells. It is positive for vascular markers (CD31, CD34, ERG, and Fli-1) and Kaposi sarcoma–associated herpesvirus/human herpesvirus 8 (KSHV/HHV8).

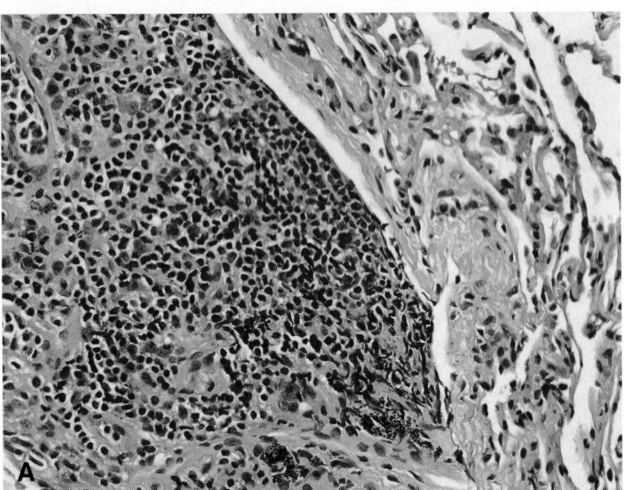

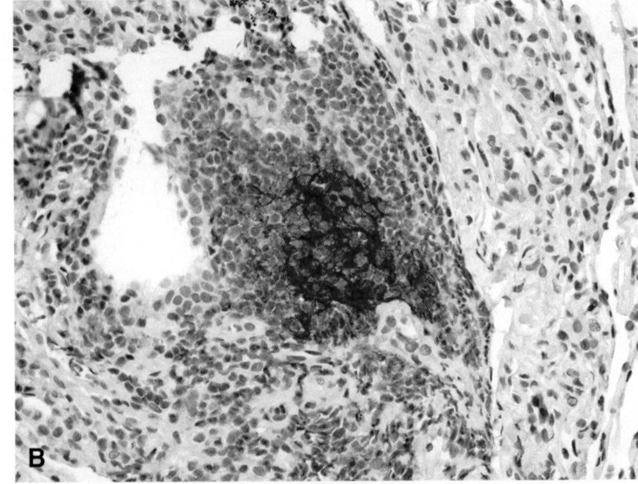

Figure 132.1 BALT, composed of small lymphocytes with several capillaries, is seen here associated with anthracotic pigment (**A**). CD21 stain highlights the central dendritic cell framework (**B**).

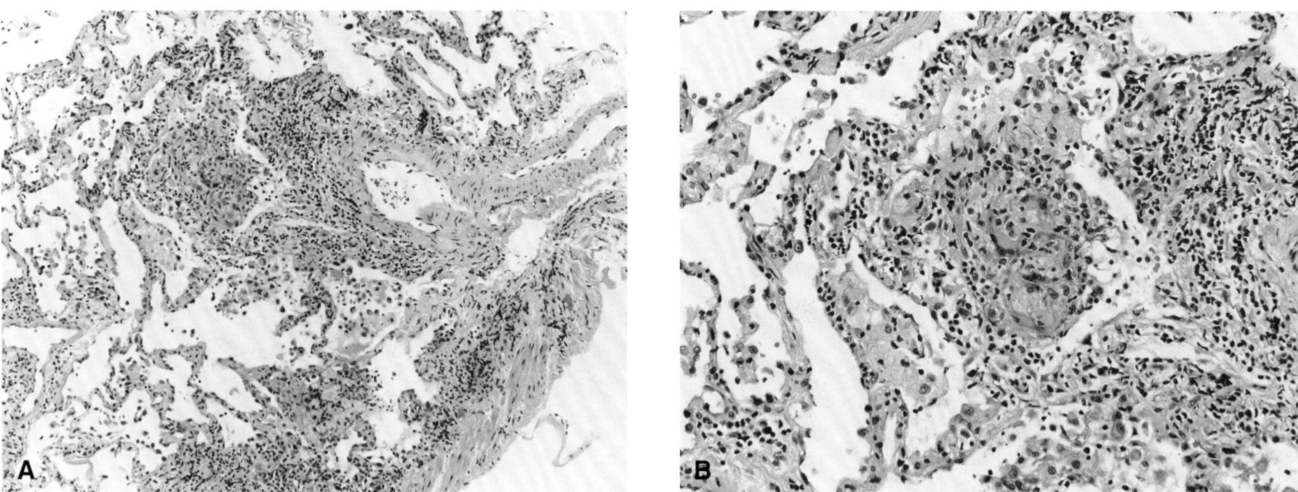

Figure 132.2 This transbronchial biopsy shows patchy interstitial chronic inflammation (**A**) and poorly formed nonnecrotizing granuloma (**B**), consistent with microaspiration.

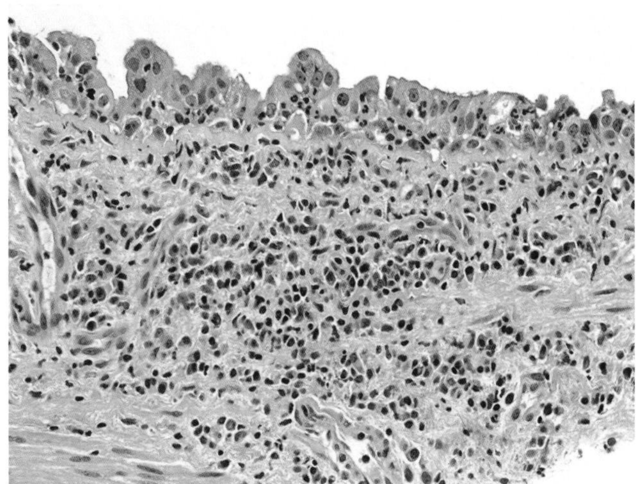

Figure 132.3 Intra-epithelial neutrophils are seen together with submucosal chronic inflammation in this transbronchial biopsy from a patient with bacterial infection posttransplant.

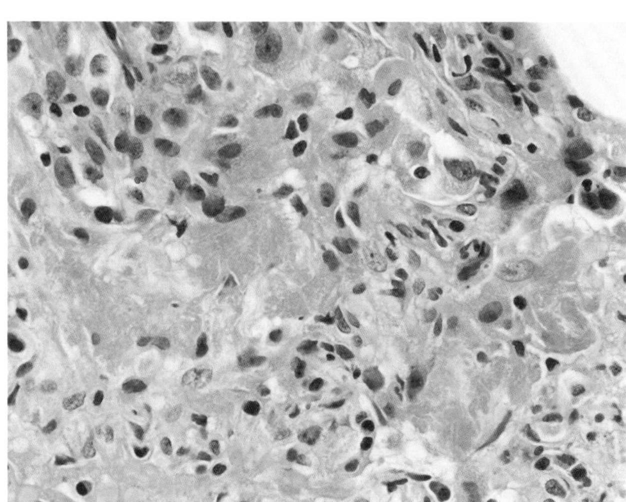

Figure 132.4 Nonspecific changes seen in this biopsy include intra-alveolar fibrin and reactive type II pneumocytes.

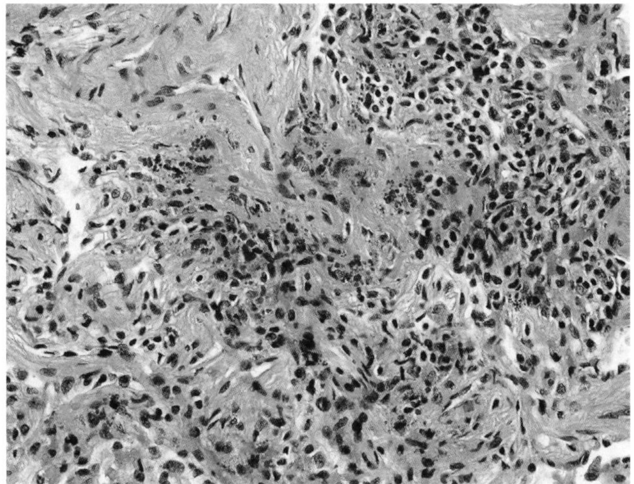

Figure 132.5 There is extensive hemosiderin in this posttransplant biopsy.

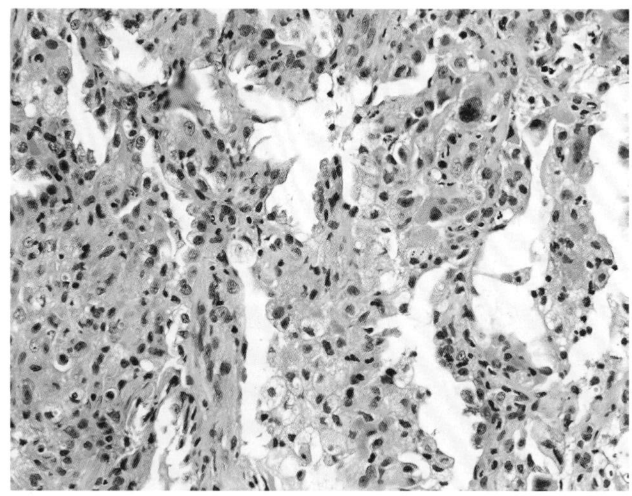

Figure 132.6 Endogenous lipoid pneumonia is seen in this biopsy with foamy macrophages and reactive type II pneumocytes.

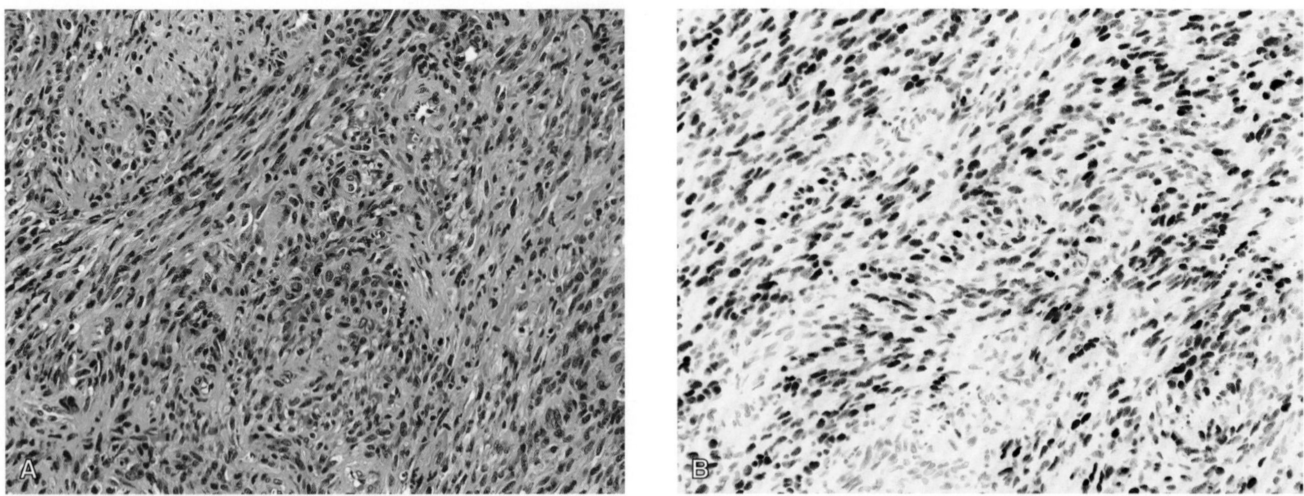

Figure 132.7 Characteristic spindle cells and extravasated red blood cells (**A**) are seen in this patient with Kaposi sarcoma. The diagnosis is confirmed by positive nuclear staining for KSHV by immunohistochemistry (**B**).

Posttransplant Lymphoproliferative Disorders

133

Aliya N. Husain

This is a spectrum of lymphoproliferative disorders that arise after both solid organ and stem cell transplantation mostly in association with Epstein–Barr virus (EBV). The incidence varies from 1% (in renal transplant patients) to 5% (in intestinal and lung transplant patients). The World Health Organization (2016) classifies posttransplant lymphoproliferative disorders (PTLDs) into plasmacytic hyperplasia PTLD, infectious mononucleosis PTLD, florid follicular hyperplasia PTLD, polymorphic PTLD, monomorphic PTLD (B- and T-/NK-cell types), and classical Hodgkin lymphoma PTLD. The early PTLD (occurring within the first year) is more likely to be polymorphic, which are likely to regress with decreased immunosuppression, in contrast to the late PTLD, which are mostly monomorphic and have a poorer prognosis. The allograft lung may be involved in addition to systemic disease.

HISTOLOGIC FEATURES

- Morphology depends on the type of PTLD. The early lesions are often not biopsied, the diagnosis being made on clinical features and rising EBV titers.
- Biopsy of the late PTLD shows a nodular infiltrate of atypical large B cells, which involve the lung parenchyma, blood vessels, and airways. Necrosis is common.

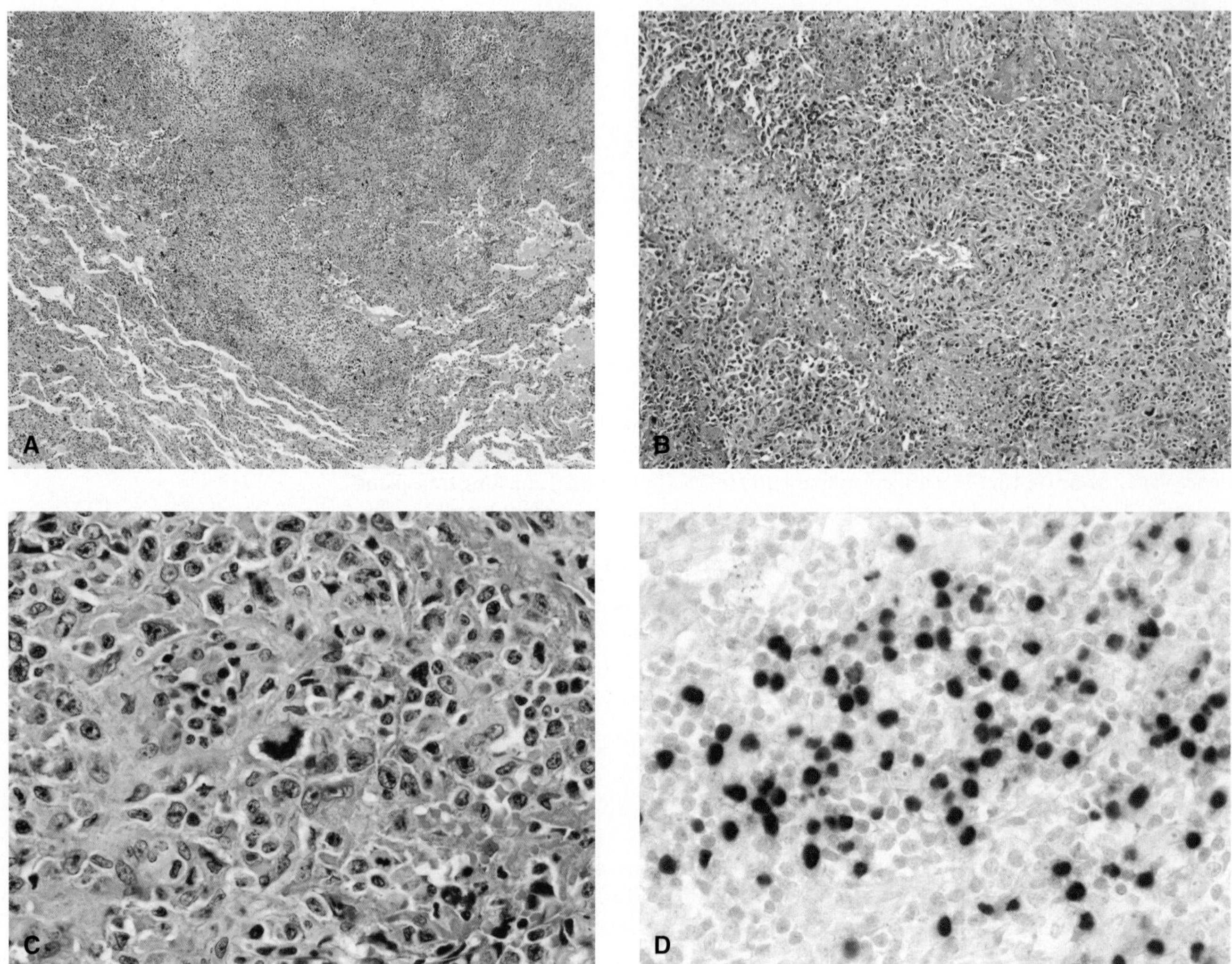

Figure 133.1 Lung wedge biopsy shows nodular infiltrate of cells (**A**), which are large and atypical and have foci of necrosis (**B and C**). In situ hybridization is positive for EBV (**D**).

Lung Pathology in Transplantation of Other Organs

134

Aliya N. Husain

In any immunocompromised host, including other organ and stem cell transplant recipients, the lungs are susceptible to infection with both opportunistic and nonopportunistic organisms as described in the sections on infection. Graft-versus-host disease (GVHD) can sometimes involve the lungs in stem cell transplant recipients (and extremely rarely after solid organ transplantation). These patients usually have GVHD of other sites, such as gastrointestinal tract and skin. Acute GVHD presents with low-grade fever, cough, and shortness of breath. Chronic GVHD manifests as progressive decrease in lung function with obstructive features.

HISTOLOGIC FEATURES

- Morphology of infection depends on the type of infection and host response.
- Extremely immunocompromised patients cannot mount an inflammatory response, and organisms grow unchecked.
- Acute GVHD shows perivascular and airway inflammation similar to that seen in acute lung transplant rejection.
- Chronic GVHD shows bronchiolitis obliterans/constrictive bronchiolitis with submucosa fibrosis of small airways, which may partially or totally obstruct the lumen.

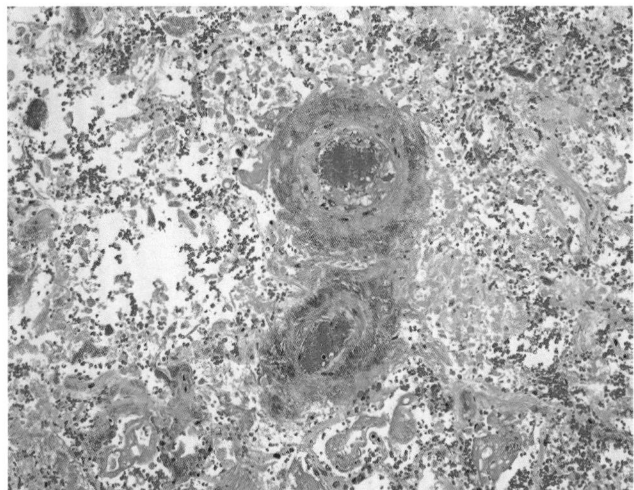

Figure 134.1 A 42-year-old man underwent stem cell transplant for progressive myelofibrosis and developed pseudomonas pneumonia seen here at autopsy. Note the extensive bacterial growth, especially around blood vessels, with no inflammatory response in the lung.

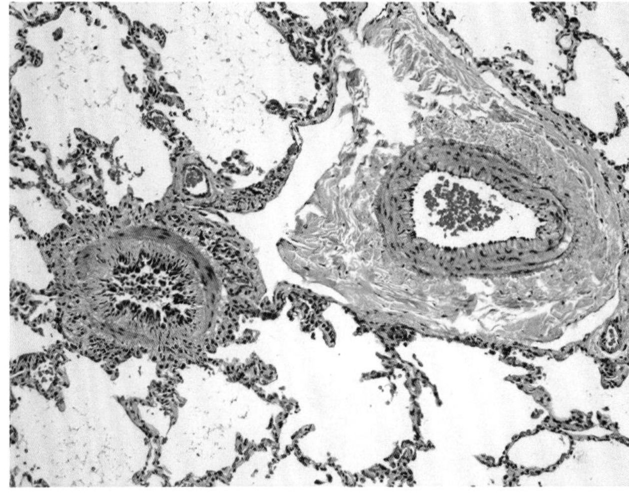

Figure 134.2 A 17-month-old child underwent stem cell transplant for severe combined immunodeficiency and developed chronic GVHD seen here as early submucosal fibrosis in a bronchiole adjacent to a normal pulmonary artery branch.

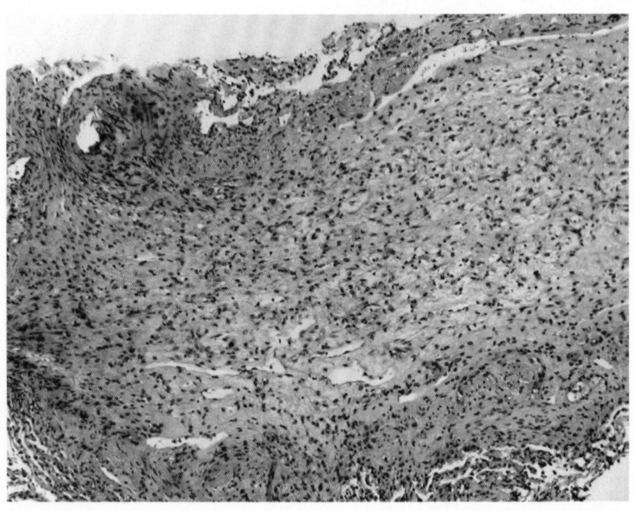

Figure 134.3 A 46-year-old man developed chronic GVHD after stem cell transplant for lymphoma. There is total occlusion of the bronchiolar lumen by granulation tissue and fibrosis.

Section 19

Lung Pathology in Collagen Vascular Diseases

Lynette M. Sholl

Lung Pathology in Collagen Vascular Diseases

135

▶ Lynette M. Sholl

The manifestations of collagen vascular diseases (CVDs) in the lung are varied both clinically and pathologically. Correlations have been observed between the pattern of interstitial lung disease and the underlying diagnosis, e.g., usual interstitial pneumonia (UIP) pattern and rheumatoid arthritis (RA), lymphocytic interstitial pneumonia and Sjogren syndrome, follicular bronchiolitis in RA and Sjogren syndrome, organizing pneumonia and autoimmune myositis, fibrotic nonspecific interstitial pneumonia (NSIP) and systemic sclerosis, and diffuse alveolar damage/hemorrhage and systemic lupus erythematosus. However, any individual pattern can be seen in a variety of CVD and multiple patterns may be observed in a single patient. Given these overlapping pathologic patterns, a diagnosis of CVD-related interstitial lung disease must be rendered in the context of a comprehensive clinical and serologic workup.

The type and severity of symptoms attributable to lung involvement reflect the pattern of disease; common features include chronic cough and dyspnea. NSIP is common in a variety of CVD diagnoses and, depending on the degree of inflammation versus fibrosis, may be at least partially reversible with immunosuppressive therapies. Organizing pneumonia presents in isolation or in tandem with NSIP and may be associated with a worse prognosis when diagnosed in the context of CVD, compared with its cryptogenic form, but should be amenable to immunosuppressive therapies. UIP pattern, the most common form of interstitial fibrosis seen in patients with RA, presents with progressive, irreversible dyspnea and a 50% 5-year mortality. UIP-pattern disease in CVD appears clinically similar to idiopathic pulmonary fibrosis, including the lack of response to immunosuppression. To date, the benefits of antifibrotic therapies have not been established for patients with UIP-pattern disease with underlying CVD.

RA, in particular, has several relatively unique pulmonary manifestations, namely follicular bronchiolitis and rheumatoid nodules. In follicular bronchiolitis, hyperplastic lymphoid tissue impinges on bronchioles and terminal airways, often leading to small airways obstruction by pulmonary function testing and air trapping visible on chest computed tomography (see also Chapter 51). Rheumatoid nodules are generally asymptomatic, but their multifocal, well-circumscribed character can mimic metastatic disease radiographically, triggering lung biopsy to rule out malignancy (see also Chapter 57). Desquamative interstitial pneumonia is reported rarely in nonsmokers in the context of CVD including RA.

Lung disease may manifest in patients with a well-established CVD diagnosis (CVD-associated interstitial lung disease); in this context, interstitial pneumonia has a better prognosis relative to its idiopathic forms. In some patients, lung involvement may be the first or only manifestation of a defined or undefined CVD (so-called lung-dominant CVD). The diagnosis of interstitial pneumonia with autoimmune features has been proposed to describe patients with an idiopathic interstitial pneumonia pattern (most commonly NSIP or UIP) and some clinical and serologic features of autoimmunity, but who fail to meet diagnostic criteria for any particular CVD. The prognostic and treatment implications of this classification have not yet been fully established.

HISTOLOGIC FEATURES

- Mixed patterns of interstitial pneumonias are common, such as cellular and/or fibrosing NSIP with organizing pneumonia or with bronchiolitis.
- Multiple compartments of the lung may be involved in an individual case, including interstitium (NSIP and UIP patterns), pleura (acute and/or organizing pleuritis), vessels (vasculitis and hypertensive vasculopathy), and airways (follicular bronchiolitis, respiratory bronchiolitis, and obliterative bronchiolitis).
- Pronounced lymphoid follicle formation in the context of fibrosing interstitial pneumonia should raise the possibility of an underlying CVD.

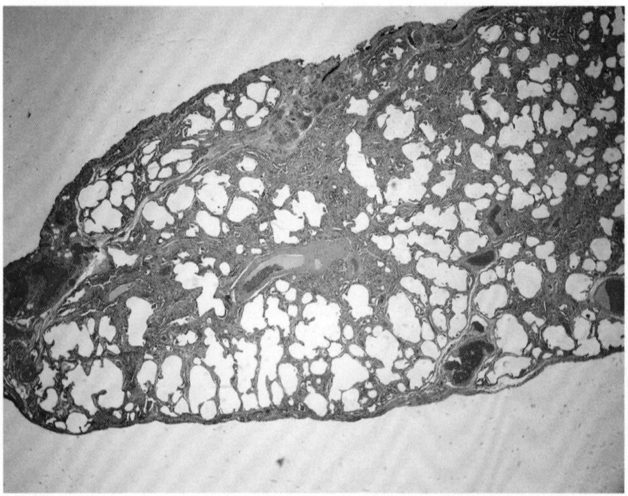

Figure 135.1 Fibrotic NSIP (scanning power) in a patient with systemic sclerosis. The interstitium is diffusely and uniformly thickened. The pleura appears fibrotic with granulation tissue formation, most evident at the *top* of the image.

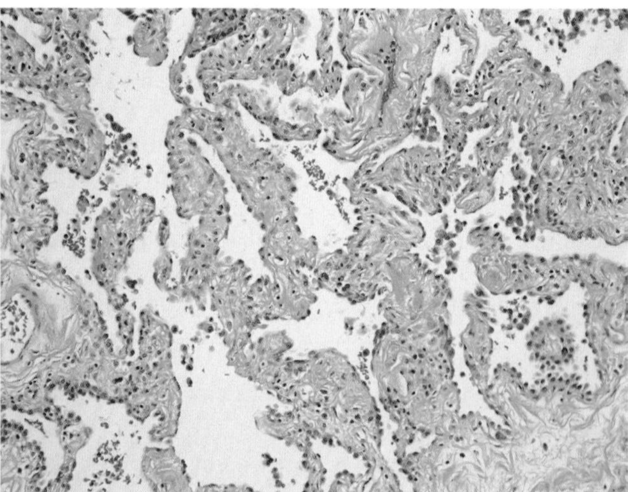

Figure 135.2 Pronounced collagen deposition and sparse inflammatory cells in the alveolar septa in fibrotic NSIP in a patient with systemic sclerosis. This type of fibrotic change is generally considered to be irreversible.

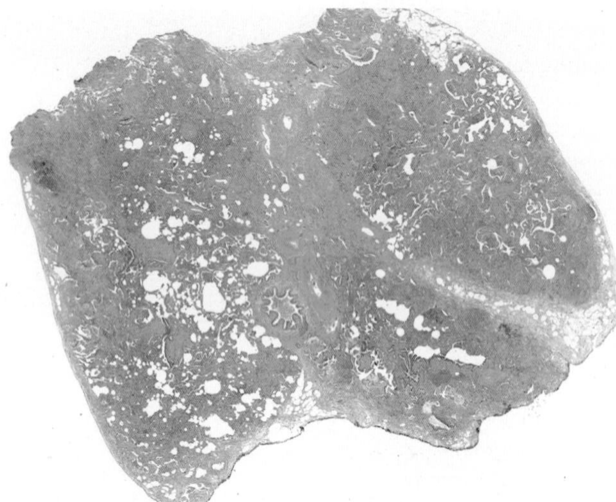

Figure 135.3 Scanning view of lung involved by NSIP combined with desquamative interstitial pneumonia in a patient with an undifferentiated CVD. The sampled lung is diffusely and homogenously infiltrated by chronic inflammatory cells, and the pulmonary arteriolar walls are significantly thickened as a result of medial hyperplasia.

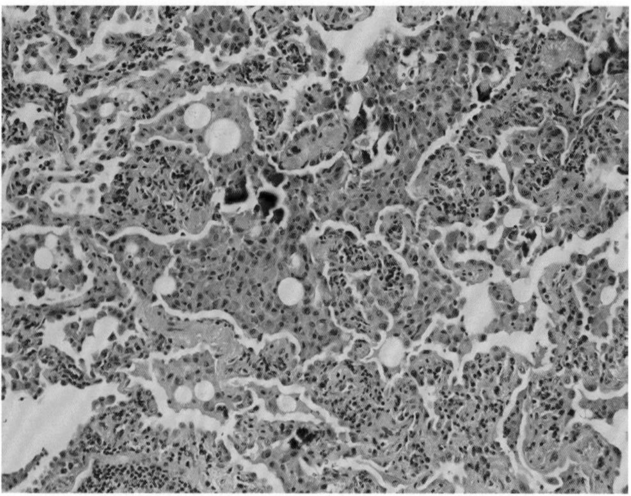

Figure 135.4 Cellular NSIP and desquamative interstitial pneumonia in CVD. There is a prominent lymphocytic infiltrate in the alveolar septa. The airspaces are filled by alveolar macrophages. Airspace calcifications are visible, likely representing aggregated endogenous cellular breakdown products.

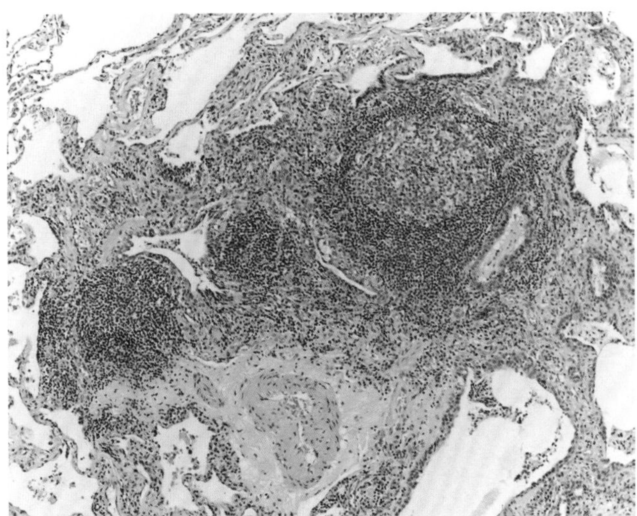

Figure 135.5 A partially obliterated respiratory bronchiole with adjacent lymphoid follicles with germinal center formation in a patient with follicular bronchiolitis in the setting of RA.

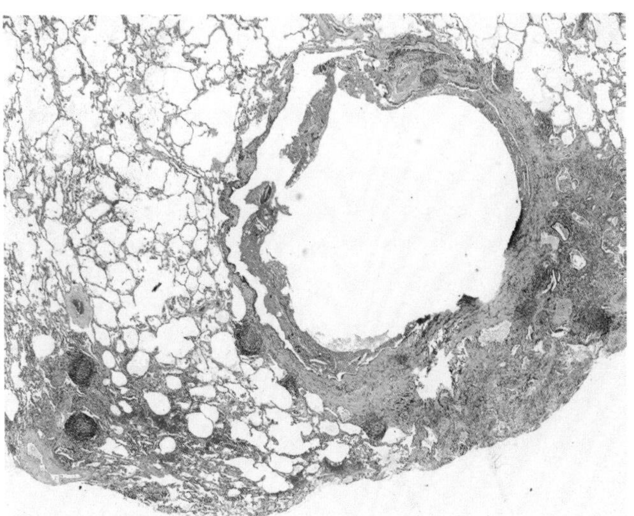

Figure 135.6 Centrilobular cyst formation at the level of the respiratory bronchiole in a patient with follicular bronchiolitis and air trapping in the setting of RA.

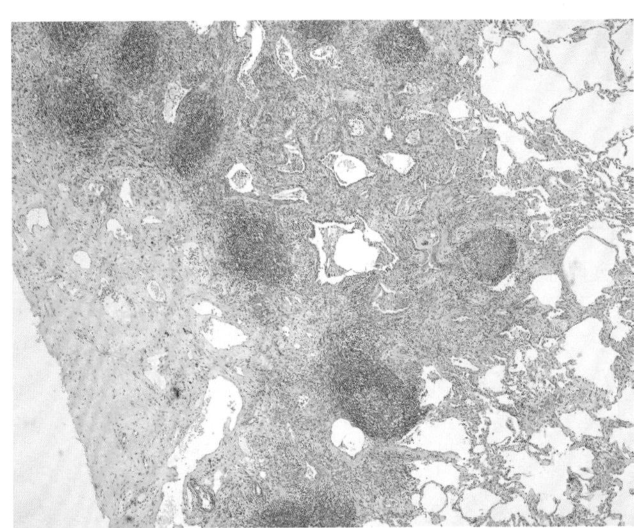

Figure 135.7 Dense subpleural fibrosis with adjacent relatively preserved lung in a patient with interstitial fibrosis in the setting of RA. Numerous lymphoid follicles are evident at the interface of the fibrosis and preserved lung. Chest computed tomography showed an idiopathic pulmonary fibrosis pattern of lung involvement.

Section 20

Therapeutic Drug Reactions and Radiation Effects

▸ Brandon T. Larsen

136 Amiodarone

Melanie C. Bois
Brandon T. Larsen

Amiodarone is a common antiarrhythmic agent and is also frequently used in congestive heart failure and ischemic heart disease to prevent sudden cardiac death. Although it is an effective antiarrhythmic agent, its clinical utility is often limited by its myriad side effects, especially pulmonary toxicity. While the risk of toxicity is directly related to the dose and duration of therapy, pulmonary toxicity may occur even with small doses and short treatment duration. Diagnosis of amiodarone lung disease is often challenging and one of exclusion, as the clinical symptoms and imaging findings are not specific. Likewise, no specific laboratory findings are diagnostic of amiodarone lung disease, and the diagnostic workup often includes evaluation of bronchoalveolar lavage fluid and/or lung biopsies. Even when characteristic features are seen microscopically, none of the histologic features are specific for amiodarone toxicity, and clinicopathologic correlation is essential, as with all therapeutic drug reactions.

CYTOLOGIC FEATURES

- Abundant finely vacuolated foamy macrophages, a feature simply representing exposure to the drug and not indicating toxicity in and of itself, often accompanied by other mixed inflammatory cells.

HISTOLOGIC FEATURES

- Organizing pneumonia with abundant intra-alveolar foamy macrophages.
- Acute or organizing diffuse alveolar damage with abundant foamy macrophages.
- Chronic interstitial pneumonitis with foamy macrophages and variable degrees of interstitial fibrosis.
- Nodular collections of foamy macrophages with central necrosis.
- Lymphoid hyperplasia with foamy macrophages.
- Eosinophilic pneumonia with foamy macrophages.
- NOTE: it should be recognized that foamy macrophages are expected with amiodarone use, and are simply a marker of exposure to the drug and are not indicative of toxicity per se, and should not be interpreted as evidence of toxicity without other supportive clinical and pathologic features and careful clinicopathologic correlation.

TRANSMISSION ELECTRON MICROSCOPIC FEATURES

- Alveolar macrophages with lamellar inclusions.

DIFFERENTIAL DIAGNOSIS

The histologic features of amiodarone lung toxicity are nonspecific and a variety of other processes enter the differential diagnosis. It should be recognized that foamy macrophages are not necessarily indicative of amiodarone toxicity and simply represent a marker of amiodarone exposure; implicating amiodarone as the cause of lung injury requires careful clinicopathologic correlation. The differential diagnosis depends on the pattern(s) of abnormalities present. If diffuse alveolar damage or organizing pneumonia is seen, an infectious etiology should be considered, including careful evaluation for viral inclusions and special stains for viruses and fungal organisms as appropriate, in addition to microbiologic cultures. Other considerations may include systemic connective tissue diseases, which can show identical patterns of injury. If significant chronic small airway pathology, mucostasis, or peribronchiolar metaplasia is present, the possibility of secondary lipid accumulation from small airways obstruction should be considered as the cause for foamy macrophage accumulation. Congestive heart failure can also result in macrophage accumulation in airspaces, although these macrophages are usually lightly pigmented (i.e., "heart failure cells") rather than foamy.

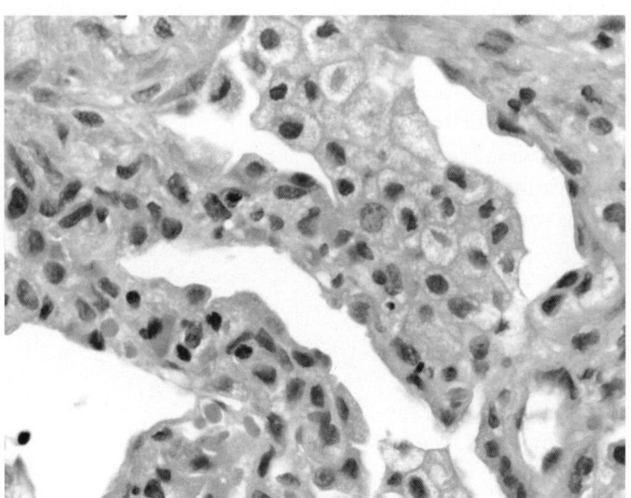

Figure 136.1 The cytologic and histopathologic hallmark of amiodarone exposure is the accumulation of foamy macrophages within alveolar spaces. Although characteristic of amiodarone exposure, this finding is not specific for amiodarone use, nor is it indicative of toxicity in and of itself.

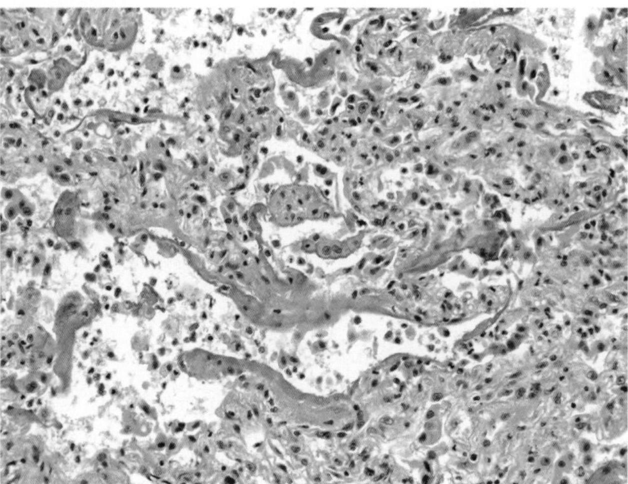

Figure 136.2 Amiodarone lung toxicity may manifest as diffuse alveolar damage, with eosinophilic proteinaceous hyaline membranes lining alveolar spaces, associated with interstitial edema, reactive type II pneumocyte hyperplasia, and intra-alveolar foamy macrophage accumulation.

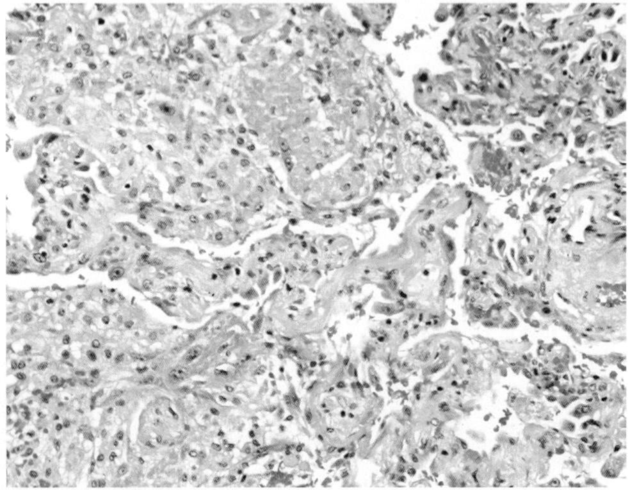

Figure 136.3 In some cases of amiodarone-induced lung toxicity, acute fibrinous lung injury can be encountered, with abundant intra-alveolar fibrin and interstitial edema accompanied by foamy macrophage accumulation.

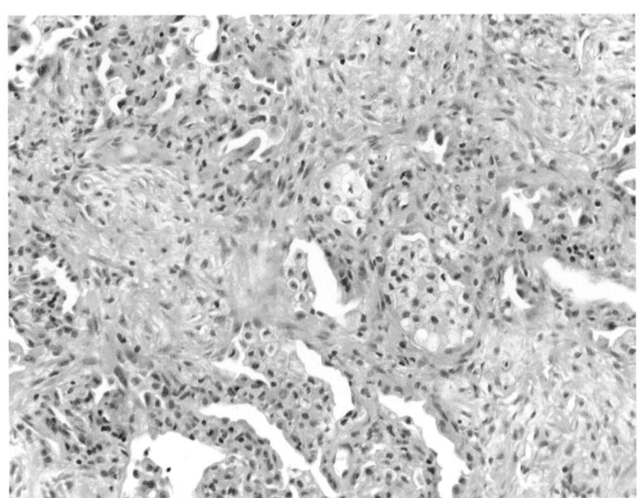

Figure 136.4 Organizing pneumonia can also be seen with amiodarone lung toxicity, especially in the more subacute setting, characterized by plugs of proliferating fibroblasts in airspaces, coupled with accumulation of foamy macrophages.

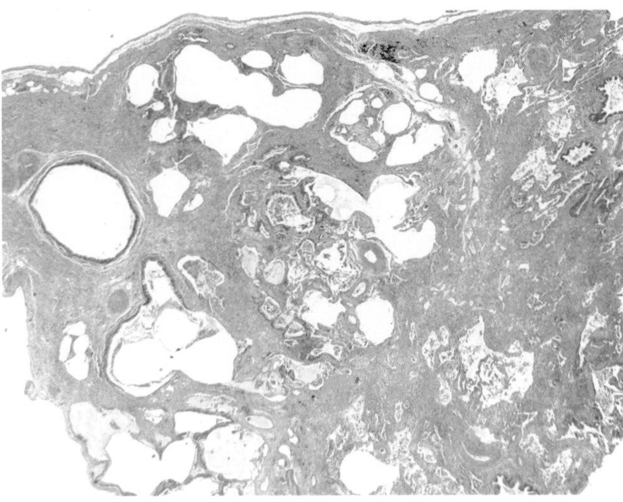

Figure 136.5 When presenting in the chronic or late stage, amiodarone lung toxicity may show interstitial fibrosis that closely mimics other forms of fibrotic interstitial lung disease.

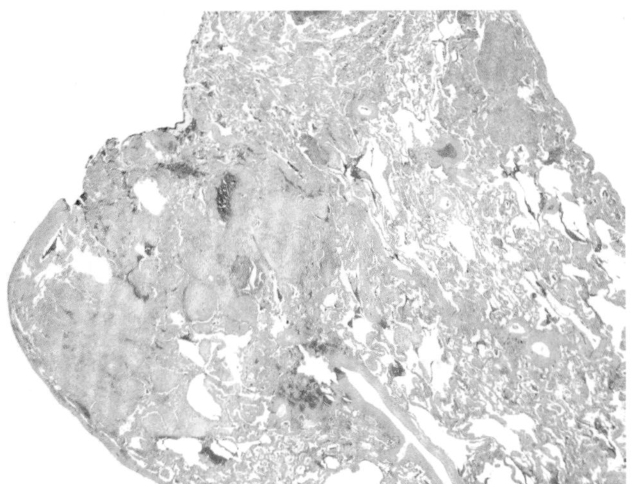

Figure 136.6 More rarely, amiodarone lung toxicity may present as pulmonary nodules, comprising foamy histiocytic collections that may mimic malignancy or other nodular processes clinically and/or histopathologically, as seen in this low-power image. Although not shown here, these nodular lesions can even undergo central necrosis in some cases.

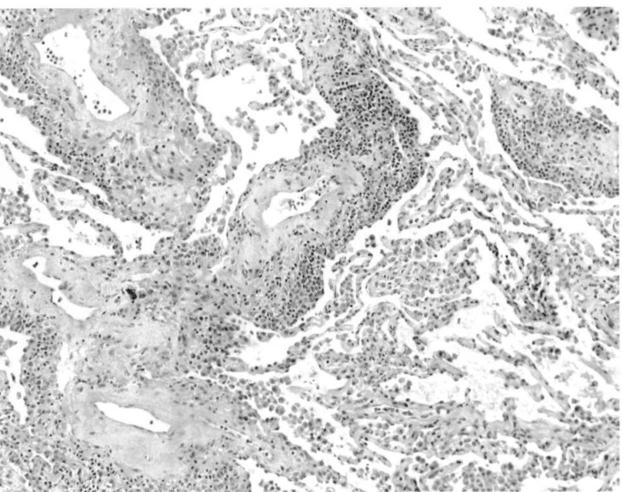

Figure 136.7 Lymphoid hyperplasia is an uncommon manifestation of amiodarone lung toxicity but can occur in a variety of patterns, including follicular bronchiolitis, a lymphoid interstitial pneumonia pattern, or even perivascular lymphoid infiltration, as illustrated here. As with other patterns of injury, foamy macrophages are typically abundant.

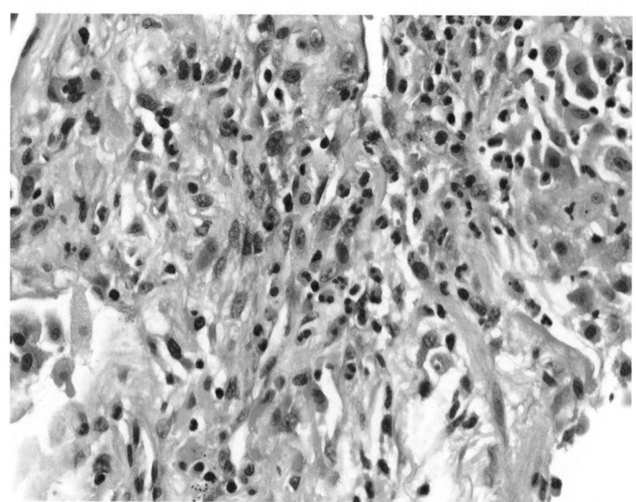

Figure 136.8 Acute and chronic eosinophilic pneumonia patterns have been associated with amiodarone lung toxicity in rare cases, histologically characterized by aggregates of eosinophils accumulating in alveolar spaces, in the presence of acute lung injury and/or organization.

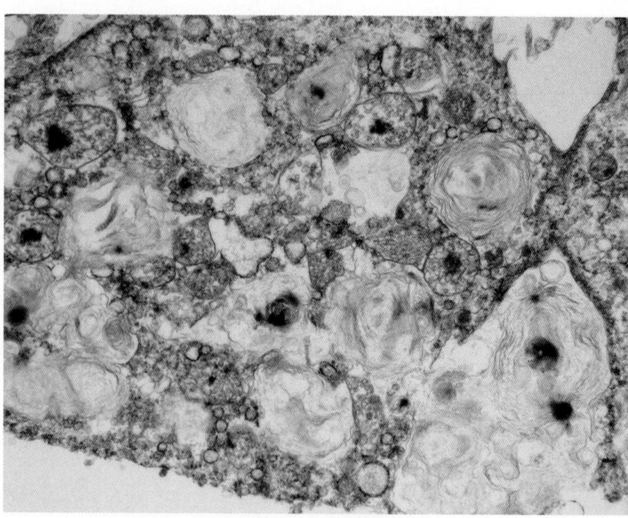

Figure 136.9 Although rarely required for diagnosis, transmission electron microscopy reveals laminated, whorled myelinoid inclusions within the cytoplasm of foamy macrophages. This feature is expected with amiodarone use and is merely a marker of exposure to the drug and is not indicative of toxicity per se.

137

Methotrexate

Melanie C. Bois
Brandon T. Larsen

Methotrexate is a folic acid antagonist that results in impaired synthesis of nucleic acids, thereby reducing cellular proliferation. These antiproliferative effects are useful for treating not only a variety of malignancies but also a multitude of autoimmune and inflammatory disorders, such as rheumatoid arthritis and psoriasis. Serious side effects of methotrexate include hepatic, pulmonary, and bone marrow toxicity. Although pulmonary toxicity most commonly occurs after chronic low-dose therapy, it can also occur acutely, especially when higher doses are utilized. Clinical manifestations are varied, and methotrexate pneumonitis can present with a variety of nonspecific pulmonary and systemic symptoms. Although most cases present in a subacute fashion, some patients may present with rapidly progressive acute respiratory failure that can be life-threatening. No specific clinical features or laboratory tests are available to diagnose methotrexate pneumonitis, and the diagnosis can be notoriously difficult to establish and requires a high index of clinical suspicion. Although a lung biopsy is not always required if the patient responds to drug discontinuation, a lung biopsy may be performed when the presentation is more acute or severe, if the etiology is uncertain, or if other disorders (e.g., infection and malignancy) are being considered.

HISTOLOGIC FEATURES

- Granulomatous interstitial pneumonia, with scattered giant cells and small poorly formed, nonnecrotizing granulomas.
- Cellular interstitial pneumonia, with variable degrees of interstitial fibrosis.
- Organizing pneumonia, with or without interstitial eosinophils.
- Diffuse alveolar damage.

DIFFERENTIAL DIAGNOSIS

Depending on the clinical scenario, the differential diagnosis of methotrexate pneumonitis typically includes infection related to immunosuppression, exacerbation of an underlying connective tissue disease, and reactions to other medications. Evaluation should always include a careful search for evidence of infection, such as viral inclusions or prominent neutrophilic inflammation, and special stains for microorganisms should also be performed when patterns of acute injury (e.g., diffuse alveolar damage and organizing pneumonia) or granulomatous inflammation are encountered. Unfortunately, there are no specific histologic features for methotrexate pneumonitis. Even when the most characteristic pattern of granulomatous interstitial pneumonia is encountered, the diagnosis requires careful clinicopathologic correlation.

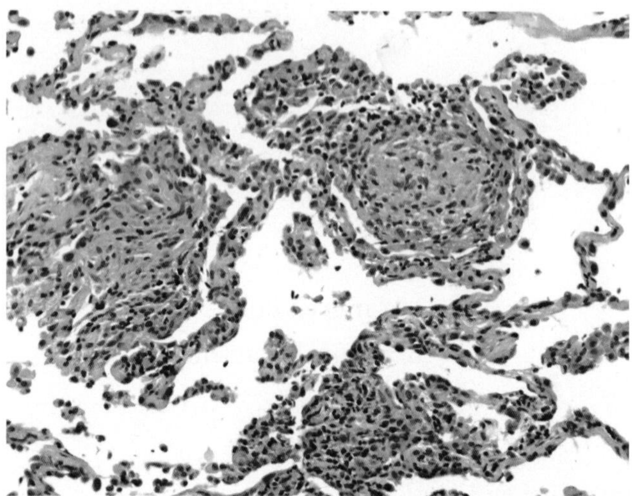

Figure 137.1 Granulomatous interstitial pneumonia is a classic manifestation of methotrexate pneumonitis, but this pattern is nonspecific and can also be encountered with infections, drug reactions, connective tissue disorders, and other causes of granulomatous inflammation.

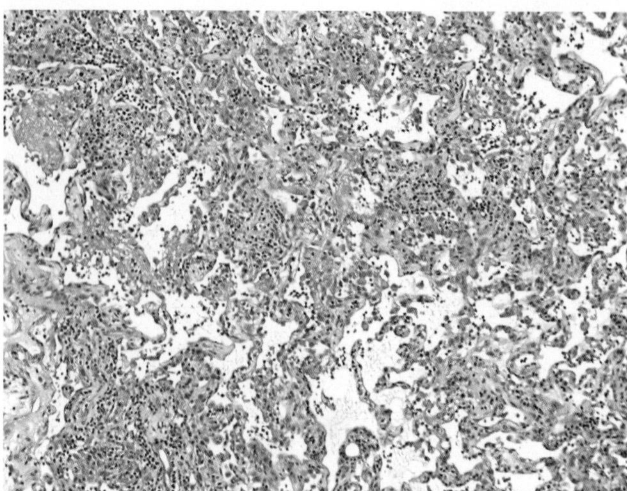

Figure 137.2 Some cases of methotrexate pneumonitis may present with a diffuse cellular interstitial pneumonia, characterized by interstitial expansion by a chronic inflammatory infiltrate, accompanied by intra-alveolar fibrin and accumulation of foamy macrophages.

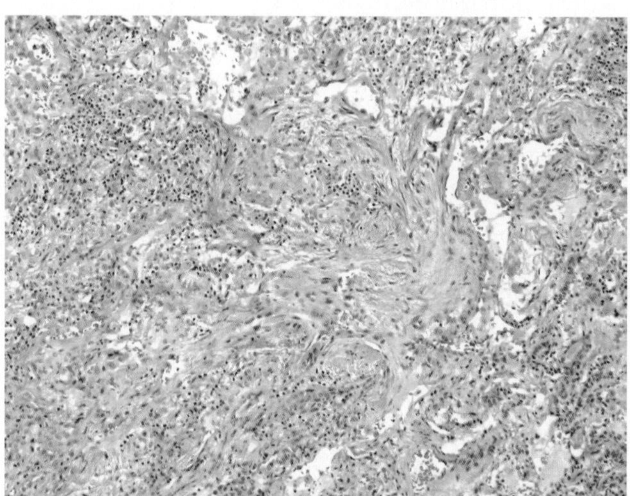

Figure 137.3 Organizing pneumonia is a nonspecific pattern of acute lung injury that may occur as a manifestation of methotrexate pneumonitis, as seen in this case, where numerous mucopolysaccharide-rich plugs of proliferating fibroblasts fill alveolar spaces.

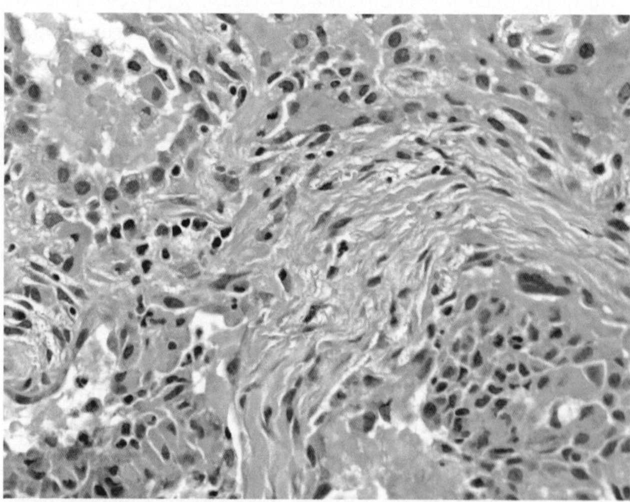

Figure 137.4 Although nonspecific, interstitial eosinophils may be present in methotrexate pneumonitis and are often a helpful clue that suggests a drug reaction.

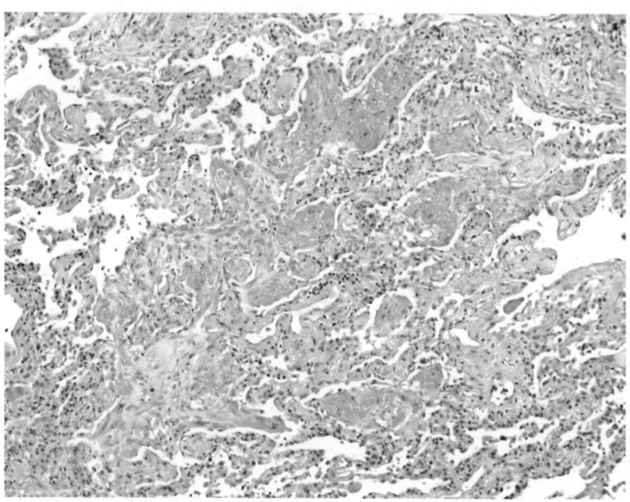

Figure 137.5 Other nonspecific patterns of acute lung injury may be encountered in methotrexate pneumonitis, as in this case where acute fibrinous and organizing pneumonia is seen; as with any acute injury pattern, the differential diagnosis includes exacerbation of the patient's underlying connective tissue disease, acute infection, and an adverse reaction to some other medication.

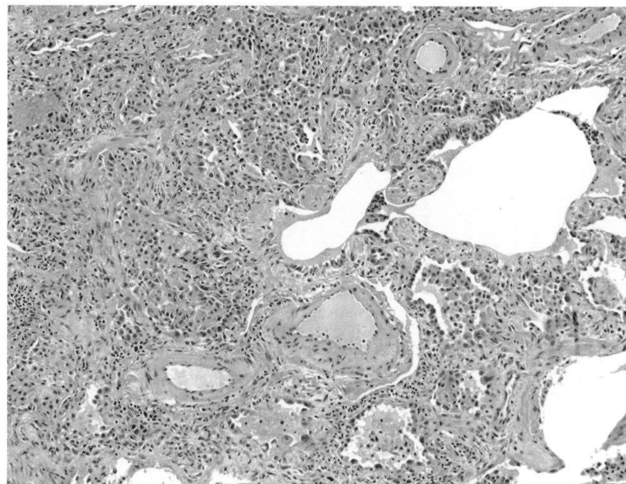

Figure 137.6 Although less common, acute and organizing diffuse alveolar damage can be seen in some cases of methotrexate-induced lung toxicity.

138 Nitrofurantoin

▶ Ying-Han (Roger) Hsu
▶ Brandon T. Larsen

Nitrofurantoin is an oral antimicrobial agent that is commonly used for the treatment of acute urinary tract infections or as prophylaxis in patients (especially women) who suffer from recurrent episodes. Although serious side effects are uncommon, pulmonary toxicity is the most feared and can present either with an acute onset after a short course of therapy or with a chronic insidious onset after months or years of therapy. Clinical manifestations include a variety of nonspecific respiratory symptoms, such as dyspnea, dry cough, and fatigue. Laboratory findings are also nonspecific but often include peripheral eosinophilia or leukocytosis. Imaging studies usually show bilateral ground-glass opacities. As with most adverse drug reactions, the diagnosis of nitrofurantoin-induced pneumonitis requires a high index of clinical suspicion, in combination with careful clinicopathologic correlation. Although a presumptive clinical diagnosis is sufficient in most cases, lung biopsies may be performed in patients with more severe disease or in whom there is higher concern for infection or malignancy.

HISTOLOGIC FEATURES

- Cellular interstitial pneumonia is common, including the cellular nonspecific interstitial pneumonia (NSIP) pattern.
- Eosinophilic pneumonia.
- Diffuse alveolar hemorrhage, sometimes with vasculitis.
- Other patterns of acute lung injury, including diffuse alveolar damage or organizing pneumonia.
- Less commonly, granulomatous interstitial pneumonia or features of giant-cell interstitial pneumonia can be seen.
- Fibrotic interstitial lung disease with chronic presentations, often indistinguishable from the usual interstitial pneumonia (UIP) pattern or fibrotic NSIP pattern.

DIFFERENTIAL DIAGNOSIS

As nitrofurantoin-induced pulmonary toxicity is associated with diverse histologic findings but no specific features, a variety of other conditions may enter the differential diagnosis, depending on the specific injury pattern(s) encountered in an individual case. Acute infections should be excluded if there is evidence of acute or subacute injury (such as diffuse alveolar damage or organizing pneumonia), and a careful evaluation for specific evidence of infection should be performed, including a search for viral inclusions and special stains for microorganisms as appropriate. A systemic connective tissue disease is another common consideration with most of these reaction patterns. Unfortunately, there are no specific histologic features to distinguish between these two possibilities, and correlation with clinical and serologic findings is essential. Hypersensitivity pneumonitis may be a consideration, if cellular interstitial pneumonia and/or granulomas are seen, and this diagnosis also requires clinicopathologic correlation. When significant fibrosis is present, other forms of chronic fibrosing interstitial pneumonia may also enter the differential diagnosis, and multidisciplinary discussion is usually required to establish the correct diagnosis.

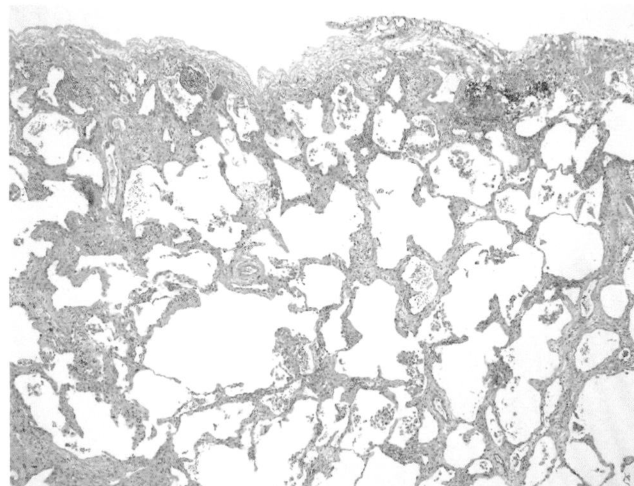

Figure 138.1 A mixed cellular and fibrotic NSIP pattern can be caused by nitrofurantoin, with relatively uniform alveolar interstitial thickening due to chronic interstitial inflammation and fibrosis, but this pattern is nonspecific and can also be seen with connective tissue diseases and hypersensitivity pneumonitis.

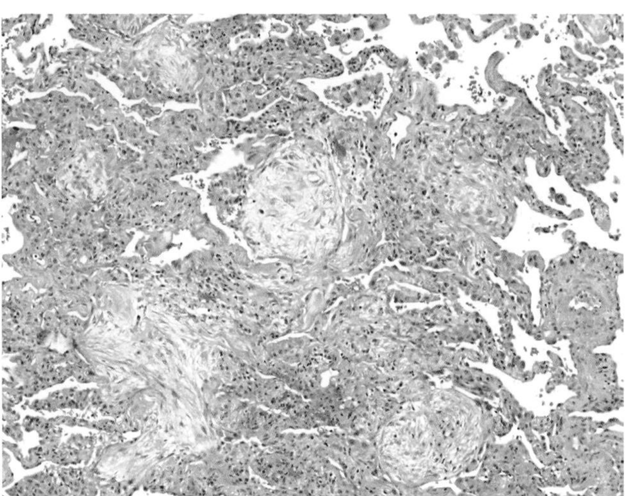

Figure 138.2 Organizing pneumonia is a nonspecific pattern of acute lung injury that can be associated with nitrofurantoin, characterized by plugs of proliferating fibroblasts within alveolar spaces along with alveolar pneumocyte hyperplasia and chronic inflammation.

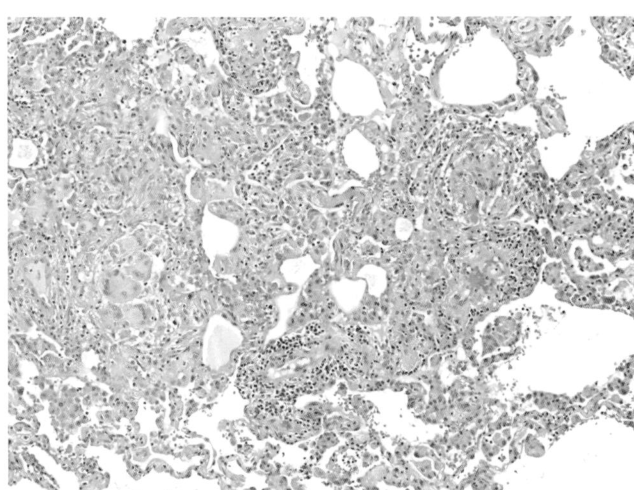

Figure 138.3 Granulomatous interstitial pneumonia is a rare histologic pattern of nitrofurantoin-induced lung toxicity, featuring chronic interstitial inflammation in combination with poorly formed nonnecrotizing granulomas and multinucleated giant cells. This pattern is nonspecific and may also be seen with chronic infections (particularly atypical mycobacterial infection), aspiration, hot tub lung, hypersensitivity pneumonitis, connective tissue diseases, and other drug reactions.

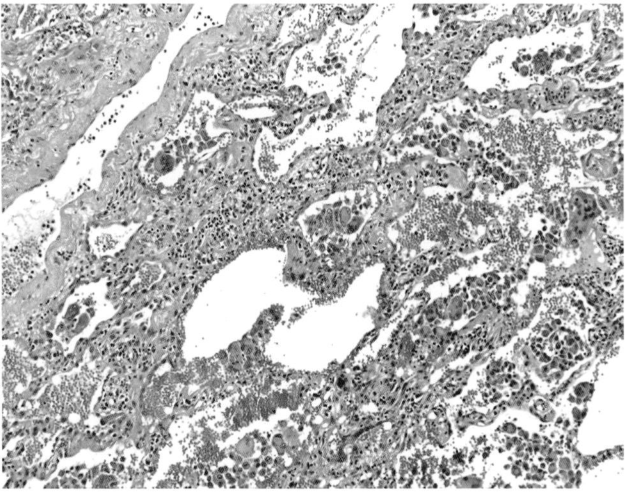

Figure 138.4 Rare cases of nitrofurantoin toxicity can show an exuberant histiocytic reaction with accumulation of giant cells and aggregates of alveolar macrophages, resembling desquamative interstitial pneumonia, as seen in smokers, or even giant-cell interstitial pneumonia associated with hard-metal exposure.

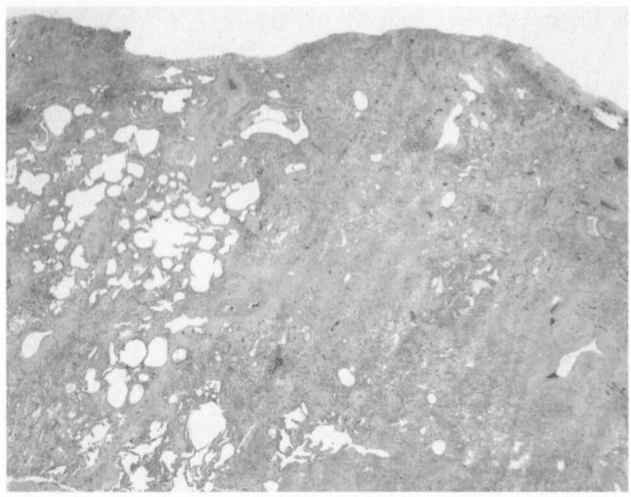

Figure 138.5 In chronic nitrofurantoin toxicity, advanced fibrosis may develop, resembling the UIP pattern or fibrotic NSIP pattern.

Fenfluramine–Phentermine ("Fen–Phen")

139

Raghavendra Pillappa
Brandon T. Larsen

Fenfluramine and phentermine are amphetamine analogues that were previously used in combination ("fen–phen") as a treatment for obesity and substance abuse disorders. Fen–phen therapy peaked in popularity in the 1990s, with the total number of prescriptions in the United States exceeding 18 million in 1996, but fen–phen was withdrawn from the United States market in 1997 after an association with development of valvular heart disease and pulmonary hypertension was recognized. These drugs target serotonergic signaling pathways to increase the bioavailability of serotonin, thereby producing appetite suppression via effects on relevant neural networks in the central nervous system. Unfortunately, elevated serotonin also induces proliferation of arterial smooth muscle cells, adventitial fibroblasts, and epithelial cells in the lung, leading to pulmonary arterial hypertension in some patients. Fen–phen has also been associated with valvular heart disease, which closely mimics carcinoid valve disease induced by serotonin-secreting gastrointestinal carcinoid tumors, likely via a similar mechanism involving serotonin.

HISTOLOGIC FEATURES

- Plexiform arteriopathy is present in about 60% of pulmonary hypertension cases associated with fen–phen.
- Fibroproliferative intimal lesions are typically present in arteries of all sizes, including large elastic conduit arteries, medium-sized muscular arteries, and small arteries.
- Diffuse and segmental medial thickening may also be present.

DIFFERENTIAL DIAGNOSIS

The differential diagnosis of pulmonary vascular changes with the use of fen–phen include other causes of plexogenic or nonplexogenic pulmonary arteriopathy, such as connective tissue diseases, heritable forms of pulmonary arterial hypertension, chronic thromboembolic pulmonary hypertension, Eisenmenger syndrome secondary to congenital heart disease, and other adverse drug reactions, among a variety of other conditions. The histologic changes are nonspecific, and distinction from these other disorders requires clinicopathologic correlation.

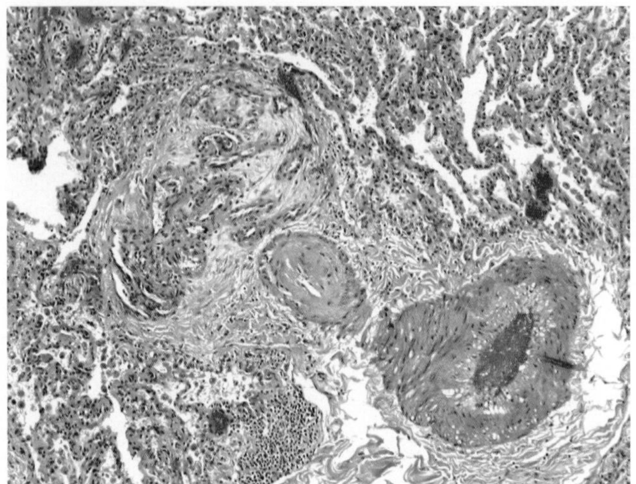

Figure 139.1 Plexogenic pulmonary arteriopathy has been associated with the use of fen–phen, characterized by plexiform proliferations of capillaries *(left of center)* near small pulmonary arteries, although this feature is nonspecific and can be seen with other forms of plexogenic pulmonary arterial hypertension.

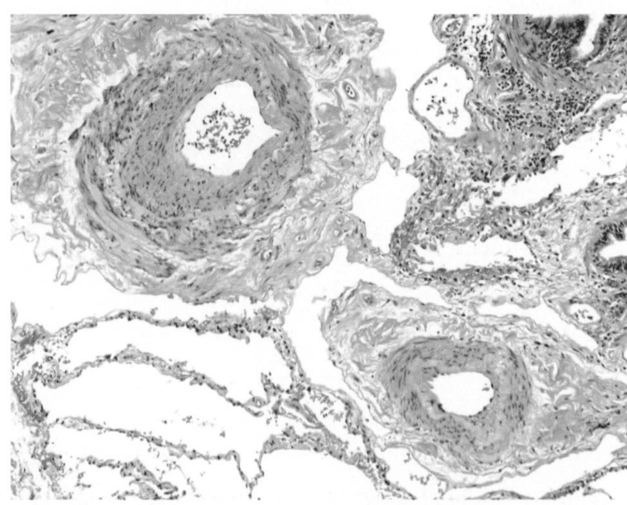

Figure 139.2 The use of fen–phen can also induce diffuse and/or segmental medial thickening in pulmonary arteries, along with fibroproliferative intimal lesions that encroach on the arterial lumen. These changes are nonspecific and can be seen with other causes of pulmonary arterial hypertension.

140 Targeted Molecular Therapies

▶ Ying-Han (Roger) Hsu
▶ Brandon T. Larsen

In recent years, there has been an explosion of new therapeutic agents targeting specific molecular pathways involved in a variety of neoplastic and nonneoplastic diseases. Among these are the tyrosine kinase inhibitors, a large and rapidly growing class of agents that target tyrosine kinases, a very large family of enzymes involved in key cell signaling pathways that regulate proliferation and differentiation. Recent years have also seen an explosion of new monoclonal antibody-based therapies, typically directed against key cell surface molecules involved in the pathogenesis of a particular disease. These highly sophisticated molecular agents are rapidly revolutionizing the treatment for many challenging diseases and offer the potential for a personalized approach to medicine. However, they are not without side effects. Many of these agents have been associated with adverse reactions in the lung, although our understanding of their effects on the lung remains incomplete and many of these reactions have not been characterized from a histopathologic standpoint, as many suspected cases are never biopsied. As with most adverse drug reactions, the diagnosis of pulmonary toxicity from one of these agents requires a high index of suspicion, in combination with careful clinicopathologic correlation. Again, it should be emphasized that the spectrum of changes that can be seen with these agents remains poorly understood, and any histologic patterns of acute or chronic injury in the lung should be viewed with suspicion if the clinical presentation suggests an adverse reaction to one of these agents.

Tyrosine kinase inhibitors are generally named with the suffix "-nib." The earliest tyrosine kinase inhibitors were approved in the early 2000s and included agents such as imatinib, gefitinib, and erlotinib, but in more recent years a number of additional inhibitors have entered the market including second- and even third-generation agents, and several dozen are now approved for clinical use with others in various stages of development. In contrast, monoclonal antibody therapies are generally named with the suffix "-mab," and include human, humanized, and chimeric forms directed against a wide variety of biologic targets. At the time of this writing, more than 70 FDA-approved monoclonal antibodies were available for clinical use, and the list is rapidly growing. Most of these agents are used for anti-inflammatory and/or antineoplastic indications. Examples include infliximab and adalimumab, which inhibit tumor necrosis factor-alpha and are used to treat disorders, such as rheumatoid arthritis and inflammatory bowel disease. Others include agents such as rituximab, which targets CD20 and is used to treat rheumatologic disorders as well as B-cell lymphoid neoplasms, and trastuzumab, which targets the HER2/neu receptor as a treatment for HER2-overexpressing breast cancers.

HISTOLOGIC FEATURES

Tyrosine Kinase Inhibitors

- Diffuse alveolar damage.
- Diffuse alveolar hemorrhage.
- Cellular interstitial pneumonia, sometimes with increased eosinophils.
- Organizing pneumonia.
- Other unusual patterns of acute or chronic injury.

Monoclonal Antibody Therapies

- Diffuse alveolar damage.
- Organizing pneumonia, with or without nonnecrotizing granulomas.
- Cellular or vaguely granulomatous interstitial pneumonia.
- Diffuse alveolar hemorrhage.
- Eosinophilic pneumonia-like reaction.
- Constrictive (obliterative) bronchiolitis.
- Pulmonary fibrosis.
- Other unusual patterns of acute or chronic injury.

DIFFERENTIAL DIAGNOSIS

When considering an adverse drug reaction in the lung, a variety of other conditions enter the differential diagnosis, depending on the histopathologic pattern(s) of injury that is present. If features of acute lung injury are seen, such as diffuse alveolar damage or organizing pneumonia, acute infection should always be considered, and special stains for microorganisms and cultures should be performed as appropriate. It should be remembered that many of these agents have anti-inflammatory properties, thereby increasing the risk of infection. If granulomas are present, the differential diagnosis may include not only granulomatous infections (especially with atypical mycobacteria) but also hot tub lung, connective tissue disorders, inflammatory bowel disease, hypersensitivity pneumonitis, berylliosis, and sarcoidosis, among other possibilities. A systemic connective tissue disease also enters the differential diagnosis in essentially all of these acute and chronic injury patterns. There are no specific histopathologic features that distinguish an adverse drug reaction from connective tissue disease, but this possibility should be suggested to clinicians so an appropriate rheumatologic workup can be performed. In patients with established rheumatologic disorders who are being treated with one of these targeted therapies, the distinction of an adverse drug reaction from an acute infection or exacerbation of the underlying rheumatologic disease can be particularly challenging and remains one of the most difficult problems in pulmonary pathology. Even after multidisciplinary discussion, an adverse drug reaction is often a presumptive diagnosis that is only made retrospectively following negative cultures and clinical improvement with empiric cessation of the agent.

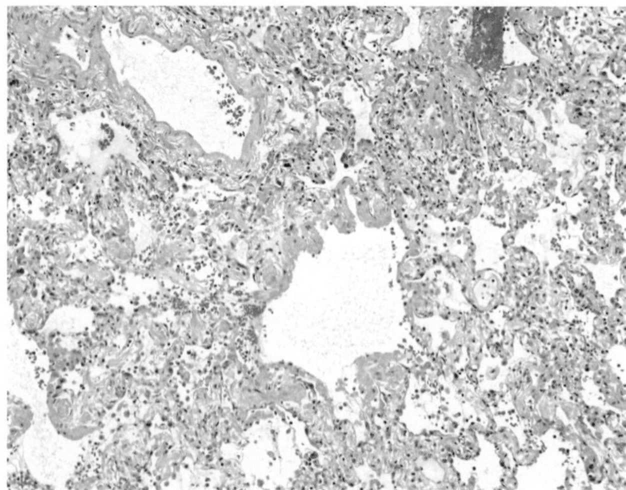

Figure 140.1 Acute and organizing diffuse alveolar damage is a common pattern of severe acute lung injury that can be encountered with targeted molecular agents, as in this example of erlotinib-induced lung toxicity, characterized by marked interstitial edema, interstitial fibroblastic proliferation, and numerous hyaline membranes.

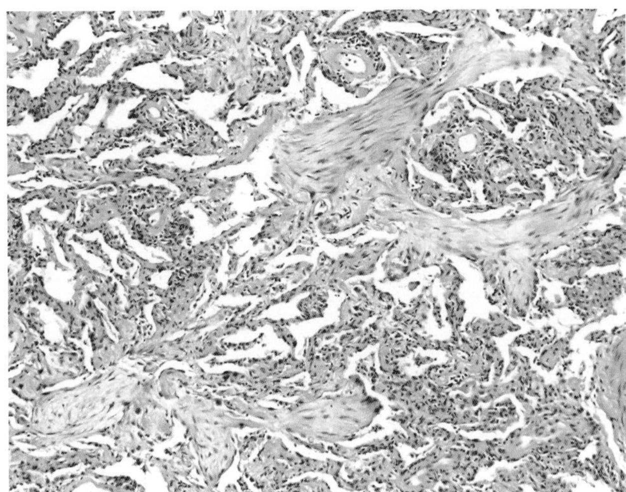

Figure 140.2 Organizing pneumonia is a nonspecific pattern of acute or subacute lung injury that can be seen with many agents, as in this case of infliximab-induced lung toxicity, featuring numerous plugs of proliferating fibroblasts in alveolar spaces.

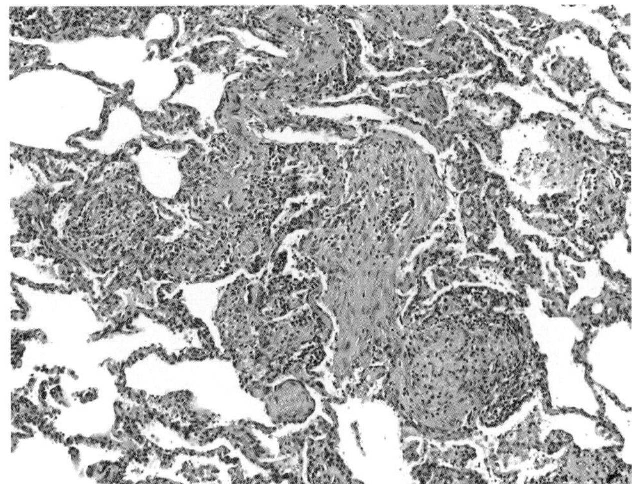

Figure 140.3 In some cases, a granulomatous organizing pneumonia pattern can occur with these agents, as in this case of adalimumab-induced lung toxicity, where vague and poorly formed nonnecrotizing granulomas are scattered throughout the interstitium and accompanied by airspace organization. When this pattern is encountered, special stains should always be performed to evaluate the infection.

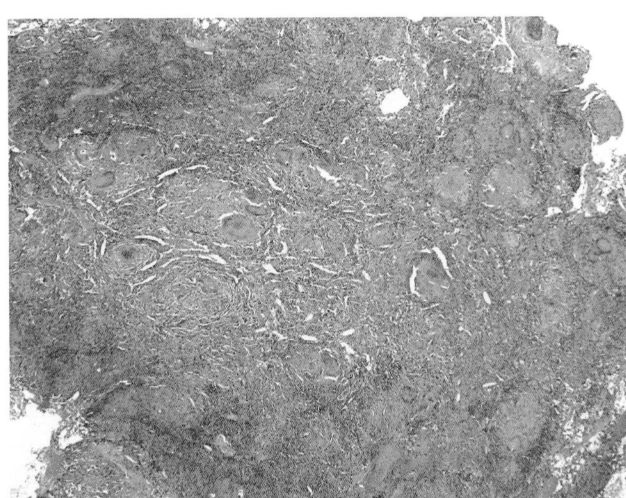

Figure 140.4 Granulomatous interstitial pneumonia is an unusual pattern that should prompt consideration of an adverse drug reaction, as in this case of etanercept-induced lung toxicity, where innumerable and nearly confluent nonnecrotizing granulomas and multinucleated giant cells expand the interstitium along with a chronic lymphocytic infiltrate. Special stains for microorganisms should always be performed when this pattern is encountered.

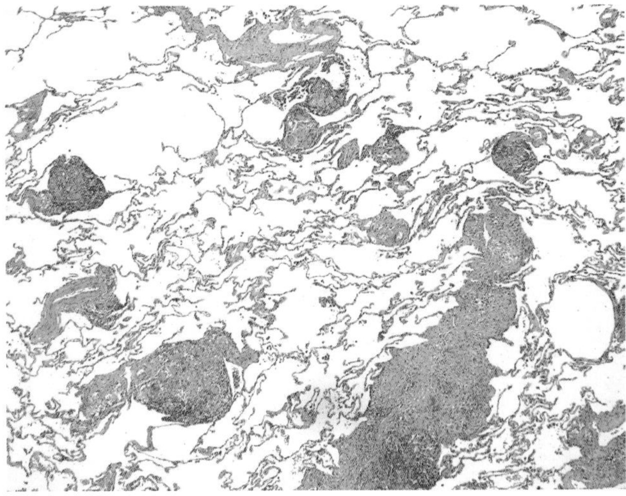

Figure 140.5 Granulomatous inflammatory reactions to some agents can closely mimic pulmonary sarcoidosis, as in this example associated with infliximab, where relatively well-formed nonnecrotizing granulomas are distributed along lymphatic routes.

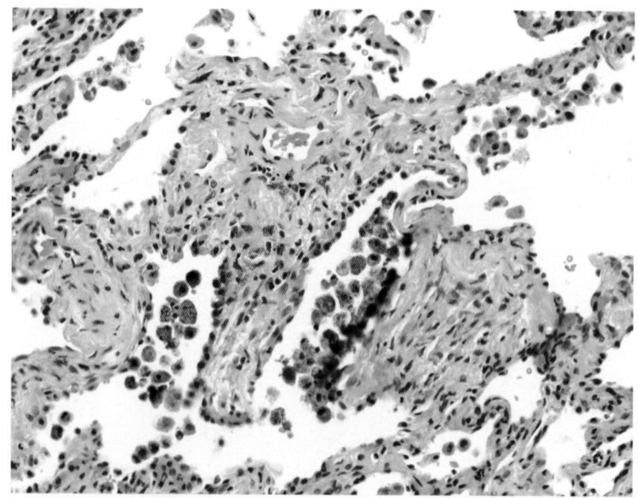

Figure 140.6 Diffuse alveolar hemorrhage is an uncommon pattern of acute lung injury that can be associated with some drugs, as in this case associated with rituximab, where accumulation of hemosiderin-laden macrophages is accompanied by resolving organization.

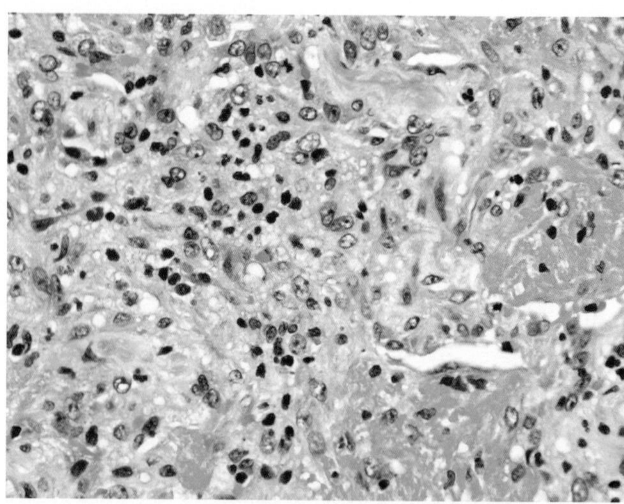

Figure 140.7 Rituximab-associated lung toxicity can occasionally present with an eosinophilic pneumonia-like reaction, featuring fibrinous exudates in the airspaces and a mixed inflammatory cell infiltrate with scattered eosinophils.

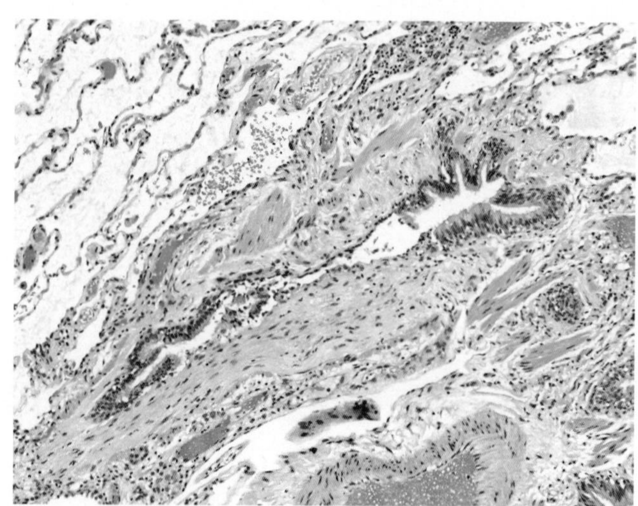

Figure 140.8 Not to be confused with the older discontinued term *bronchiolitis obliterans* organizing pneumonia or BOOP, the constrictive (obliterative) bronchiolitis pattern is characterized by mild chronic bronchiolitis with marked subepithelial fibrosis, resulting in luminal narrowing and small airways obstruction, a nonspecific pattern of injury that can be caused by some medications, as in this case associated with the use of rituximab.

141

Other Drugs

▶ Robert W. Ricciotti
▶ Brandon T. Larsen

In addition to the medications already profiled in previous chapters, a wide variety of other drugs and therapeutic agents can injure the lung. Some of the more common drugs associated with lung toxicity include chemotherapeutic agents, particularly when used in combination regimens. The instance of pulmonary toxicity with these agents varies widely, as do their clinical manifestations and latency periods. The histologic manifestations also vary widely and are often incompletely understood, as most patients with a presumed drug reaction will not be biopsied, and even if they are biopsied, the histologic changes are nonspecific and the diagnosis is generally only made in a retrospective and presumptive fashion, after other potential causes of injury have been ruled out. Drugs that have been associated with lung toxicity number in the hundreds, and illustration and discussion of all potential reactions is beyond the scope of this atlas, although it should be recognized that the Internet is a powerful tool when a drug reaction is suspected. One of the most helpful online resources is the Drug-Induced Respiratory Disease Website, more commonly known as "Pneumotox" (http://www.pneumotox.com), an online database of reported adverse reactions in the lung from a wide variety of agents, including not only their clinical patterns of presentation but also any reported histopathologic patterns of injury.

CYTOLOGIC FEATURES

- Cellular atypia is common, especially with chemotherapeutic agents, including large and hyperchromatic nuclei with coarse granular or smudged chromatin.
- Intranuclear vacuoles, binucleation, or multinucleation can also be seen.
- NOTE: it should be recognized that cytologic changes are expected with chemotherapy agents, are simply a marker of exposure to the drug, are not indicative of toxicity per se, and should not be interpreted as evidence of toxicity without other supportive clinical and pathologic features.

HISTOLOGIC FEATURES

Cyclophosphamide

- Diffuse alveolar damage and/or organizing pneumonia, often with marked interstitial edema, may be present.
- Occasionally, diffuse alveolar hemorrhage can occur.
- Fibrosing interstitial pneumonia.

Bleomycin

- Acute lung injury, presenting either as diffuse alveolar damage or organizing pneumonia, typically with marked interstitial edema and marked reactive atypia and hyperplasia of type II pneumocytes.
- Cellular interstitial pneumonia, sometimes evolving to fibrotic lung disease resembling other patterns of fibrosing interstitial pneumonia.

Busulfan

- Organizing diffuse alveolar damage.
- Interstitial fibrosis.

Sulfasalazine

- Eosinophilic pneumonia.
- Cellular interstitial pneumonia with interstitial edema.
- Organizing diffuse alveolar damage.
- Fibrosing interstitial pneumonia.

Statins

- Cellular interstitial pneumonia, evolving to fibrosis resembling the mixed cellular and fibrotic nonspecific interstitial pneumonia (NSIP) pattern.
- Marked vacuolization of pneumocytes and accumulation of foamy macrophages in airspaces.

Radioembolization (Yttrium-90) Microspheres

- Changes consistent with radiation pneumonitis (see Chapter 142).
- Scattered purple microspheres (30 to 40 μm in diameter), in areas of acute injury.

Levamisole-Adulterated Cocaine

- Diffuse alveolar hemorrhage, often p-antineutrophilic cytoplasmic antibody–associated.
- Interstitial fibrosis.

DIFFERENTIAL DIAGNOSIS

As with any putative drug reaction in the lung, the differential diagnosis will include other causes of acute and/or chronic lung injury. Considerations may vary based on the pattern or patterns of injury or fibrosis that are present. Generally, if patterns of acute injury (e.g., diffuse alveolar damage, organizing pneumonia, and acute fibrinous pneumonitis) are encountered, the specimen should be carefully evaluated for infection with an appropriate workup, including GMS stains and cultures. When marked cytologic atypia is present, as often seen with chemotherapeutic agents, the differential diagnosis will also include viral infection. Immunohistochemical stains for viral agents, viral cultures, and appropriate molecular studies can be helpful in this distinction. When interstitial fibrosis is encountered, the differential diagnosis will include other fibrosing interstitial pneumonias, including connective tissue disease–associated interstitial lung disease, chronic hypersensitivity pneumonitis, and idiopathic pulmonary fibrosis, among other possibilities. Distinction from a drug reaction typically requires careful correlation with clinical, imaging, and laboratory studies, preferably via multidisciplinary discussion.

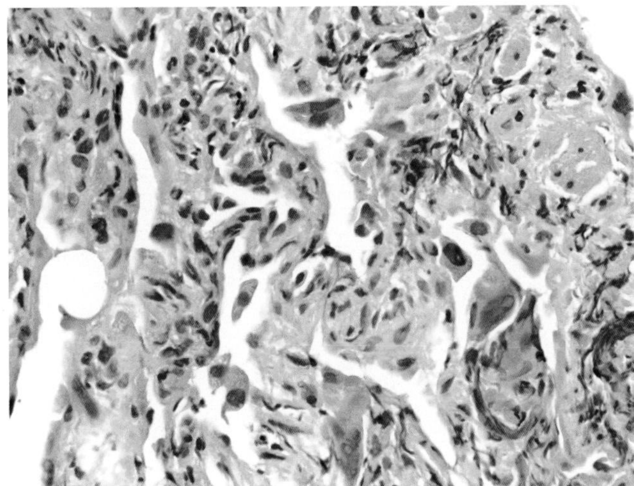

Figure 141.1 Lung toxicity due to chemotherapeutic agents often shows cellular atypia in the form of hyperchromatic nuclei with coarse or smudged chromatin as seen in this example of toxicity following the administration of multiagent chemotherapy.

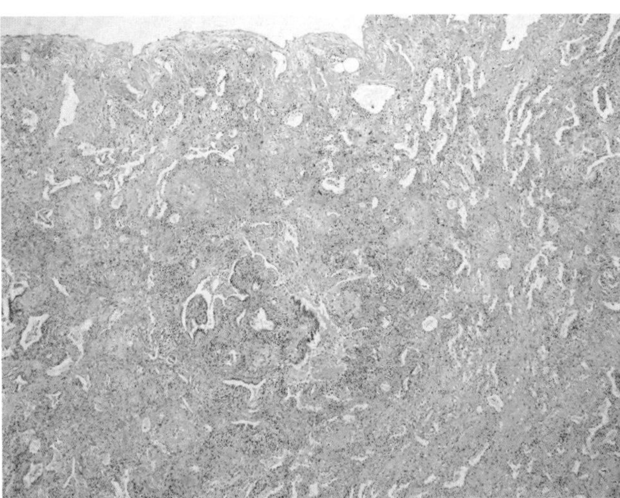

Figure 141.2 While cyclophosphamide toxicity may present with an acute lung injury pattern (i.e., diffuse alveolar damage or organizing pneumonia), it may also result in fibrosing interstitial pneumonia as seen in this example. The pattern of fibrosis is nonspecific and requires clinical correlation to exclude other potential causes of fibrosis.

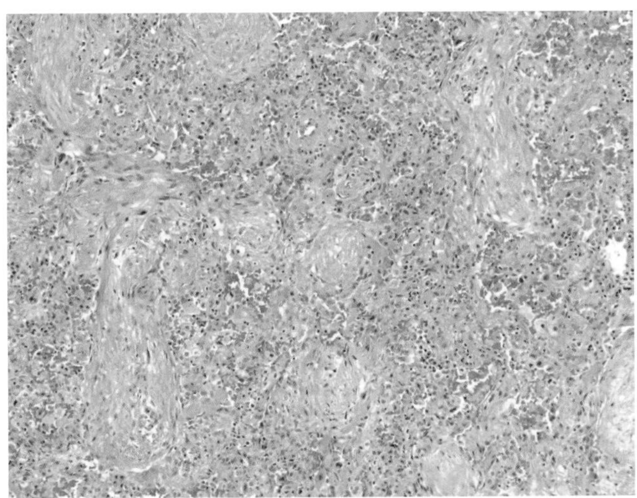

Figure 141.3 Bleomycin lung toxicity often shows an acute lung injury pattern including organizing pneumonia with fibroblast plugs filling airspaces, associated chronic inflammation, and reactive type II pneumocyte hyperplasia.

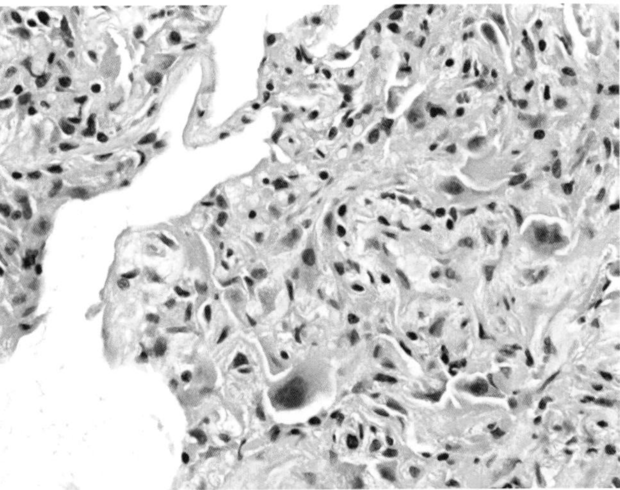

Figure 141.4 As with other chemotherapeutic agents, bleomycin may result in cellular atypia with enlarged, hyperchromatic, smudged nuclei potentially mimicking viral cytopathic changes.

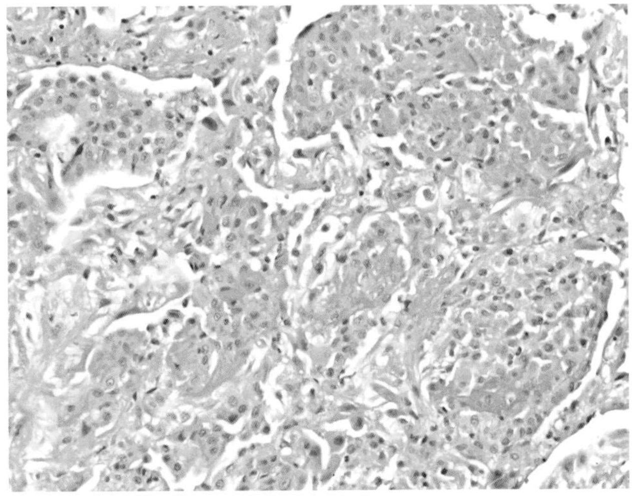

Figure 141.5 Busulfan-induced acute lung toxicity may show acute fibrinous lung injury with intra-alveolar fibrin deposition, interstitial edema, and accumulation of numerous foamy macrophages.

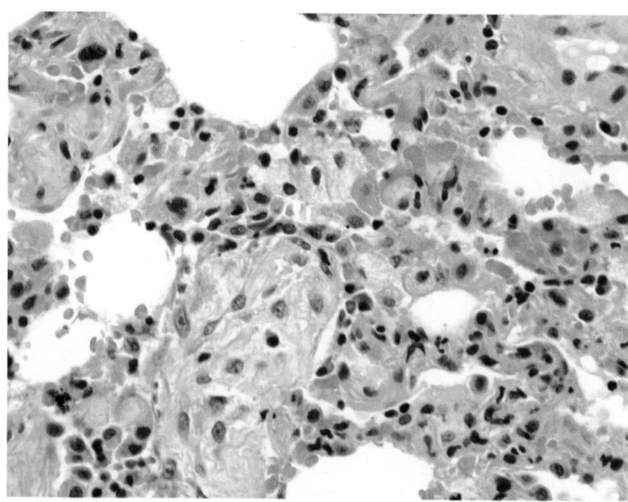

Figure 141.6 Lung injury due to atorvastatin may show features of acute lung injury in the form of organizing pneumonia with fibroblast plugs within airspaces, foamy macrophages, and reactive type II pneumocyte hyperplasia.

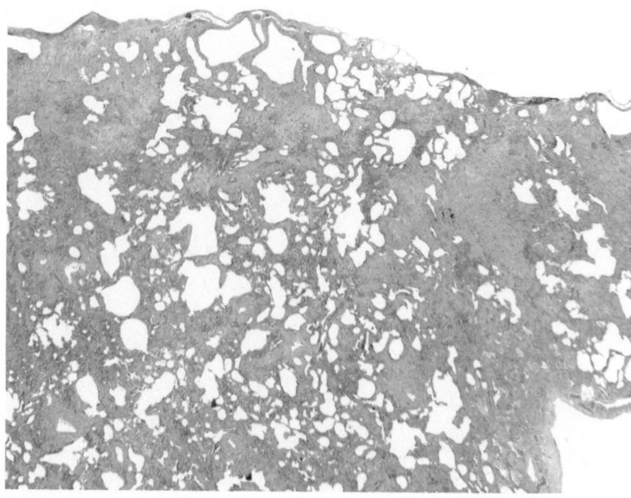

Figure 141.7 Statin-induced lung injury may show features of interstitial pneumonia, mimicking interstitial lung disease of other causes, such as this example having the appearance of the mixed cellular and fibrotic NSIP pattern.

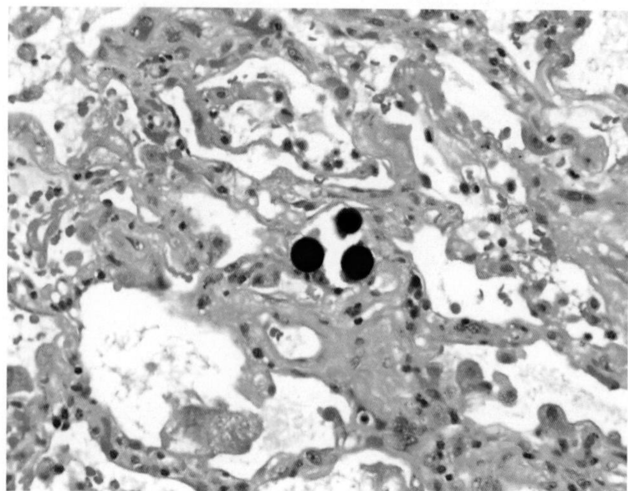

Figure 141.8 Toxicity due to radioembolization with yttrium-90 shows characteristic purple microspheres measuring 30 to 40 μm in diameter. The microspheres are typically found in areas of acute lung injury (i.e., diffuse alveolar damage) typical of radiation pneumonitis (see Chapter 142).

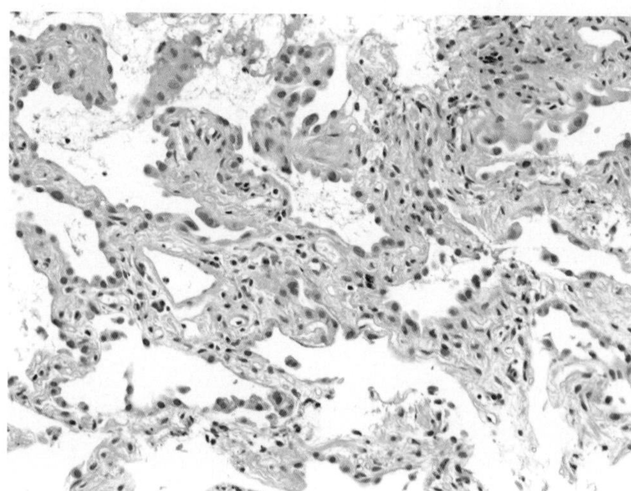

Figure 141.9 Lung injury due to levamisole-adulterated cocaine use resulting in interstitial changes resembling the cellular NSIP pattern, a few scattered eosinophils, and prominent reactive type II pneumocyte hyperplasia.

Radiation Pneumonitis

Raghavendra Pillappa
Brandon T. Larsen

Ionizing radiation is commonly used as a treatment for breast, lung, and hematologic malignancies. Radiation-induced lung damage is often the dose-limiting factor in these patients and can present either as acute pneumonitis or as chronic fibrotic lung disease. The effects of radiation on the lung may be potentiated by chemotherapy and infections, which are also important causes of acute lung injury. Patients with acute radiation pneumonitis typically present 3 to 12 weeks following radiation exposure with dyspnea, a nonproductive cough, low-grade fever, chest pain, and/or malaise, along with pulmonary infiltrates. Patients with chronic or late radiation pneumonitis typically present many months or even years after exposure with pulmonary fibrosis. Diagnosis requires clinical correlation between the onset of symptoms and the timing of radiotherapy, after exclusion of other causes of acute or chronic lung injury, such as infections, tumor progression, other adverse drug reactions, and thromboembolic disease, among others. The diagnostic process usually involves bronchoscopy with bronchoalveolar lavage, sometimes in combination with a transbronchial biopsy or even a surgical lung biopsy in problematic cases.

CYTOLOGIC FEATURES

- Single cells or sheets of cells with markedly increased cell size, but with a preserved nuclear to cytoplasmic ratio.
- Degenerative or smudgy nuclear chromatin, with occasional nuclei and abundant cytoplasm.

HISTOLOGIC FEATURES

- Acute radiation pneumonitis typically shows acute and organizing diffuse alveolar damage, but this may evolve to an organizing pneumonia pattern in the subacute phase.
- Large bizarre cells with "radiation atypia," characterized by enlarged hyperchromatic and degenerative smudgy nuclei and abundant eosinophilic cytoplasm, with a low nuclear to cytoplasmic ratio.
- Markedly atypical type II pneumocytes with enlarged hyperchromatic nuclei and vacuolated cytoplasm.
- Squamous metaplasia of airway epithelium.
- Interstitial edema can be present, with a mononuclear inflammatory cell infiltrate.
- Platelet thrombi and microemboli in small blood vessels.
- Chronic radiation pneumonitis typically presents with interstitial fibrosis that can mimic the usual interstitial pneumonia (UIP) or fibrotic nonspecific interstitial pneumonia (NSIP) patterns, or it can present with other mixed or unclassifiable fibrotic patterns.
- Medial thickening and/or hyalinization in pulmonary arteries, often with plump endothelial cells.
- Foamy cells in the thickened intima and/or media of pulmonary arteries and veins.

DIFFERENTIAL DIAGNOSIS

A variety of other conditions may enter the differential diagnosis, depending on whether the patient is presenting acutely or chronically. When diffuse alveolar damage or organizing pneumonia is encountered, a careful search for evidence of infection should be undertaken, including a search for viral inclusions and neutrophilic infiltrates, and a GMS stain should also be performed, as *Pneumocystis* and fungal infections can be very subtle on an hematoxylin and eosin–stained slide. Recognition of cells with bizarre radiation-related cytologic atypia and degenerative smudgy chromatin is often helpful, but these cells can closely mimic virally infected cells, and immunohistochemistry for viruses and correlation with viral cultures can aid in this distinction. When fibrosis predominates, a variety of other fibrotic lung diseases may enter the differential diagnosis, although recognition of residual bizarre stromal cells with radiation atypia and abnormal vessels with characteristic foam cells can be helpful. As with all forms of fibrotic lung disease, clinicopathologic correlation via multidisciplinary discussion may be required to establish a definitive diagnosis.

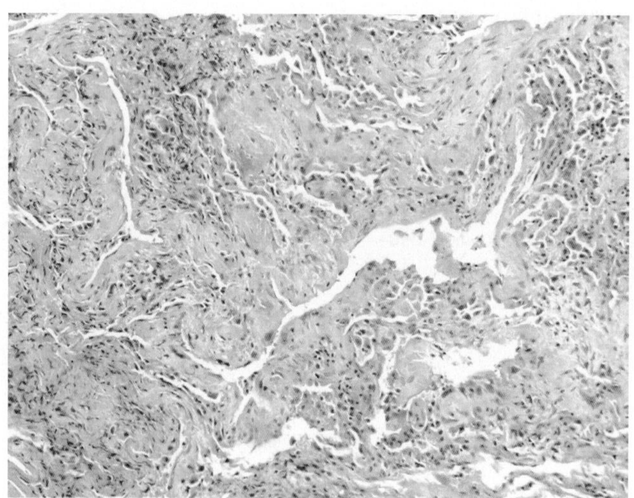

Figure 142.1 By the time a biopsy is performed, acute radiation pneumonitis often shows diffuse alveolar damage in the organizing phase with residual hyaline membranes, exuberant fibroblastic proliferation and edema, and marked reactive type II pneumocyte hyperplasia.

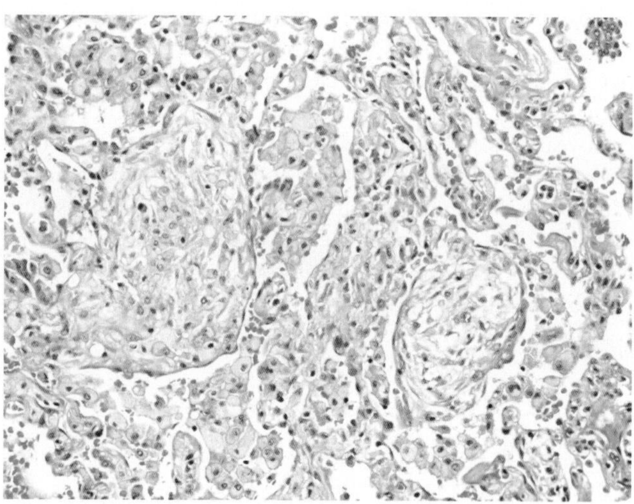

Figure 142.2 Radiation pneumonitis in the subacute stage often shows an organizing pneumonia pattern, characterized by plugs of proliferating fibroblasts in alveolar spaces.

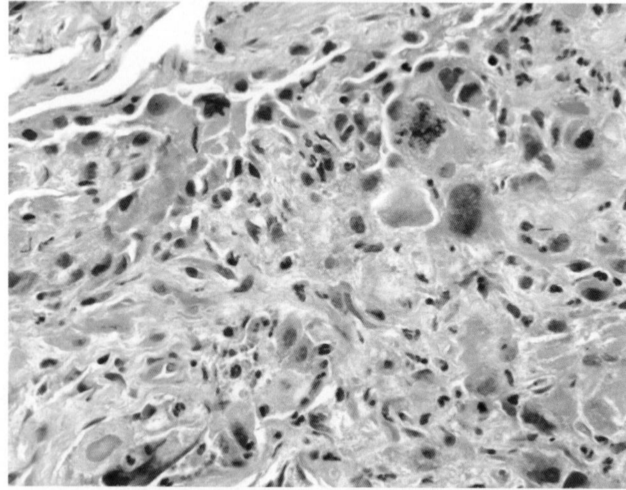

Figure 142.3 At high-power magnification, radiation pneumonitis often shows scattered frankly bizarre cells with "radiation atypia," characterized by marked nuclear enlargement but with preservation of the nuclear to cytoplasmic ratio and degenerative smudgy chromatin. These cells can closely mimic virally infected cells.

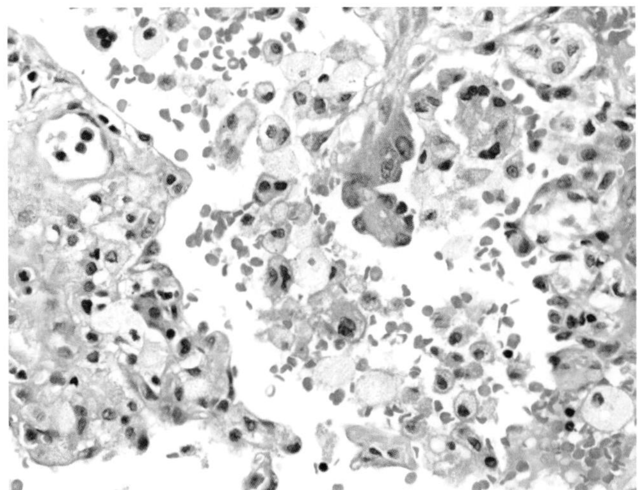

Figure 142.4 Radiation pneumonitis is sometimes associated with prominent vacuolization of pneumocytes and alveolar macrophages, a nonspecific change that can also be encountered with other drugs, such as amiodarone and statins, and with other conditions, such as proximal bronchial obstruction.

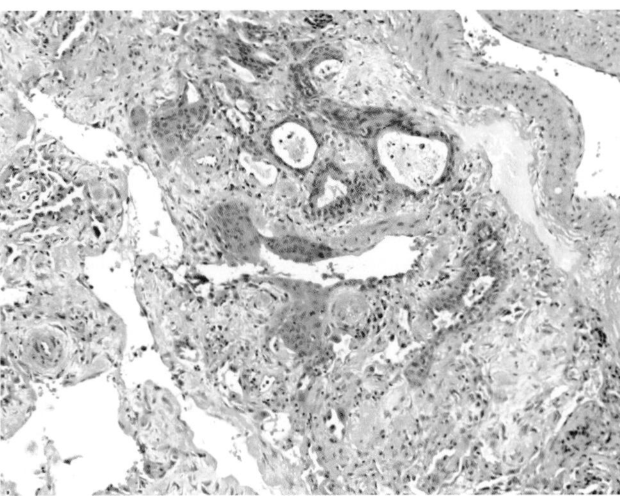

Figure 142.5 Squamous metaplasia of bronchiolar epithelial cells is a nonspecific change that often accompanies diffuse alveolar damage and may be encountered with radiation pneumonitis and other causes of severe acute lung injury.

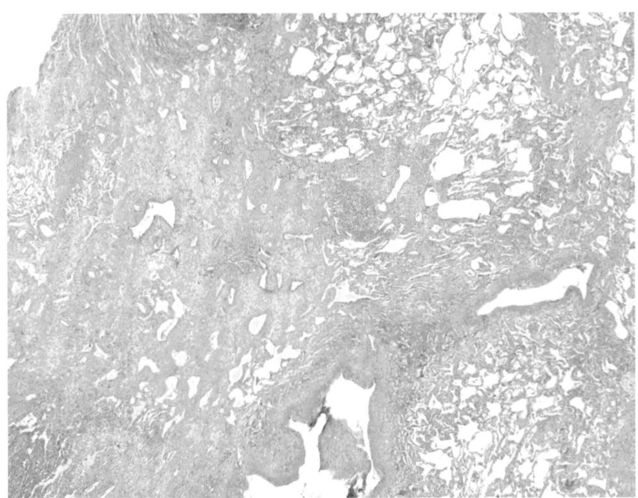

Figure 142.6 Interstitial fibrosis is the hallmark of chronic radiation pneumonitis, which can present with advanced fibrotic changes that resemble the fibrotic NSIP pattern or even the UIP pattern, as in this case.

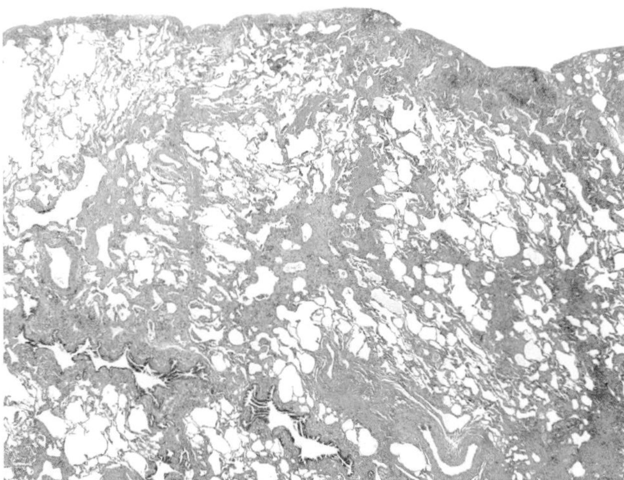

Figure 142.7 Chronic radiation pneumonitis can also present with unusual or unclassifiable patterns of lung fibrosis, where the extent and distribution of fibrotic change is difficult to characterize and does not conform to any of the recognized patterns of fibrotic interstitial lung disease.

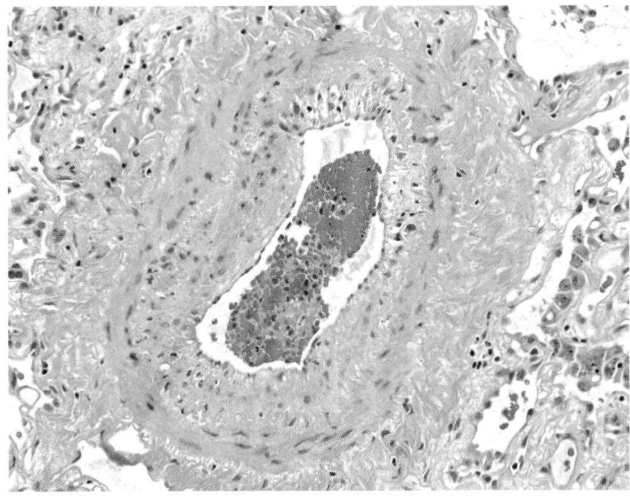

Figure 142.8 Vasculopathy is a common feature of chronic radiation pneumonitis and is characterized by medial and/or intimal thickening, often with foamy cells in the abnormal intima and plump endothelial cells.

Section 21

Pneumoconioses

► Timothy C. Allen

143 Asbestosis

Timothy C. Allen
Richard Attanoos
Maxwell L. Smith

Asbestosis is a lung disease caused by the inhalation of a large number of asbestos fibers. Asbestos, a fibrous silicate, has been used predominantly as an insulator and fire retardant and is categorized as serpentine (which includes chrysotile asbestos) and amphibole (which includes, among others, amosite and crocidolite asbestos). Individual asbestos exposure can be roughly gauged by the number of asbestos bodies identified, as the number of asbestos bodies found corresponds to the number of asbestos fibers inhaled. Electron microscopic examination of a known weight of lung tissue after digestion allows for a count of asbestos bodies and a calculation of the concentration of asbestos fibers in an individual patient's lung.

Asbestos exposure in and of itself is not diagnostic of asbestosis; essentially all people without occupational asbestos exposure have inhaled some asbestos fibers from ambient air, mostly in urban areas, in quantities insufficient to cause asbestosis. Asbestos exposure is indicated by the identification of asbestos fibers or asbestos bodies. Asbestos bodies may be seen in occupationally asbestos-exposed individuals who show no lung fibrosis. By definition, the diagnosis of asbestosis required the identification of lung fibrosis in association with asbestos bodies and asbestos fibers. Asbestosis has a latency of approximately 20 to 40 years from initial exposure, occasionally longer.

Asbestosis exhibits a dose–response relationship and is dependent on host susceptibility. As such, each asbestosis patient must reach a threshold amount of asbestos exposure before assuming a risk of developing asbestosis. Individuals exposed to identical asbestos levels will not all develop asbestosis. Overall, the risk of developing asbestosis increases with increased exposure above the individual's threshold.

Fibrosis in asbestosis patients starts in the first tiers of alveolar septa and progresses in the development of interstitial fibrosis until ultimately developing end-stage lung disease and honeycombing. Radiologically, asbestosis shows similar findings as usual interstitial pneumonia, with disease predominantly involving the periphery of the lower lung lobes. On gross examination, lungs show dense fibrosis and honeycombing with the most severe disease involving the periphery of the lower lung lobes. The pleura may be thickened and show pleural plaques; however, pleural thickening and pleural plaques are not diagnostic of asbestosis and are not required for the diagnosis of asbestosis. Pleural plaques may be identified in patients without parenchymal fibrosis.

Because asbestos fibers may be identified in sputum and bronchoalveolar lavage specimens in asbestos-exposed individuals, whether or not there is asbestosis, it is not diagnosable by cytology. Small, limited biopsies, such as needle core biopsies and transbronchial biopsies, do not contain enough lung tissue for either the exclusion or diagnosis of asbestosis. A wedge biopsy, or larger specimen, is necessary for the appropriate evaluation of lung tissue and accurate diagnosis of asbestosis.

HISTOLOGIC FEATURES

- Diagnosis of asbestosis requires both the presence of asbestos bodies and the characteristic pattern of lung fibrosis.
- The fibrosis is worse in the lower lung zones and at the peripheries; fibrosis that is focal, unilateral, or worse in the upper lung lobes is not diagnostic of asbestosis.
- Aside from characteristic fibrosis, diagnosis of asbestosis requires the identification of at least two asbestos bodies, to avoid overdiagnosis when finding an occasional asbestos body in an individual without sufficient asbestos exposure.
- Typically, the increasing number of identified asbestos bodies reflects increasing severity of fibrosis.
- Asbestos bodies represent only asbestos exposure; they do not represent the interstitial lung disease of asbestosis.
- Asbestos fibers are clear; however, many, termed *asbestos bodies*, have an iron-containing proteinaceous coat that stains golden yellow to brown, giving them a barbell-like shape.
- Iron stain emphasizes the bright blue iron coatings of asbestos bodies against a pale pink background, making them more identifiable.
- Ferruginous bodies must be distinguished from asbestos bodies, which are only one type of ferruginous body.
- Particles and fibers in the lung that become iron-coated are also ferruginous bodies; they must be distinguished from asbestos bodies.
- Asbestos bodies may become partially encased by alveolar macrophages.
- The identification of asbestos bodies in routine tissue sections from persons typically signifies some exposure to asbestos above a background level in an individual.
- Because of its long latency, fibrosis in asbestosis is composed of mature collagen.
- Granulation tissue, as identified with acute lung injury, is not a diagnostic criterion of asbestosis.
- Early interstitial fibrosis, involving the first tiers of alveolar septa, must be distinguished from smoking-related respiratory bronchiolitis.
- Fibrosis of asbestosis progresses to include more alveolar septa, progressing ultimately to end-stage lung disease and honeycombing.
- Nonasbestosis-related lung changes may be present and may make the diagnosis of asbestosis more difficult to exclude or confirm; these changes include tobacco-related changes, superimposed mixed-dust pneumoconiosis, tuberculosis or other infections, and desquamative interstitial pneumonia-like changes.

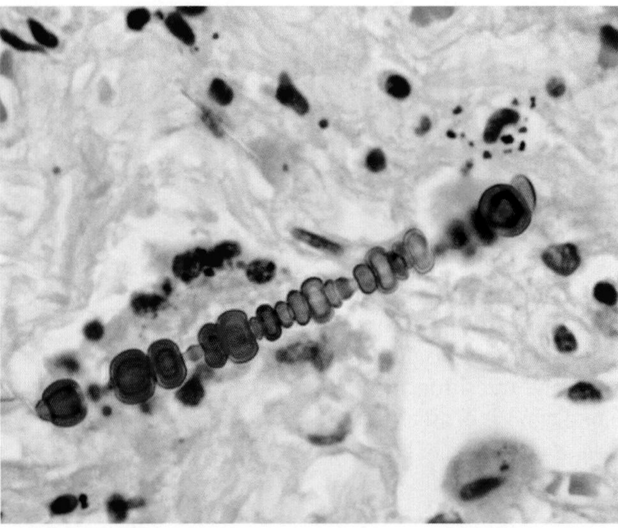

Figure 143.1 Asbestos body with characteristic dumbbell shape and clear central fibrous core.

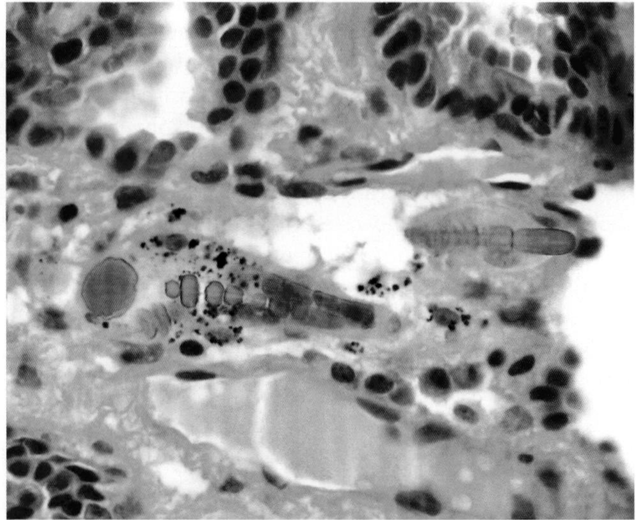

Figure 143.2 Multiple asbestos bodies seen in one field are indicative of very high exposure to asbestos.

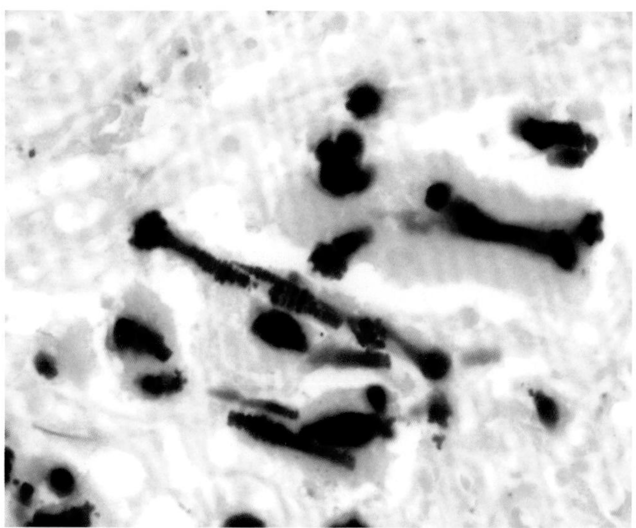

Figure 143.3 Iron stain highlights the iron coatings of asbestos bodies, assisting in their identification.

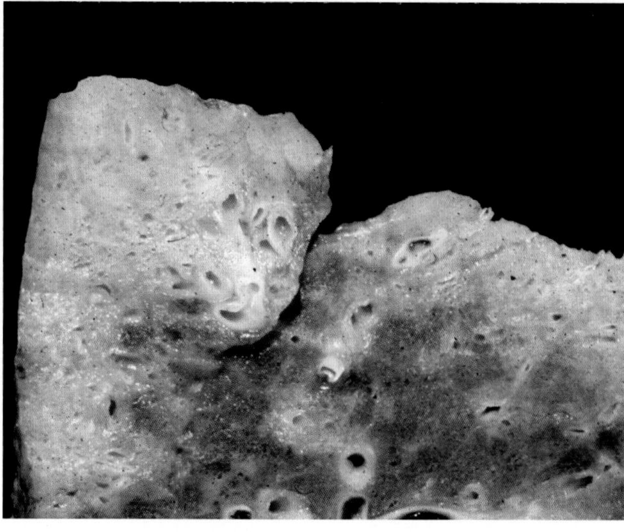

Figure 143.4 Gross image of severe asbestosis showing marked fibrosis.

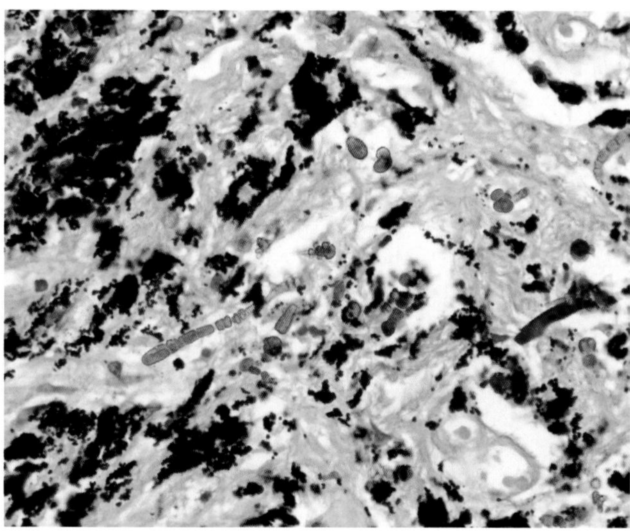

Figure 143.5 Abundant black carbon particulates, asbestos bodies, and ferruginous bodies are present; ferruginous bodies should not be interpreted as asbestos bodies.

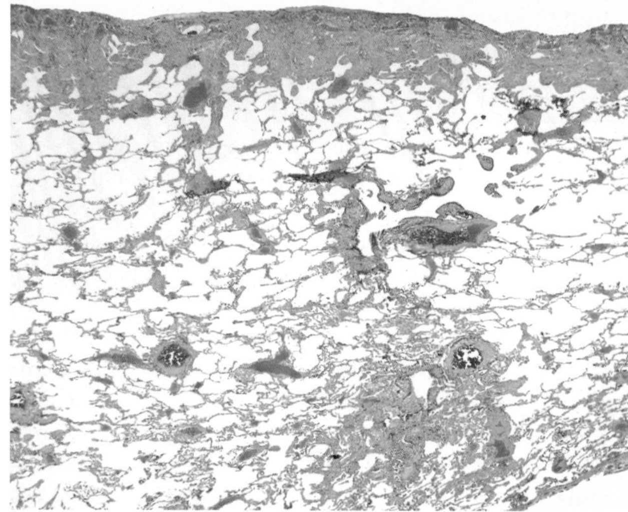

Figure 143.6 Early asbestosis showing predominantly peripheral and peribronchiolar fibrosis.

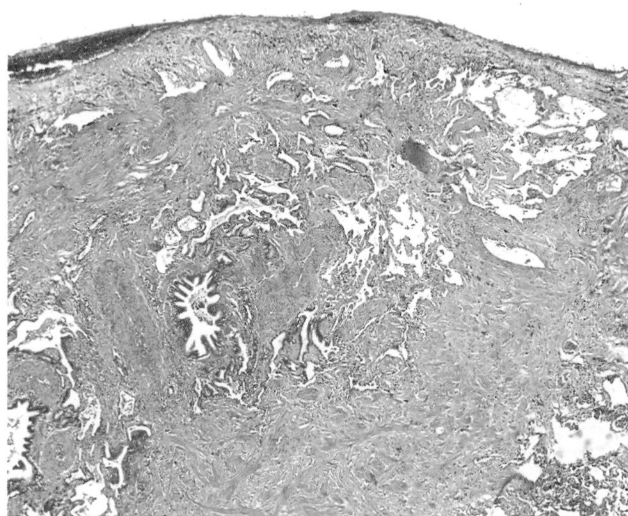

Figure 143.7 Peripheral fibrosis, predominantly in the lower lung lobes, is a characteristic feature of asbestosis; however, it may be seen in other interstitial lung diseases, such as usual interstitial pneumonia.

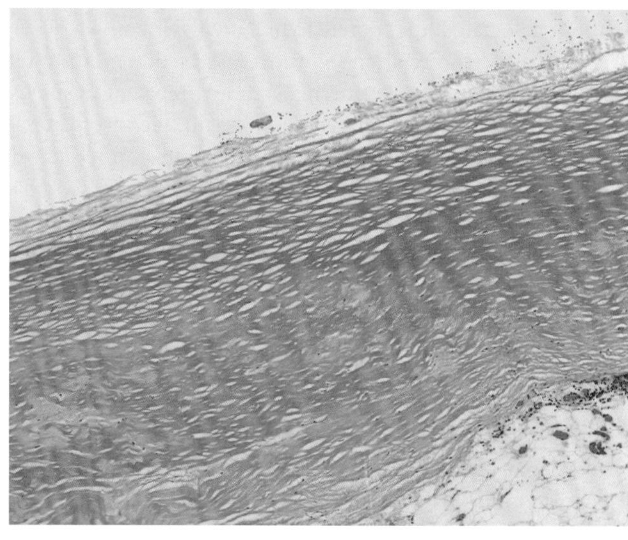

Figure 143.8 Pleural plaques may be identified in patients with asbestosis; however, they are not diagnostic, they are not required for the diagnosis, and they may be seen in individuals without asbestosis.

144

Silicosis

▶ Timothy C. Allen
▶ Richard Attanoos
▶ Maxwell L. Smith

Silicosis is caused by inhalation of large amounts of crystalline silica (quartz) particles; patients often have a high occupational exposure from sandblasting, mining, glass-making, stone working, and quarry mining. Patients are often asymptomatic; however, conglomerate silicosis patients frequently develop dyspnea and hypoxemia. Some patients die due to cor pulmonale and resultant respiratory failure. Simple silicosis, also termed *nodular silicosis* or *chronic silicosis*, has a prolonged latency period, usually between 20 and 40 years from the patient's initial exposure; disease may progress after exposure ends. In rare cases, accelerated silicosis may develop, usually within 3 to 10 years after initial exposure. Also, in cases with extreme, overwhelming silica exposure, acute silicosis may occur, showing a histologic pattern of pulmonary alveolar proteinosis. Silicosis, in contrast to asbestosis, has an upper lung lobe predilection.

Silicotic nodules are the characteristic lesion in patients with silicosis; the numbers and distribution of the nodules vary widely among patients. Simple silicosis is defined as the presence of multiple silicotic nodules less than 1 cm in diameter. Some of these patients will progress to develop conglomerate silicosis, also termed *progressive massive fibrosis*, which is defined as a confluence of silicotic nodules greater than 2 cm in diameter. Silicosis increases a patient's susceptibility to mycobacterial and fungal infections; cavitation, often associated with concurrent tuberculosis, may arise in confluent nodules.

Grossly, silicotic nodules are sharply circumscribed and, on cut section, show a whorled arrangement of slate gray hyalinized collagen. Nodules may be calcified. Silicotic nodules are frequently found in the subpleural areas of the upper lung lobes; however, they can be found throughout the lungs. Pleural nodules, typically involving visceral pleura, also occur and have been termed *candle wax lesions* or *pleural pearls* because of their slate gray nodular appearance. Although not silicosis, silicotic nodules may be identified in hilar lymph nodes without associated lung parenchymal involvement.

Laboratory studies often show increased sedimentation rate, antinuclear antibodies, and immune complexes. Scleroderma is more prevalent in silicosis patients.

In patients with accelerated silicosis, nodules are generally more poorly formed, with more interstitial fibrosis, than in patients with simple silicosis.

Differential diagnosis includes mixed-dust pneumoconiosis and other pneumoconioses. With polarization, silica particles may be confused with endogenous calcium oxalate crystals and other incidental particles. Also, small collections of dust-laden macrophages containing anthracotic pigment and birefringent particles seen in smokers may be confused with silicosis.

HISTOLOGIC FEATURES

- Silica nodules are typically found in upper lung lobe bronchovascular bundles, interlobular septa, and pleura; however, they may be identified throughout the lung parenchyma.
- Silica nodules are often seen in bronchial and hilar lymph nodes.
- Nodules begin as small collections of dust-laden macrophages containing anthracotic pigment, with little or no obvious fibrous component.

- As nodules advance, they become centrally fibrotic and acellular, with whorled collagen and with peripheral collections of dust-laden macrophages.
- Nodules ultimately develop into rounded to oval masses of hyalinized collagen, with central and peripheral collections of anthracotic pigment and with peripheral collections of dust-laden macrophages.
- Mature silica nodules may contain calcifications.
- With parenchymal nodules, surrounding focal emphysema due to adjacent parenchymal fragmentation.
- On polarization, there are weakly birefringent small, approximately 2-micron silica crystals, usually scattered among larger, more strongly birefringent, more obvious accompanying silicate particles.

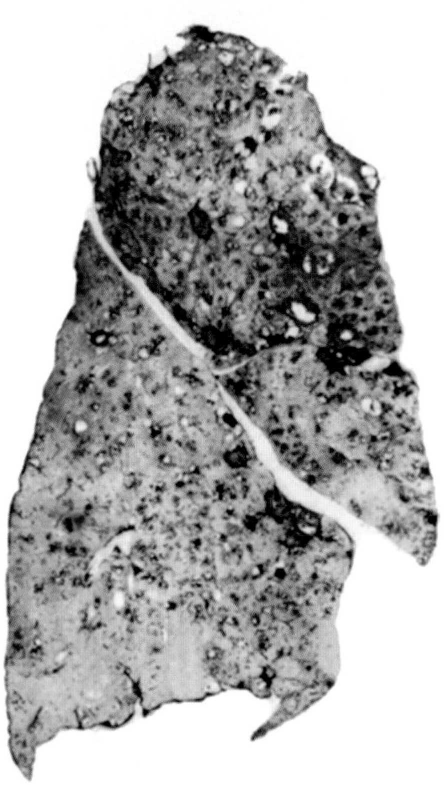

Figure 144.1 Whole lung section of silicosis, showing silicotic nodules involving predominantly upper lobe.

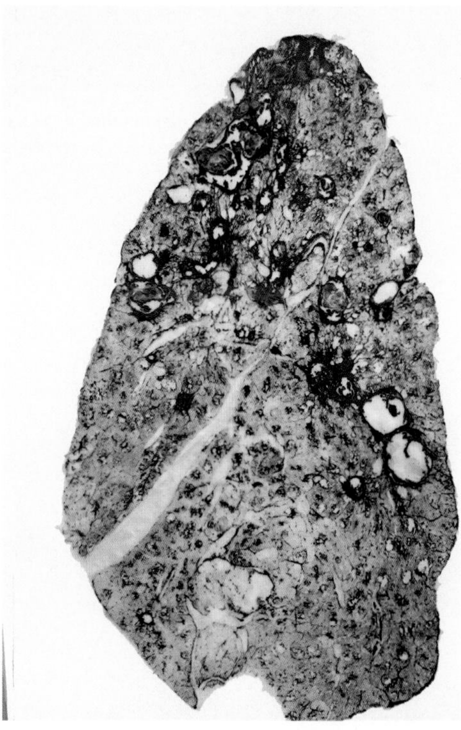

Figure 144.2 Whole lung section of nodular silicosis from a slate worker; note rounded to oval masses of hyalinized collagen.

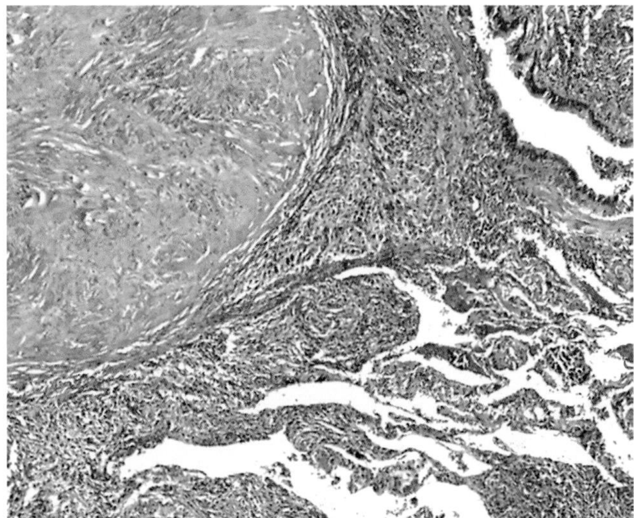

Figure 144.3 Silicotic nodule showing central whorl of almost acellular hyalinized collagen and anthracotic pigment and peripheral dust-laden macrophages.

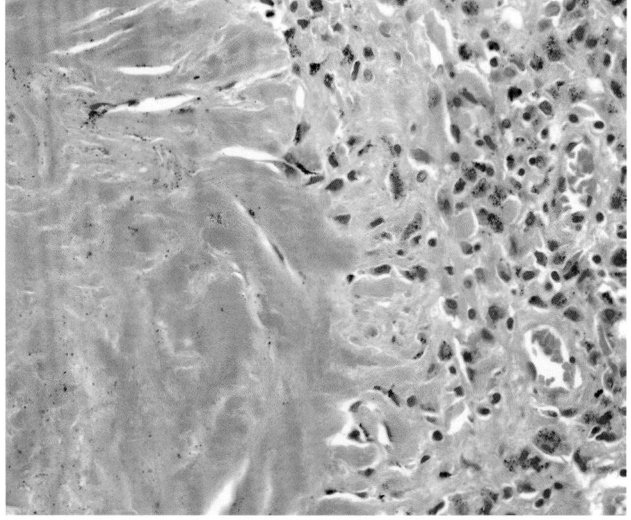

Figure 144.4 Edge of a silicotic nodule, shown under polarized light in Figure 144.5.

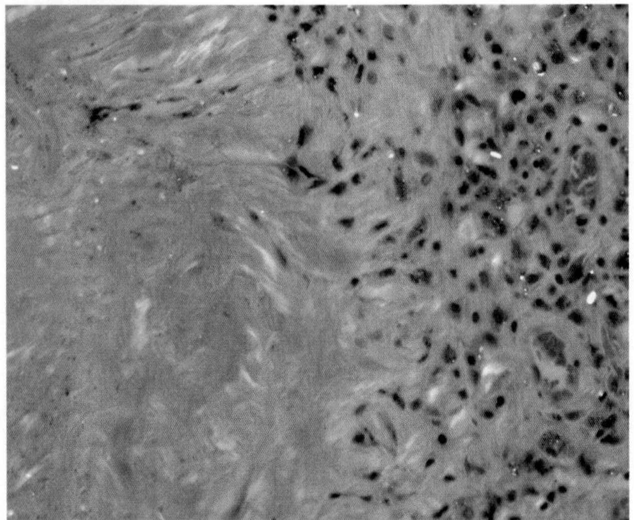

Figure 144.5 On polarized light, a silicotic nodule contains a mixture of tiny, weakly birefringent silica particles admixed with larger brightly birefringent silicate particles.

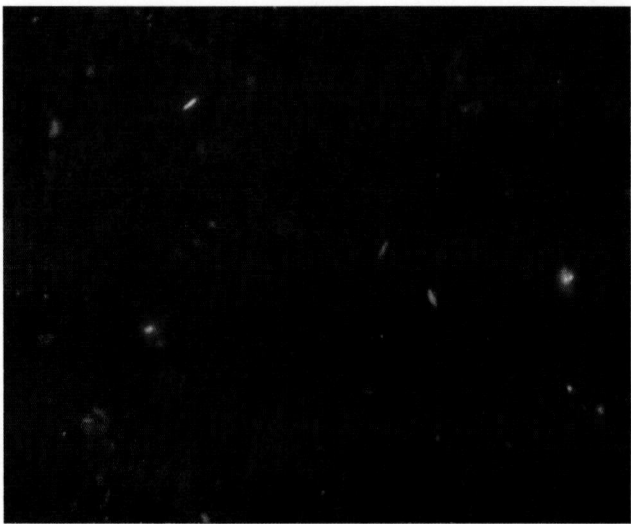

Figure 144.6 Higher power view of silicotic nodule showing, on polarized light, tiny, weakly birefringent silica particles admixed with larger more strongly birefringent silicate particles.

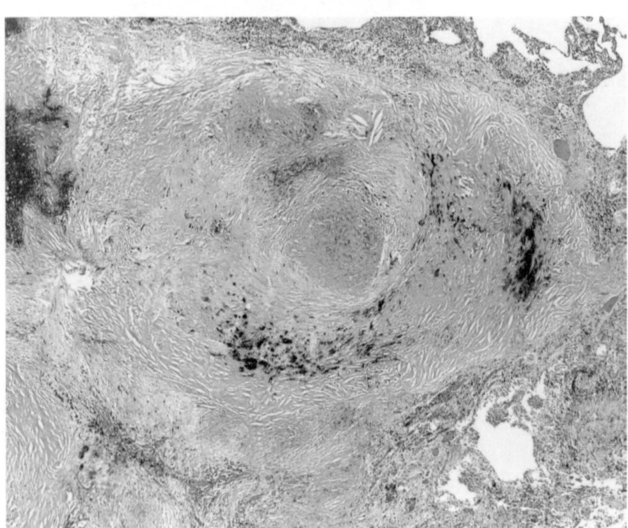

Figure 144.7 Complicated silicosis, also termed *progressive massive fibrosis*, with large confluent advanced silicotic nodules.

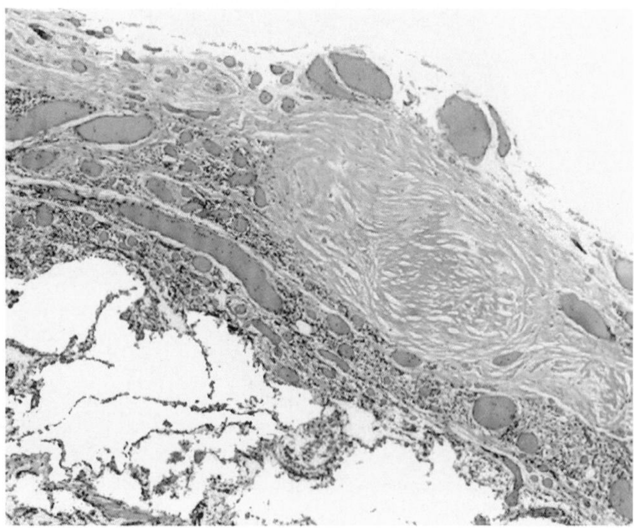

Figure 144.8 Acellular collagenous nodules with "whorled" appearance present in the pleura; these appear externally as "candle wax" lesions.

145

Silicatosis

Timothy C. Allen
Richard Attanoos
Maxwell L. Smith

Silicatosis, caused by silicate inhalation, is usually seen in patients with occupational exposures of talc, kaolinite, mica, vermiculite, and other silicates from mines and quarries. Most patients are asymptomatic; however, in patients with widespread pulmonary fibrosis, dyspnea is common. Silicatosis is uncommon in comparison with asbestosis and silicosis. Silicates may be contaminated with silica or asbestos in certain settings, and these contaminating materials are often responsible for greater contribution to the lung disease than the nonasbestos silicates in these circumstances.

HISTOLOGIC FEATURES

- Silicatosis is characterized by the perivascular and peribronchiolar deposition of birefringent silicate particles, lying within variably sized collagen deposits.
- There are six different lesions that may be present: macules, nodules, fibrosis, and dust deposits within bronchiolar walls, foreign body granulomas, interstitial fibrosis, and massive fibrosis.
- Silicate macules are nonpalpable collections of dust-laden macrophages within respiratory bronchiole walls; there is little or no associated fibrosis.
- Silicate nodules are hard, fibrotic nodular lesions measuring 2 to 10 mm, generally found in the upper and middle lung zones.
- Nodules are made up of dust-laden macrophages lying within haphazard bundles of collagen; multinucleated giant cells may be present.
- The hyalinized collagen is likely secondary to silica contamination.
- Fibrosis and dust deposits may occur within the walls of membranous (terminal) bronchioles, respiratory bronchioles, and alveolar ducts; they represent a form of mineral dust–induced small airway disease.
- Foreign-body granulomas may occur in silicatosis patients.
- Interstitial fibrosis may be found in more advanced disease and exhibits interstitial pneumonia with fibrosis with abundant dust particles, with or without giant cells.
- Massive fibrosis is seen in advanced silicatosis and is characterized by marked fibrosis, likely due to nodule coalescence, with innumerable dust particles; there may be associated pleural thickening.

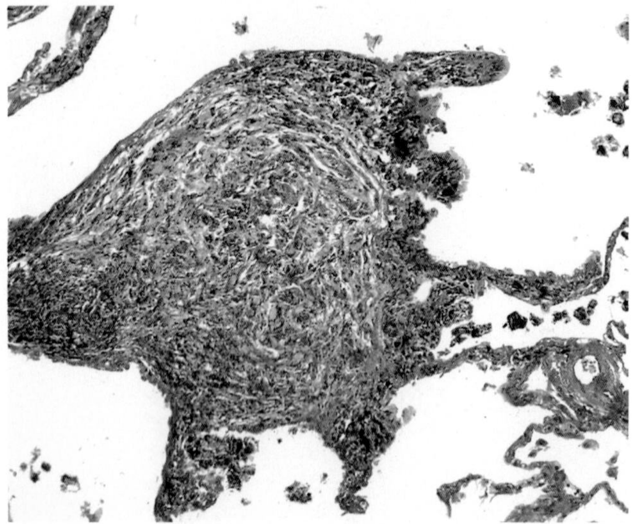

Figure 145.1 Silicate nodule, with collagen bundles and dust-laden macrophages.

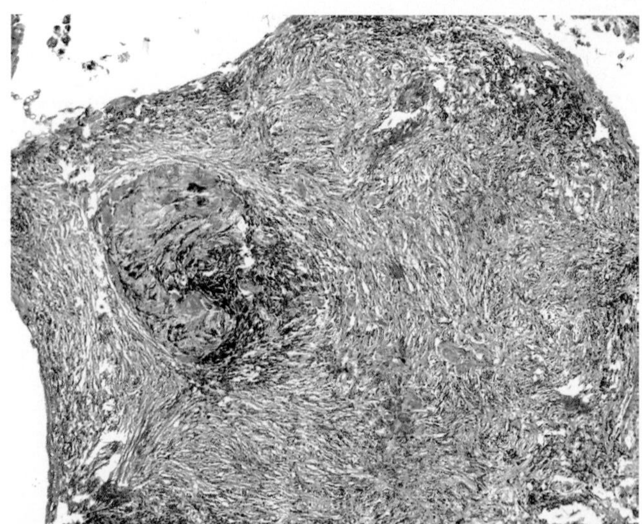

Figure 145.2 Focus of massive fibrosis with diffuse collections of dust-laden macrophages.

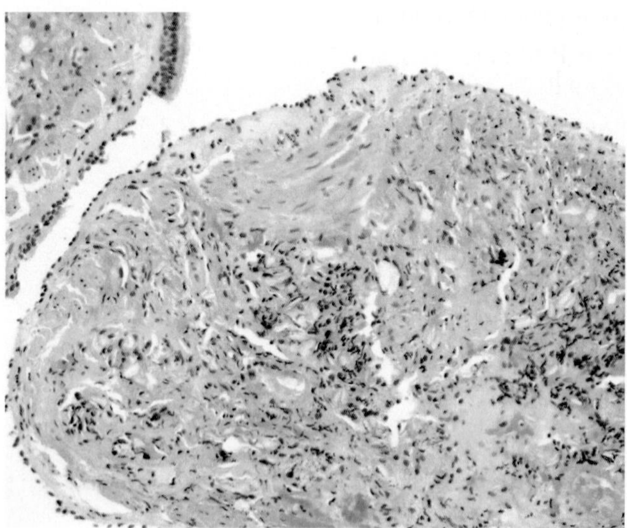

Figure 145.3 Bronchiole wall containing fibrosis and associated dust deposits.

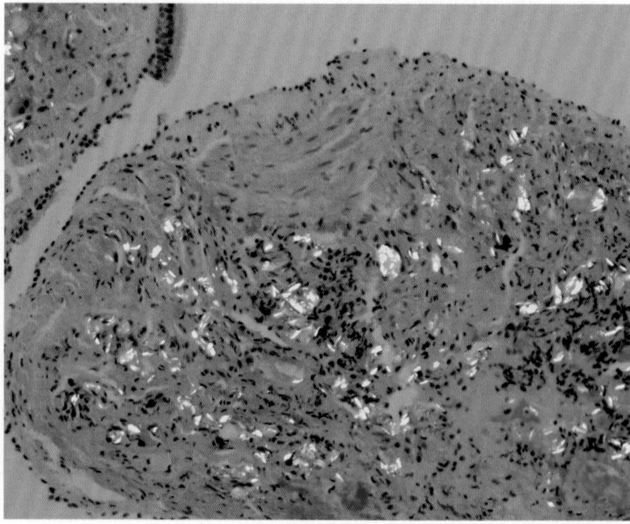

Figure 145.4 On polarization, the fibrotic area within the bronchiolar wall shows bright birefringent silicate particles.

Mixed Pneumoconiosis and Mixed-Dust Pneumoconiosis

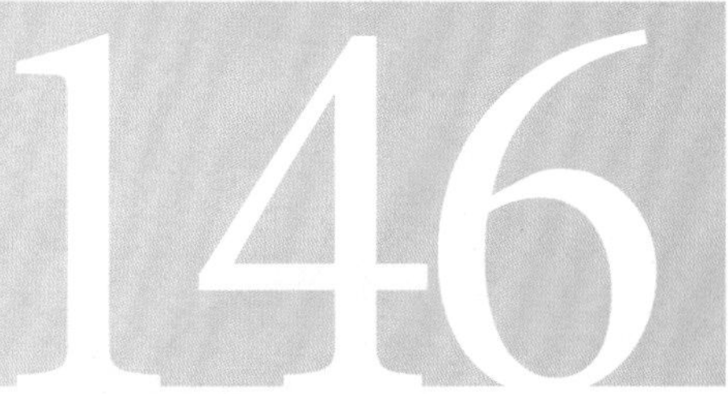

Timothy C. Allen
Richard Attanoos
Maxwell L. Smith

Mixed pneumoconiosis and mixed-dust pneumoconiosis are characterized by macules or fibrotic lesions, which may or may not have accompanying silicotic nodules, with a clinical history of mixed-dust exposure. The majority of industrial dust exposures are mixed-dust exposures; however, it is a diagnosis of exclusion after eliminating other pneumoconioses from the differential diagnosis. The two diagnoses are similar; however, they are distinct. Mixed pneumoconiosis has distinctive histologic features of two separate pneumoconioses, such as asbestosis, with its characteristic pattern of fibrosis and asbestos bodies, and silicosis, with its characteristic silicotic nodules. Mixed-dust pneumoconiosis, in contrast, involves dust exposures with more than one component, producing hybrid lesions that are not classic for either of the dusts. Exposure to silicates contaminated with silica, for example, might produce pulmonary lesions that are neither silicotic nodules nor pure silicate nodules, but instead a hybrid lesion. Patients present generally with dyspnea and cough and show variable pulmonary function test results. Prognosis is also variable, with some patients relatively unaffected and others progressing to end-stage lung disease and ultimately death. X-ray often shows irregular and small round opacities; with reticular and reticulonodular opacities often seen on CT scan.

HISTOLOGIC FEATURES

- Distinct histologic features of more than one dust exposure.
- Hybrid lesions, showing histologic features of two distinct dust, may be present.
- Varying combinations of macules, mixed-dust fibrotic nodules, and silicotic nodules.
- Macules show accumulations of dust-laden macrophages with little fibrous stroma.
- Macules are typically peribronchiolar and perivascular.
- Mixed-dust fibrotic nodules are often stellate, "medusa head" lesions with central whorled hyalinized collagen and surrounding collections of dust-laden macrophages that extend into lung parenchyma.
- Silicotic nodules are firm discrete round lesions of paucicellular whorled hyalinized collagen.
- Polarized light shows birefringent needles of crystalline silica, as well as birefringent plates of silicates.
- Nonspecific interstitial pneumonia may be seen.

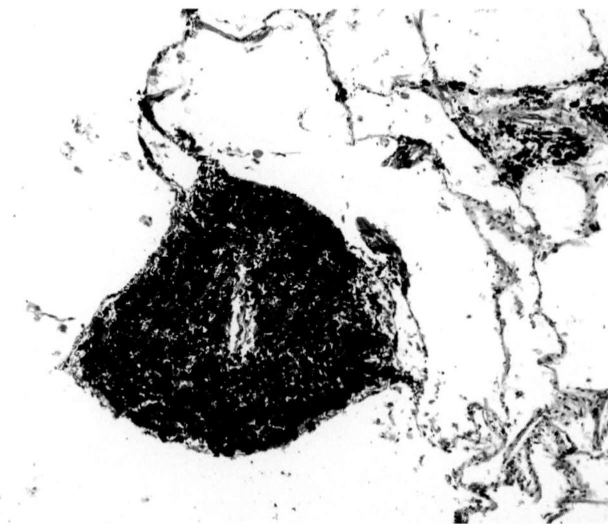

Figure 146.1 Dust-laden macule in a silicate- and silica-exposed patient with mixed-dust pneumoconiosis.

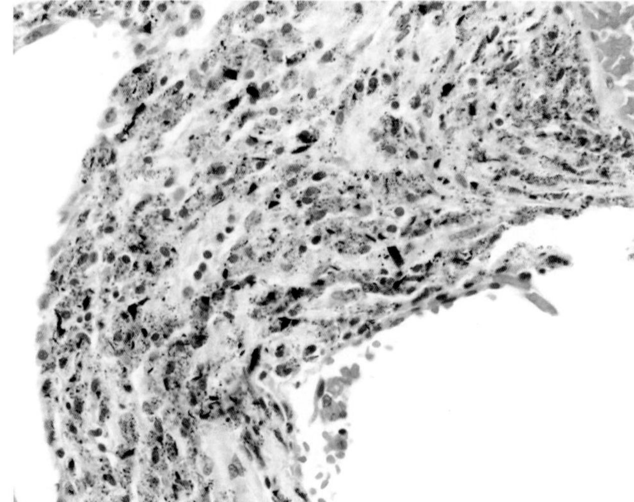

Figure 146.2 Dust-laden fibrotic nodule containing dust-laden macrophages, anthracotic pigment, and irregular fibrosis in a patient with mixed-dust pneumoconiosis.

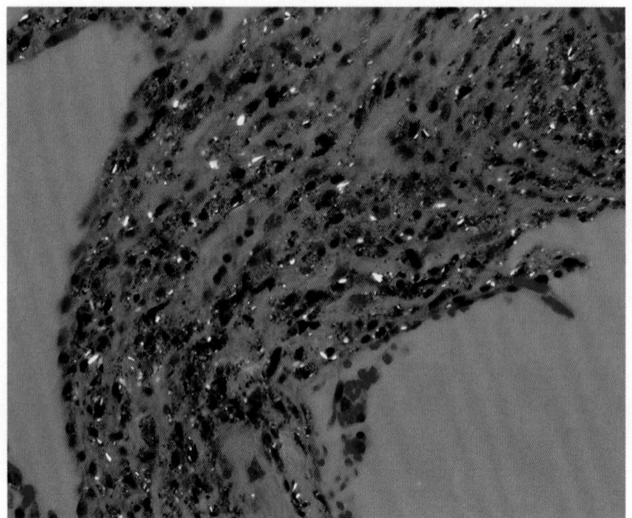

Figure 146.3 On polarized light, the fibrotic nodule shows smaller, weakly birefringent needle-like silica particles and larger, irregular, more strongly birefringent plate-like silicate particles.

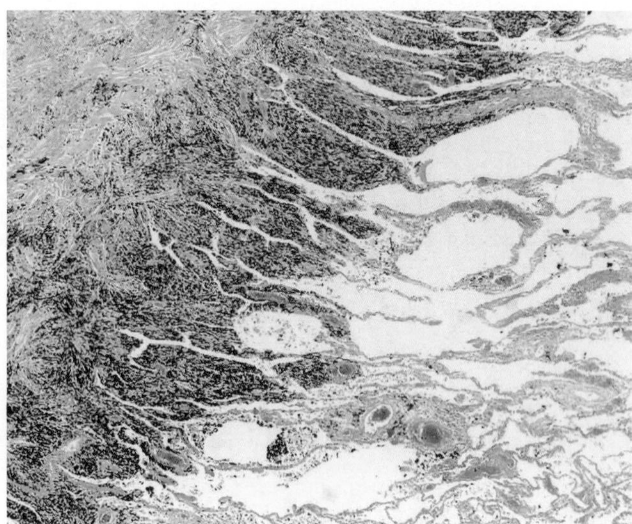

Figure 146.4 Rounded silicotic nodule in a patient with mixed-dust pneumoconiosis, with an irregular stellate "medusa head" edge of dust-laden macrophages extending into surrounding lung parenchyma, and central hyalinized collagen.

Coal Worker's Pneumoconiosis

147

▶ Timothy C. Allen
▶ Richard Attanoos
▶ Allen R. Gibbs
▶ Maxwell L. Smith

Coal dust is predominantly made up of noncrystalline carbon, as well as varying amounts of quartz (crystalline silica), mica, and kaolin. Coal worker's pneumoconiosis, commonly known as *black lung disease*, is found in coal miners; the intensity of the disease is related to exposure level and duration. Patients may be asymptomatic; however, patients with progressive massive fibrosis may have severe dyspnea and hypoxemia, may progress to cor pulmonale, and may die of disease. The amount of quartz making up the coal dust varies among coal types and significantly effects the degree of lung change. Radiologically, coal worker's pneumoconiosis shows bilateral small round upper lobe opacities. Grossly, coal dust nodules may be identified, primarily in the upper lung lobes. Coal dust nodules are primarily a mixture of coal dust and quartz silica and, therefore, a lesion of mixed-dust pneumoconiosis. The amount of quartz silica present determines the amount of hyalinized collagen present in the coal dust nodule. Coal dust nodules may be further divided into micronodules (up to 7 mm) and macronodules (7 to 2 cm). With advanced disease, progressive massive fibrosis occurs, with confluent areas of fibrosis 2 cm and larger, and is seen predominantly in the upper lung lobes. If the confluent areas show cavitation, concomitant tuberculosis must be considered. Differential diagnosis includes cigarette-related and environment-related anthracotic pigment deposition.

HISTOLOGIC FEATURES

- Aggregates of dust-laden macrophages with little attendant fibrosis, termed *coal dust macules*, are seen predominantly in the upper lung lobes, with associated focal emphysema.
- Coal dust macules lie within the walls of respiratory bronchioles, alveolar ducts, and adjacent alveoli.
- Fibrotic nodules containing dust-laden macrophages, termed *coal dust nodules*, evolve from coal dust macules and may be found in respiratory bronchioles.
- Coal dust nodules may show a central area made up of whorls of dense hyalinized collagen, with surrounding dust-laden macrophages, imparting a "medusa head" appearance to the nodule.
- Coal dust nodules may also be found in the interlobular septa and in peribronchial and subpleural connective tissue.
- Coal dust nodules are usually seen in association with coal dust macules; both are predominantly found in the upper lung lobes.
- Simple coal worker's pneumoconiosis involves coal dust macules and/or coal dust nodules.
- Nodules may coalesce, causing progressive massive fibrosis.

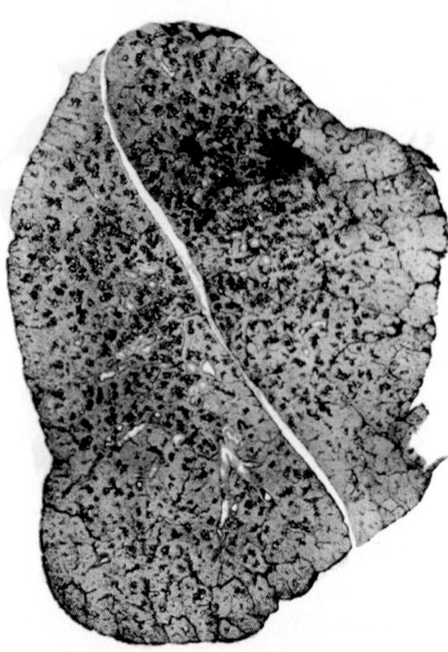

Figure 147.1 Whole lung section of simple coal worker's lung showing coal dust macules, predominantly involving the upper lung lobe. (Gough-Wentworth whole section by Dr. Jethro Gough and Dr. I.E. Wentworth courtesy of Dr. Allen R. Gibbs and Dr. Richard Attanoos.)

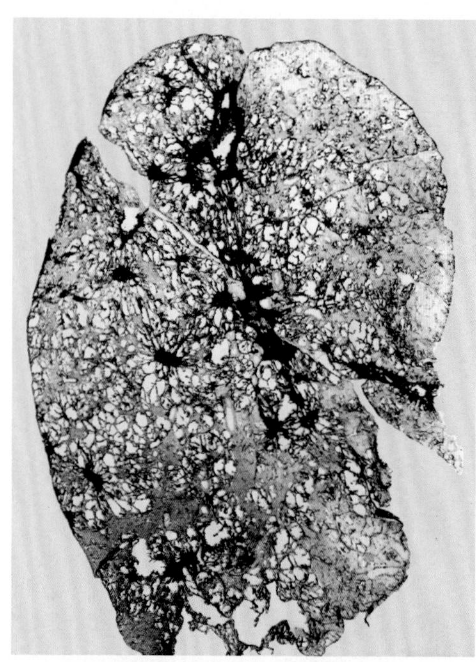

Figure 147.2 Whole lung section of coal worker's lung with coalescing nodules, forming progressive massive fibrosis. (Gough-Wentworth whole section by Dr. Jethro Gough and Dr. I.E. Wentworth courtesy of Dr. Allen R. Gibbs and Dr. Richard Attanoos.)

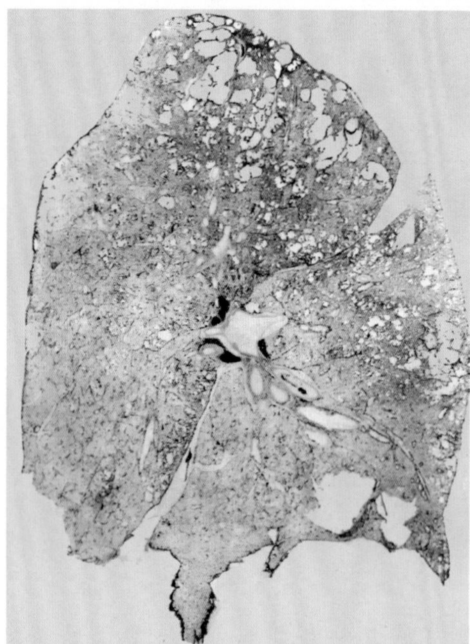

Figure 147.3 Whole lung section of coal worker's lung with marked apical and posterior centrilobular emphysema. (Gough-Wentworth whole section by Dr. Jethro Gough and Dr. I.E. Wentworth courtesy of Dr. Allen R. Gibbs and Dr. Richard Attanoos.)

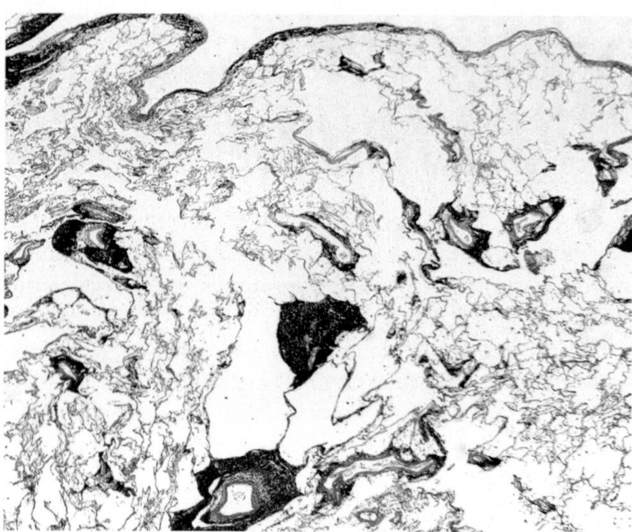

Figure 147.4 Lung parenchyma containing coal dust macules consisting of abundant coal particles, with associated focal emphysema.

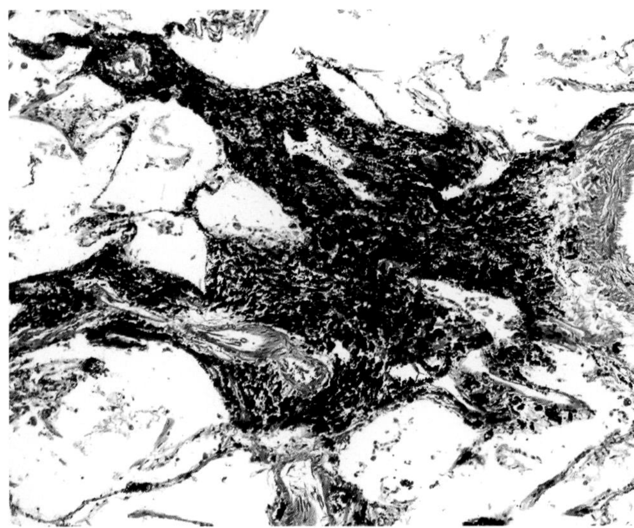

Figure 147.5 Coal dust macule containing coal dust-laden macrophages involving alveolar walls; fibrous tissue is apparent, and there is no fibrosis.

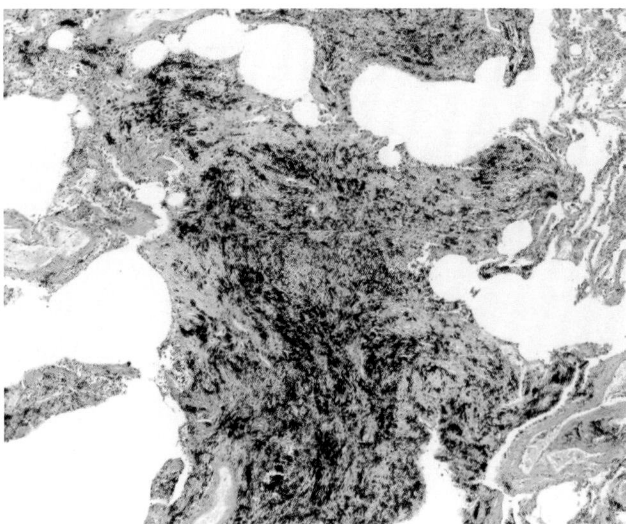

Figure 147.6 Coal dust nodule with dust-laden macrophages and fibrosis.

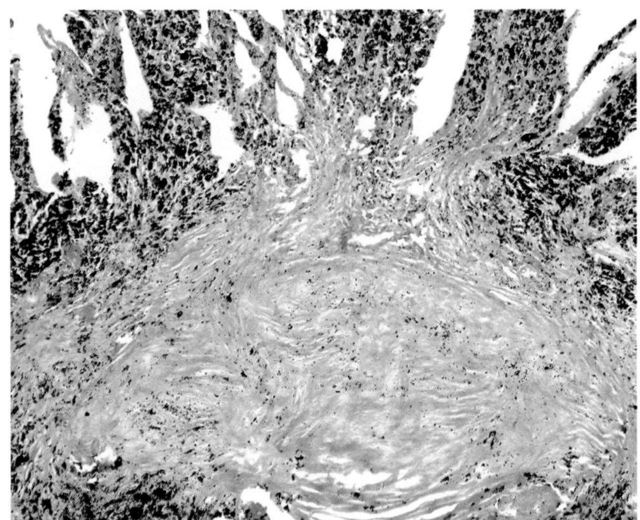

Figure 147.7 Coal dust nodule with dust-laden macrophages and fibrosis, showing whorls of dense hyalinized collagen, denoting exposure to coal dust containing quartz silica, and a "medusa head" of surrounding dust-laden macrophages.

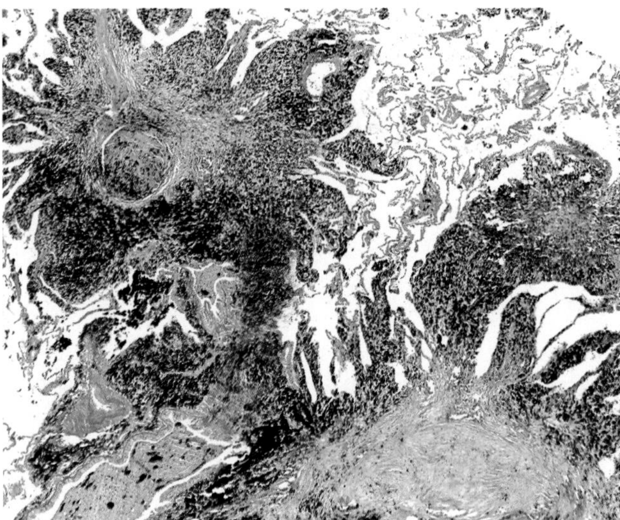

Figure 147.8 Coal dust nodules may coalesce, ultimately resulting in progressive massive fibrosis with confluent areas of fibrosis 2 cm and larger.

Giant-Cell Interstitial Pneumonia/Hard-Metal Pneumoconiosis

148

Timothy C. Allen
Richard Attanoos
Maxwell L. Smith

Giant-cell interstitial pneumonia is the histologic correlate of the clinical diagnosis of hard-metal pneumoconiosis. Patients inhale hard metals, typically cobalt, occupationally, in industries such as the alloy and ceramics industries, and tool, drilling equipment, and armament manufacturing industries. Patients present with increasing dyspnea and are found to have restrictive changes and small lung volume by pulmonary function testing. Radiologically, there is prominent interstitial thickening diffusely. As less than 1% of occupationally exposed individuals develop disease, it is thought that hypersensitivity plays a pathogenic role. Grossly, lungs are small and fibrotic. Differential diagnosis includes other interstitial lung diseases, such as desquamative interstitial pneumonia (DIP), usual interstitial pneumonia (UIP), nonspecific interstitial pneumonia (NSIP), and hypersensitivity pneumonitis. Occupational history and testing via analytic electron microscopy, energy-dispersive x-ray elemental analysis, or other techniques assist in the accurate diagnosis of giant-cell interstitial pneumonia.

HISTOLOGIC FEATURES

- Thickened, fibrotic alveolar septa, with associated type II pneumocyte hyperplasia, a variable chronic inflammatory cell infiltrate, and collections of alveolar macrophages.
- Multinucleated giant cells in alveoli, containing up to 20 to 30 nuclei, are a characteristic finding.
- The multinucleated giant cells may exhibit emperipolesis.
- The collections of alveolar macrophages may mimic a DIP-like pattern.
- Fibrous alveolar septa may expand, eventually mimicking a UIP-like or NSIP-like pattern of lung fibrosis.
- Dust deposits are not obvious.

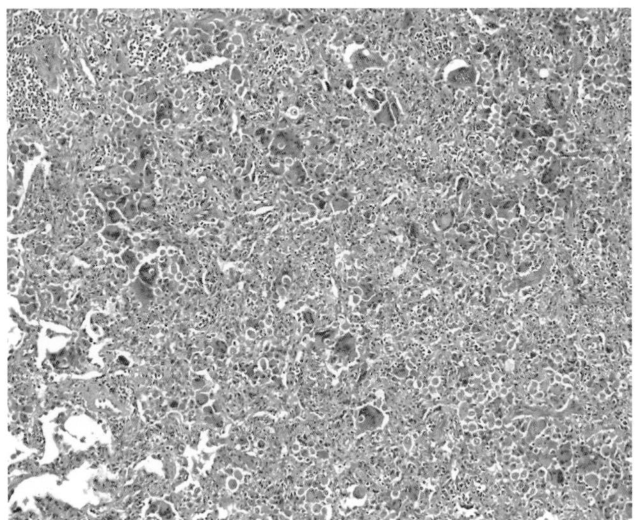

Figure 148.1 Thickened alveolar septa and a DIP-like pattern of alveolar macrophages; multinucleated giant cells are prominent.

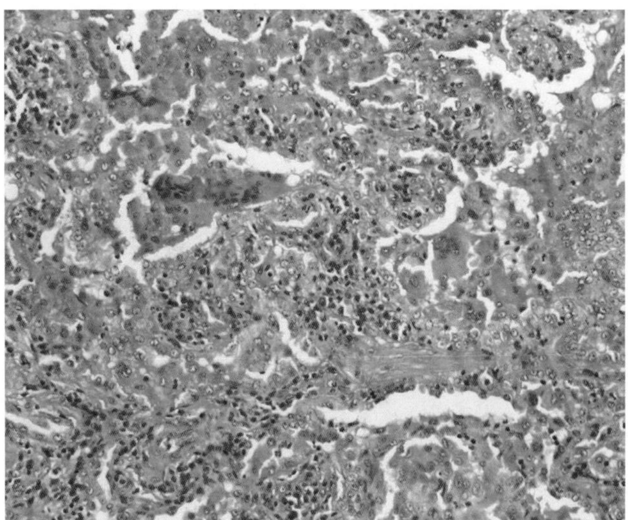

Figure 148.2 Higher power magnification showing alveolar septal widening and scattered multinucleated giant cells.

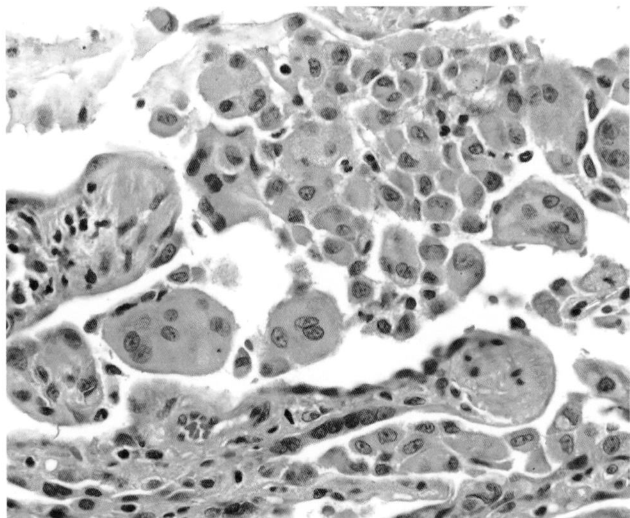

Figure 148.3 Alveolar macrophages may exhibit a DIP-like pattern.

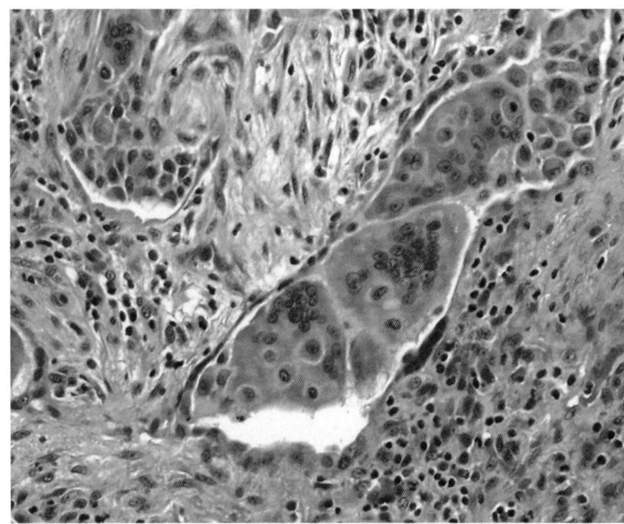

Figure 148.4 Giant cells often contain numerous nuclei.

149

Siderosis

Timothy C. Allen
Richard Attanoos
Maxwell L. Smith

Pulmonary siderosis, generally a disease of iron foundry workers, welders, steel mill workers, and miners, is characterized by the buildup in lung parenchyma of exogenous iron particles. Iron is minimally fibrinogenic and has been termed an *inert mineral*; siderosis patients typically may be asymptomatic even while showing radiologic changes of pulmonary fibrosis. Even so, extremely heavy exposures to iron may cause small airway fibrosis and fibrous nodules. In comparison, silicosiderosis, caused by workplace exposure to both iron and silica, is a mixed-dust pneumoconiosis. In other mixed-dust pneumoconioses, iron may be present but contribute little to the disease clinically. Differential diagnosis, aside from silicosiderosis and other mixed-dust pneumoconioses, is chronic passive congestion. Chronic passive congestion shows large numbers of hemosiderin-laden macrophages in airspaces. Although both iron deposits and hemosiderin stain positively with iron stain such as Prussian blue, only iron deposits show the black to dark brown centers within the pigment deposits and the golden halo surrounding them.

HISTOLOGIC FEATURES

- Peribronchiolar and perivascular iron pigment deposition is characteristic of siderosis.
- Iron, which is generally iron oxide, exhibits an oval to round, reddish brown to reddish black dust in lung parenchyma.
- Deposits show black or dark brown cores with golden halos.
- Iron deposition may be in lung interstitium and macrophages, with little fibrotic response.
- Ferruginous bodies may occasionally be seen.
- Iron deposits are nonbirefringent on polarization.
- Macules, made up of perivascular and peribronchiolar deposits of iron, iron-laden macrophages, and ferruginous bodies, with little fibrotic response, may occur.
- Nodules, made up of parenchymal deposits of iron, iron-laden macrophage, and ferruginous bodies, with little fibrotic response, may be seen.
- In patients with silicosiderosis, increased fibrosis with frequently dense hyalinized collagen is seen.

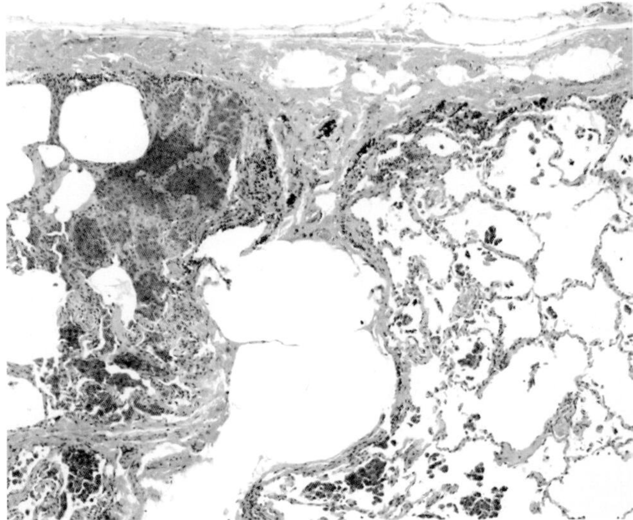

Figure 149.1 Perivascular and alveolar macrophage deposition of iron.

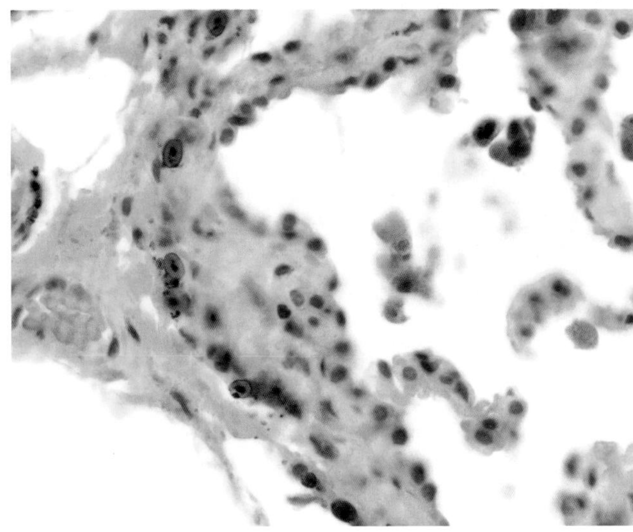

Figure 149.2 Alveolar septal deposition of iron.

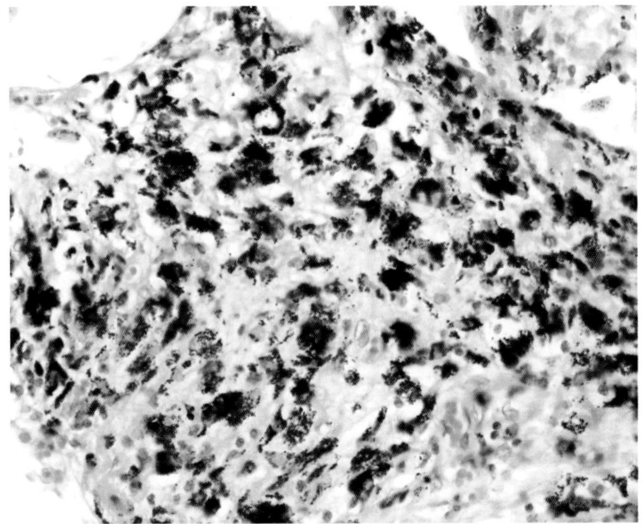

Figure 149.3 Macule containing brown to black iron pigment.

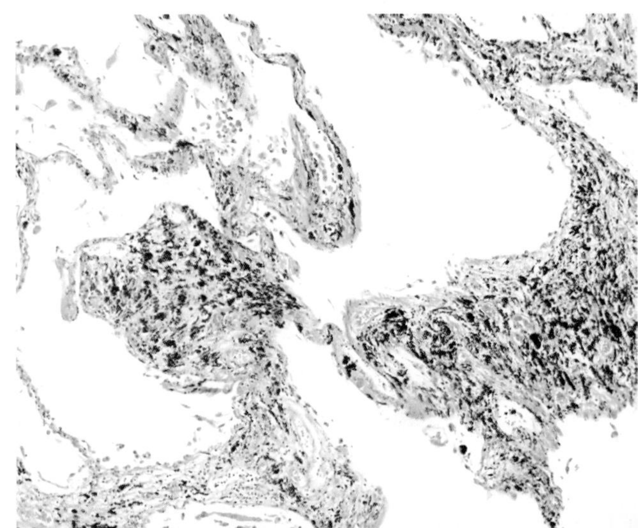

Figure 149.4 Siderotic nodules within lung parenchyma.

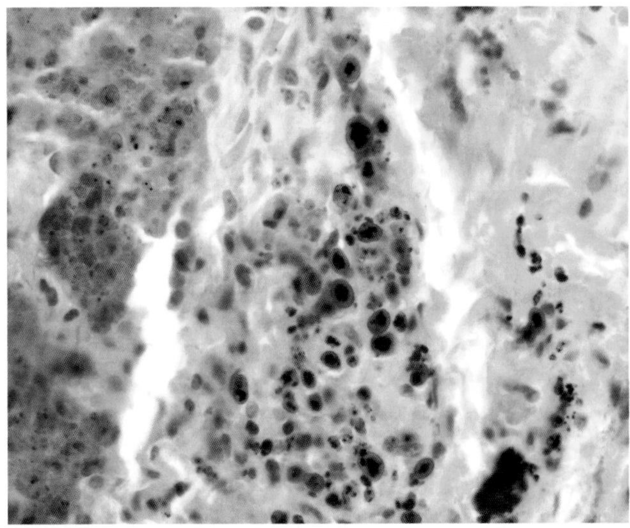

Figure 149.5 Iron oxide pigment, with brown to black cores and surrounding golden halo.

150

Aluminosis

▶ Timothy C. Allen
▶ Richard Attanoos
▶ Maxwell L. Smith

Aluminosis, also termed *aluminum pneumoconiosis*, is a rare interstitial fibrotic lung disease considered to be due to industrial aluminum hydroxide exposure occurring in the production of aluminum powders by the substitution of nonpolar lubricants for stearin, as well as aluminum arc welding, aluminum smelting, and aluminum polishing. Inhalation of dust containing aluminum is thought to induce a hypersensitivity reaction manifested clinically by restrictive lung changes and progressive dyspnea. Grossly, lungs may show areas of fibrosis within lung parenchyma and may have a grayish metallic sheen; however, some cases show grossly normal lungs. Differential diagnosis includes other pneumoconioses, pulmonary alveolar proteinosis, and sarcoidosis. The disease may cause death.

HISTOLOGIC FEATURES

- Peribronchiolar and perivascular collections of dust-laden macrophages containing grayish or gray-brown refractile dust particles.
- The refractile material is not birefringent with polarized light and is negative for iron on iron stain.
- Some cases show little or no tissue reaction, whereas others show fibrosis; occasional cases have reported granulomatous inflammation, a pulmonary alveolar proteinosis-like reaction, or a desquamative interstitial pneumonia-like change.
- Fibrotic areas are often in a lymphangitic distribution within pleura and bronchovascular bundles and may contain dust-laden macrophages.

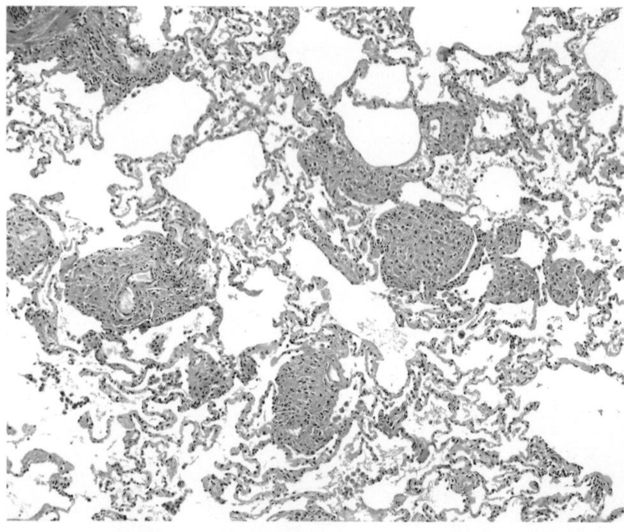

Figure 150.1 Nests of dust-laden macrophages within lung parenchyma.

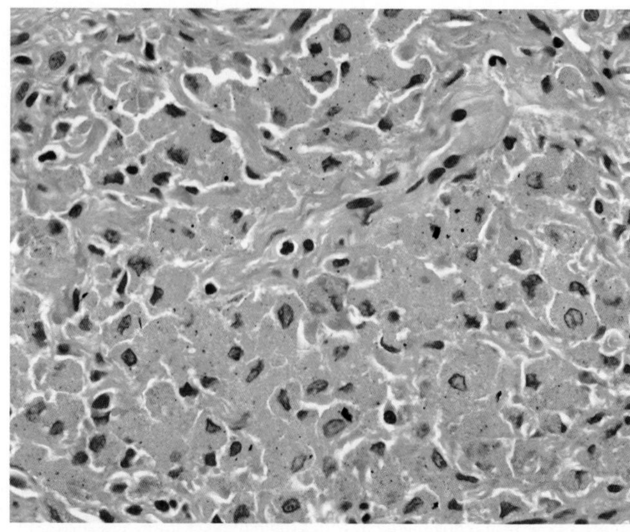

Figure 150.2 Brownish-gray pigment fills the macrophages.

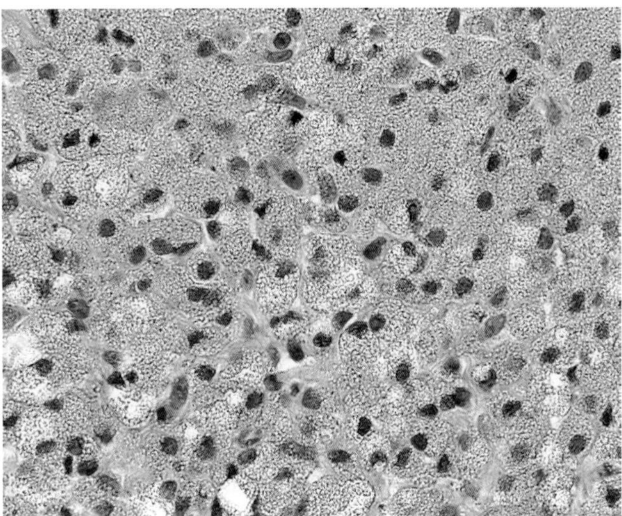

Figure 150.3 The pigment within the macrophages is refractile; however, it does not birefringent by polarized light.

Section 22

Metabolic Disorders/Storage Diseases

▸ Timothy C. Allen

151

Pulmonary Alveolar Microlithiasis

▸ Timothy C. Allen
▸ Maxwell L. Smith

Pulmonary alveolar microlithiasis, a rare infiltrative lung disease, consists of alveolar deposition of innumerable spherical calcium phosphate microliths, termed *calcospherites*. Pulmonary alveolar microlithiasis is an autosomal recessive disease with high penetrance, resulting from a mutation in the *SLC34A2* gene, which codes for a sodium phosphate IIb transporter protein. Alveolar type II pneumocytes are unable to clear phosphate ions, leading to microlith deposition. Patients may present at any age; however, most present in the second to fourth decades. The disease has a male:female ratio of 3:2. Patients often have mild symptoms until the development of cor pulmonale, despite striking radiologic findings. Microliths may occasionally be identified in a bronchoalveolar lavage specimen. Grossly, the lungs are hard and gritty. The primary differential diagnosis is corpora amylacea and intra-alveolar lamellar bodies, features seen frequently in patients with left-sided heart failure; however, corpora amylacea do not show calcification. Additional differential diagnoses include other diseases showing a military pattern on radiology, such as tuberculosis, sarcoidosis, amyloidosis, and pneumoconiosis. Treatment is generally limited to lung transplant. Transbronchial biopsy often establishes the diagnosis.

HISTOLOGIC FEATURES

- Microliths are variably sized rounded concentrically laminated concretions, often with an identifiable granular center, measuring approximately 50 to 1,000 μm.
- Microliths can show an "onionskin" appearance.
- Microliths show periodic acid–Schiff positivity.
- Alveolar walls may be normal; however, some cases show interstitial fibrosis.

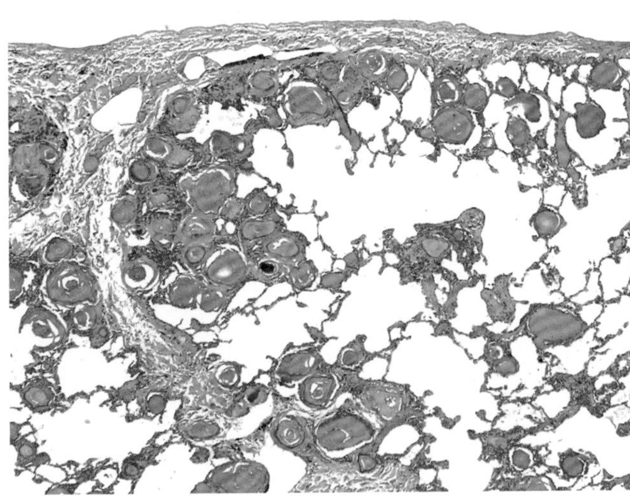

Figure 151.1 Lung parenchyma showing alveoli filled with microliths.

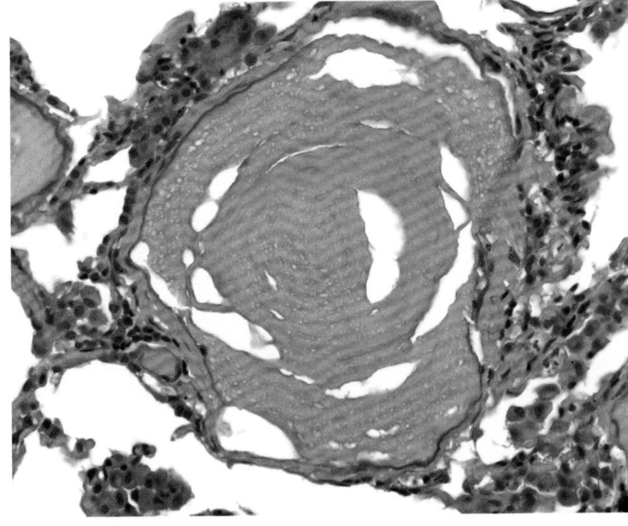

Figure 151.2 Laminated microlith showing an "onionskin" appearance.

152 Pulmonary Metastatic Calcification/Calcinosis

Timothy C. Allen
Maxwell L. Smith

Pulmonary metastatic calcification, also termed *pulmonary calcinosis*, is characterized by the deposition of calcium salts in lung parenchyma. It is caused by increased serum calcium levels; it is most typically identified in patients with chronic renal insufficiency undergoing dialysis. It may also be seen in patients with paraneoplastic syndromes, systemic sclerosis, sarcoidosis, hypervitaminosis D, hyperthyroidism, and cancers with extensive bone involvement. Disease typically diffusely involves the lung parenchyma. Patients are usually asymptomatic. Differential diagnosis includes dystrophic calcification, a more common type of pulmonary calcification generally identified in necrotic tissue and scars.

HISTOLOGIC FEATURES

- Pulmonary metastatic calcification is characterized by the deposition of granules and plates of basophilic material within alveolar septa, bronchiolar walls, and vessel walls.
- Metaplastic bone formation, termed *ossification*, and parenchymal fibrosis may occur.
- Von Kossa stain, a calcium stain, highlights the granules and plates.

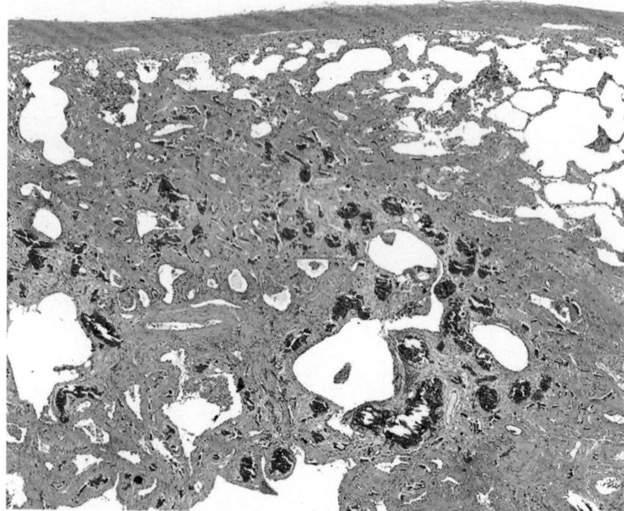

Figure 152.1 Granules and plates of basophilic material, with associated fibrosis, involve lung parenchyma.

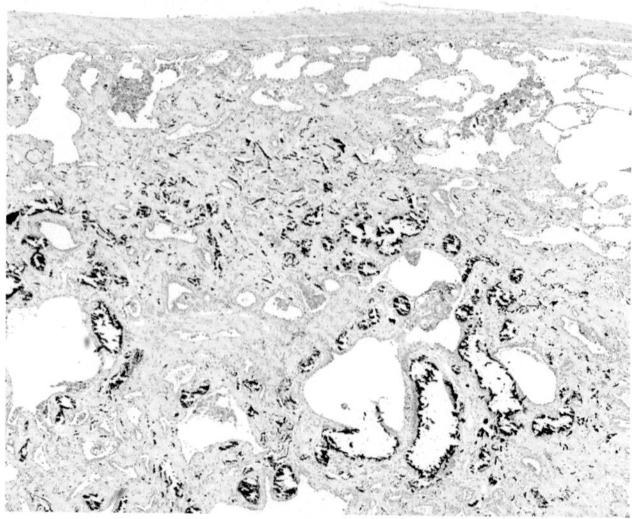

Figure 152.2 Pulmonary metastatic calcification deposits are highlighted by von Kossa stain.

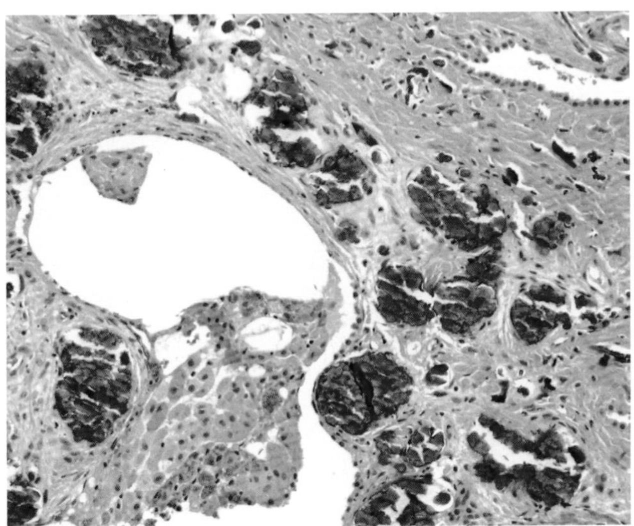

Figure 152.3 Granular deposits of calcium.

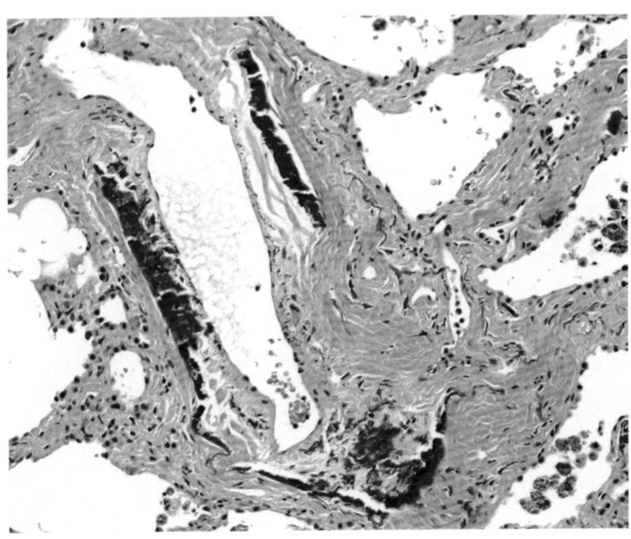

Figure 152.4 Plates of basophilic calcium.

153 Storage Diseases

▶ Timothy C. Allen
▶ Maxwell L. Smith

Storage diseases can cause significant lung disease. Patients may present with diffuse interstitial lung disease; however, in many cases, lung involvement is asymptomatic, with the patient's symptoms arising from extrapulmonary disease. Storage diseases involving the lung include Niemann–Pick disease, Gaucher disease, and cholesteryl ester storage disease (CESD). Patients often show diffuse or finely nodular reticular infiltrates on chest x-ray. Many cases of storage disease are diagnosed by their clinical features and via blood testing; however, in cases where the disease manifests itself in the lung early, lung biopsy may be critical for diagnosis.

Niemann–Pick disease is characterized by the deficiency or absence of acid sphingomyelinase. Patients with type A disease usually die within a few years of birth; however, patients with type B disease often live to adulthood and show progressive pulmonary infiltration, causing significant morbidity and often leading to death. Gaucher disease is characterized by lysosomal β-glucosidase deficiency and the accumulation of glucocerebroside. Infantile, juvenile, and adult forms occur, with the adult form lacking neurologic involvement. CESD is a rare storage disease characterized by a deficiency of acid lipase, with the accumulation of neutral lipids, predominantly cholesterol esters. CESD patients often show extensive systemic atherosclerosis with pulmonary hypertension.

HISTOLOGIC FEATURES

Collections of foamy macrophages are a characteristic of lung involvement with storage diseases. They are located in the pleura, septa, airspaces, and interstitium, in comparison with predominantly airway-centered foamy macrophages seen in cases of obstruction and aspiration. When necessary, electron microscopy may assist in accurate diagnosis.

Niemann–Pick Disease

- Interstitial and alveolar collections of foamy macrophages containing uniformly arranged lipid droplets forming a "mulberry-like" pattern.
- On electron microscopy, the macrophages contain cytoplasmic giant lamellar structures.

Gaucher Disease

- Foamy macrophages have eccentric nuclei and contain lipid forming a "wrinkled tissue paper" or "striated small rod-like" pattern.
- The foamy macrophages are periodic acid–Schiff positive.

Cholesteryl Ester Storage Disease

- Alveolar and interstitial macrophages contain cytoplasmic lipid deposits.
- There are concentric intimal deposits of foam cells, with extracellular lipid and reactive fibrosis, within pulmonary arteries.

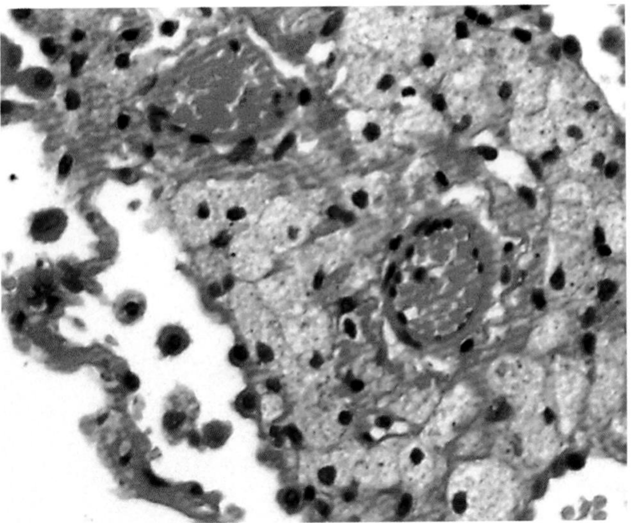

Figure 153.1 Interstitial collection of foamy macrophages in a patient with pulmonary involvement with Niemann–Pick disease.

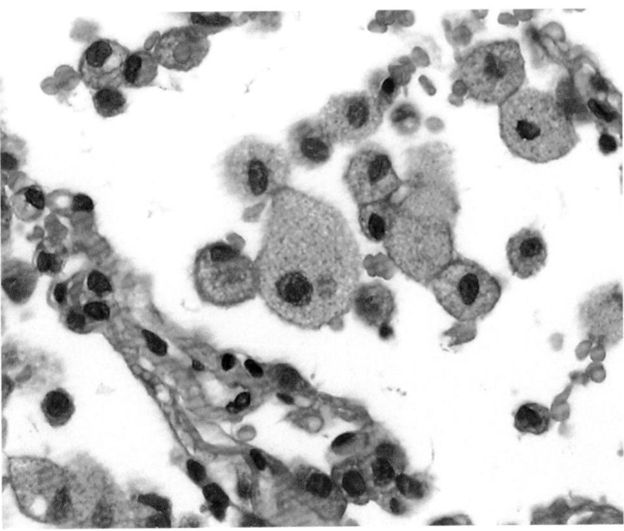

Figure 153.2 Mulberry-like pattern of lipid in the foamy macrophages in Niemann–Pick disease.

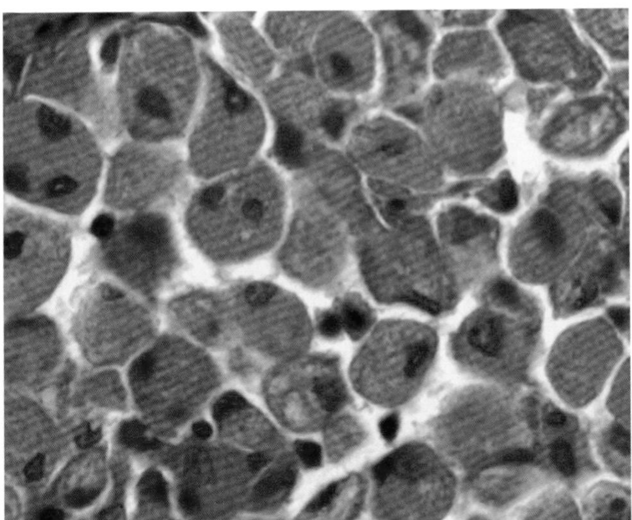

Figure 153.3 "Striated small rod-like" or "wrinkled tissue paper" pattern in a patient with pulmonary involvement with Gaucher disease.

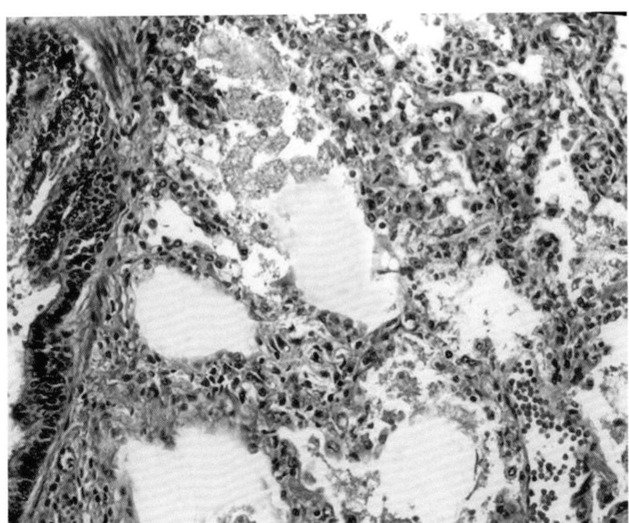

Figure 153.4 Collections of interstitial and alveolar macrophages in a patient with pulmonary involvement with CESD.

Section 23

Nonneoplastic Lesions of the Pleura

▸ Ross A. Miller

Fibrinous and Fibrous Pleuritis

154

Ross A. Miller
Philip T. Cagle

Inflammation of the pleura is termed *pleuritis*. Pleuritis can resolve; however, continued inflammation can result in a fibrinous exudative process involving the visceral and/or parietal surfaces known as *fibrinous pleuritis*. Fibrinous pleuritis can become organized, which is characterized by the formation of granulation-type tissue, sometimes referred to as *organized fibrinous pleuritis*. With further development and/or resolution of the inflammatory process at this stage, fibrosis can occur resulting in a thickened and fibrotic pleura in the area affected, which is termed *fibrous pleuritis*. In certain cases, the fibrous tissue may become well developed and organize into a plaque—a thick, firm, grossly identifiable white–yellow to tan lesion of the visceral and/or parietal pleura surfaces. A variety of etiologies can lead to the development of fibrinous and fibrous pleuritis including inflammatory conditions involving or adjacent to the pleura (pneumonia, pericarditis, hepatitis, peritonitis, and pancreatitis), connective tissue disorders, drug reactions, and malignancy. Pleural plaques can form as a result of infections, surgery, trauma, apical caps, and asbestos exposure. Pleural plaques occurring from asbestos exposure are often bilateral and symmetrical involving the lower lung fields.

Microscopically, fibrinous material with its accompanying inflammation is seen along the pleura in fibrinous pleuritis. The mesothelial layer is oriented along the pleural surface which may show reactive and/or hyperplastic change (mesothelial hyperplasia). Lymphoid aggregates are often seen in the pleural and subpleural tissues. When granulation tissue is present, the proliferating capillaries and fibroblasts present may bring sarcomatous or desmoplastic mesothelioma into diagnostic consideration. Fibrinous and fibrous pleuritis is generally limited to and oriented along pleural surfaces; the malignant cells of mesothelioma will involve the entire surface and invade into adjacent tissues. Keratin immunohistochemical stains can be helpful to identify the location and orientation of the mesothelial cells in both conditions. In addition, the blood vessels seen with granulation tissue tend to be parallel to each other and perpendicular to the pleural surface. Fibrous pleuritis is characterized by a fibrous pleura; occasional scattered inflammatory cells are often seen. Pleural plaques consist of virtually acellular collagen bundles, often in a characteristic basket weave pattern.

HISTOLOGIC FEATURES

- Fibrinous pleuritis consists of fibrinous material with accompanying inflammatory cells. The mesothelial layer is oriented along the pleural surface.
- The mesothelium can be reactive; accompanying mesothelial hyperplasia can be seen.
- As fibrinous pleuritis becomes more organized, granulation tissue is seen.
    - The mesothelial cells should be oriented along the pleural surface (can be highlighted with immunohistochemical stains for keratin markers).
    - Blood vessels of granulation tissue are parallel to each other and perpendicular to the pleural surface.
- Lymphoid aggregates may be present in pleural or subpleural tissues.
- Fibrous pleuritis is characterized by the development of fibrous tissue.
- As fibrous tissue becomes well developed a plaque may form, characterized by virtually acellular collagen bundles in a basket weave pattern.

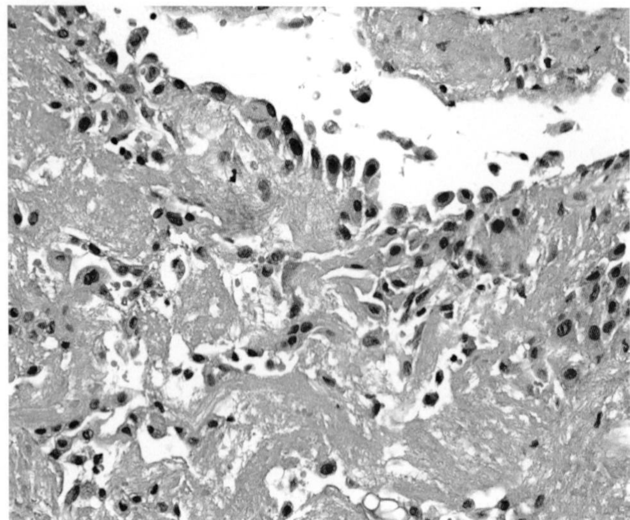

Figure 154.1 Fibrinous pleuritis: fibrinous material with accompanying inflammatory cells and mesothelial cells oriented along the pleural surface.

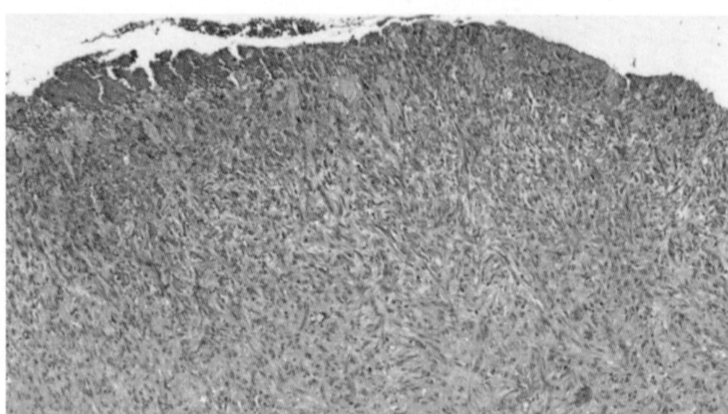

Figure 154.2 As fibrinous pleuritis becomes more organized, granulation tissue forms. The small blood vessels that are present are parallel to one another and perpendicular to the surface of the pleura.

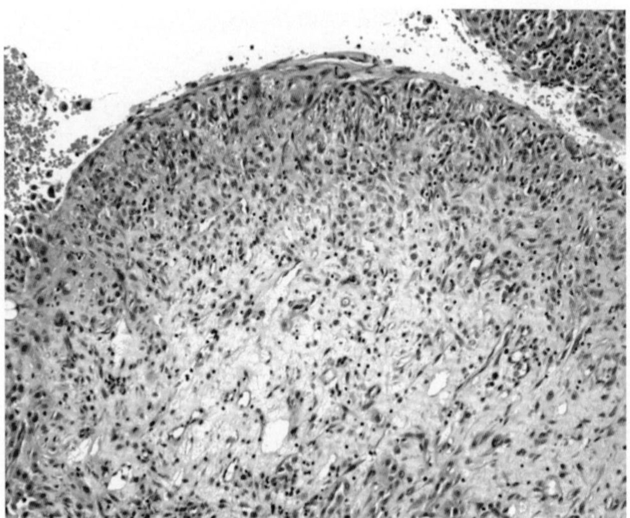

Figure 154.3 Organized fibrinous pleuritis with granulation tissue formation.

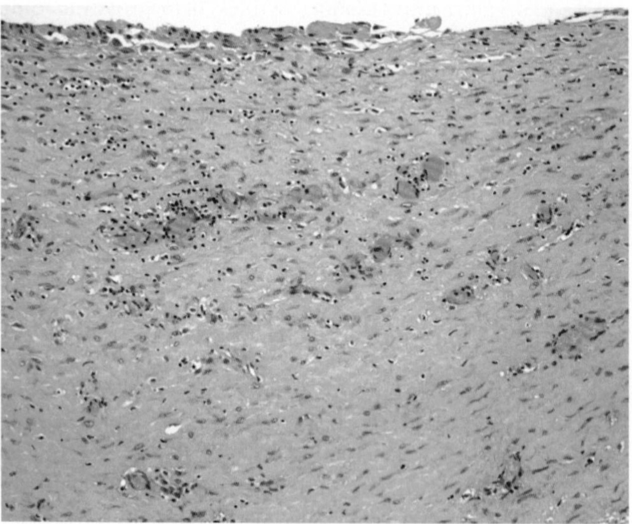

Figure 154.4 Fibrous pleuritis is characterized by well-formed fibrosis tissue. Scattered inflammatory cells can be seen.

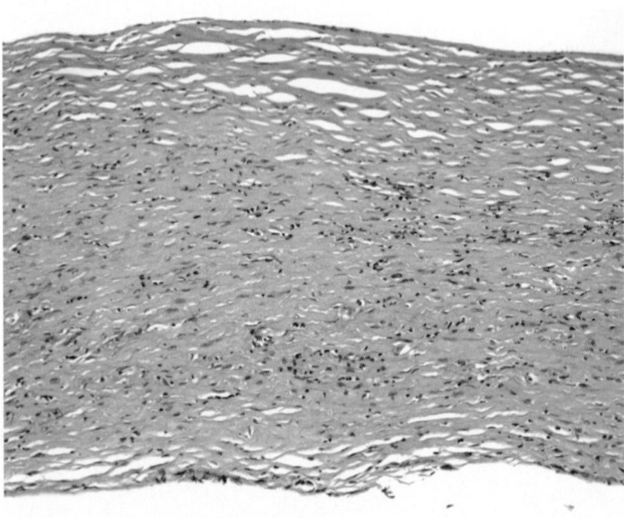

Figure 154.5 Fibrous pleuritis with early plaque formation; note the basket weave collagen bundles at the *top* of the image.

155

Specific Forms of Pleuritis

Ross A. Miller
Philip T. Cagle

Similar to the descriptive terminology used with fibrinous and fibrous pleuritis, descriptive terms have been used to characterize other forms of pleuritis with particular microscopic findings.

Eosinophilic pleuritis is characterized by numerous eosinophils in the pleural fluid and/or tissue and tends to occur with pneumothorax or hemothorax (i.e., exposure to air and/or blood, which can be iatrogenic). Given the association, it is not surprising that eosinophilic pleuritis is also often seen following pleurectomy or surgery to excise blebs and bullae. The cause of eosinophilic pleuritis is not limited to air and/or blood exposure as it has been described with certain infections (parasite, tuberculosis, fungus, and some bacteria), drug reactions, and can be seen in women of child-bearing age having lung tissue affected by lymphangioleiomyomatosis.

Granulomatous pleuritis is characterized by granulomatous inflammation and/or well-defined granulomas with or without necrosis involving the pleura. Associations included certain infections (particularly fungus and tuberculosis), sarcoidosis, granulomatosis with polyangiitis (formerly known as *Wegener granulomatosis*), and secondary to foreign-body material. Foreign-body material is sometimes instilled into the pleural space in efforts to treat recurrent pleural effusions by obliterating the potential pleural space.

CYTOLOGIC FEATURES

Eosinophilic Pleuritis

- Numerous eosinophils; often, reactive changes can be seen within mesothelial cells.

HISTOLOGIC FEATURES

Eosinophilic Pleuritis

- Eosinophils infiltrating pleural tissue; associated reactive mesothelium, histiocytes, lymphocytes, and giant cells are often seen.
- Adjacent lung tissue may have scattered eosinophils, particularly within small vessels.
- Underlying or adjacent lung may show bullae, honeycomb change, or lymphangioleiomyomatosis.

Granulomatous Pleuritis

- Granulomatous inflammation and/or well-formed granulomas with or without necrosis involving the pleura.

- Special stains for fungal (for example, Gomori methenamine silver) or acid-fast (Kinyoun or auramine) organisms can help identify microorganisms; it is important to remember that a negative stain does not exclude the presence of organisms.
- Sometimes, foreign material may be identified, particularly with polarization; foreign material is sometimes used to obliterate the potential pleural space to prevent and treat recurrent pleural effusions.

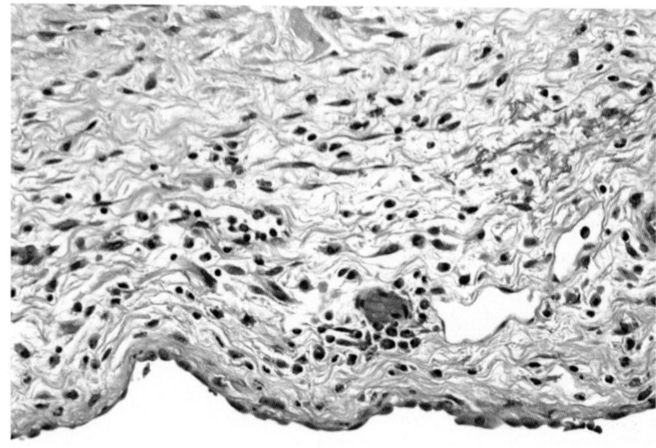

Figure 155.1 Eosinophilic pleuritis: eosinophils can be seen within the pleural tissue along with scattered histiocytes and chronic inflammatory cells.

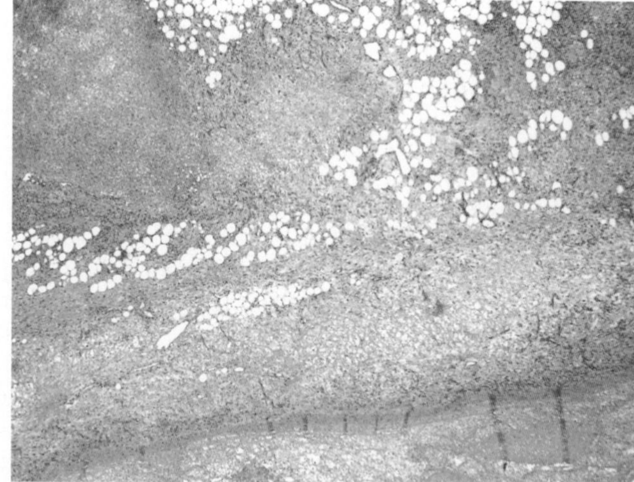

Figure 155.2 Pleuritis with areas of necrosis and reactive changes.

156 Eosinophilic Pseudovasculitis

Ross A. Miller
Armando E. Fraire*

Eosinophilic pseudovasculitis is a subpleural infiltration of vascular walls by eosinophils. It was first described by Luna et al. and originally given the name reactive eosinophilic vascular infiltration. There is a described association with pneumothorax; however, the exact etiology is not known. One proposed theory is a defect in vascular transport of eosinophils migrating toward injured pleura. Typically, the eosinophilia seen is most pronounced in vessels close to the pleura and diminishes in those moving away from the pleural surface. Correctly identifying the process mitigates one from unnecessarily working up a patient for other conditions associated with eosinophils (Churg–Strauss, Langerhans-cell histiocytosis, parasite infections, eosinophilic vasculitis, etc.).

HISTOLOGIC FEATURES

- Transmural infiltration of eosinophils in vessels near the pleura; diminishing quantity of eosinophils in vessels moving away from the pleura.
- No necrosis is seen and no granulomatous inflammation is identified.

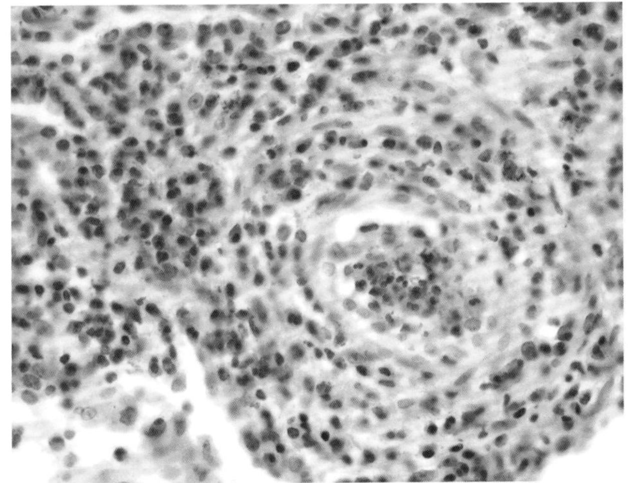

Figure 156.1 Note blood vessel cut at right angle showing transmural infiltration of its wall by numerous eosinophils. Note also the absence of necrosis and a cluster of eosinophils within the vascular lumen.

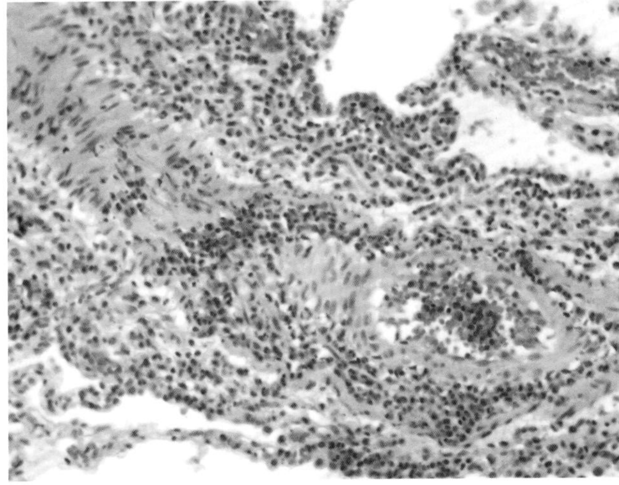

Figure 156.2 A neighboring blood vessel, cut somewhat obliquely, shows similar dense eosinophilic infiltration of its wall. Note also eosinophilia of the adjacent lung parenchyma.

*The author would like to acknowledge the work of Dr. Fraire, who contributed to the previous edition.

157 Reactive Mesothelial Hyperplasia

Ross A. Miller
Philip T. Cagle

The mesothelium can become reactive and undergo hyperplasia in response to a variety of conditions including pleural effusion, infections, pneumothorax, surgery, trauma, connective tissue disease, and drug reactions. When present, reactive mesothelial cells can be abundant in pleural fluid cytology specimens showing significant cytologic atypia and even mitotic figures. When hyperplasia is also present, papillary tufts and other three-dimensional structures can be seen. Surgical biopsy specimens can also be quite challenging, particularly when mesothelial proliferations are entrapped by overlying fibrinous and/or fibrous pleuritis which can mimic invasion. Often, a multimodality approach is needed to correctly classify the process taking clinical, radiographic, and pathologic findings into account. Small biopsy and cytology specimens can be quite problematic sometimes requiring multiple different samples before definitive classification is made.

CYTOLOGIC FEATURES

- Mesothelial cells are typically cuboidal to round with variable cell and nuclear size/shape.
- Cytoplasm can be vacuolated to foamy or dense; the peripheral clear rim or "skirt" appearance (resulting from long microvilli processes visible by electron microscopy) helps to appropriately classify the cells.
- Adjoining cells or small cellular clusters are typically separated by a small space, sometimes referred to as a *window* (also due to long microvillus processes extending from the cells).
- Binucleation, multinucleation, and even mitotic figures can be seen.
- Cellularity tends to decrease with additional fluid specimens in a stepwise fashion.
- Mesothelial clusters typically have scalloped borders.
- With marked reactive processes, there is often a spectrum of "normal" to "markedly reactive" mesothelial cells.
- Reactive mesothelial cells have overlapping features with metastatic malignancies and mesothelioma; certain features tend to favor one process over the other.
  - Metastatic malignancy: typically a "second" population of malignant cells can be seen; clusters usually have smooth borders; lack the "spectrum" of change seen in reactive mesothelial processes. Immunohistochemistry can be very helpful: two mesothelial markers (for example, calretinin and D2-40) and two markers for the malignancy being considered (for example, in carcinoma: BerEP4 and MOC31).
  - Mesothelioma: very cellular (cellularity tends to persist, even with repeat samples), cell clusters are large (typically greater than 15 cells), marked cytologic atypia, lack spectrum of change, sometimes fluorescence in situ hybridization can be helpful (for example, loss of 9p21 harboring the p16 gene).

HISTOLOGIC FEATURES

- Entrapment of proliferating and reactive mesothelial cells by fibrinous material, granulation tissue, and/or fibrous tissue can mimic malignancy. Features favoring a benign process include a linear arrangement of cells parallel to the overlying pleural surface and lack of invasion into deeper or surrounding tissues.
- Keratin immunohistochemical stains can be helpful to identify the location and orientation of the mesothelial cells.

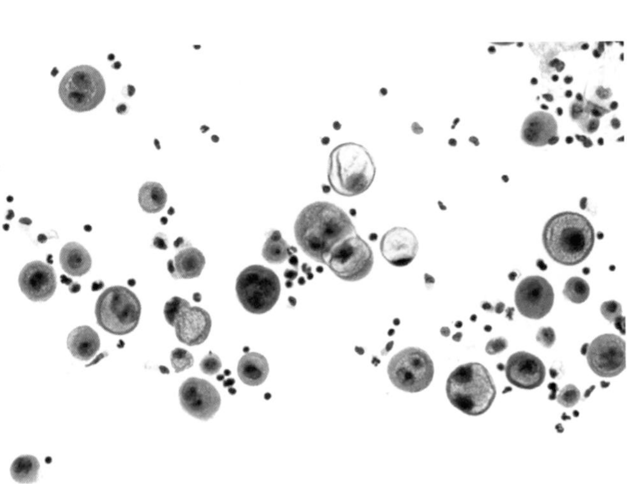

Figure 157.1 Reactive mesothelial cells on cytologic preparation; note the "window" between the two cells in the *middle* of the image and the peripheral cytoplasmic "skirt."

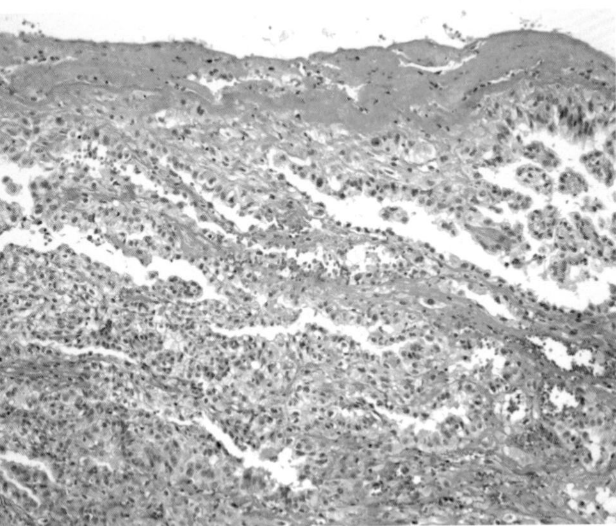

Figure 157.2 Reactive and proliferating mesothelial cells, with overlying fibrinous material.

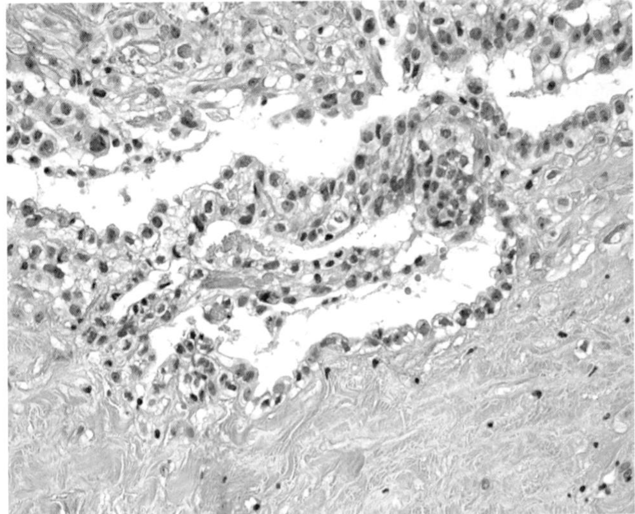

Figure 157.3 Higher power view of reactive and proliferating mesothelial cells, with overlying fibrinous material.

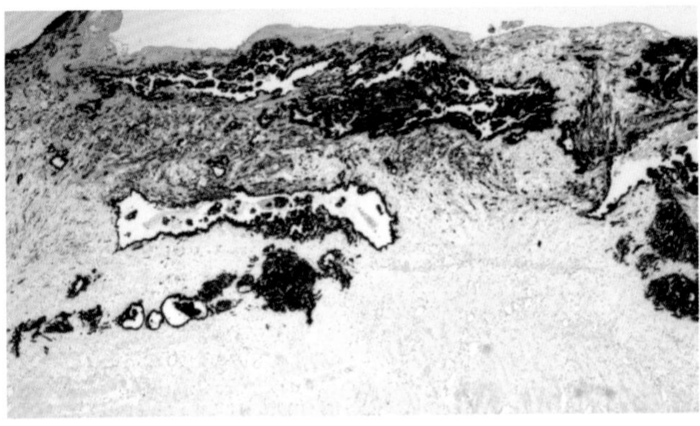

Figure 157.4 Pankeratin stain highlighting reactive mesothelial cells; note the linear arrangement; no infiltration is seen.

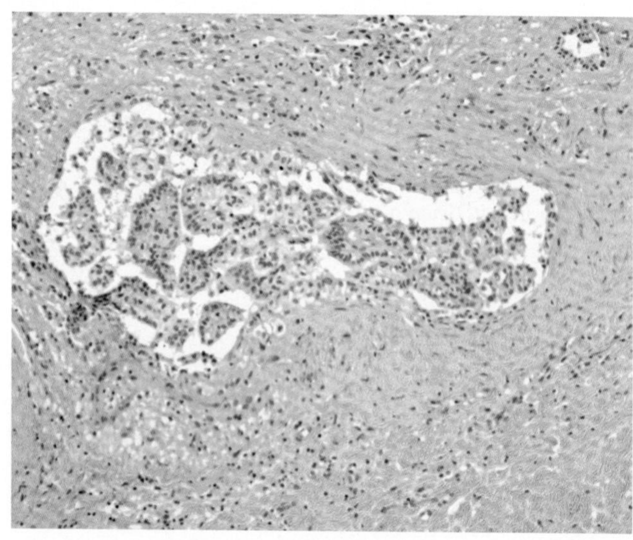

Figure 157.5 Entrapped mesothelial cells can mimic an invasive front.

158

Endometriosis

Ross A. Miller
Rodolfo Laucirica*

Endometriosis, defined as extrauterine endometrial tissue and characterized by endometrial glands with surrounding endometrial stroma, can occur in a variety of places throughout the body including the pleura. The glands appear like those in proliferative phase endometrium; as such, mitotic figures can be seen. Owing to the appearance, sometimes other entities including pleuropulmonary blastoma, biphasic pulmonary blastoma, adenocarcinoma, and biphasic mesothelioma may be diagnostic considerations. Usually, considering the possibility of endometriosis and correlating with clinical information can lead one to correct classification. Symptoms can include shortness of breath, cough, pleuritic pain, and hemoptysis. Pneumothorax and effusions have been described. Often, the symptom severity is cyclical, corresponding to the menstrual cycle.

CYTOLOGIC FEATURES

- Benign columnar cells and glands.
- Endometrial-type stroma.
- Background blood and/or hemosiderin.
- Decidual changes can be seen.

HISTOLOGIC FEATURES

- Endometrial glands surrounded by endometrial-type stoma.
- Often associated with inflammation, hemorrhage, and hemosiderin-laden macrophages.
- Decidual changes can be seen.

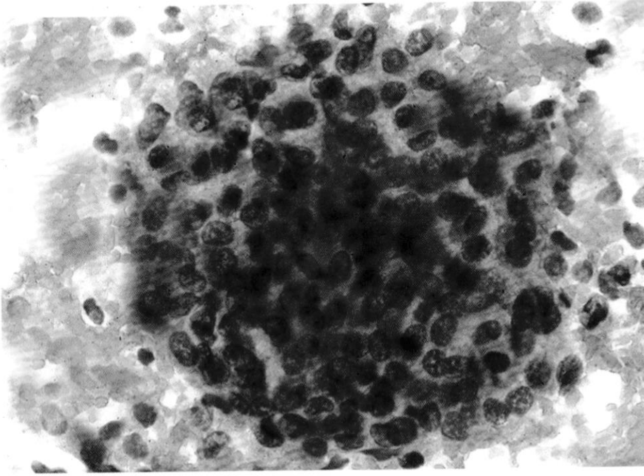

Figure 158.1 Cytology figure of pleural fluid showing endometrial glands and blood in a patient with endometriosis of the pleura.

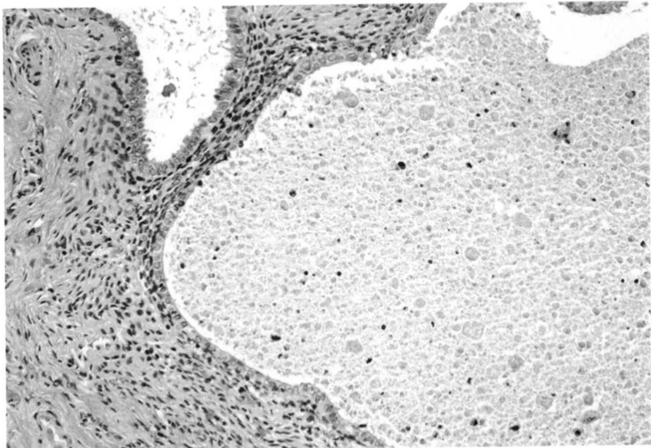

Figure 158.2 Biopsy of pleura showing endometrial glands filled with hemosiderin, blood, and debris in endometriosis of the pleura.

*The author would like to acknowledge the work of Dr. Laucirica, who contributed to the previous edition.

159 Splenosis

Ross A. Miller

Thoracic splenosis is rare and can occur when splenic tissue is seeded into the pleura or lung parenchyma following trauma. Most often, thoracic splenosis presents as a pleural-based nodule and may be mistaken for metastasis on imaging studies.

CYTOLOGIC FEATURES

- Lymphoid tissue with abundant blood.

HISTOLOGIC FEATURES

- Nodules of splenic tissue with characteristic red and white pulp.

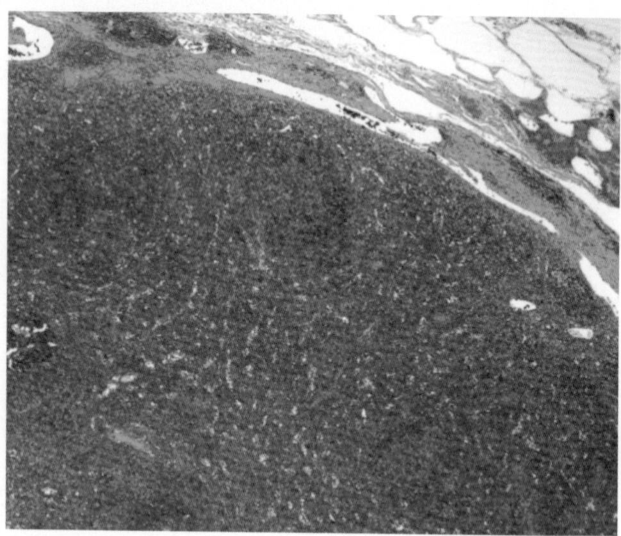

Figure 159.1 A nodule of splenic tissue with adjacent lung parenchyma.

160 Ectopic Hepatic Tissue

Ross A. Miller

Ectopic liver tissue is uncommon and, if present, is typically seen in the abdominal cavity. Although extremely rare, it has been described in the lung and/or the pleura. The cause is typically attributed to a liver developmental abnormality occurring congenitally or secondary to trauma or surgery. Often, the liver tissue is thought to be a pulmonary lesion and the patient will undergo a surgical procedure.

CYTOLOGIC FEATURES

- Polygonal hepatocytes, cuboidal to low columnar bile epithelium, and occasional Kupffer cells.

HISTOLOGIC FEATURES

- Liver parenchyma with central veins and portal tracts.
- Adjacent lung and/or pleural tissue.

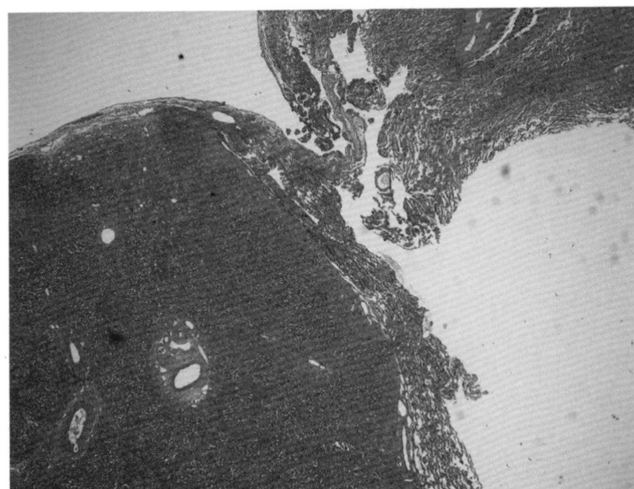

Figure 160.1 Ectopic liver with adjacent lung and pleura in a 9-week-old infant.

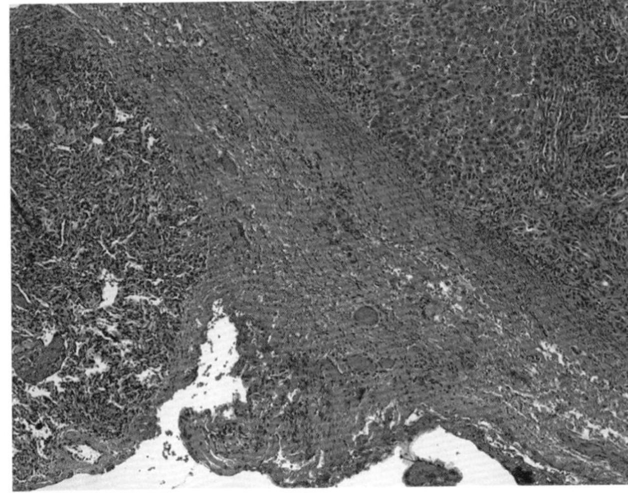

Figure 160.2 Higher power view: lung seen in the *lower left* of the image, liver in the *upper right*, and pleura between the two.

Nodular Histiocytic Hyperplasia

161

Ross A. Miller
Anna Sienko*

Nodular histiocytic hyperplasia has been described in a variety of tissue sites including the pleura, pericardium, peritoneum, and in hernia sacs. It is typically found incidentally on microscopic examination of tissue and consists of a benign proliferation of histiocytes (which can be highlighted with immunohistochemical stains for CD68 or CD163) admixed with mesothelial cells (positive for mesothelial markers such as calretinin, D2-40, or WT-1). The finding is considered a reactive process; neoplastic processes (both primary and metastatic) are often diagnostic considerations and correct classification can be potentially challenging, particularly in small biopsies.

HISTOLOGIC FEATURES

- Nodular histiocyte aggregates; histiocytes are typically polygonal cells with eosinophilic to slightly foamy cytoplasm and round to angulated nuclei.
- Some histiocytes may have a signet ring–like appearance.
- Admixed inflammatory cells and mesothelial cells.
- Immunohistochemistry:
  - Histiocytes: positive for CD68 and CD163.
  - Mesothelial cells: positive for calretinin, D2-40, WT-1, or other mesothelial markers.

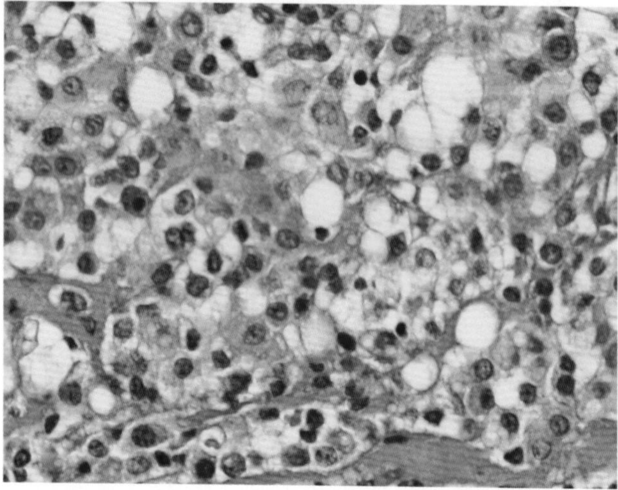

Figure 161.1 Many cells demonstrate "bubbly" and clear-appearing cytoplasm.

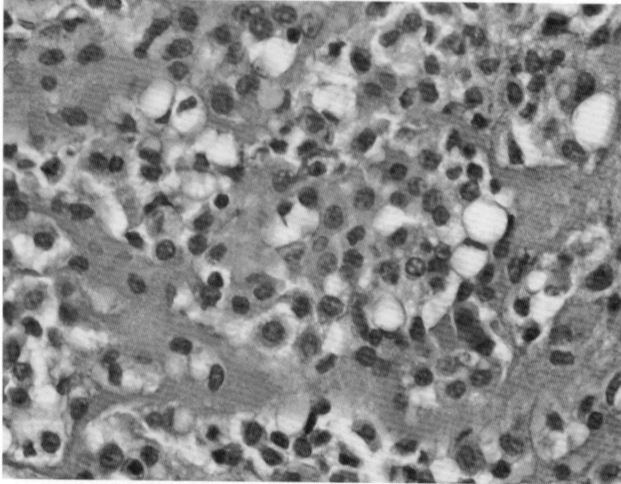

Figure 161.2 Cells showing signet ring–like morphology.

*The author would like to acknowledge the work of Dr. Sienko, who contributed to the previous edition.

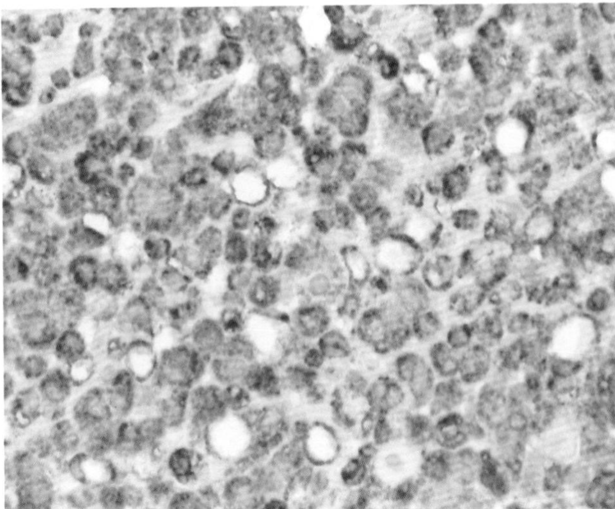

Figure 161.3 Uniform diffuse staining of cytoplasm with CD68 (KP1) consistent with histiocytes.

Section 24

Pediatric Pulmonary Pathology

▶ Aliya N. Husain

Congenital Pulmonary Airway Malformation Type 1

162

▶ Jennifer Pogoriler
▶ Aliya N. Husain

A number of pathologic classification schemes have been proposed for congenital cystic lung lesions, including the commonly used Stocker types of congenital pulmonary airway malformation (CPAM), the fetal groups, and the "small cyst"/"large cyst" classifications. Although most lesions can be classified using these systems, the occasional case remains difficult to categorize.

The Stocker type 1 lesion ("large cyst") type of CPAM was historically identified as the most common type of lesion; however, this is likely due to the fact that most of these lesions are large and cause respiratory and/or hemodynamic compromise. With increasing resection of asymptomatic, prenatally detected lesions, this type is now known to be relatively rare. Intrauterine therapy for fetuses with symptomatic lesions may include thoracoamniotic shunt if cysts are large.

HISTOLOGIC FEATURES

- Cysts are usually large (≥2 cm), although they may be multicystic.
- "Cysts" always connect to smaller airspaces/alveolar parenchyma.
- Cyst wall is relatively thick with smooth muscle.
- Epithelium is columnar and often has papillary projections.
- Alveoli surrounding the cysts are enlarged and may show immature features.
- Differential diagnosis includes bronchogenic cyst (does not connect to surrounding small airways and alveoli and contains cartilage and submucosal glands) and cystic pleuropulmonary blastoma.
- Airway mucin/muciphages are rare—these lesions have not been associated with bronchial atresia.
- Squamous cells may be present in the cysts and airspaces of neonates.
- Pleura nodosum may be present on the pleural surface of patients treated with thoracoamniotic shunts.
- Clusters of mucous cells may be present within the large cysts or extending into surrounding airspaces. Terminology for these clusters is poor defined.
- Mucinous adenocarcinoma can arise in unresected or incompletely resected type 1 CPAM, and complete resection is recommended.

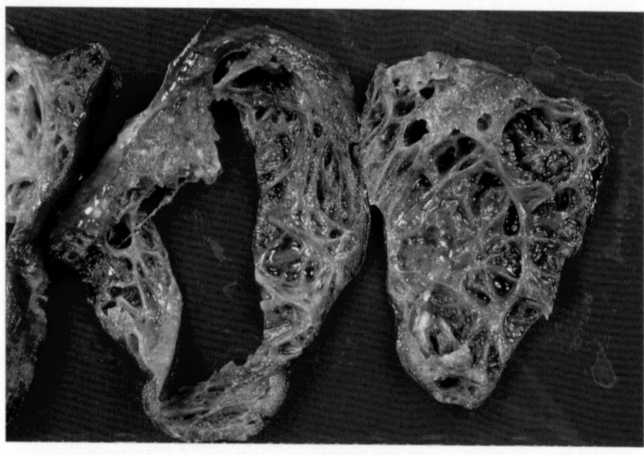

Figure 162.1 The typical gross morphology consists of a large, often multiloculated cyst involving the majority of the lobe.

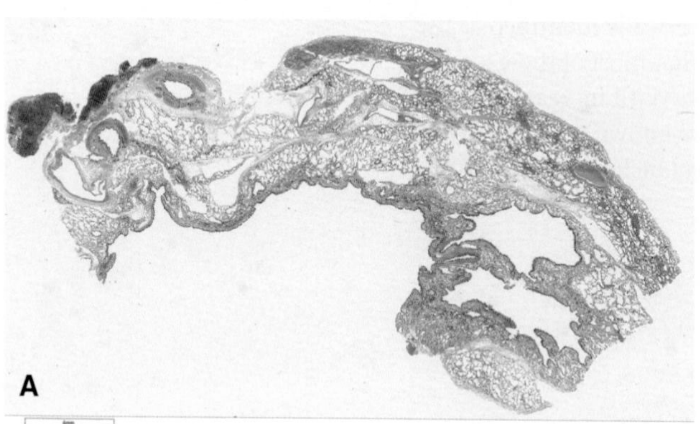

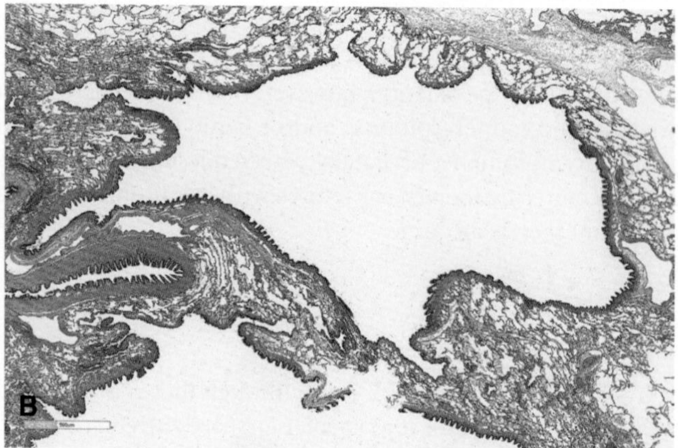

Figure 162.2 This CPAM type 1 shows multilocular cysts (**A**), and higher power magnification (**B**) shows connections to the alveolar parenchyma.

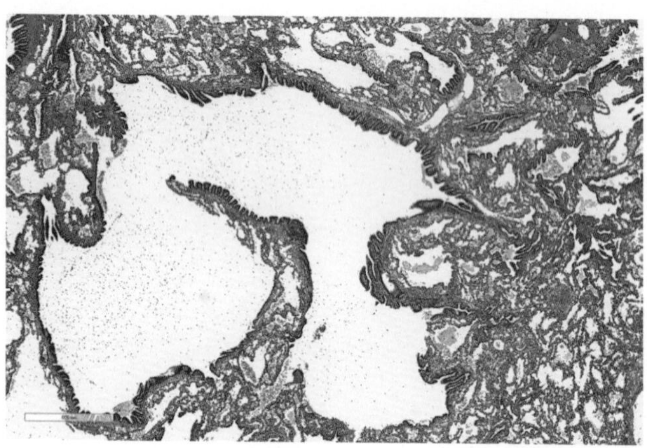

Figure 162.3 This CPAM type 1 shows epithelium of the large cyst forming prominent papillary structures.

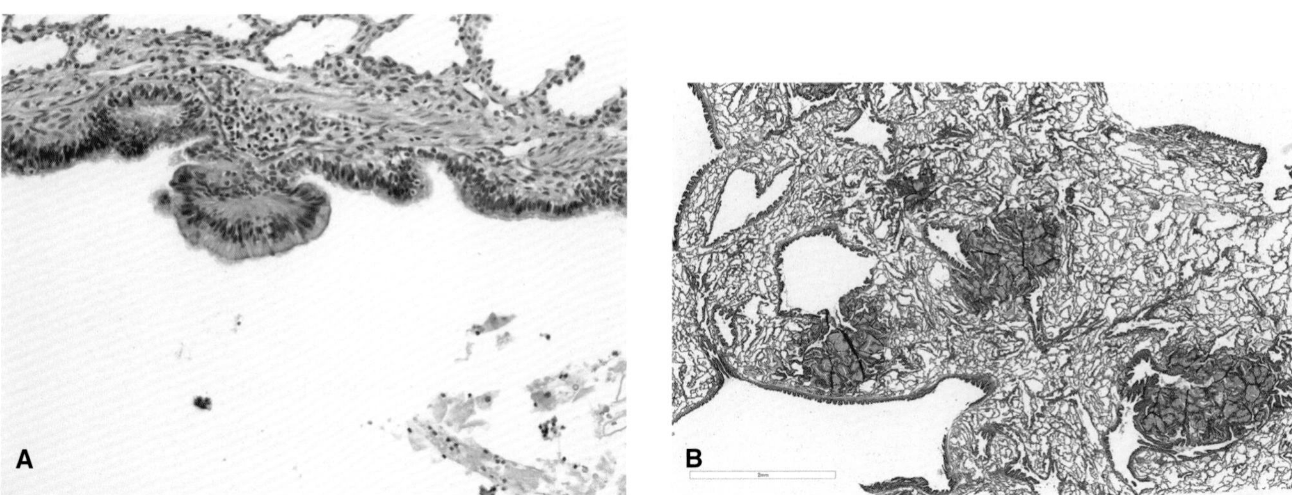

Figure 162.4 Type 1 CPAM often has mucinous cells, which may form small clusters within the large cysts (**A**) or more extensively involve the alveoli surrounding the dominant cyst (**B**).

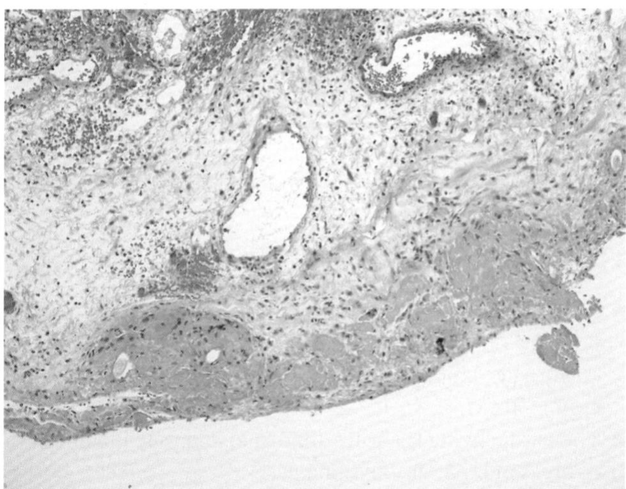

Figure 162.5 CPAMs treated with thoracoamniotic shunt may show hair and/or squamous cells embedded in reactive cells on the pleural surface ("pleura nodosum").

Developmental Abnormalities Associated with Bronchial Obstruction

163

▸ Jennifer Pogoriler
▸ Aliya N. Husain

Although historically considered as separate entities, numerous reports have linked the pathogenesis and demonstrated the overlapping morphology of bronchial atresia, type 2 ("small cyst") congenital pulmonary airway malformation (CPAM) and congenital lobar overinflation (previously termed *congenital lobar emphysema*). The term *bronchial atresia sequence* may be used to encompass this spectrum of lesions. Most type 2 CPAMs were previously identified when they became infected or were incidentally discovered in workup for other developmental anomalies, but the majority are now identified during routine prenatal ultrasound without other associated malformations. Resection of asymptomatic lesions may be performed to prevent infection and remove any possibility of malignancy.

HISTOLOGIC FEATURES

- Bronchial atresia can be grossly identified by the presence of a mucocele distal to the point of obstruction. The dilated bronchus adjacent to the point of obstruction may create a cystic space larger than 2 cm, but this should not be confused with type 1 ("large cyst") CPAM.
- The parenchyma is always abnormal and may include areas of classic type 2 CPAM and/or areas of lobar emphysema.
- Congenital lobar emphysema/congenital lobar overinflation refers to a radiologic finding of hyperlucency and may be due to an increased number of alveoli (polyalveolar lobe) or overdistended alveoli. Either finding may be seen in cases with grossly obvious bronchial atresia and may be adjacent to cases of type 2 CPAM.
- Cysts of type 2 CPAM are relatively small (usually <1 cm) with low cuboidal-type epithelium ("back-to-back" bronchioles) with variable intervening enlarged alveoli.
- In contrast to the often distended bronchioles in the same specimen, the cysts are unaccompanied by a pulmonary artery.
- Rarely, skeletal muscle fibers ("rhabdomyomatous dysplasia") may be seen between the cysts of type 2 CPAMs.
- Other areas of the lesion are often less clearly cystic but consist of malformed parenchyma with dilated bronchioles and enlarged alveoli ("congenital lobar emphysema").
- Features of obstruction (airway mucus and muciphages) are common, and numerous studies have shown that careful gross microdissection can identify areas of atresia in small bronchi in most of these lesions.

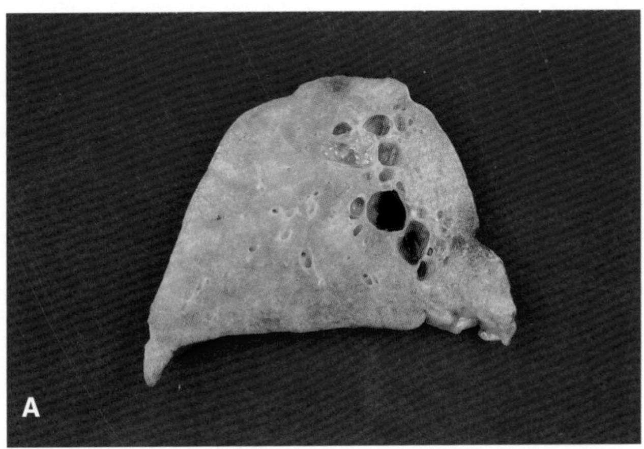

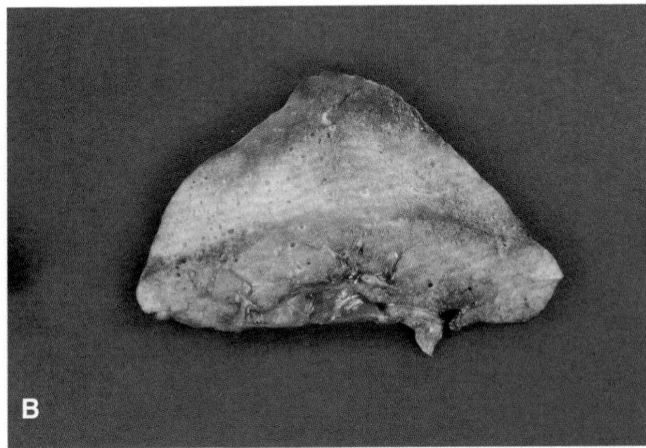

Figure 163.1 These gross images of type 2 CPAMs show the variable but small cysts. **A:** Small cystic spaces are present to the right of the few larger (<1 cm) dilated bronchi. **B:** The majority of this lobe has scattered minute cystic spaces.

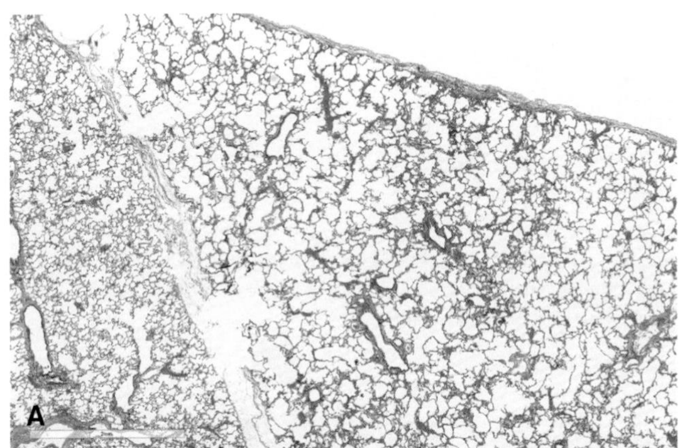

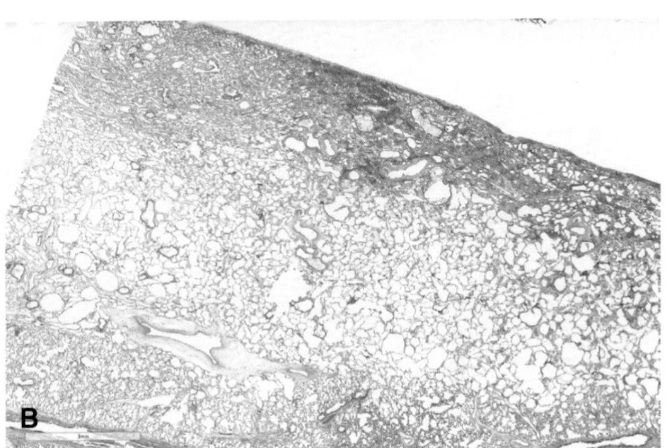

Figure 163.2 In bronchial atresia sequence **(A)** the alveoli are markedly enlarged *(right)* compared with normal parenchyma *(left)*. In other cases **(B)** the bronchi are markedly dilated *(center)* and filled with mucin *(top)*, compared with normal parenchyma at the bottom.

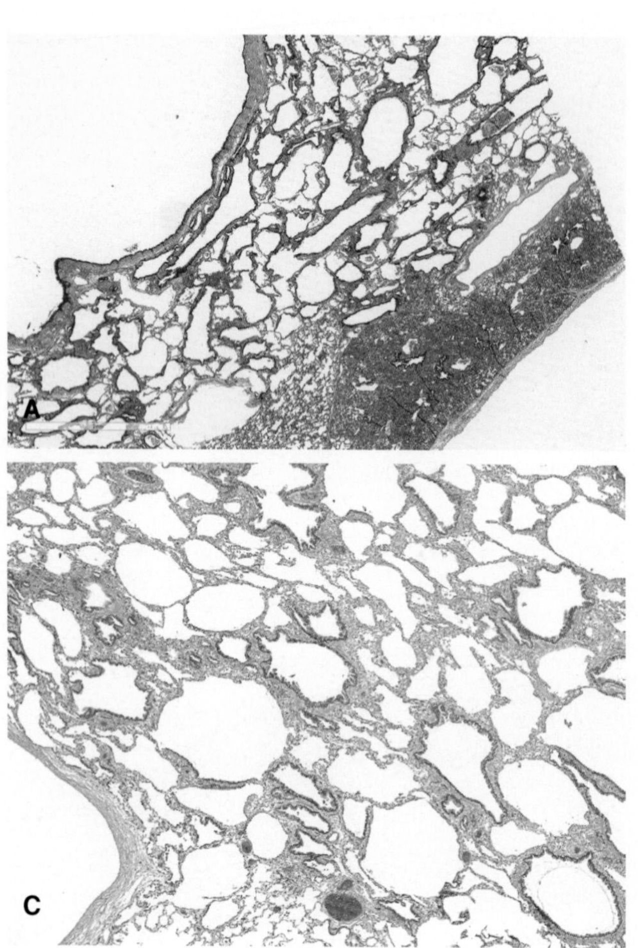

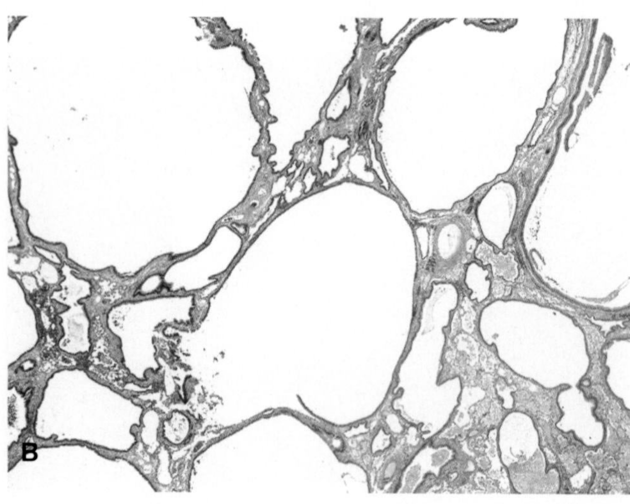

Figure 163.3 In these examples of type 2 CPAM, the area of cystic dilation may be very focal (**A**) or more widespread with "back-to-back" bronchioles, some of which contain mucin (**B**), or increased bronchiolar-like cystic spaces with intervening alveoli (**C**).

Congenital Pulmonary Airway Malformation Type 3

▸ Jennifer Pogoriler
▸ Aliya N. Husain

Congenital pulmonary airway malformation (CPAM) type 3 was originally described in the Stocker classification as a rare type of CPAM encompassing virtually the entire lobe. In contrast to the cystic types of CPAM, type 3 was predominantly not cystic (other than small dilated bronchi at the center of the lesion) and instead was composed of markedly immature-type parenchyma reminiscent of the pseudoglandular stage of development.

Because of the early age of many of these infants, some have suggested that this lesion is essentially hyperplasia of the entire lobe of lung in an immature infant. However, the description of type 3 lesions also bears striking similarity to a subset of CPAMs resected during fetal development with immature cuboidal to columnar lining and occupying virtually the entire lobe. The epithelium of the CPAM in these cases is often markedly more immature than expected for gestational age. This diagnosis remains controversial.

HISTOLOGIC FEATURES

- No cysts or rare dilated airways.
- The vast majority of the lobe is involved.
- Cuboidal epithelium lining airspaces with increased loose mesenchyme between the alveolar sacs and occasional flattened epithelium at the periphery.

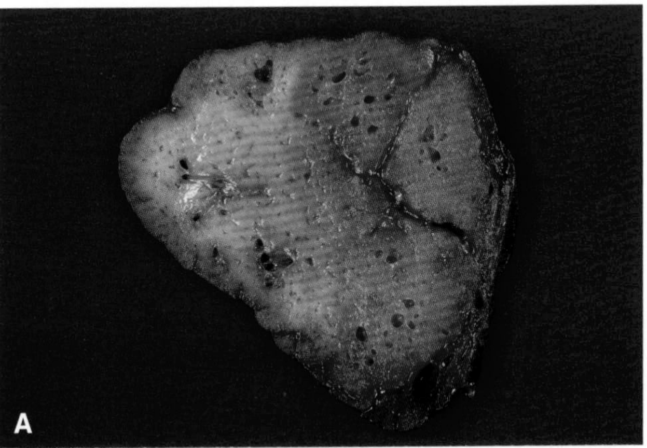

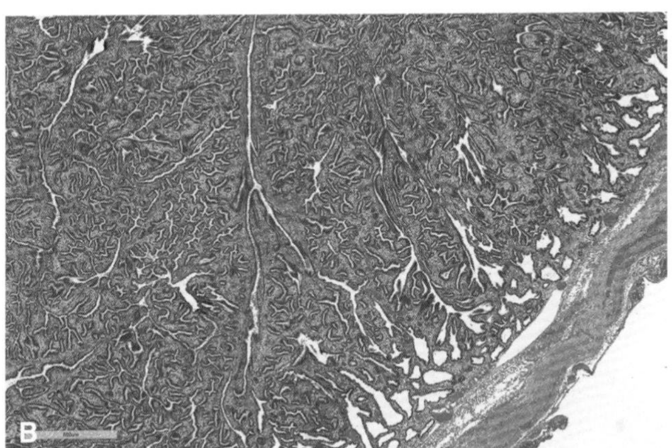

Figure 164.1 This CPAM resected at 30 weeks involves virtually the entire lobe (**A**) without some dilated bronchi; no significant cysts were observed. (**B**) The histology shows markedly immature-type lung with expanded mesenchyme lined by cuboidal cells.

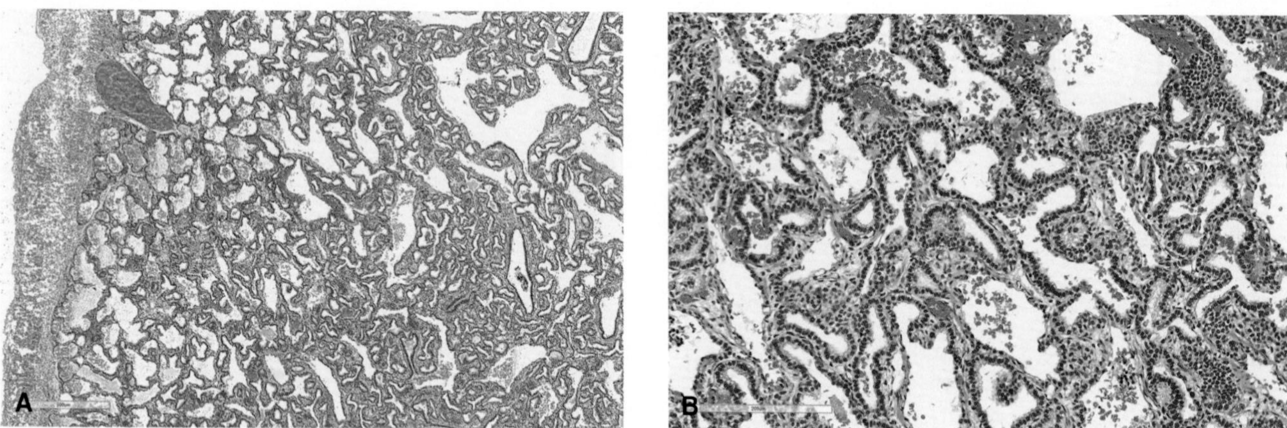

Figure 164.2 This CPAM resected at 32 weeks of gestation shows a similar pattern with markedly immature parenchyma extending almost to the periphery of the lung (**A**) and alveolar spaces lined by cuboidal cells (**B**).

165

Pulmonary Sequestration

Jennifer Pogoriler
Aliya N. Husain

Pulmonary sequestration refers to a segment of lung that receives its blood supply from a systemic artery. It may be extralobar or intralobar. An extralobar sequestration is invested in a separate pleura from the remainder of the lung and does not connect to the tracheobronchial tree. Rarely, there may be an aberrant connection to the gastrointestinal tract.

Intralobar sequestration is almost always found in the lower lobe of the lung with its blood supply derived from branches of the aorta. A strict definition of intralobar sequestration requires that the airway does not connect to the tracheobronchial tree, and often a large bronchus is identified histologically at an aberrant "hilum" where the systemic vessel enters the lung. However, the term is commonly used to refer to any segment of lung with a systemic vessel without pathologic documentation of aberrant airway.

HISTOLOGIC FEATURES

- Because sequestrations lack normal connections to the tracheobronchial tree, lung development is always abnormal on the spectrum of other cases of bronchial atresia/type 2 congenital pulmonary airway malformation (CPAM).
- "Hybrid lesion" has been used to describe sequestrations with parenchyma that is markedly cystic (similar to type 2 CPAM).
- Aberrant skeletal muscle fibers ("rhabdomyomatous dysplasia") may be found in the cystic areas of type 2 CPAM.
- The systemic arteries of sequestrations are typically much thicker than normal pulmonary arteries. Sequestrations removed from older patients may show prominent pulmonary hypertensive changes as well as chronic inflammation and fibrosis.
- Lymphangiectasia may be present in a subset of sequestrations.

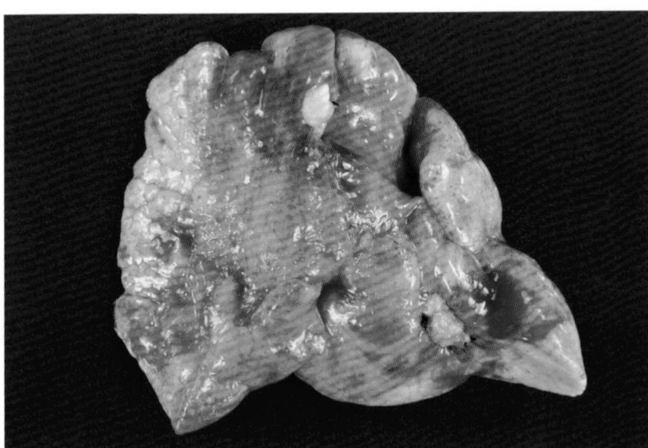

Figure 165.1 This intralobar sequestration shows the normal hilar structures tied off *(right lower edge)* and an aberrant systemic artery tied off near the *top* of the specimen.

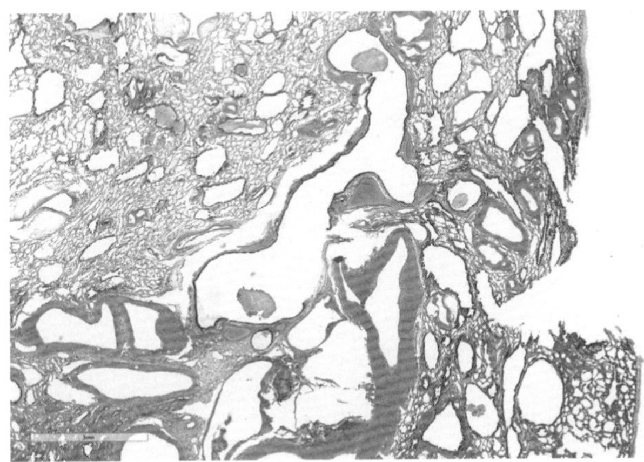

Figure 165.2 The section taken near the entrance of the aberrant systemic artery shows a large bronchial structure consistent with an "aberrant hilum" and suggests that there is a lack of connection to the tracheobronchial tree. There is mucous plugging of multiple airways, which are mildly increased, and marked enlargement of the alveoli.

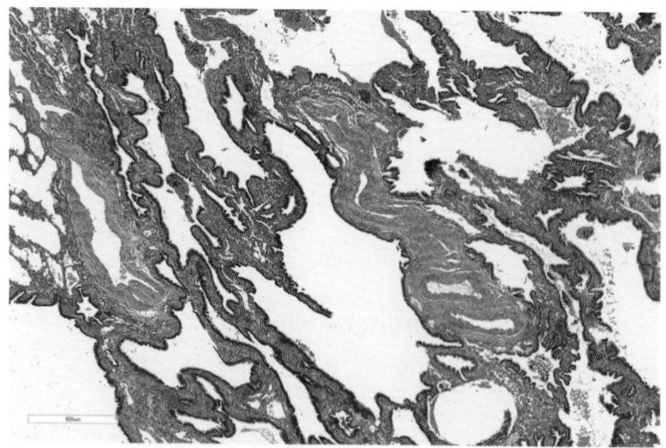

Figure 165.3 This intralobar sequestration shows areas of "back-to-back" bronchioles, and the term *hybrid lesion* can be applied. The pulmonary arteries are derived from the systemic supply and have a thicker media than would be expected in pulmonary arteries.

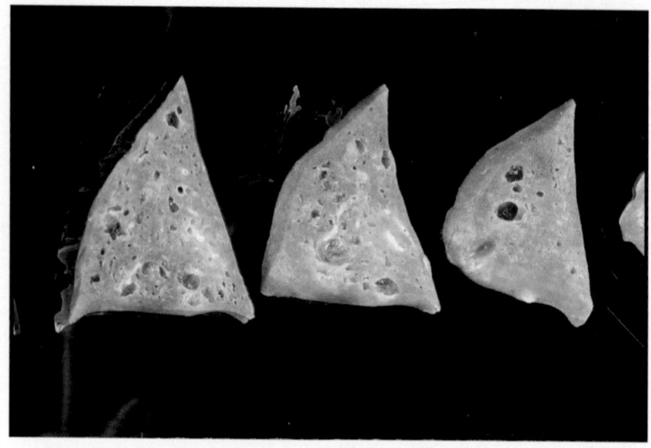

Figure 165.4 This extralobar sequestration shows numerous small cystic spaces, many of which are filled by mucous plugs.

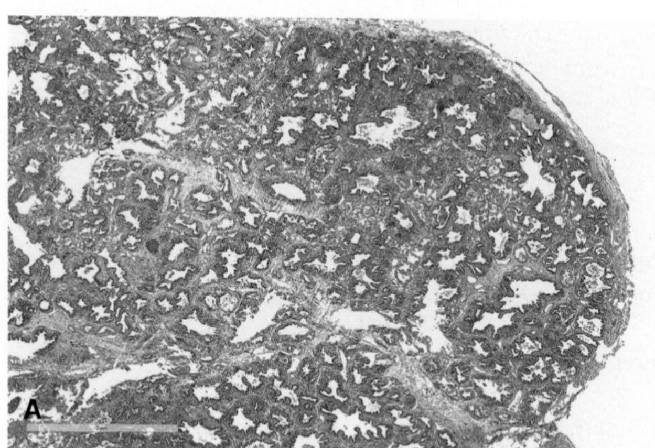

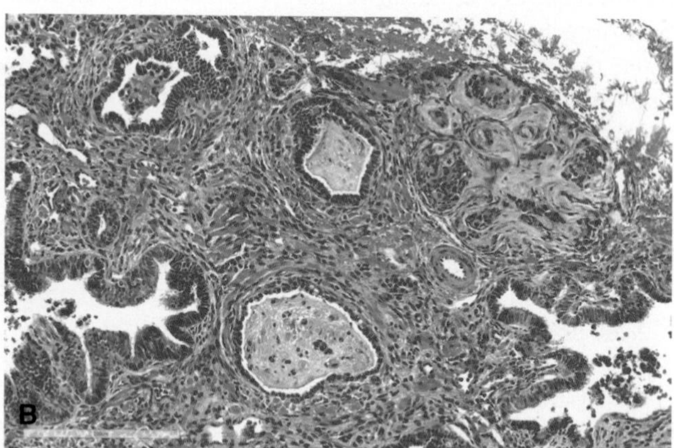

Figure 165.5 Histology of this extralobar sequestrations shows large numbers of bronchial structures (**A**), some of which are filled by mucin *(top right)*. Higher power magnification (**B**) shows aberrant striated skeletal muscle fibers.

166 Bronchogenic Cyst

Jennifer Pogoriler
Aliya N. Husain

Bronchogenic cyst is a common anomaly that may present in the mediastinum attached to the trachea or bronchus or less frequently within the parenchyma of the lung itself. It is usually unilocular but may be multilocular. It is a true cyst that is not connected to the tracheobronchial tree; although if it causes obstruction during development, it may be associated with parenchymal malformation.

HISTOLOGIC FEATURES

- Although typically lined by respiratory type epithelium, it may have squamous epithelial lining.
- Bronchogenic cyst should have cartilage and smooth muscle and may have submucosal glands in the wall.
- The differential diagnosis includes esophageal duplication cyst (squamous or enteric epithelium with smooth muscle and absence of cartilage) and neurenteric cyst (associated with the spine, usually with enteric-type epithelium).
- Bronchogenic cyst that is located within the lung itself may be mistaken for a congenital pulmonary airway malformation (CPAM) type 1. In contrast to CPAM type 1, bronchogenic cyst does not communicate with the adjacent alveoli.

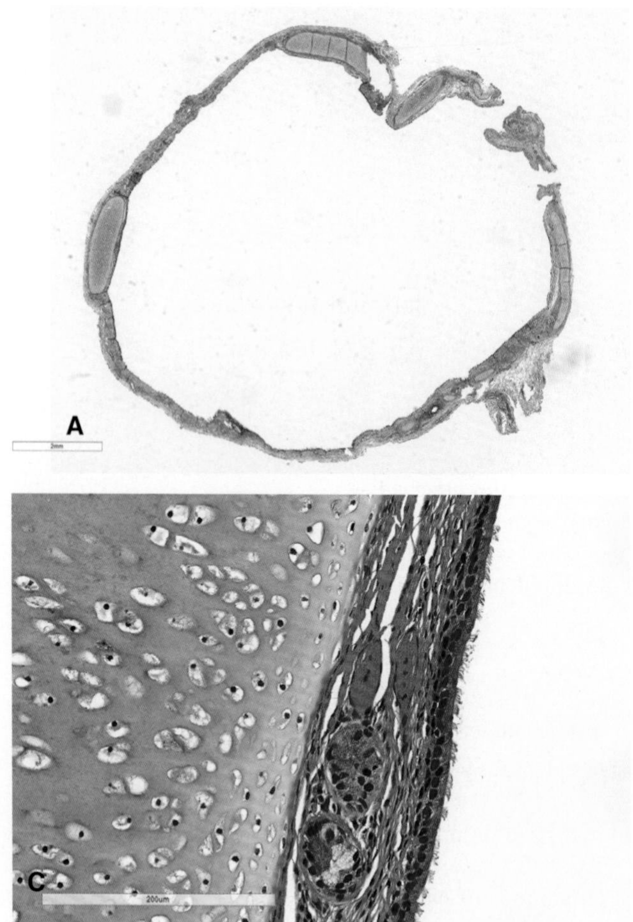

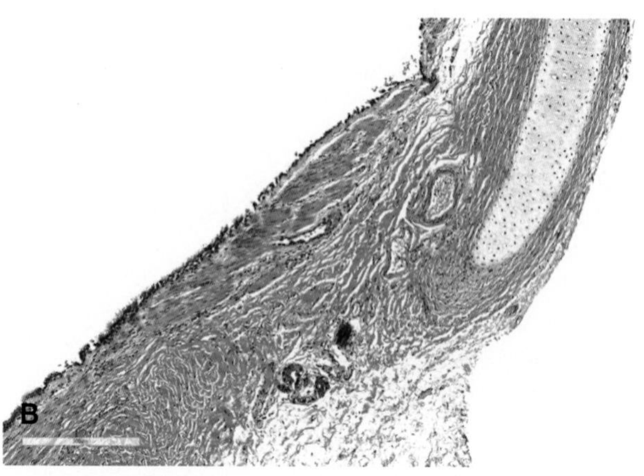

Figure 166.1 Unilocular bronchogenic cyst (**A**) with cartilage and rare submucosal glands (**B**). The epithelium is variably attenuated, but intact areas show ciliated columnar epithelium (**C**).

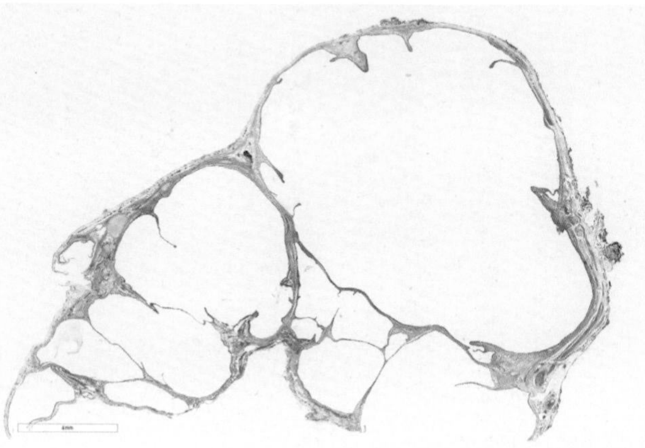

Figure 166.2 Multiloculated bronchogenic cyst with cartilage in airway.

167 Pulmonary Growth Abnormalities

▸ Jennifer Pogoriler
▸ Aliya N. Husain

Appropriate development of pulmonary parenchyma is dependent on the flow of fluid in and out of the lung during gestation.

PULMONARY HYPERPLASIA

Pulmonary hyperplasia is seen in a variety of circumstances due to obstruction of lung fluid during development. Congenital high airway obstruction syndrome due to obstruction of the larynx or trachea prevents fluid from escaping from the lungs and results in diffuse hyperplasia. Localized hyperplasia may be due to obstruction of a single lobe resulting in polyalveolar lobe where the number of alveoli is greater than expected for the stage of development. It is unknown why a subset of obstructed lobes may develop polyalveolar lobe while others develop lobar overinflation or congenital pulmonary airway malformation–type changes, but it may depend on the timing and degree of obstruction.

Histologic Features

- Pulmonary hyperplasia often involves an increase in the number of alveoli (polyalveolar lobe) and overexpansion.

PULMONARY HYPOPLASIA

Pulmonary hypoplasia is classically seen in cases of oligohydramnios when there is insufficient fluid to stimulate development. Other causes of pulmonary hypoplasia include a reduction in thoracic volume and impaired fetal breathing. This is best diagnosed based on pulmonary weight or volumes relative to controls. Alveolar development may be impaired but is often approximately appropriate for gestational age.

Histologic Features

- Pulmonary hypoplasia is best defined by weight or volume criteria.
- Histologic findings may be normal but can show alveolar simplification.

Alveolar growth abnormalities are also a common diagnosis in biopsy of infants with prematurity, congenital heart disease, chromosomal anomalies, and congenital diaphragmatic hernia. In these cases the alveoli are enlarged and simplified. These patients have often been intubated, and there may be some degree of interstitial fibrosis or extension of smooth muscle into the alveolar septa, reflecting chronic ventilation.

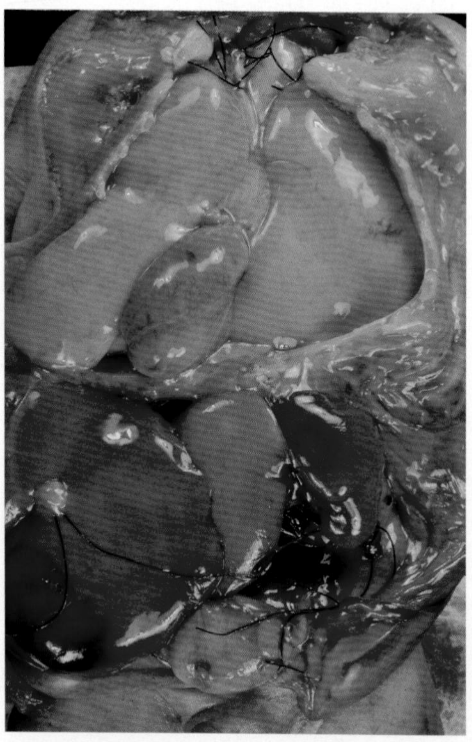

Figure 167.1 This case of congenital high airway obstruction shows marked pulmonary hyperplasia with flattening of the diaphragms and bilaterally enlarged lungs relative to the size of the heart.

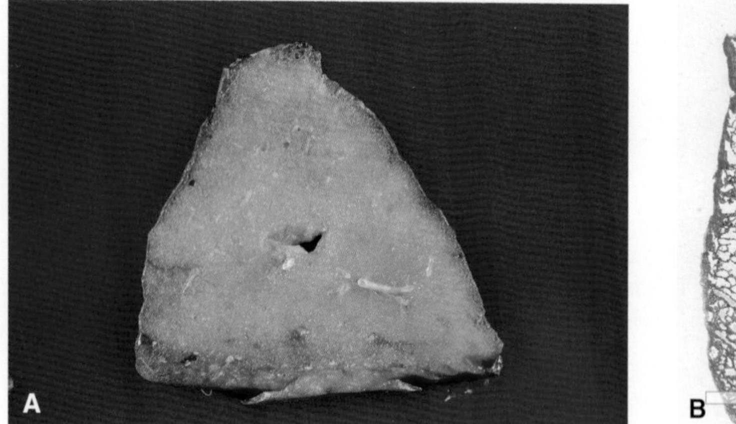

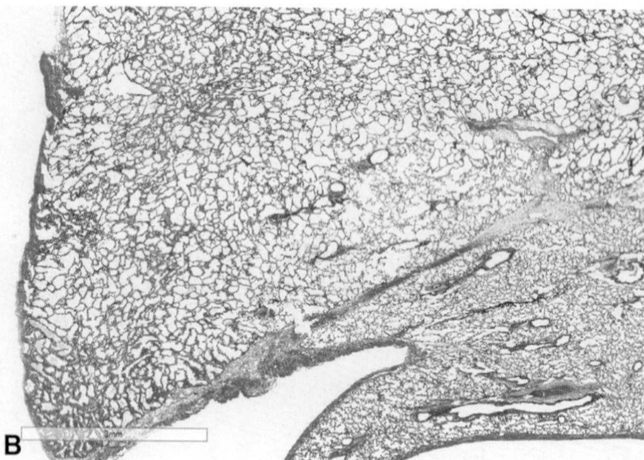

Figure 167.2 This case of polyalveolar lobe shows uniform enlargement of the lobe without cysts (**A**) and a combination of increased numbers of alveoli and mild airspace enlargement (**B**).

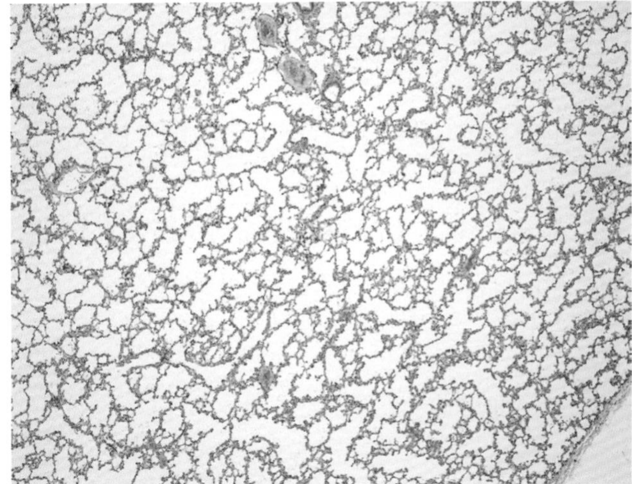

Figure 167.3 This section from a pneumonectomy of a term infant shows increased numbers of alveoli.

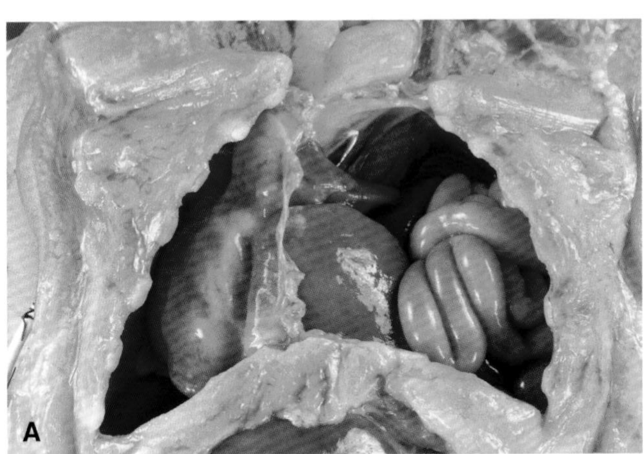

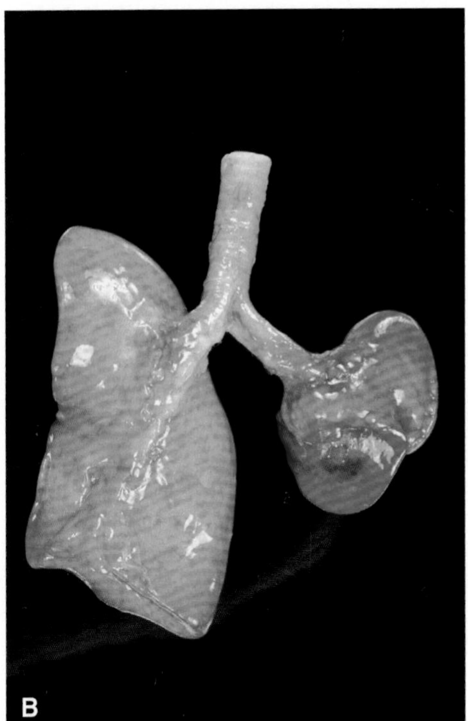

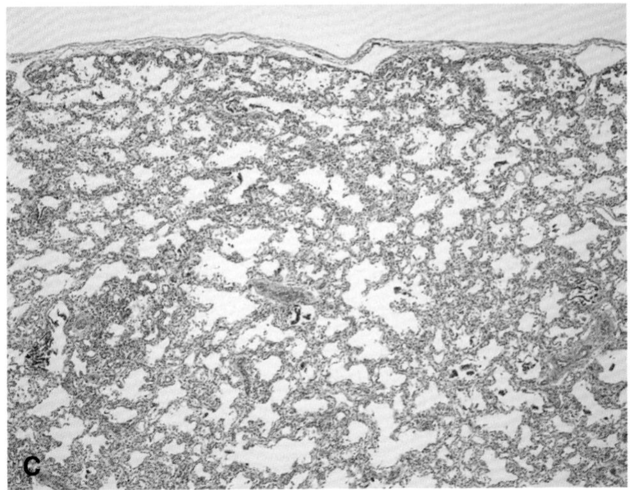

Figure 167.4 A 2-week-old, ex-35-week-gestation infant with congenital diaphragmatic hernia has bilateral pulmonary hypoplasia with a minute left lobe visible in the thorax above the herniated liver (**A**). The right lobe is also hypoplastic but larger than the left lobe (**B**). Histology (**C**) shows mild alveolar simplification with terminal bronchioles reaching almost to the pleural surface and mildly expanded mesenchyme.

168

Neuroendocrine Hyperplasia of Infancy

▸ Jennifer Pogoriler
▸ Aliya N. Husain

Neuroendocrine hyperplasia of infancy (persistent tachypnea of infancy) is a rare, poorly understood disorder presenting in the first year of life. Infants are otherwise healthy but present with tachypnea and retractions and CT findings of central ground-glass opacities. In the presence of typical CT findings and clinical presentation, biopsy is not required for diagnosis. Treatment is supportive, and the symptoms generally improve over years.

HISTOLOGIC FEATURES

- Hematoxylin and eosin (H&E) stain shows normal or near-normal lung parenchyma.
- Mild airway inflammation, alveolar macrophages, or mildly increased smooth muscle or airway fibrosis may be present.
- Neuroendocrine cells are increased, particularly in respiratory bronchioles, but the distribution of neuroendocrine cells may be highly variable within the same patient, and at least 10 to 15 airways should be evaluated.
- Neuroendocrine cells may be identifiable by light microscopy as clear cells in the airway epithelium.
- Neuroendocrine cells are best demonstrated by bombesin immunohistochemistry. Other neuroendocrine markers have been shown to be less sensitive.
- Neuroendocrine cells should be present in at least 70% of airways and should involve at least 10% of the airway epithelial cells in at least one airway.
- Clusters of neuroendocrine cells (neuroendocrine bodies) are present in some alveolar ducts.
- Neuroendocrine cells are often increased in other chronic lung diseases of infancy, and the diagnosis should not be made in this context.

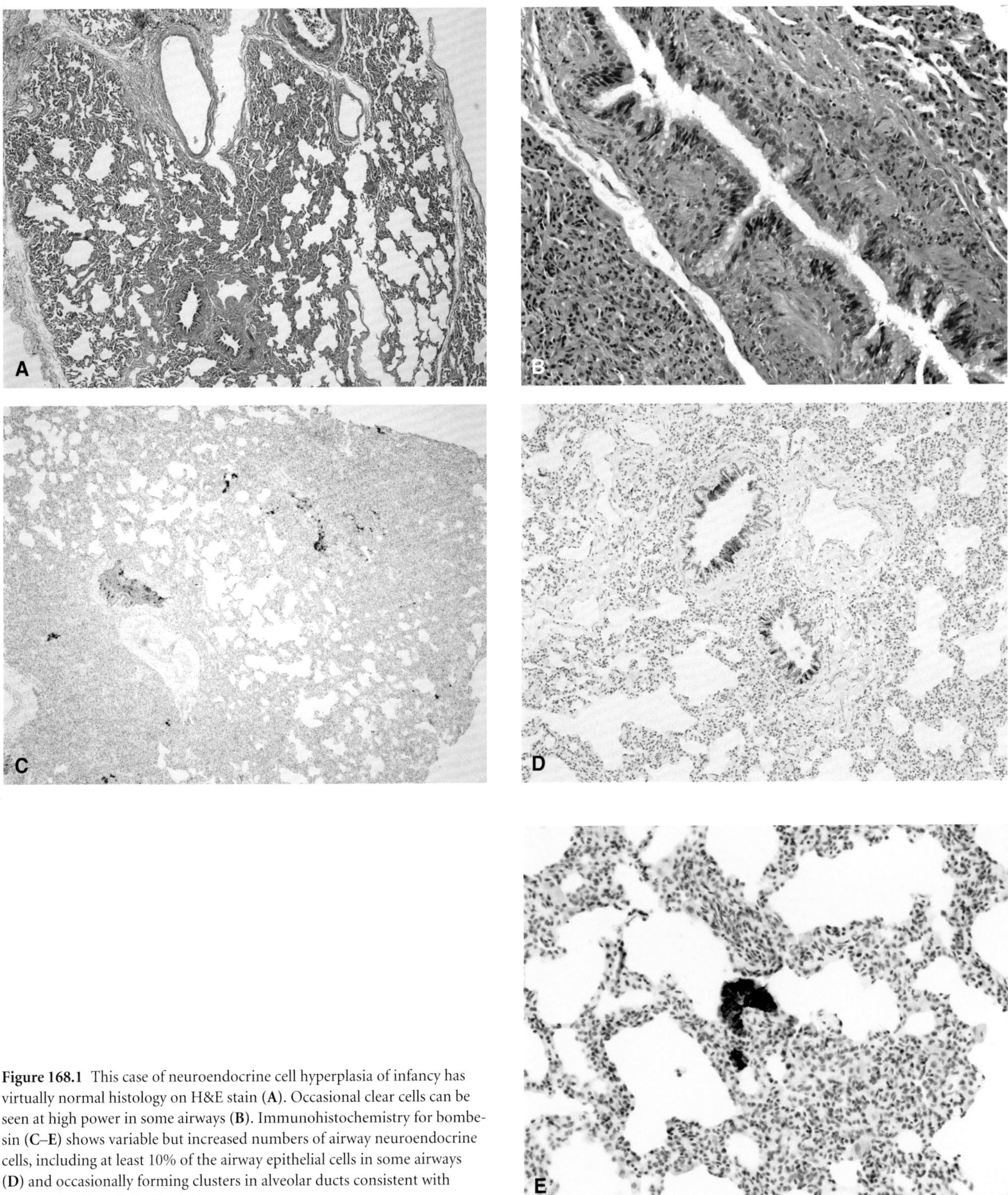

Figure 168.1 This case of neuroendocrine cell hyperplasia of infancy has virtually normal histology on H&E stain (**A**). Occasional clear cells can be seen at high power in some airways (**B**). Immunohistochemistry for bombesin (**C–E**) shows variable but increased numbers of airway neuroendocrine cells, including at least 10% of the airway epithelial cells in some airways (**D**) and occasionally forming clusters in alveolar ducts consistent with neuroendocrine cell bodies (**E**).

169 Pulmonary Interstitial Glycogenosis

▸ Jennifer Pogoriler
▸ Aliya N. Husain

Pulmonary interstitial glycogenosis (PIG), as an isolated disorder, is an extremely rare disorder of infancy. However, patchy PIG is often found as a component of other lung disorders of infancy, including in biopsies for alveolar growth abnormalities due to prematurity or vascular disease. The significance of the expansion of mesenchymal cells is unclear, but some cases may respond to steroids; however, the overall prognosis may depend on the other abnormalities in the biopsy.

HISTOLOGIC FEATURES

- Expansion of interstitium by bland spindle cells with prominent clear cytoplasm.
- PIG often occurs in a patchy form in the context of other chronic lung disease of infancy.
- Cells show small amounts of finely granular periodic acid–Schiff (PAS)-positive, diastase-sensitive material in the cytoplasm.
- Cells are positive for vimentin but negative for smooth muscle actin (SMA) or CD68.
- The differential diagnosis includes storage disorders, which may be differentiated by electron microscopy.

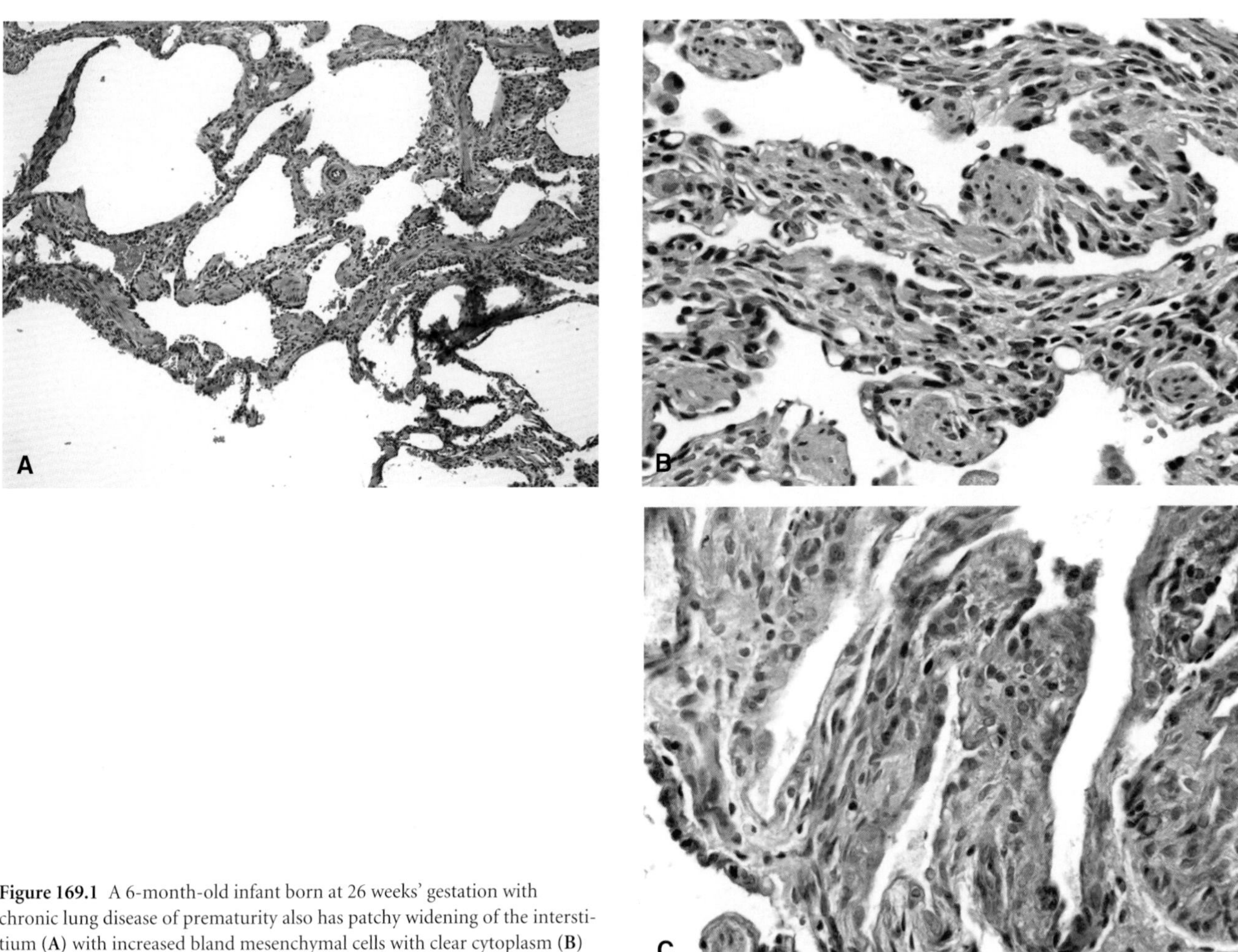

Figure 169.1 A 6-month-old infant born at 26 weeks' gestation with chronic lung disease of prematurity also has patchy widening of the interstitium (**A**) with increased bland mesenchymal cells with clear cytoplasm (**B**) that has very fine PAS-positive granules (**C**).

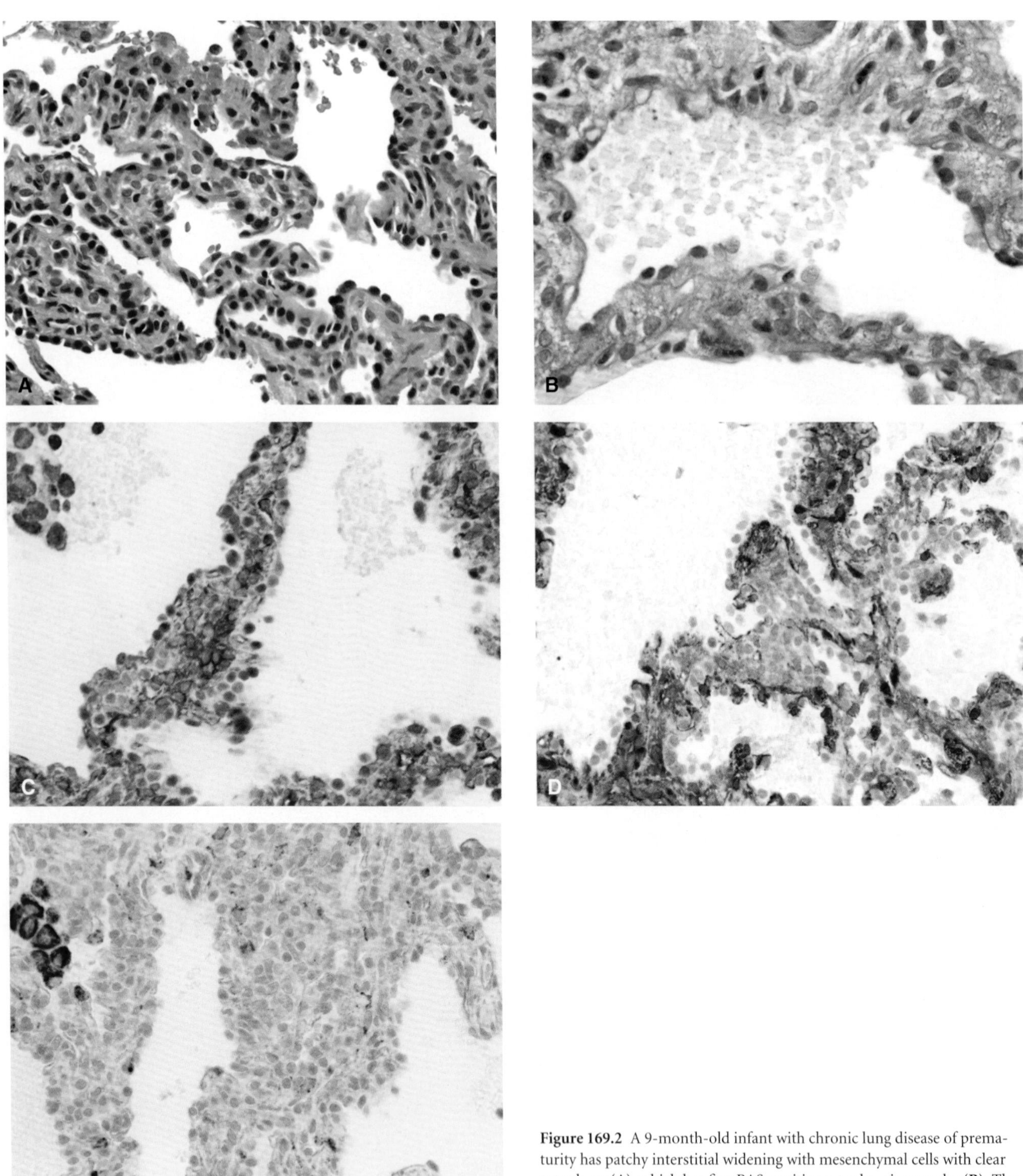

Figure 169.2 A 9-month-old infant with chronic lung disease of prematurity has patchy interstitial widening with mesenchymal cells with clear cytoplasm (**A**), which has fine PAS-positive cytoplasmic granules (**B**). The cells are positive for vimentin (**C**) but negative for SMA (**D**) and CD68 (**E**).

Genetic Disorders of Surfactant Metabolism

170

Jennifer Pogoriler
Aliya N. Husain

Although pediatric patients with profound immune abnormalities (connective tissue disease or acute leukemia) can present with adult-type pulmonary alveolar proteinosis, in this age group the usual clinical concern is for genetic abnormalities in surfactant proteins (surfactant protein B or C), the expression (NKX2-1) or their production (ABCA3). Rarely disorders in GMCSF receptors cause abnormal uptake. The most common of these is *ABCA3* mutation. Originally described as presenting in early infancy with respiratory failure, the much wider clinical spectrum has since been described including adults who present with interstitial fibrosis. Genetic patterns vary from autosomal recessive (SFPTB, ABCA3) to autosomal dominant (SFPTC, NKX2-1, GMCSFR).

HISTOLOGIC FEATURES

The histologic features depend on the mutation and likely the age at which the biopsy is performed but often include alveolar periodic acid–Schiff (PAS)–positive proteinaceous material (which may be very patchy or even focal), foamy macrophages and cholesterol clefts, prominent reactive pneumocytes, and interstitial expansion and inflammation.

- The pattern of lung disease depends on the mutation and likely partially depends on the age at which the patient is biopsied.
- Congenital pulmonary alveolar proteinosis is most commonly associated with surfactant B and *ABCA3* mutations.
- Chronic pneumonitis of infancy pattern shows much more patchy alveolar material with pneumocyte hyperplasia and marked interstitial widening.
- The desquamative interstitial pneumonia pattern shows macrophages diffusely filling airspaces with mild interstitial thickening.
- Older patients may show highly variable patterns of fibrosis and cystic disease, although intra-alveolar PAS-positive material can often be found at least focally, along with cholesterol clefts and foamy macrophages.
- Immunohistochemistry (IHC) may be useful to demonstrate the absence of surfactant protein B, but abnormal, IHC-positive protein products may accumulate and a normal pattern of IHC does not exclude surfactant deficiency.
- A subset of surfactant mutation may lead to abnormal surfactant production, particularly ABCA3, which causes central densities in surfactant bodies, but normal electron microscopy does not exclude surfactant deficiency.
- Genetic testing is often useful to confirm the diagnosis (Table 170.1).

Table 170.1. **Genetic, Clinical, And Pathologic Features of Genetic Disorders of Surfactant Metabolism**

Gene	SFTPB	SFTPC	ABCA3	NKX2-1	GMCSFR
Inheritance pattern	Autosomal recessive	Autosomal dominant	Autosomal recessive	Autosomal dominant	Autosomal recessive
Presentation	Severe, infancy	Variable from infancy to adulthood	Variable from infancy to childhood	Variable from infancy to childhood, brain and thyroid abnormalities	Variable from infancy to childhood
Common histologic patterns	Congenital pulmonary alveolar proteinosis	Chronic pneumonitis of infancy, nonspecific interstitial pneumonia, and other nonspecific patterns of fibrotic lung disease in older patients	Congenital pulmonary alveolar proteinosis, desquamative interstitial pneumonia, and nonspecific interstitial pneumonia	Varies from normal to mild cystic disease	Pulmonary alveolar proteinosis
Common electron microscopy findings	Disorganized, vesicular inclusions	Variable but may be normal	"Fried egg" density at the center of lamellar body	None	None

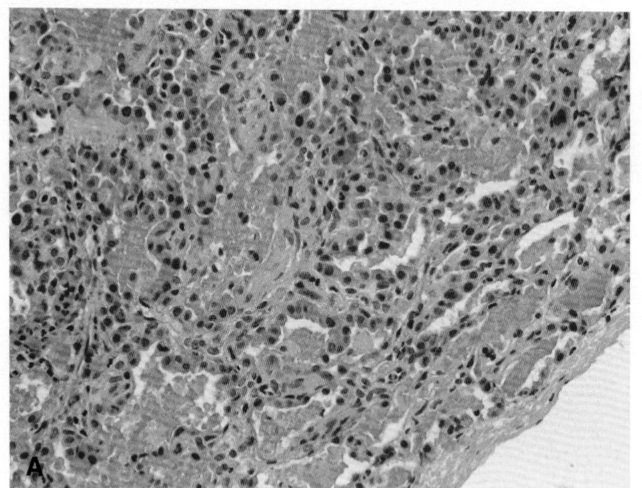

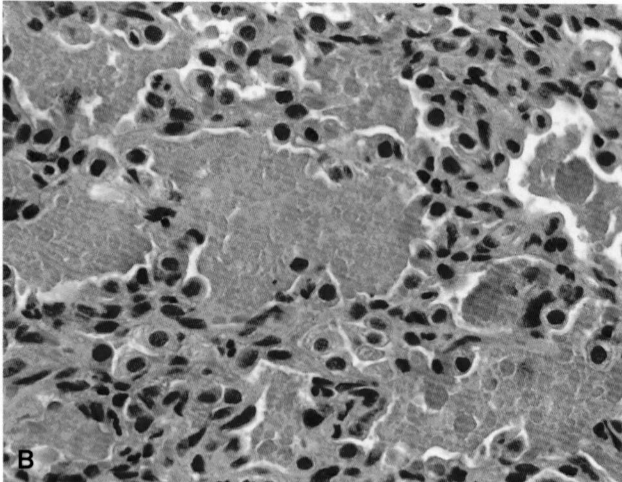

Figure 170.1 Lung biopsy from an infant with congenital increased work of breathing shows diffuse, prominent alveolar proteinaceous material (**A**) with prominent type II pneumocytes (**B**) consistent with a pattern of congenital alveolar proteinosis.

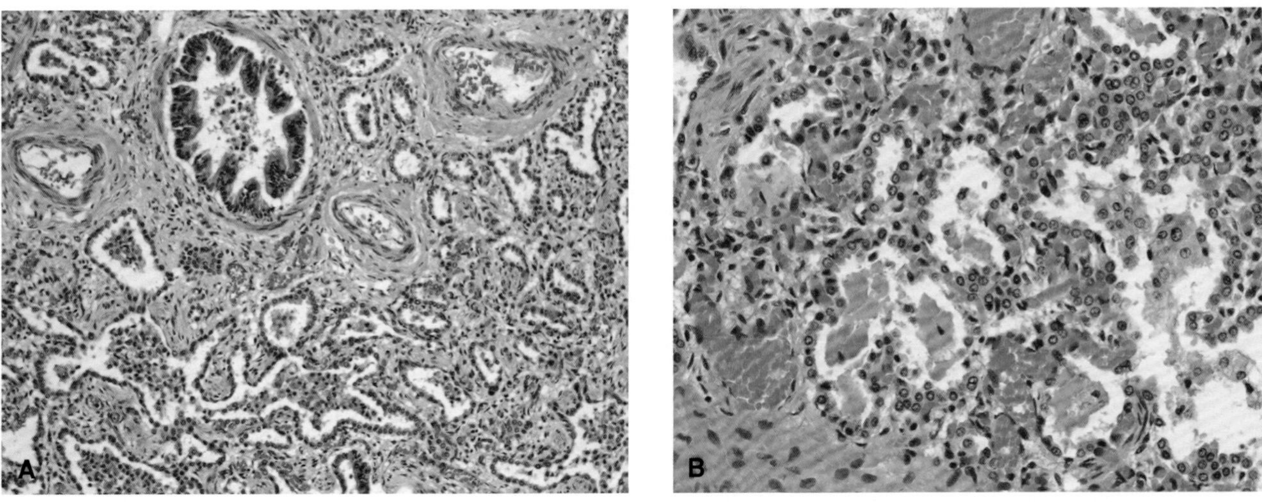

Figure 170.2 Lung biopsy from an infant with an *ABCA3* mutation shows a patchy widened mesenchyme and prominent type II pneumocytes with intra-alveolar macrophages filling the alveoli in a desquamative interstitial pneumonia pattern (**A**) and only focal proteinaceous material (**B**).

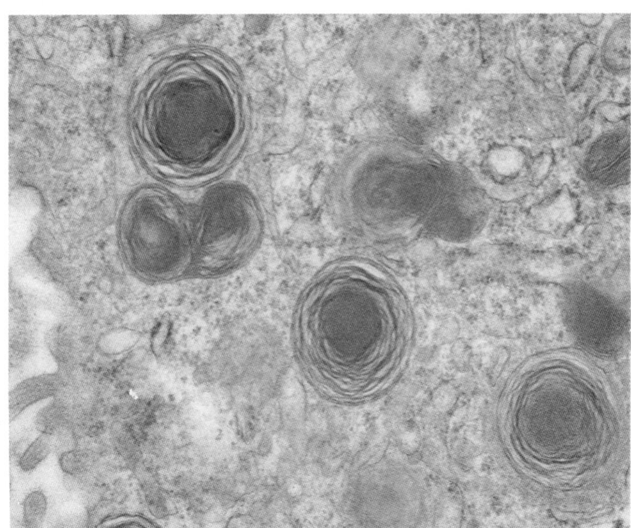

Figure 170.3 Electron micrograph of the lung biopsy from an infant with *ABCA3* mutation deficiency shows a central electron-dense deposit with a "fried egg" appearance.

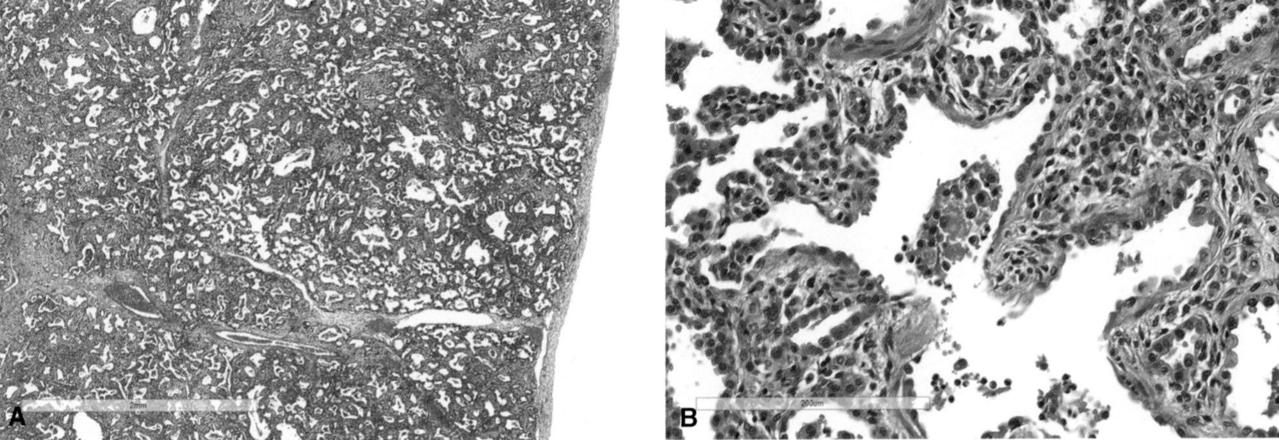

Figure 170.4 This explant for *ABCA3* mutation with chronic pneumonitis of infancy pattern shows diffuse mesenchymal widening and type II pneumocyte hyperplasia but minimal airspace filling (**A**). Higher power view reveals rare granular proteinaceous material (**B**).

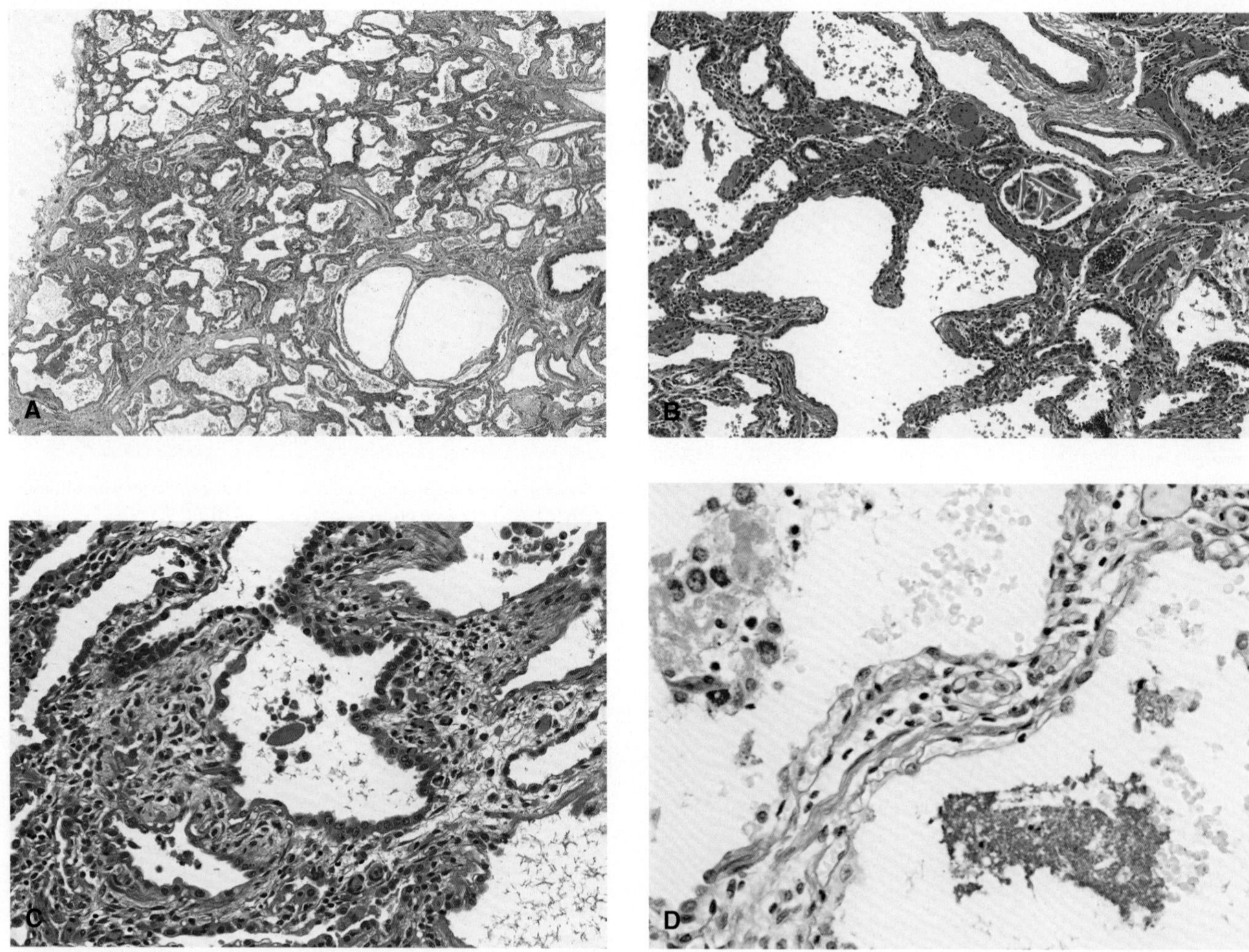

Figure 170.5 This explant for surfactant C deficiency shows fibrosis and markedly enlarged airspaces with prominent type II pneumocytes and interstitial inflammation (**A**). Variable airspace filling with foamy macrophages with cholesterol clefts (**B**) and rare proteinaceous material (**C**) that is PAS-D-positive (**D**) is consistent with abnormalities in processing of surfactant.

171

Cystic Fibrosis

▸ Jennifer Pogoriler
▸ Aliya N. Husain

Cystic fibrosis is a relatively common pediatric lung disorder caused by autosomal recessive mutations in the cystic fibrosis transmembrane conductance regulator transporter. Bronchiectasis begins in infancy and is most severe in the upper lobes. Pathology specimens are predominantly seen as explant or at autopsy. Inability to clear thickened secretions leads to repeated infection and bronchiectasis.

HISTOLOGIC FEATURES

- Widespread bronchiectasis with associated chronic inflammation, ulceration, and reactive epithelial features, including squamous metaplasia and increased goblet cells, can be seen. Submucosal glands may be prominent.
- Thick, eosinophilic mucin is often adherent to the airways.
- Infection is most commonly bacterial, but fungal or nontuberculous mycobacterial infection may also occur.

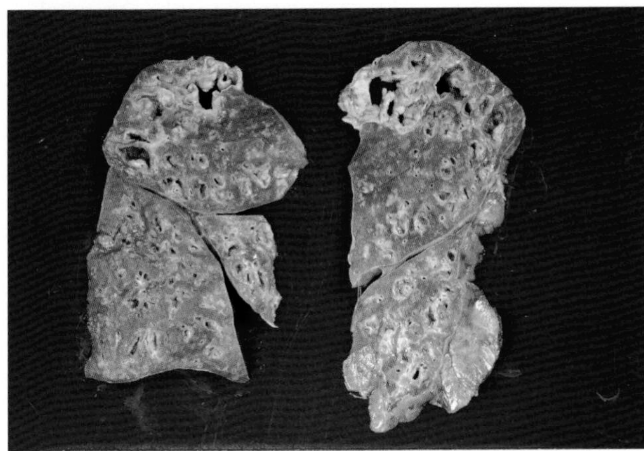

Figure 171.1 These autopsy lungs from a patient with cystic fibrosis show marked bronchiectasis and a bronchiectatic cyst in the upper lobe.

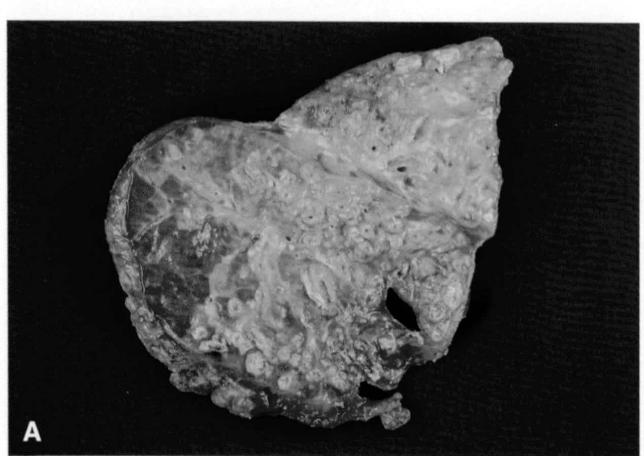

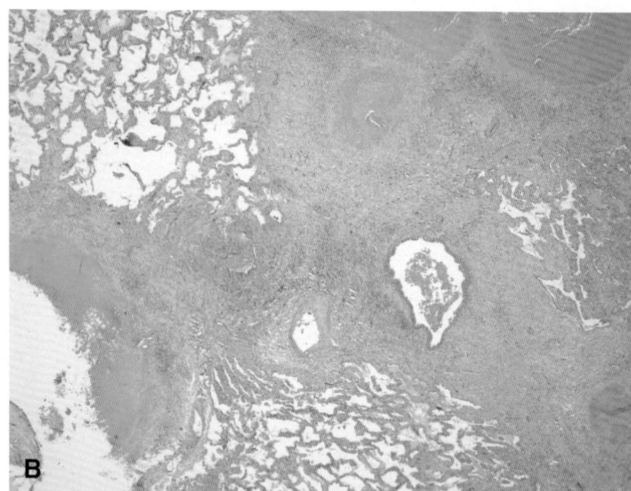

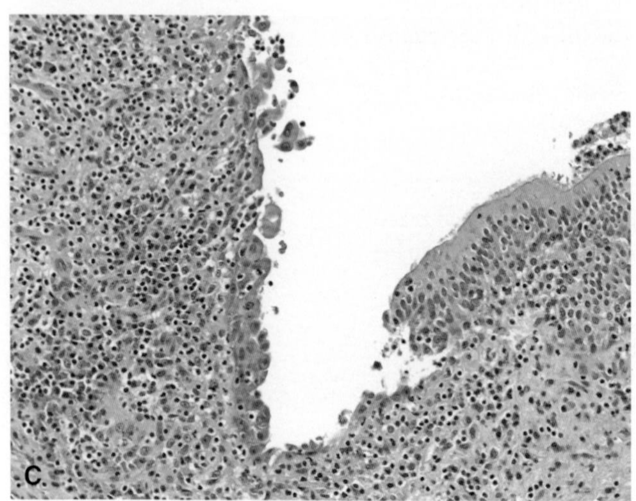

Figure 171.2 This explant from a patient with cystic fibrosis (**A**) shows marked inflammation around the bronchioles with necrotizing granulomas (**B**) that were positive for *Mycobacterium avium intracellulare*. Reactive epithelial cells (**C**) line many of the bronchi.

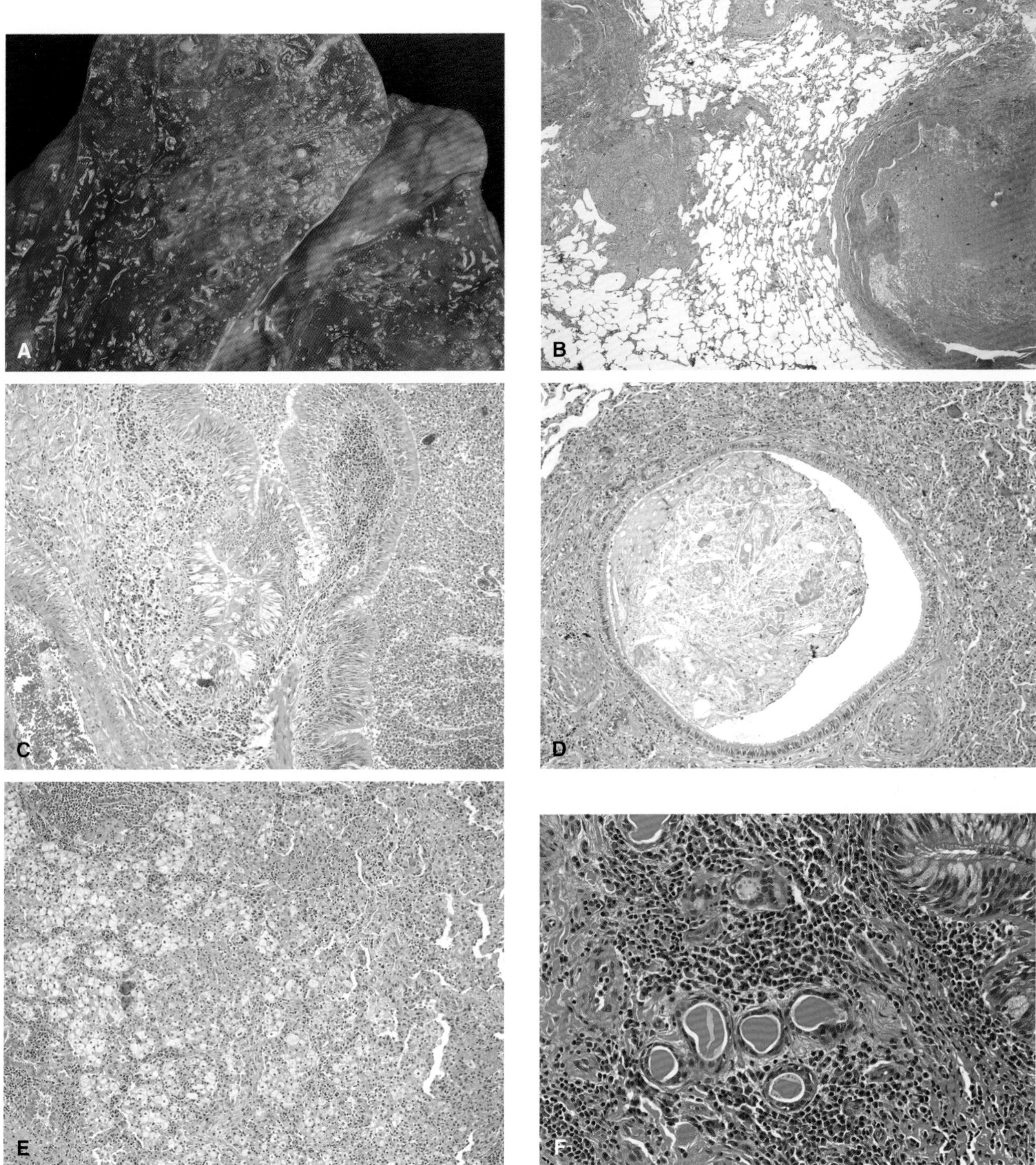

Figure 171.3 This explanted lung with cystic fibrosis shows extensive mucus obstructing the airways (**A**) with bronchiectasis (**B**), reactive airway epithelial cells with increased goblet cells (**C**), bronchiolectasis with dense eosinophilic mucus and pulmonary hypertensive changes (**D**), and adjacent endogenous lipoid pneumonia (**E**). Dense eosinophilic mucus is also present in submucosal glands (**F**).

Primary Ciliary Dyskinesia

172

▶ Jennifer Pogoriler
▶ Theodore J. Pysher
▶ Aliya N. Husain

Primary ciliary dyskinesia (PCD) is a spectrum of disorders due to mutations in motile cilia that result in abnormal ciliary movement. Nearly half of affected patients have Kartagener syndrome (situs inversus, recurrent sinusitis, and bronchiectasis), whereas others have situs solitus with recurrent ear, sinus, and lung infections, and 6% to 12% have heterotaxy. Male patients are often infertile, and female patients may have subfertility or ectopic pregnancy. Surgical pathology findings are nonspecific, and resection is rare, except for bronchiectasis with recurrent infection. Diagnosis may be made by genetic testing and/or electron microscopy. So far, approximately 35 genes have been identified that account for approximately two-thirds of cases of PCD. Approximately two-thirds of patients with PCD will have abnormal ultrastructural findings, so the two methods of evaluation are complementary. Measurement of nasal nitric oxide is a relatively new clinical technique that is approved as an alternative diagnostic measurement in older children.

HISTOLOGIC FINDINGS

- Bronchiectasis is the most common finding in surgical lung specimens.
- Defects diagnosable by electron microscopy include dynein arm deficiencies, central pair (transposition) defects, and radial spoke defects.
- Dynein arm deficiencies result in near-complete absence of recognizable outer and/or inner arms in 100% of cilia. Fewer than two outer or one inner average number of arms are present.
- Outer dynein arm defects are the most common anomaly seen by ultrastructural evaluation.
- Central apparatus defects result in a subset of abnormal cilia, lacking a central pair. Often one of the outer doublets is transposed into the center (microtubular disorientation) (8 + 1 arrangement). These features may be seen in patients with missing inner dynein arms. Similar disorganization is seen in patients with mutations affecting radial spokes.
- Because central pair and radial spoke defects only affect a subset of cilia (and non-PCD biopsies can show small percentages of abnormal cilia), this diagnosis requires evaluation of numerous cilia from more than one cell.
- Reactive abnormalities that are not diagnostic of PCD include compound cilia, disorientation, and occasional accessory or single microtubules.

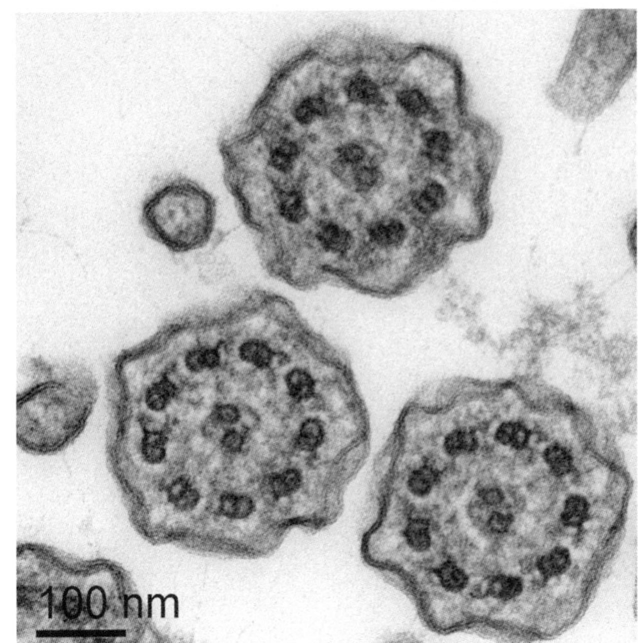

Figure 172.1 This electron micrograph shows a normal cilium with nine outer doublets and one central pair (9 + 2). Several complete inner and outer dynein arms can be identified in each cilium. The central pairs are all in a parallel orientation. (Images courtesy of University of Utah Electron Microscopy Core Laboratory.)

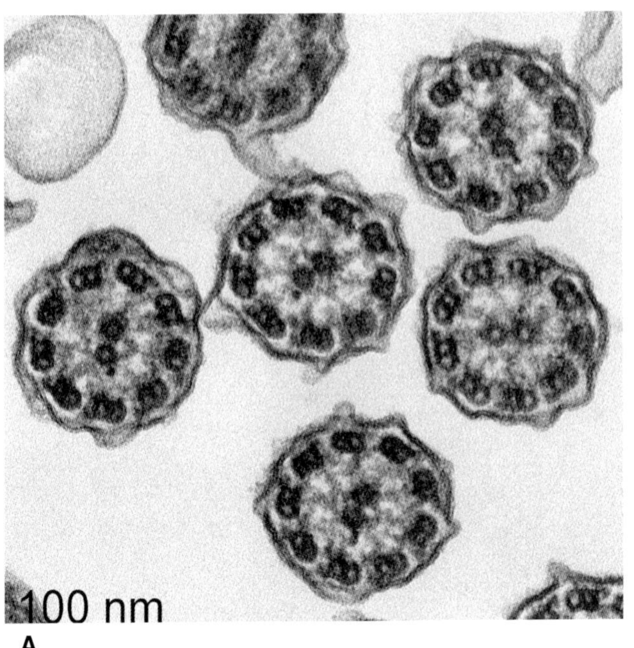

A

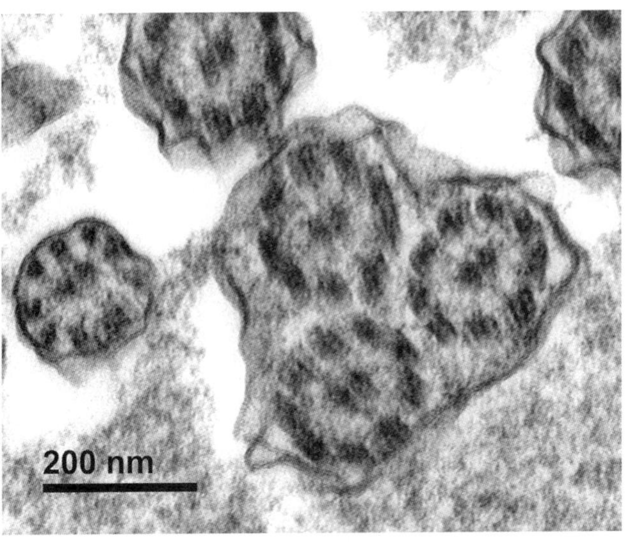

B

C

Figure 172.2 Nonspecific cilial ultrastructural abnormalities can be seen secondary to recurrent infection, including ciliary disorientation (**A**) where the central pair is not oriented in parallel, compound cilia (**B**), and loss of microtubules (**C**), and are not considered diagnostic for PCD. (Images courtesy of University of Utah Electron Microscopy Core Laboratory.)

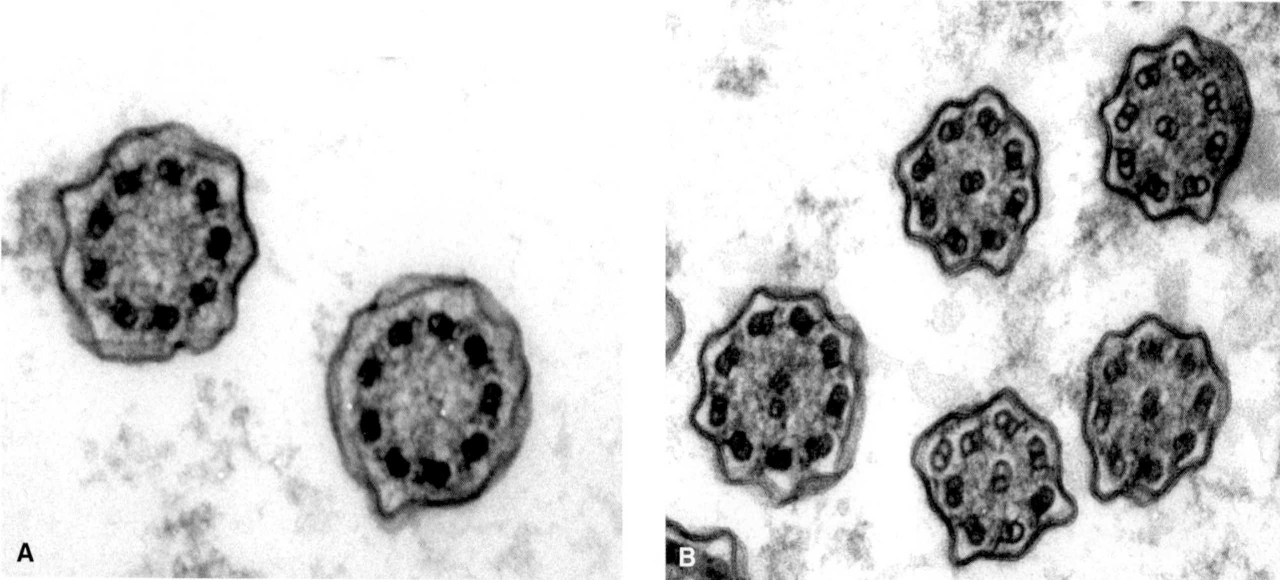

Figure 172.3 Electron micrograph of the sample from a PCD patient with a central apparatus defect shows an absence of central microtubules in some cilia (**A**) and displacement of one of the outer doublets into the center of the cilia in others (**B**). (Images courtesy of University of Utah Electron Microscopy Core Laboratory.)

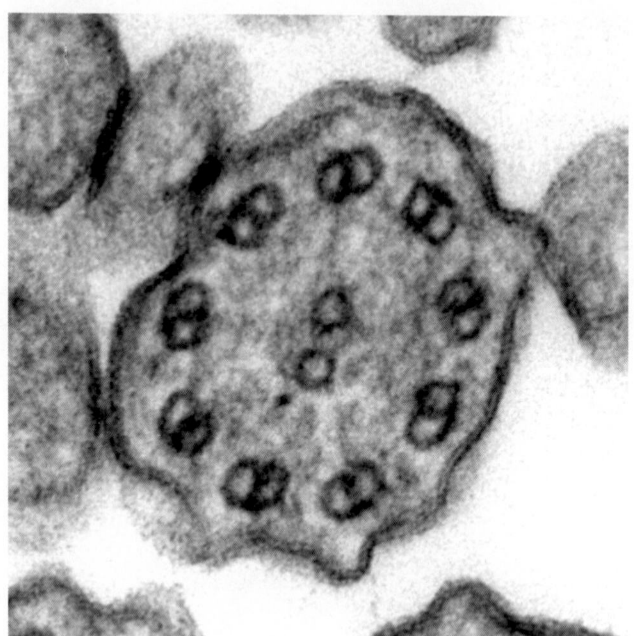

Figure 172.4 Electron micrograph of the sample from a PCD patient shows an absence of both inner and outer dynein arms. (Images courtesy of University of Utah Electron Microscopy Core Laboratory.)

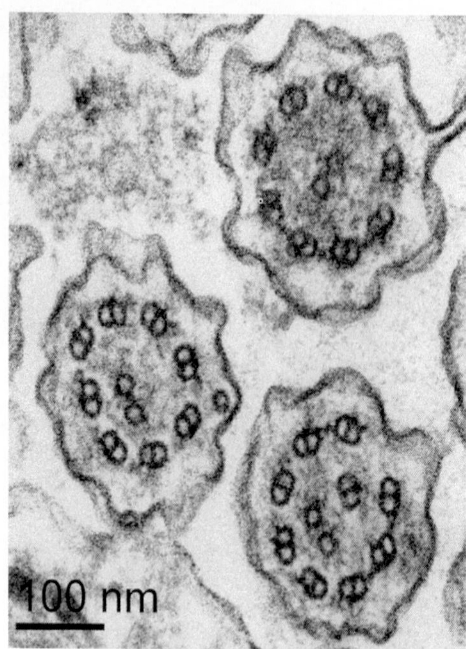

Figure 172.5 Electron micrograph of the sample from a PCD patient with a radial spoke defect shows two abnormal cilia with disorganization. The left cilium has eight outer doublets with a single microtubule, whereas the bottom right cilium has eight outer doublets and one doublet and central pair irregularly placed in the center. (Images courtesy of University of Utah Electron Microscopy Core Laboratory.)

Chronic Granulomatous Disease

173

▶ Jennifer Pogoriler
▶ Aliya N. Husain

Chronic granulomatous disease (CGD) is due to defects in the nicotinamide adenine dinucleotide phosphate (NADPH) oxidase pathway, resulting in ineffective killing of organisms by phagocytic cells and recurrent infection. Most cases are X-linked, but autosomal recessive inheritance patterns are also possible. The lungs are a common site of infection, and biopsy may be performed if sputum or bronchoalveolar lavage culture fails to determine the cause of infection.

HISTOLOGIC FEATURES

- Lung biopsy may show scattered granulomas, but diffuse and confluent mixed granulomatous and acute and chronic inflammation is more typical.
- Some lung biopsies may show nonspecific patterns of chronic inflammation and fibrosis without granulomas.
- Granulomas are usually microscopic in size.
- CGD granulomas vary from nonnecrotizing granulomas, granulomas with a central neutrophilic microabscess surrounded by palisading histiocytes, to classic necrotizing granulomas.
- Giant cells and/or eosinophils may be present within the granulomas.
- Large macrophages with finely granular pale yellow pigment may be present in a subset of cases but are not common.
- Culture and special stains to evaluate for infection are required for all cases.

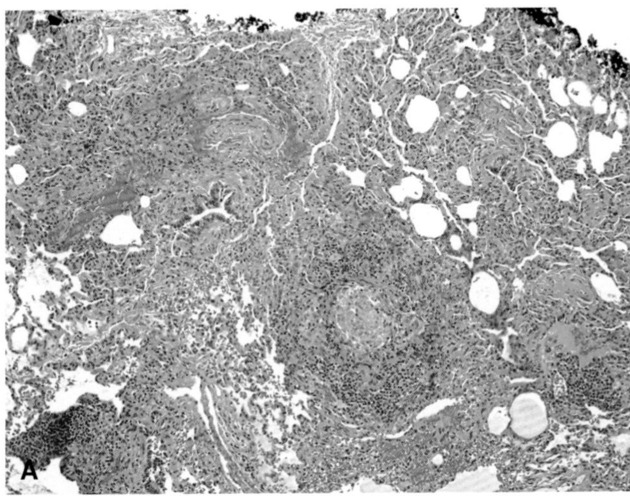

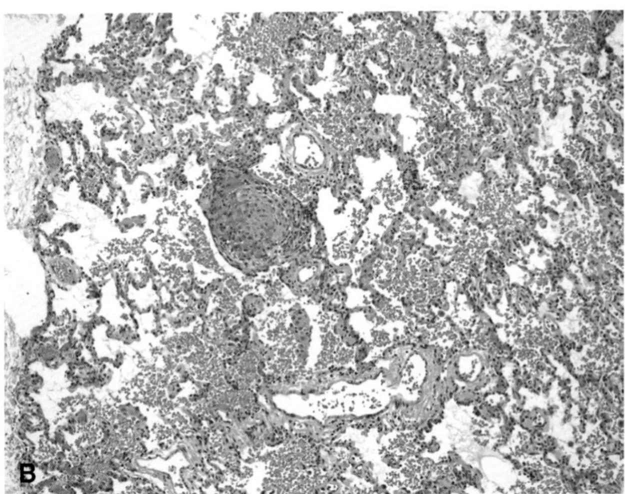

Figure 173.1 This toddler without active infection had rare minute noncaseating granulomas near small airways (**A**) and in the interstitium (**B**).

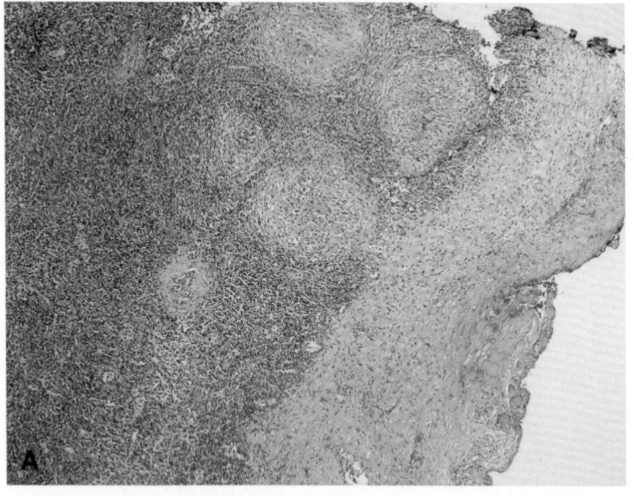

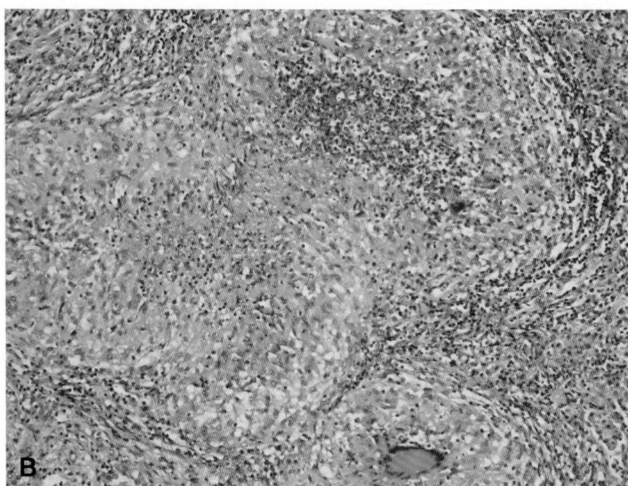

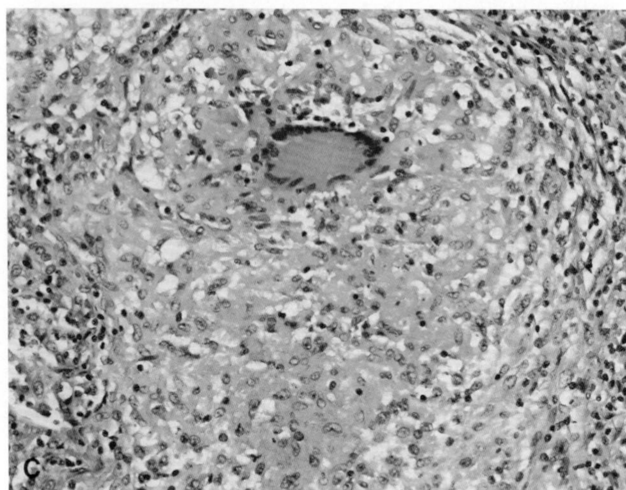

Figure 173.2 This patient with CGD shows more marked chronic inflammation with subpleural granulomas (**A**) that are necrotizing (**B**) with occasional giant cells (**C**).

Alveolar Capillary Dysplasia with Misalignment of Pulmonary Veins

Jennifer Pogoriler
Aliya N. Husain

Alveolar capillary dysplasia with misalignment of pulmonary veins (ACDMPV) was initially described in neonates with respiratory distress and pulmonary hypertension, but multiple case reports have described sudden onset of symptoms in older infants who were previously healthy, implying a wider array of phenotypes than previously reported. A subset of patients with ACDMPV have other developmental anomalies, most commonly hypoplastic left heart syndrome or other congenital heart disease, malrotation of the intestines, Hirschsprung disease, or genitourinary anomalies.

Mutations in the *FoxF1* gene have been described in a subset of patients, some of which are familial and usually maternally inherited. Phenotypic expression is highly variable, and prolonged survival has been reported in some patients with aggressive supportive therapy, allowing a bridge to transplant.

HISTOLOGIC FEATURES

- Alveoli are typically markedly simplified with a widened interstitium containing decreased numbers of capillaries, which are centrally located, resulting in a deficient air–blood interface.
- Features are usually diffuse but may be patchy, and the severity of alveolar abnormalities is variable.
- Aberrant thin-walled vessels with smooth muscle are present in the bronchovascular bundles, now known to correspond to aberrantly dilated bronchial veins that shunt blood from the pulmonary arteries to pulmonary veins.
- Pulmonary veins are present in the interlobular septa.
- Small venules around the airways are often markedly congested.
- Features of pulmonary hypertension, including pulmonary artery medial hypertrophy and muscularization of arterioles, are often present.
- Lymphangiectasia may be present.

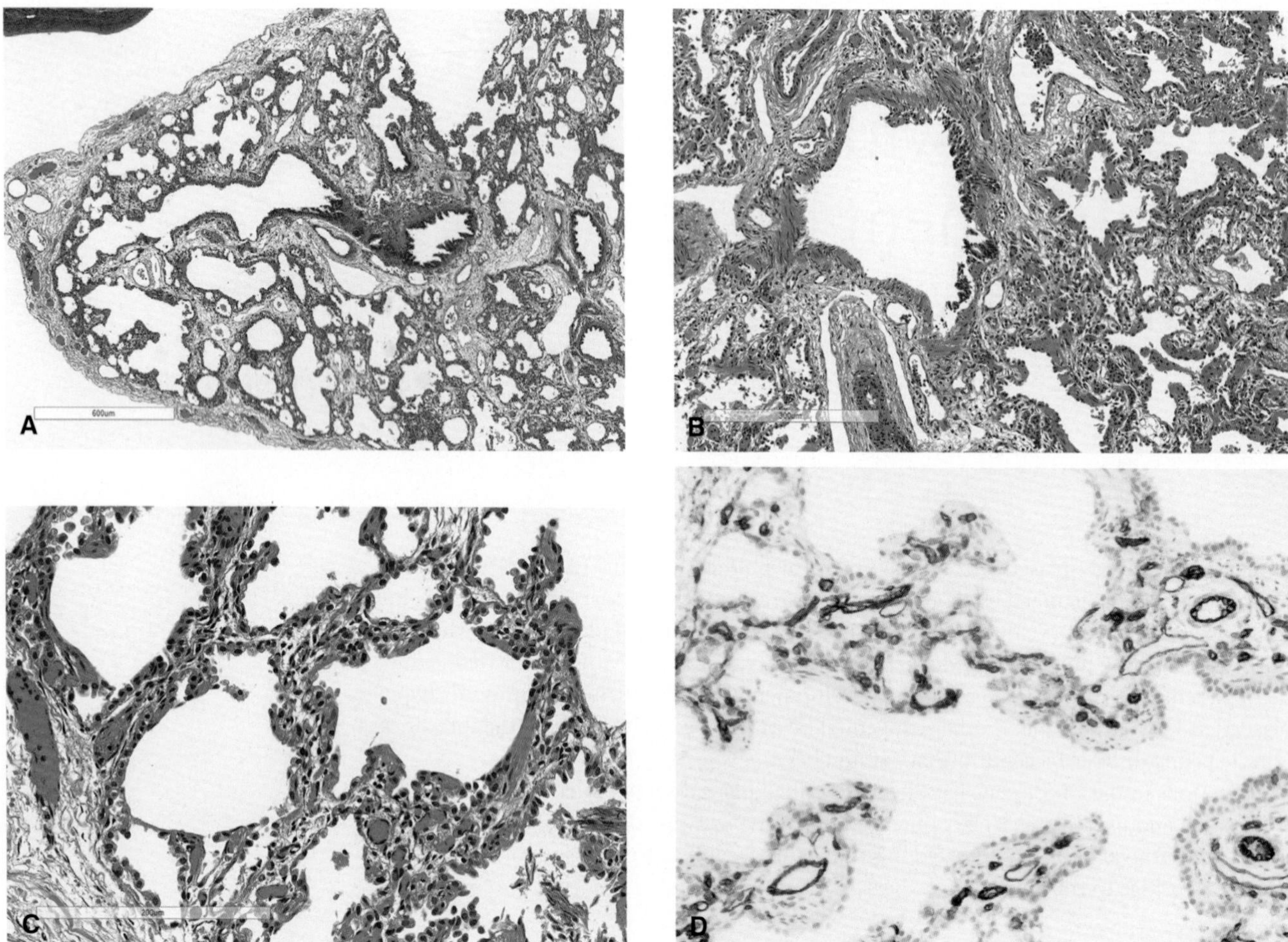

Figure 174.1 **A:** This wedge biopsy shows simplified alveolar architecture with an expanded mesenchyme. The central airway has one thicker walled pulmonary artery above and a thinner walled aberrant muscular vein below. In another bronchovascular bundle (**B**), thick-walled arteries are above and below the airway, whereas a thin-walled muscular vessel is to the upper right. The expanded mesenchyme has a few capillaries in the alveolar septa (**C**), but they are often located away from the epithelial interface and are reduced as seen by immunohistochemistry for CD31 (**D**).

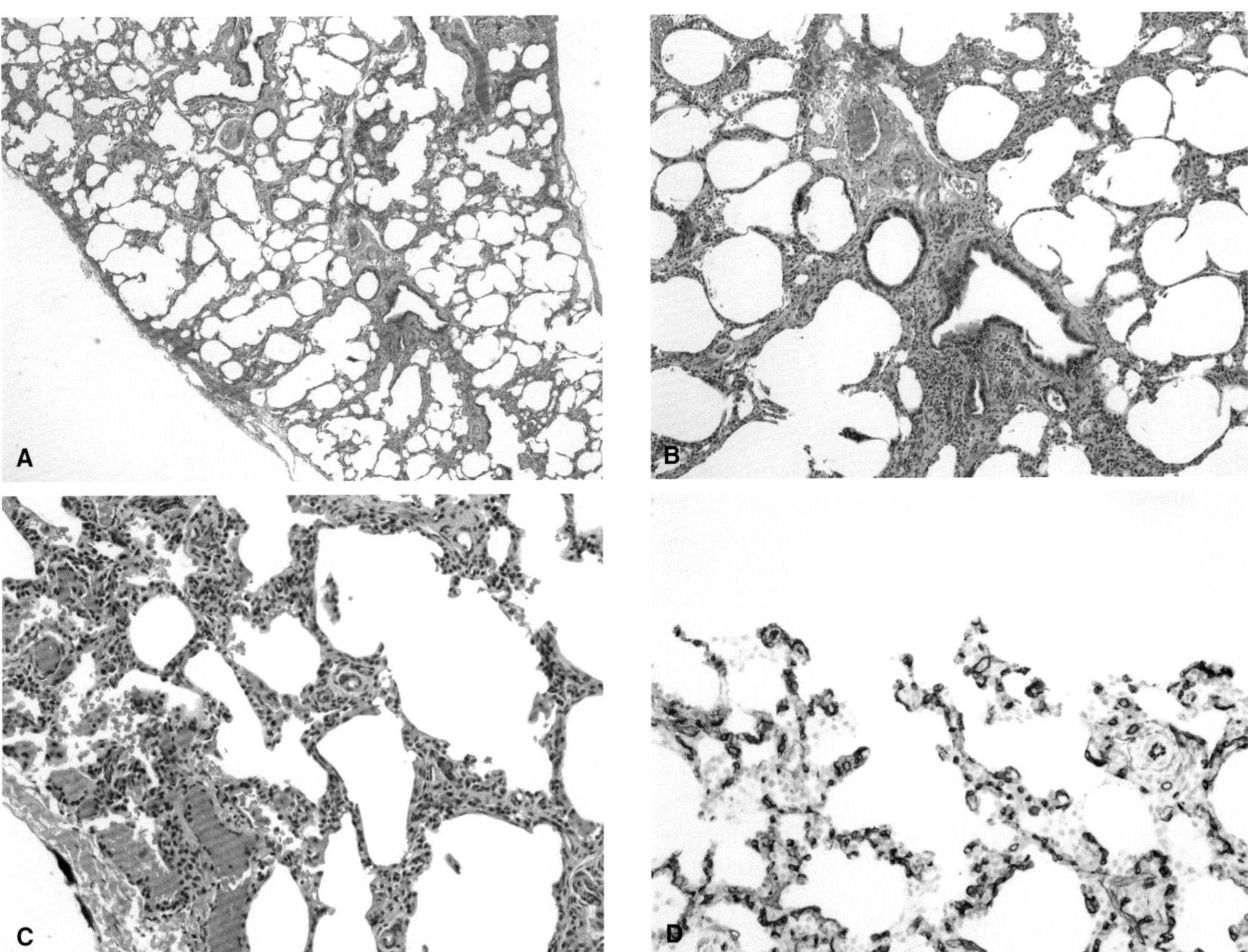

Figure 174.2 In this example of ACDMPV presenting in an older infant, the alveolar septa are thinner, but alveolar are large and simplified (**A**). Aberrant thin-walled muscular veins are present in the bronchovascular bundles (**B**) and muscularization of arterioles is prominent (**C**). Immunohistochemistry for CD34 (**D**) shows an abnormal double layer of capillaries in the alveolar septa.

175

Acinar Dysplasia

▶ Jennifer Pogoriler
▶ Aliya N. Husain

Acinar dysplasia is an extremely rare lung disease presenting in neonates as inability to ventilate. Recent genetic studies have reported mutations in *TBX4* and *FGFR2* genes in a subset of patients with this disorder. It is considered to be universally lethal, and biopsy diagnosis of this disorder allows for alterations in aggressive postnatal treatment.

HISTOLOGIC FEATURES

- Grossly hypoplastic lungs.
- Diffuse, bilateral marked underdevelopment of terminal bronchioles and alveoli. The disorder has been compared with the pseudoglandular or saccular stage of lung development.
- Bronchioles extend to the pleural surface, and cartilage may be identified in the pleura.
- A few poorly developed sac-like "airspaces" surround airspaces, but normal alveoli are not present.

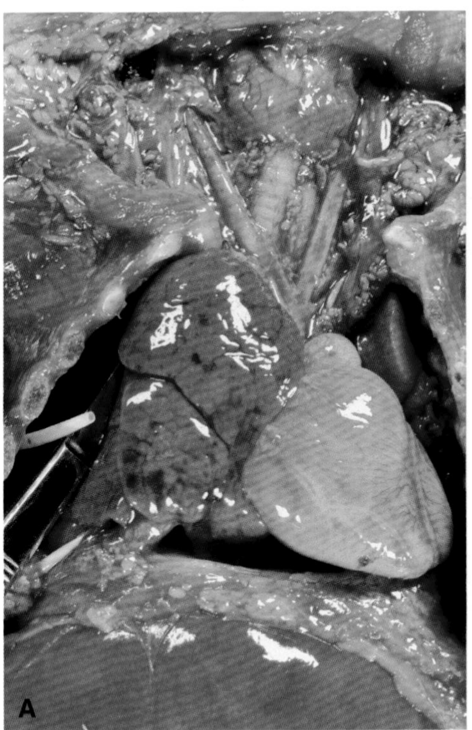

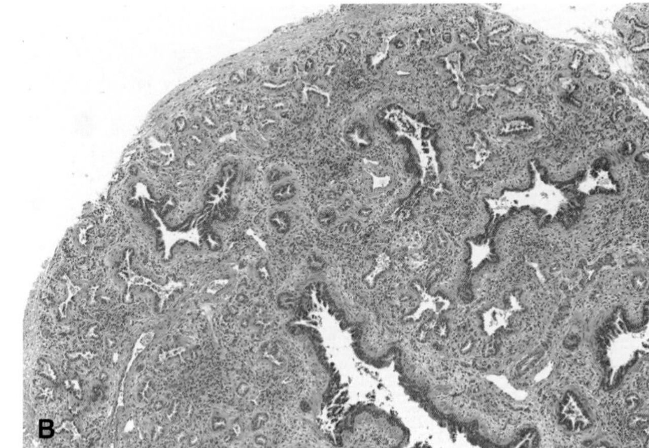

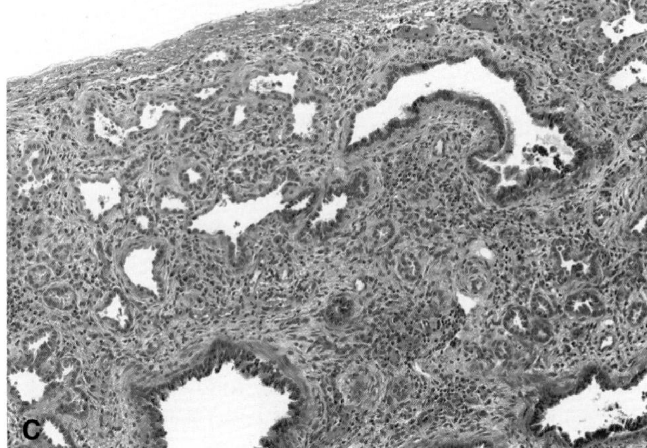

Figure 175.1 The lungs of this infant with acinar dysplasia are markedly hypoplastic compared with the normal-sized heart (**A**). Premortem biopsy showed numerous bronchioles separated by a few poorly developed air sacs with prominent mesenchyme and without any normal alveolar development (**B**). Bronchioles extended to the pleural surfaces (**C**).

176 Complications of Prematurity

Jennifer Pogoriler
Aliya N. Husain

Complications of prematurity include hyaline membrane disease, chronic lung disease of prematurity, and pulmonary interstitial emphysema.

HYALINE MEMBRANE DISEASE

With surfactant treatment, hyaline membrane disease has become rare in preterm infants. It is histologically similar to diffuse alveolar damage seen in other ages and may range from isolated hyaline membranes to early organization depending on the timing.

Histologic Features

- In acute cases, typical features of hyaline membranes, superimposed on immature lung architecture, are seen including eosinophilic acellular membranes lining airspaces, reactive type II pneumocytes, and various stages of organization (depending on timing).
- Airway injury may be present characterized by necrosis of the epithelium or later by regenerative or metaplastic features.

CHRONIC LUNG DISEASE OF PREMATURITY

Chronic lung disease of prematurity following treatment with surfactant shows alveolar enlargement and simplification similar to that seen in some patients with congenital heart disease or chromosomal anomalies. The alveoli may be mildly thickened with a double layer of capillaries.

Histologic Features

- Historic features of chronic lung disease of prematurity (bronchopulmonary dysplasia), including alternating areas of lung collapse and overexpansion, are rarely seen in the era of surfactant administration.
- Chronic lung disease of prematurity now typically presents with uniform alveolar simplification and enlargement.
- Although fibrosis is often scant, small smooth muscle bundles often extend into the alveolar walls.
- Secondary pulmonary hypertensive changes are common, with muscularization of arterioles and muscular hypertrophy of pulmonary arteries.

INTERSTITIAL EMPHYSEMA

Interstitial emphysema is most commonly seen in ventilated preterm infants, although it may rarely occur in full-term babies.

Histologic Features

- Air rupture into the interstitial connective tissue of the bronchovascular bundles create spaces unlined by endothelium or epithelium.
- Air may rupture into the lymphatics, creating confusion with lymphangiectasia.
- In cases of persistent interstitial emphysema, foreign body–type giant cells may partially line the airspaces.

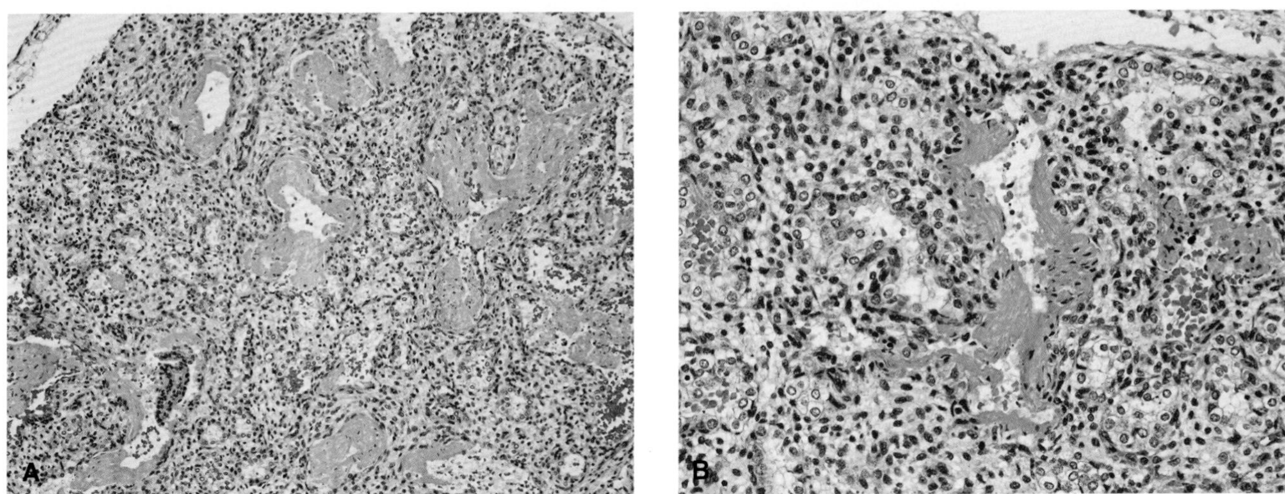

Figure 176.1 A and B: In this infant born at 24 weeks' gestation who died several days after birth, hyaline membranes are prominent.

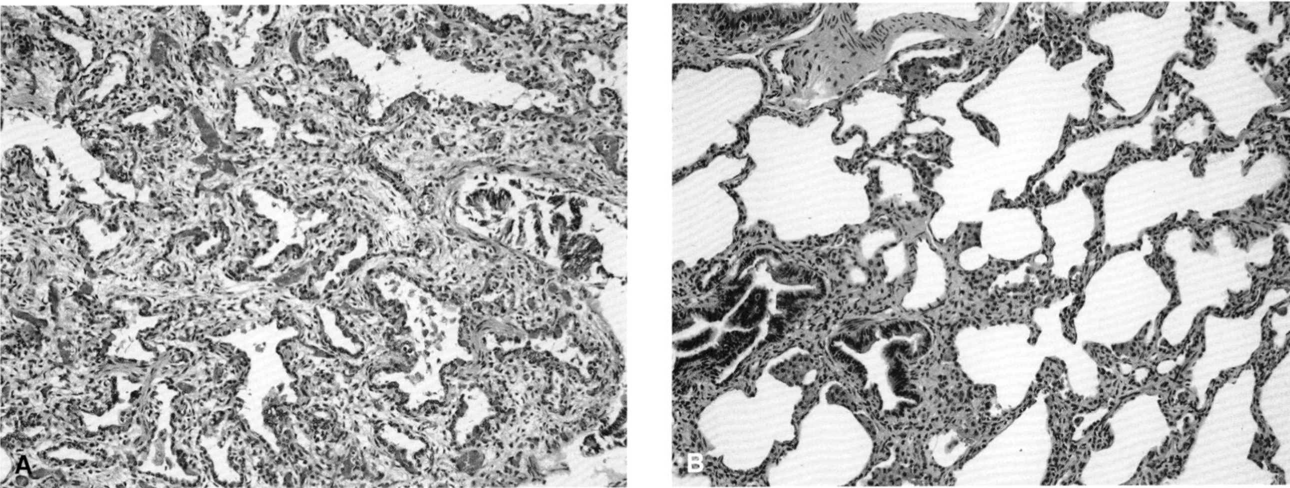

Figure 176.2 In this infant born at 24 weeks' gestation who survived for 7 weeks, there is alveolar simplification and variable interstitial thickening by mesenchymal cells with clear cytoplasm (**A**), whereas other areas have thinner alveolar walls (**B**). Reactive pneumocytes remain prominent (**A**), suggesting ongoing injury.

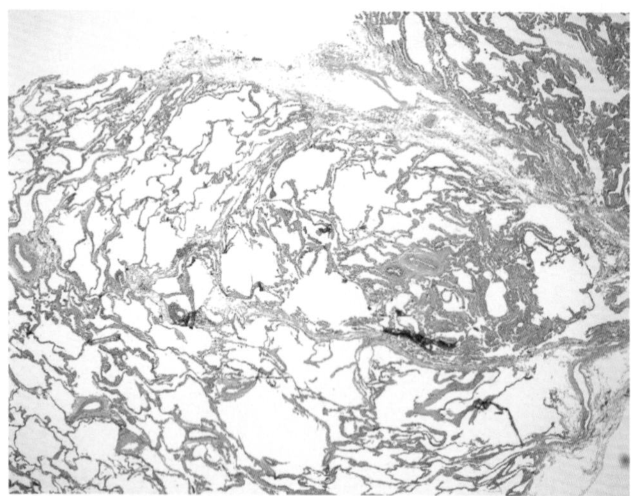

Figure 176.3 This preterm infant at 6 months has widespread alveolar simplification. Although many of the alveolar septa are thin, patchy pulmonary interstitial glycogenosis was present.

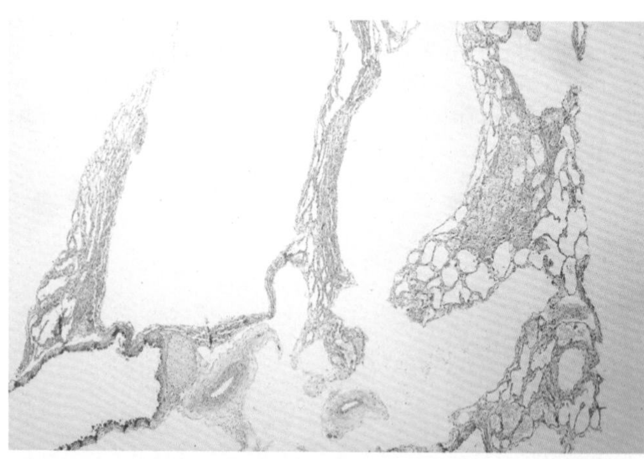

Figure 176.4 In this preterm infant who was ventilated, large empty spaces dissect into the interstitium of the bronchovascular bundles. These areas are not lined by lymphatic endothelium.

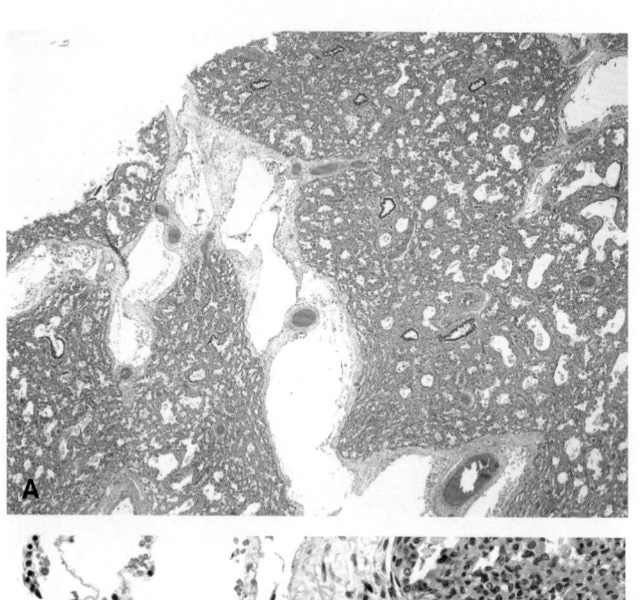

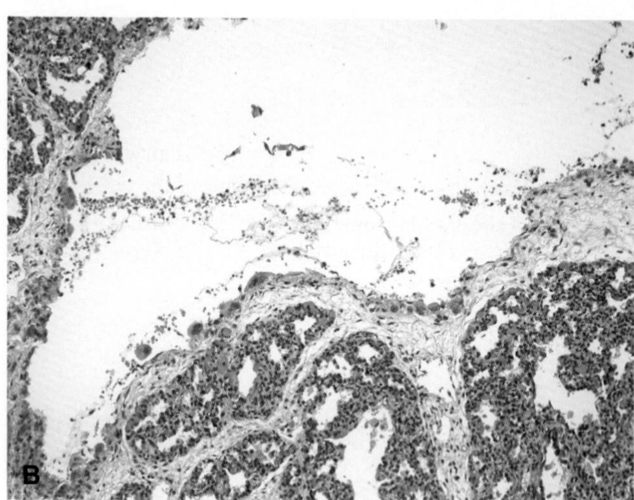

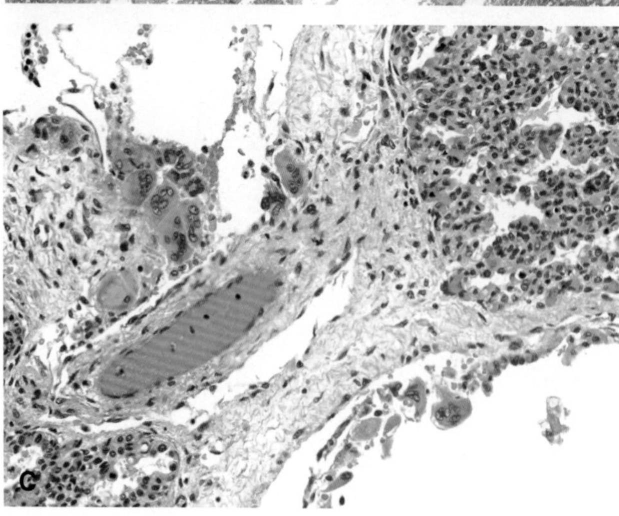

Figure 176.5 In this patient with persistent pulmonary interstitial emphysema, large cystic spaces are seen spreading along the bronchovascular bundles (**A**). They are partially lined by reactive macrophages and giant cells (**B and C**).

177 Meconium Aspiration

Jennifer Pogoriler
Aliya N. Husain

Only a small subset of infants born with meconium-stained amniotic fluid develop meconium aspiration syndrome characterized by respiratory distress and, in severe cases, by pulmonary hypertension. The pathogenetic mechanisms may include airway obstruction, inflammation, inactivation of surfactant, and pulmonary hypertension. The diagnosis is usually made clinically, but biopsy may be performed to rule out other causes of pulmonary hypertension in the newborn.

HISTOLOGIC FEATURES

- Widespread blue-tinted mucin throughout airways.
- Extensive squamous and acellular eosinophilic debris.
- Pigmented material in macrophages may be rare.
- Acute or organizing diffuse alveolar damage may be present.
- Chronic intrauterine meconium aspiration has been reported to cause infarcts and granulomatous inflammation.

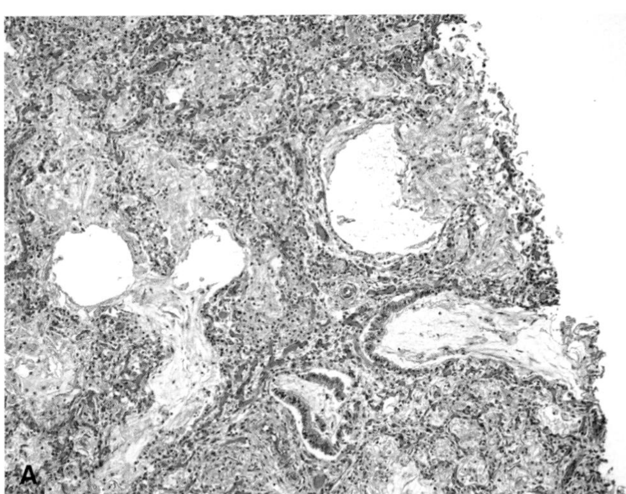

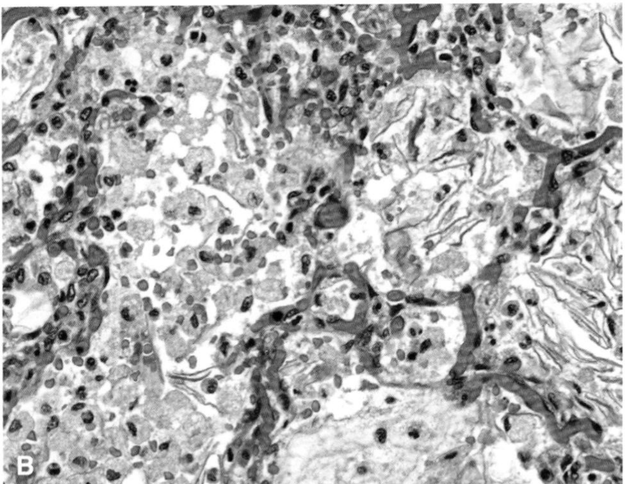

Figure 177.1 In this infant with meconium aspiration, extensive blue mucin (**A**) is present in airways along with aspirated squamous cells and rare pigmented material (**B**).

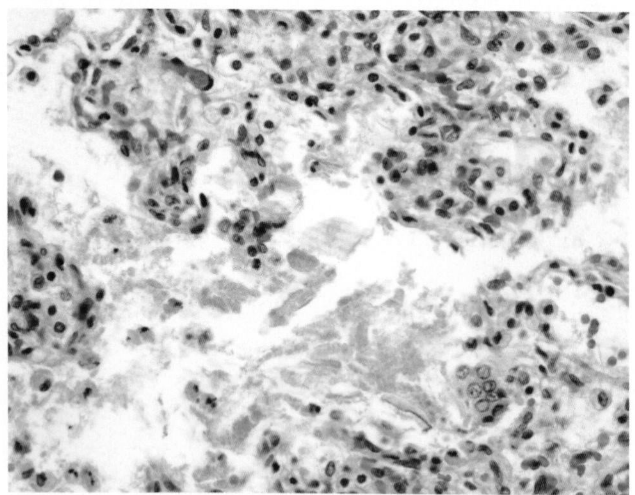

Figure 177.2 In this infant there is eosinophilic and finely pigmented tan-yellow material free in alveolar spaces and in rare macrophages. Aspirated squamous cells are also present.

178

Lymphatic Disorders

▶ Jennifer Pogoriler
▶ Aliya N. Husain

The most common lymphatic disorder in infants is lymphangiectasia. This may rarely be a primary disorder, which can be generalized or confined to the lungs, but is more commonly seen secondary to congenital heart disease. Lymphangiectasia may be a component of other disorders of the lung, such as sequestrations or congenital pulmonary airway malformations. In contrast, lymphangiomatosis refers to increased, abnormally anastomosing lymphatic spaces in the bronchovascular bundles and pleura. Localized lymphangioma of the lung is extremely rare.

HISTOLOGIC FEATURES

- Distended lymphatics are present in bronchovascular bundles and in the pleura.
- If necessary, they can be highlighted with immunohistochemistry for podoplanin (D2-40), although they are usually obvious on hematoxylin and eosin stain.
- Artifactual dilation of lymphatics can be produced by perfusion of the lung even via the airways, and care should be taken in making this diagnosis.
- Lymphangiomatosis has increased, abnormally anastomosing channels in the pleura and septa.
- Kaposiform lymphangiomatosis has a spindle-cell component that is D2-40 positive.
- Lymphangioma is a localized vascular malformation with a regional increase in number.

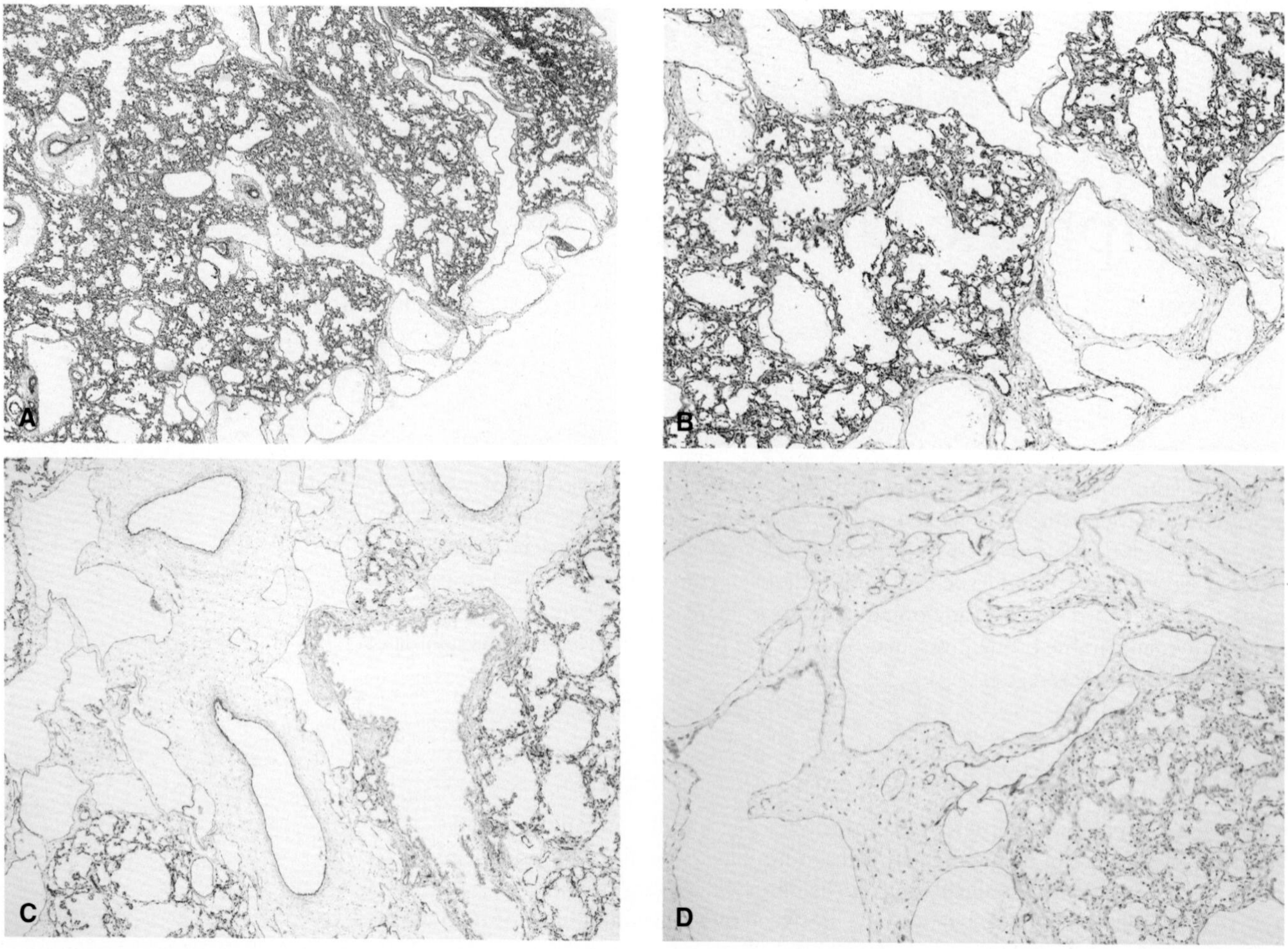

Figure 178.1 In this patient with hypoplastic left heart syndrome, expanded lymphatics are present around bronchovascular bundles, in interlobular septa, and along the pleura (**A**). The dilated spaces are surrounded by an endothelial lining without muscle in the wall (**B**). The endothelial lining can be highlighted by vascular marker CD31 (**C**) or lymphatic marker D2-40 (**D**).

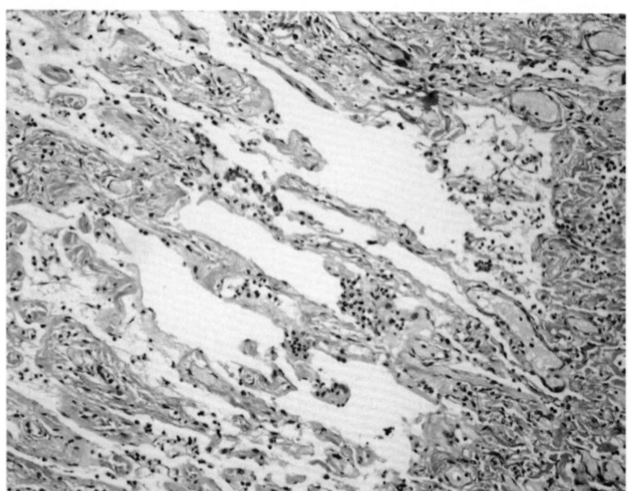

Figure 178.2 In this patient with lymphangiomatosis, septal lymphatics are increased and form abnormal anastomosing channels.

Juvenile Respiratory Papillomatosis

179

Aliya N. Husain
Jennifer Pogoriler

Juvenile respiratory papillomatosis usually presents in young children with hoarseness. An adult form is morphologically similar. This is a rare disorder due to infection of the respiratory tract of an infant by human papilloma virus (HPV), most commonly low-risk type 6 or 11. Papillomas most commonly involve the larynx and often recur requiring multiple surgical procedures. Rarely, the papillomas may extend to the lower respiratory tract, including the alveoli where they grow along the alveolar surface. Malignant transformation to squamous carcinoma is unusual in children (<1%).

HISTOLOGIC FEATURES

- Squamous papillomas are usually confined to the upper airways, and lung involvement is rare.
- HPV positive, which can be demonstrated by in situ hybridization.
- Benign papillomatosis may involve the lungs, filling and replacing the alveoli.
- Dysplasia and progression to squamous-cell carcinoma are extremely rare events.

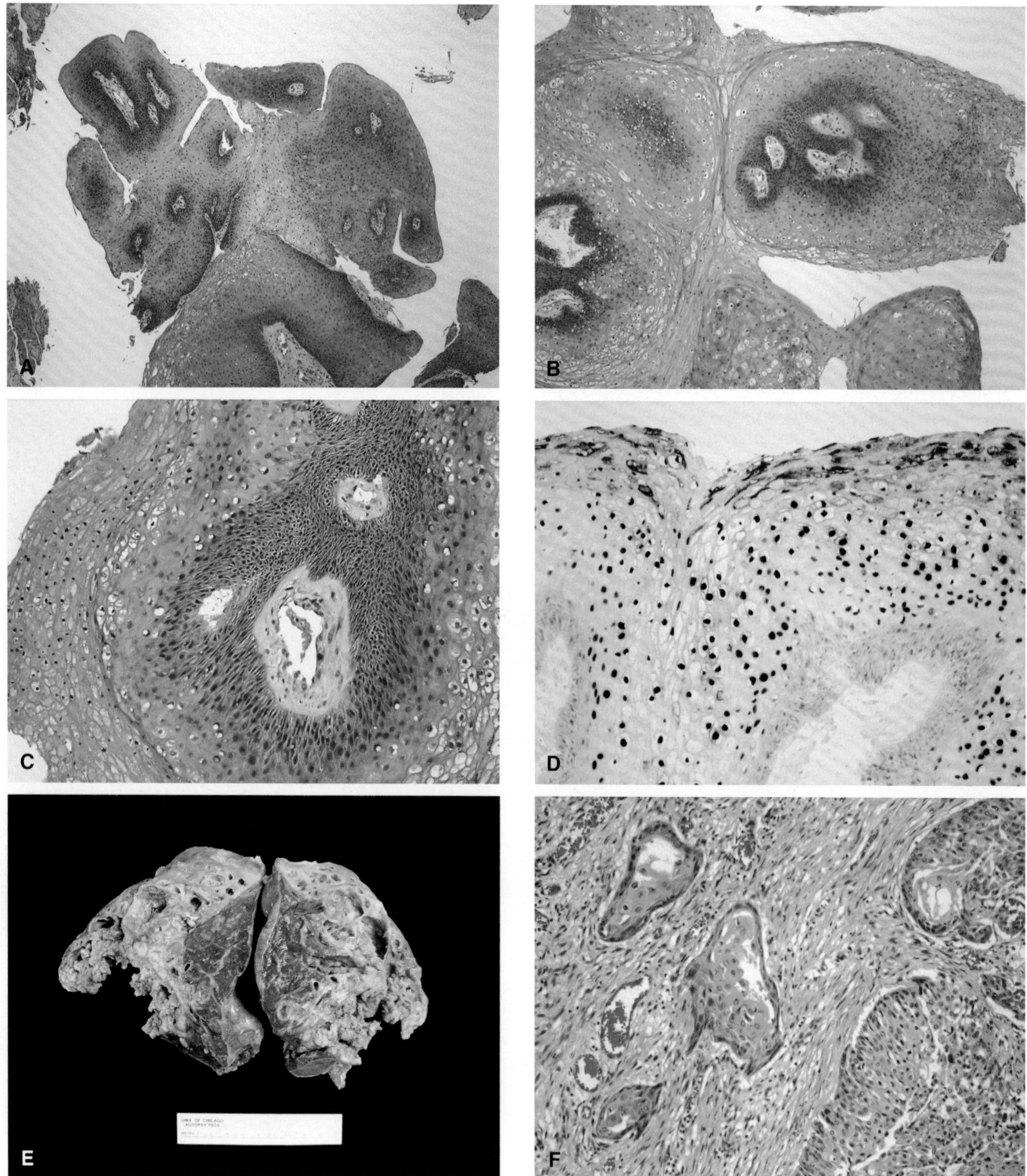

Figure 179.1 This patient had multiple laryngeal squamous papillomas starting at the age of 18 months, which were excised 54 times over his life. This low-power picture was from his 21st excision at the age of 9 years (**A**). This was the 25th excision at the age of 10 years (**B**), higher power of which shows only mild dysplasia (**C**). In situ hybridization was positive for HPV6 (**D**). His disease progressed to involve the lungs grossly seen here at autopsy at the age of 13 years (**E**). Microscopic examination showed well-differentiated squamous-cell carcinoma (**F**).

180 Pleuropulmonary Blastoma

Jennifer Pogoriler
Aliya N. Husain

Pleuropulmonary blastoma (PPB) classically presents in infants or very young children with a cystic or solid lung mass that may cause pneumothorax. Biallelic mutations in *DICER1* are found in this tumor, with approximately two-thirds of patients having a germ line mutation. The DICER1 syndrome also includes (among other tumors) cystic nephroblastoma, cervical rhabdomyosarcoma, Sertoli–Leydig cell tumor of the ovary, nasal chondromesenchymal hamartoma, ciliary body medulloepithelioma, and nodular hyperplasia of the thyroid with papillary thyroid carcinoma.

PPB is known to progress from cystic (type I) to solid (type III) gross morphology by an intermediate type II (partly cystic, partly solid) with correspondingly higher risk with each progressive stage. A subset of patients with type I tumors will apparently spontaneously regress, and type Ir PPB is defined as a cystic lesion without immature cells. These patients are important to identify because of the risk of other tumor development in themselves or affected family members.

HISTOLOGIC FEATURES

Type I PPB

- Type I PPB is grossly multicystic, although microscopic thickening of septa may be seen.
- There is an abrupt transition from adjacent normal lung to cystic spaces composed of variably thin septa.
- Focal or continuous layer of immature mesenchymal cells forms a cambium layer.
- Rhabdomyoblastic differentiation may be seen.

Regressed Type Ir PPB

- Regressed type Ir PPB shows similar cystic features without immature cells.
- Areas of hemorrhage or calcification may be present.
- Because the primitive cells may be focal in type I PPB, the cyst must be completely submitted for microscopic examination to make a diagnosis of type Ir.

Type II and Type III PPB

- Type II PPB is grossly composed of solid and cystic areas.
- Type III PPB is solid.
- The malignant areas of types II and III are composed of mixtures of sarcomatous patterns including rhabdomyoblastic, spindled areas, blastemal areas, immature cartilaginous areas, and markedly atypical cells.

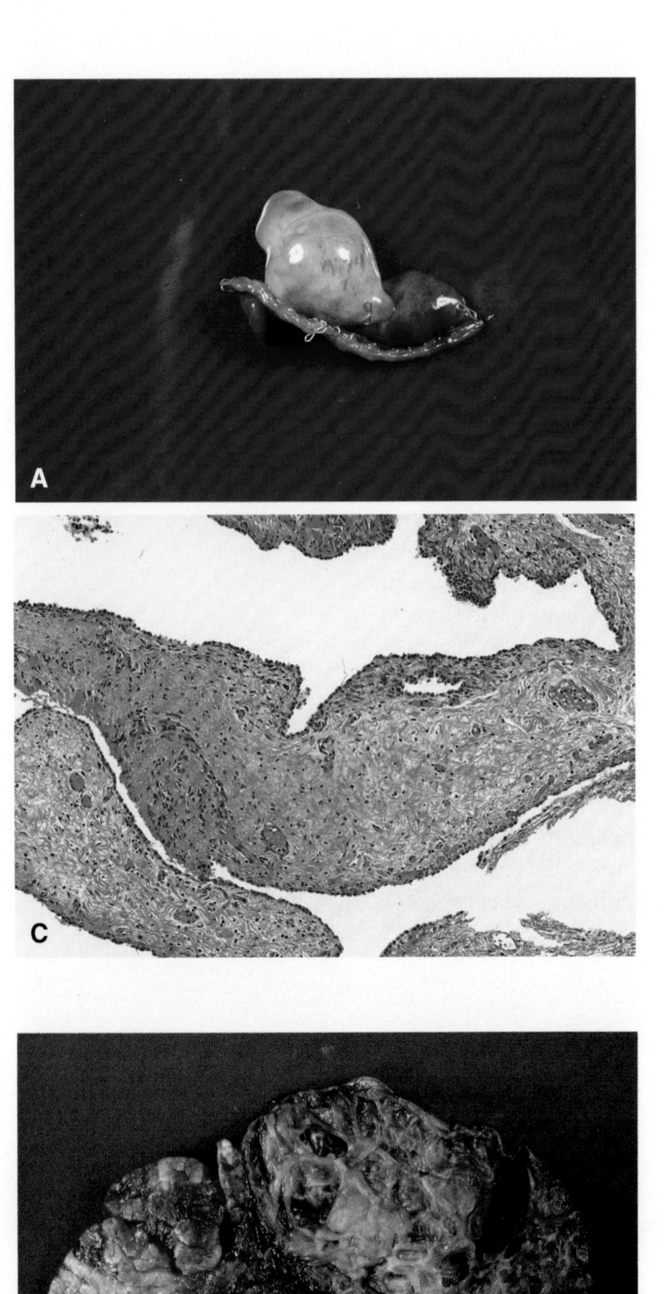

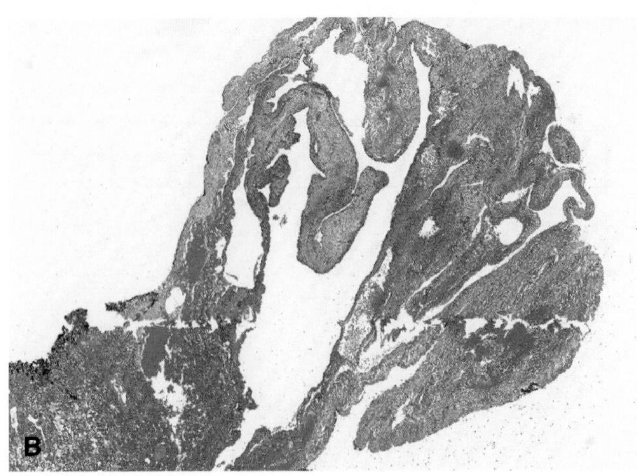

Figure 180.1 Regressed PPB with a thin-walled cyst at the periphery of the lung (**A**). The collapsed cyst has a variably thick fibrous wall (**B**) lined by flattened to cuboidal epithelium (**C**).

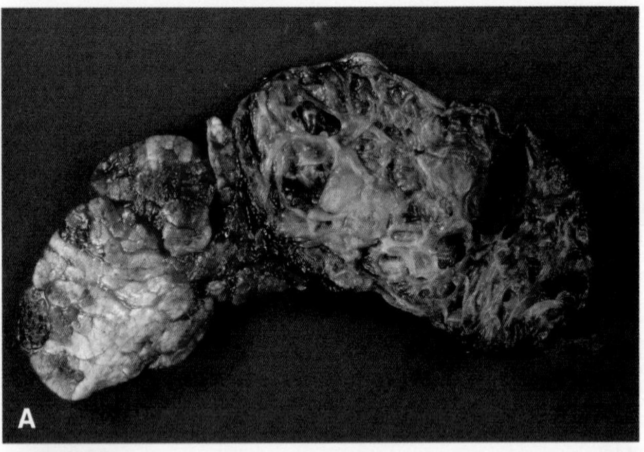

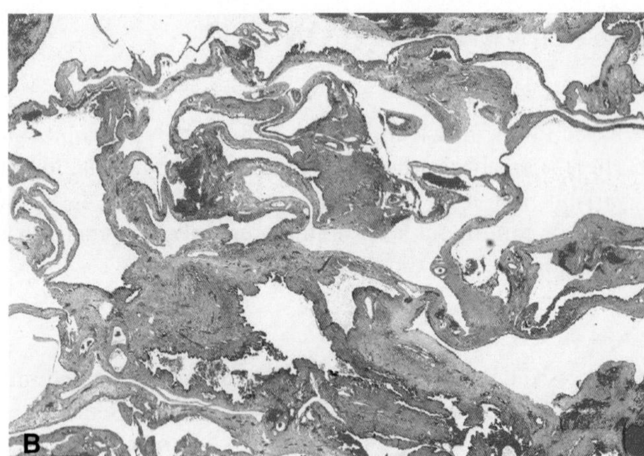

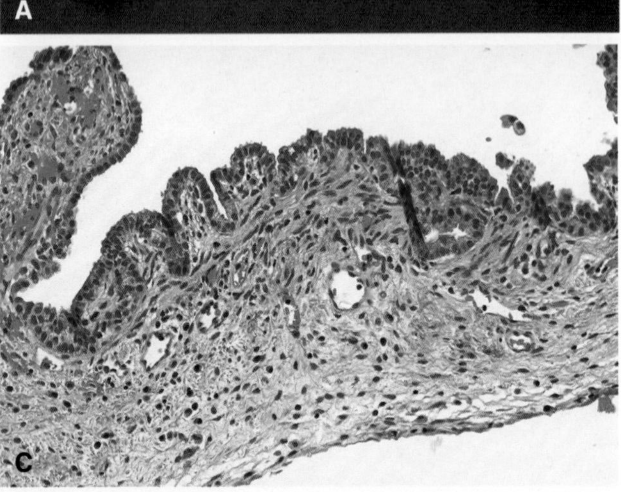

Figure 180.2 Type I (cystic) PPB (**A**) having variable fibrous cyst walls lined by flattened to cuboidal epithelium (**B**) with focal condensation of mesenchymal cells (**C**) under the epithelium.

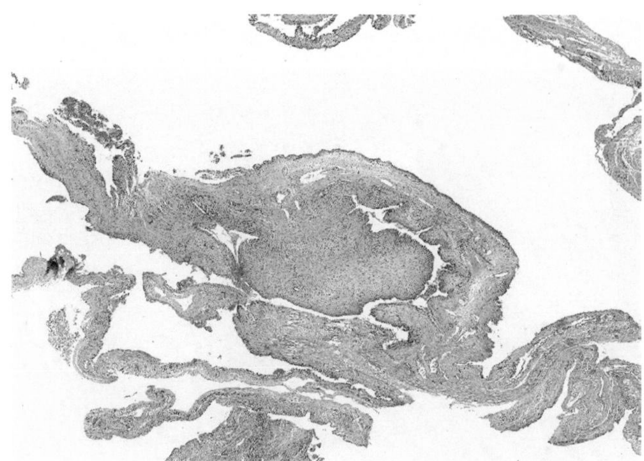

Figure 180.3 Type I PPB having fibrous walls with focal expansion composed of fine spindle cells with increased cellularity.

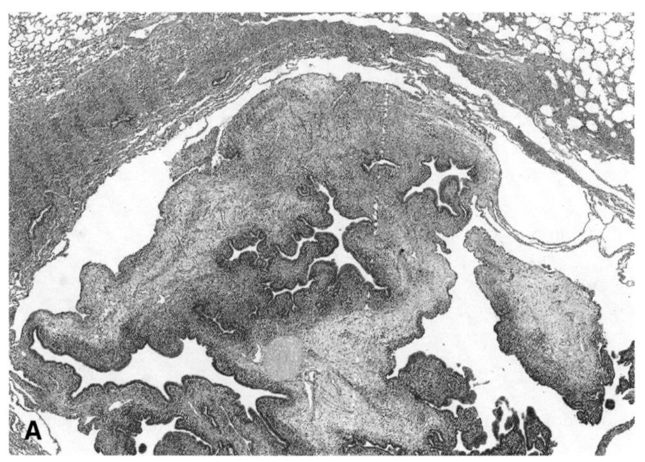

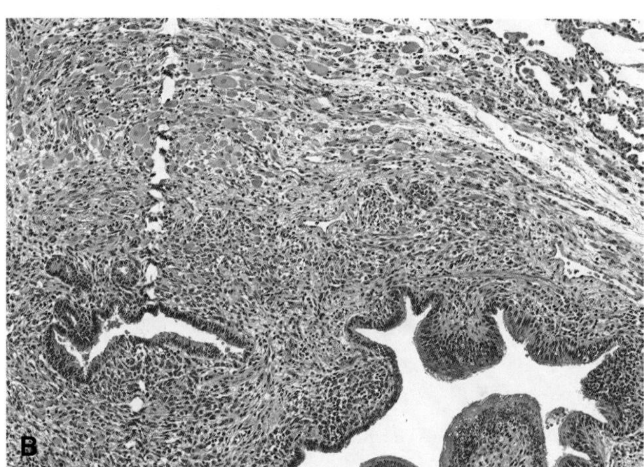

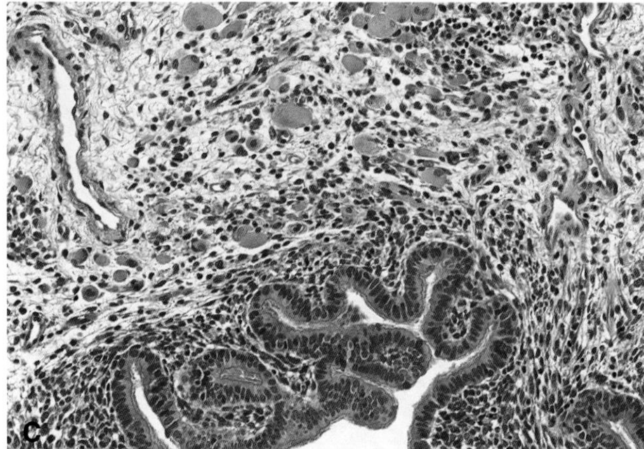

Figure 180.4 PPB progressing from cystic to solid. The epithelium varies from columnar to flattened, and there is a small nodule of cartilage formation (**A**). Mesenchymal cells are condensed below the epithelium with clear skeletal muscle differentiation (**B and C**).

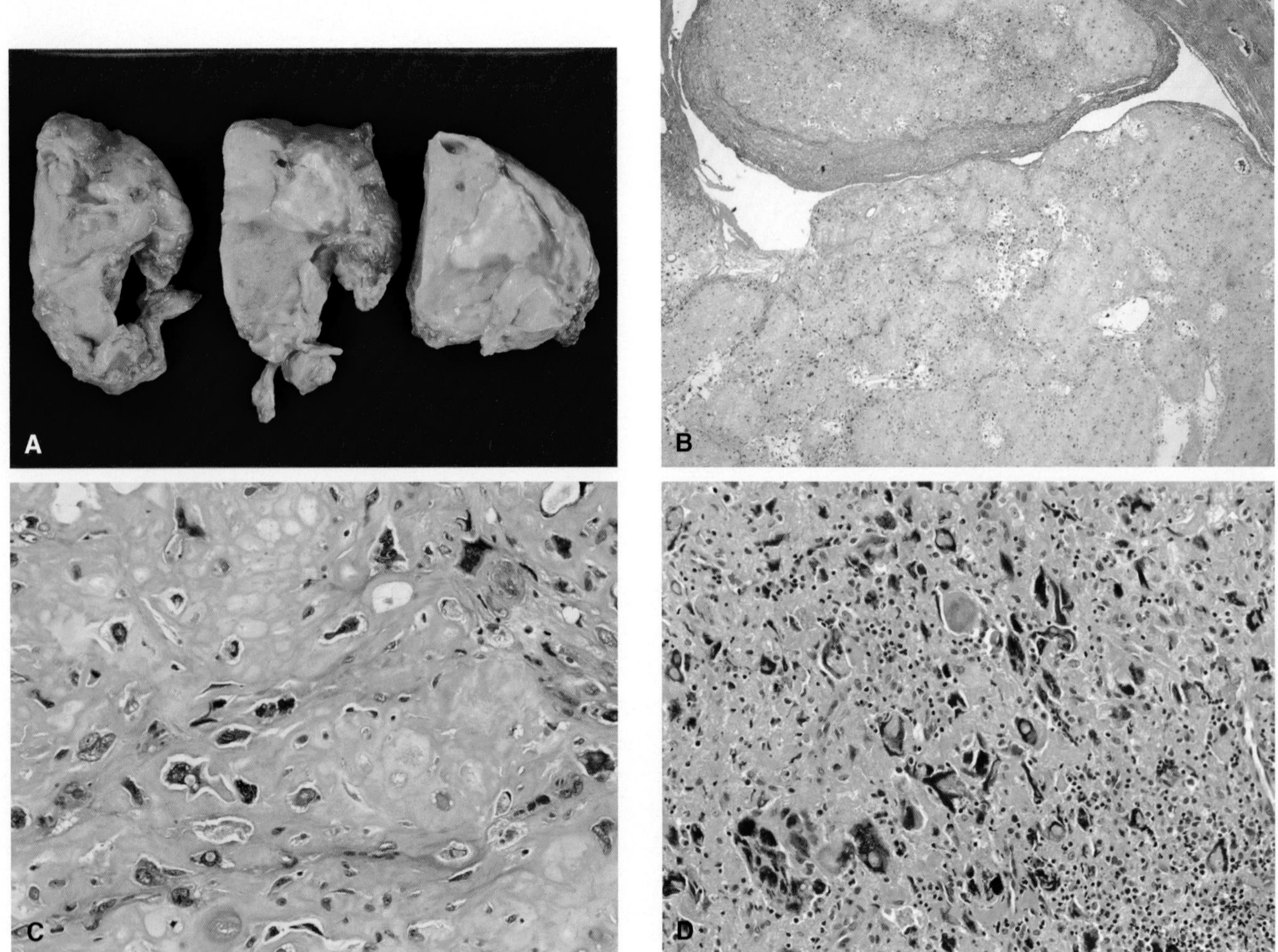

Figure 180.5 Solid PPB (**A**) having extensive atypia and areas of cartilaginous differentiation (**B and C**), as well as possible skeletal muscle differentiation (**D**).

181 Other Primary Lung Tumors in Children

Jennifer Pogoriler
Aliya N. Husain

Primary lung tumors in children are rare and most commonly include inflammatory myofibroblastic tumor, carcinoid tumor, and salivary gland–type carcinomas. Carcinoid and salivary gland tumors are morphologically identical to their adult counterparts and are not further illustrated here. Other tumors that may occur in children as primary lung tumors include leiomyoma, myofibroma, and synovial sarcoma and have the same histologic features as elsewhere in the body. Infantile hemangioendothelioma may present in infants as a bronchial mass with features similar to those seen in the skin and subcutaneous tissue of the head and neck. Fetal lung interstitial tumor and congenital peribronchial myofibroblastic tumor are tumors that are specific to the pediatric lung.

INFLAMMATORY MYOFIBROBLASTIC TUMOR

Histologic Features

- Most common primary lung tumor in children.
- These may present as a solid peripheral or hilar mass.
- Nodular collection of spindled cells with variable amounts of admixed inflammatory cells.
- Usually positive for smooth muscle actin (SMA) with a "tram track" myofibroblast appearance.
- Approximately 50% harbor ALK1 translocations.
- ALK1 immunohistochemistry is a useful surrogate, but staining may not perfectly correlate with rearrangement status.
- The majority of inflammatory myofibroblastic tumors in children have a translocation, most commonly ALK1 and ROS1. Other reported translocations include RET and PDGFRB.

CONGENITAL PERIBRONCHIAL MYOFIBROBLASTIC TUMOR

As the name suggests, this rare entity has been diagnosed in perinatal or neonatal patients. Previously this was called *congenital leiomyosarcoma* or *congenital fibrosarcoma*; mortality may be high owing to the size of the tumor and development of cardiac failure and hydrops in the fetus. However, in patients who survive to resection, malignant behavior has not been reported.

Histologic Features

- Mass formed by sheets of spindled cells in fascicles, often with extensive cartilaginous plates.
- Peripheral spread along bronchovascular bundles.

- Variable staining for muscle-specific actin, SMA, or desmin may be present but is often negative.
- Mitotic activity may be brisk, and necrosis can be present.
- Degree of proliferation and differentiation may vary with the stage of development.
- No consistent underlying genetic anomalies have been reported to date.

FETAL LUNG INTERSTITIAL TUMOR

This rare tumor presents prenatally or within the first few months of life.

Histologic Features

- Sharply demarcated from adjacent normal parenchyma.
- Variably sized airspaces with thickened septa filled by bland ovoid cells with clear cytoplasm.
- Cytoplasm is periodic acid–Schiff positive/diastase sensitive, consistent with glycogen.
- No condensation into cambium layer, mitosis, or necrosis.
- Primitive cells and rhabdomyoblastic differentiation are not present.
- Small bronchovascular-like bundles may be present within the mass.
- Variable SMA-positive and desmin-positive staining.
- Positive for vimentin.
- Single report of an ALK translocation was recently published.

INFANTILE HEMANGIOENDOTHELIOMA

Histologic Features

- Rare benign tumor usually associated with the large airways.
- Similar histology to tumors more commonly seen in the skin and liver: small vessels with plump endothelium.
- Mitotic figures may be present.
- Immunohistochemistry is positive for GLUT1 and endothelial markers (CD34 and CD31).

SYNOVIAL SARCOMA

Histologic Features

- Synovial sarcoma can rarely present as a pleural mass in children or young adults and, in a cystic form, can cause spontaneous pneumothorax.
- The genetic and histologic features are similar to those found elsewhere, although occasionally the areas of typical cellularity are not diffuse.

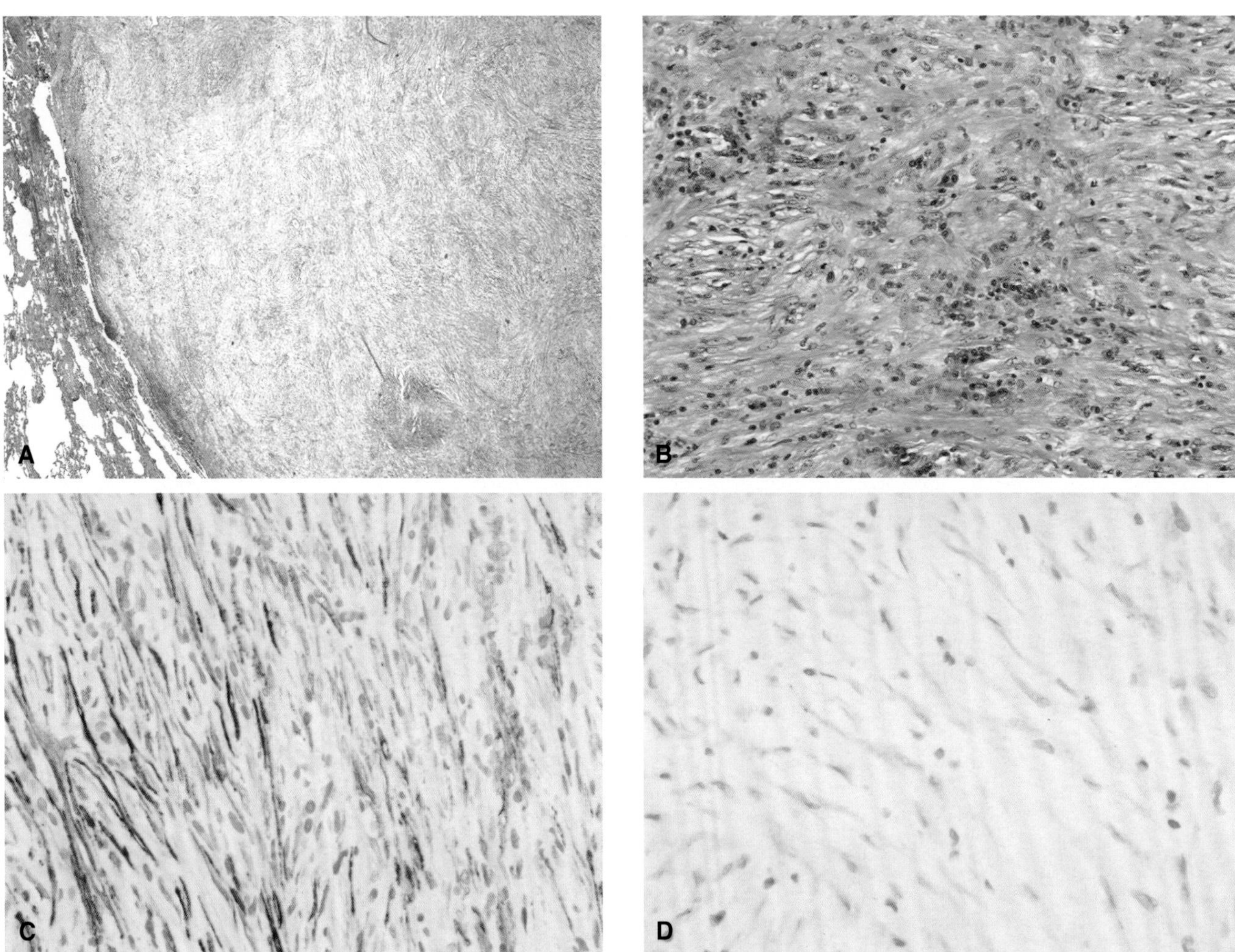

Figure 181.1 Inflammatory myofibroblastic tumor presented as a well-circumscribed nodule (**A**) composed of bland spindled cells with intermixed lymphocytes and plasma cells (**B**). The myofibroblasts are positive for SMA (**C**) and weakly positive for ALK1 (**D**) in this ALK1 translocation–positive tumor.

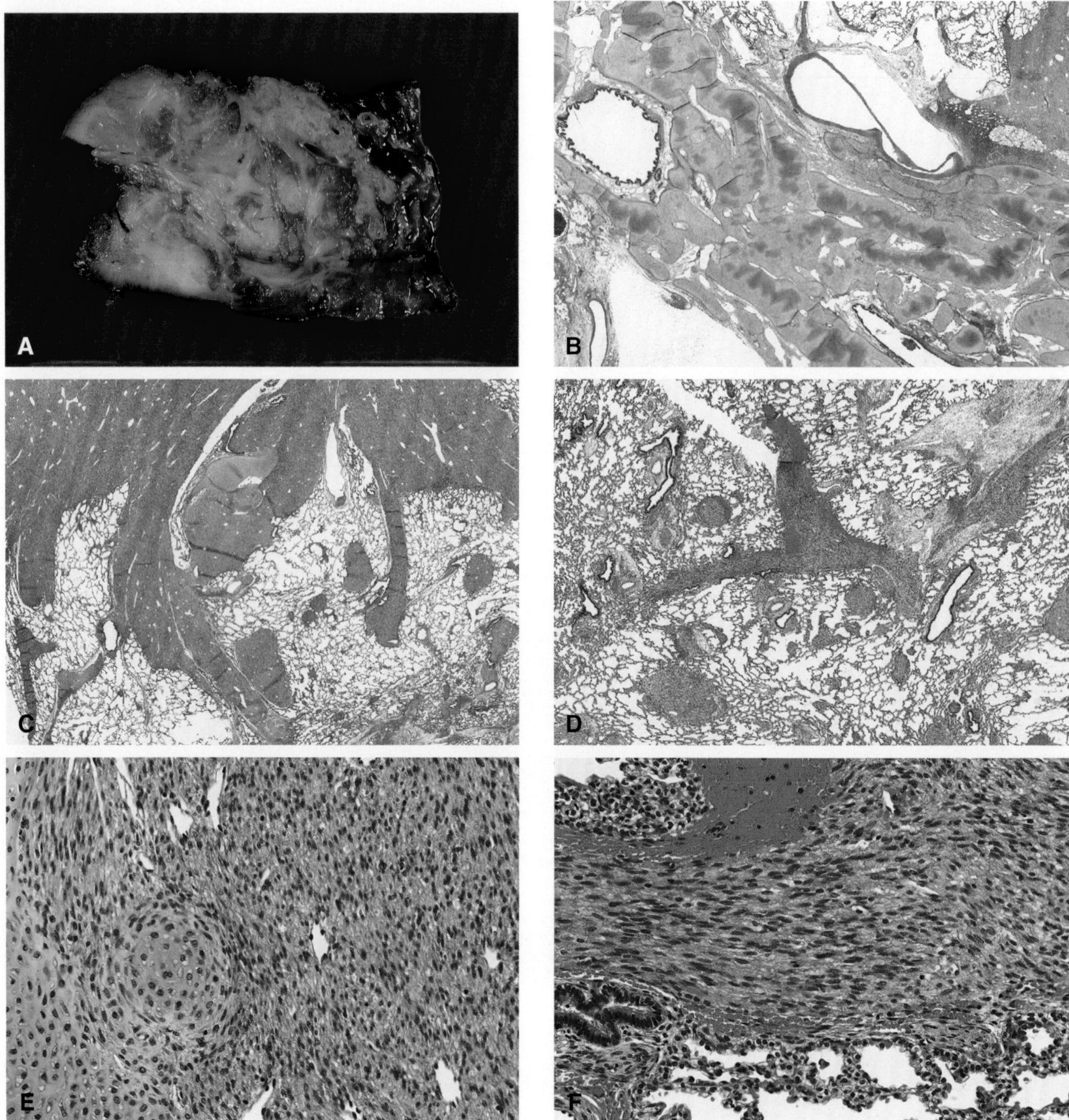

Figure 181.2 This congenital peribronchial myofibroblastic tumor grossly shows areas of glistening cartilage as well as nodules and sweeping fascicles of fibrous tissue (**A**). At low power, a combination of cellular but well-differentiated cartilage and spindled cells are seen (**B and C**), although in relatively different amounts in different areas of the tumor. Extension of the tumor is seen along bronchovascular bundles (**D**). The spindled cells and cartilaginous areas are cellular, but the nuclei are low grade. Mitotic activity is variable (**E and F**).

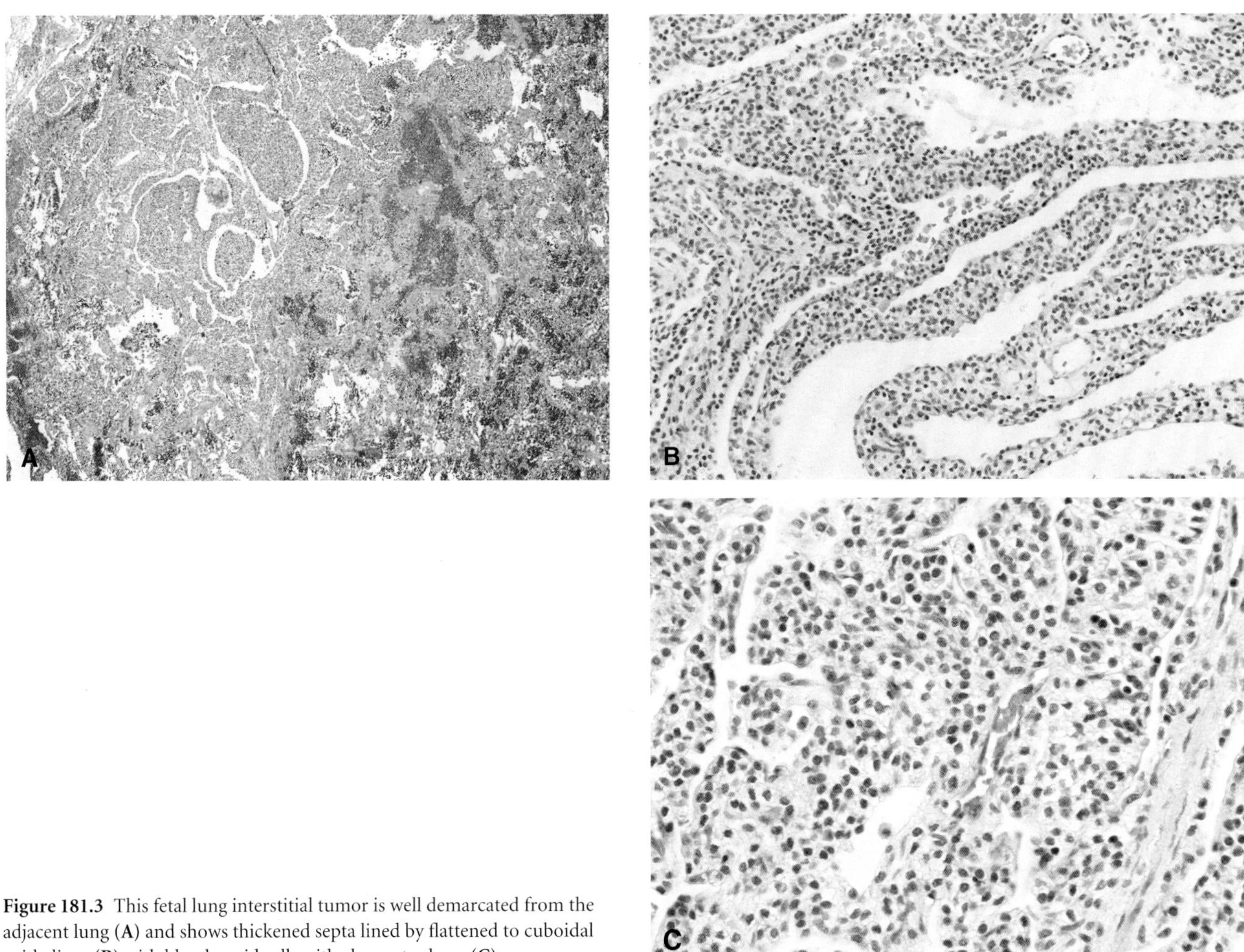

Figure 181.3 This fetal lung interstitial tumor is well demarcated from the adjacent lung (**A**) and shows thickened septa lined by flattened to cuboidal epithelium (**B**) with bland ovoid cells with clear cytoplasm (**C**).

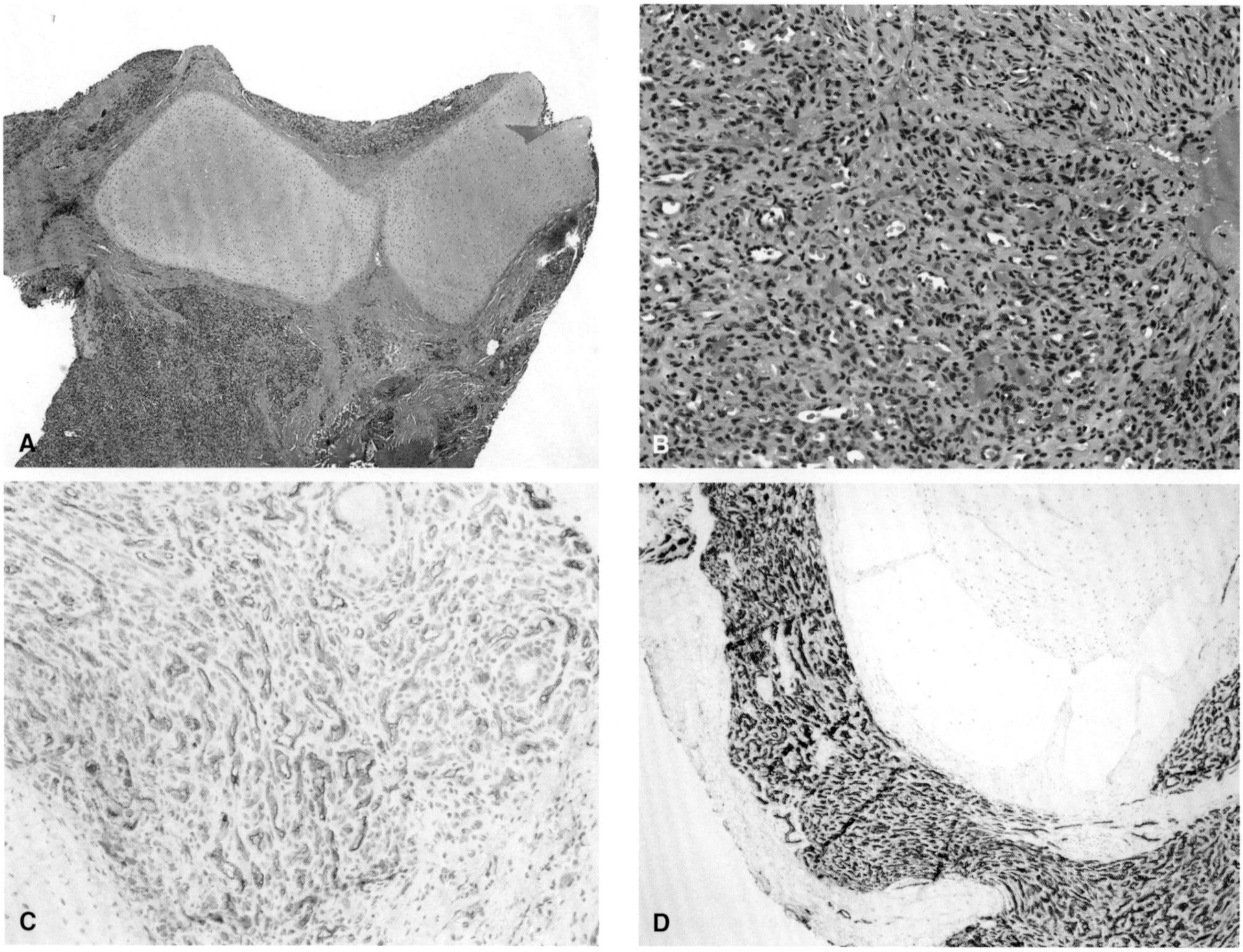

Figure 181.4 This infantile hemangioma intimately encircles bronchial cartilage bundles (**A**) and is composed of closely packed small vessels (**B**) that are positive for CD31 (**C**) and GLUT1 (**D**).

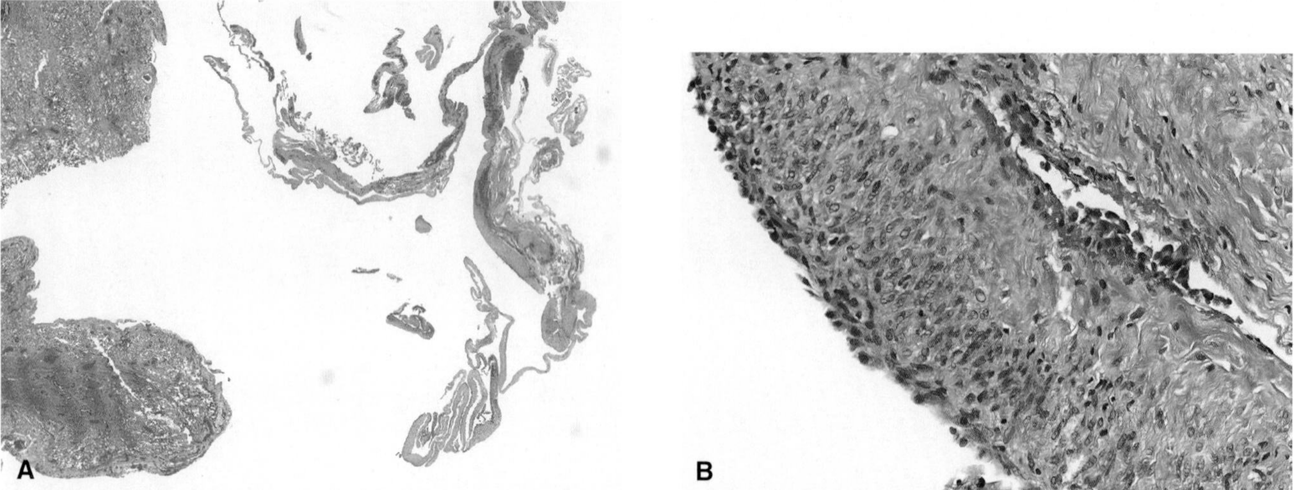

Figure 181.5 Translocation-positive synovial sarcoma presented as a cystic pleural lesion (**A**) in a 15-year-old. The majority is hypocellular with only small hypercellular foci of spindled cells (**B**).

Pediatric Tumors Metastatic to the Lung

182

Jennifer Pogoriler
Aliya N. Husain

The most common metastatic solid tumors in children are Wilms tumor, osteosarcoma, Ewing sarcoma, and rhabdomyosarcoma. Removal of metastasis may be part of treatment for disease, not just for staging or diagnosis. Involvement of the lung by hematologic malignancies, especially Hodgkin lymphoma and large B-cell lymphoma, is common and is covered in the adult section.

HISTOLOGIC FEATURES

- Metastatic tumors usually have the same features, as the original tumor and the diagnosis is often known or suspected prior to resection, although occasionally the lung lesion may be the first pathologic specimen.
- Posttherapy changes are frequent, especially in Wilms tumor and osteosarcoma.

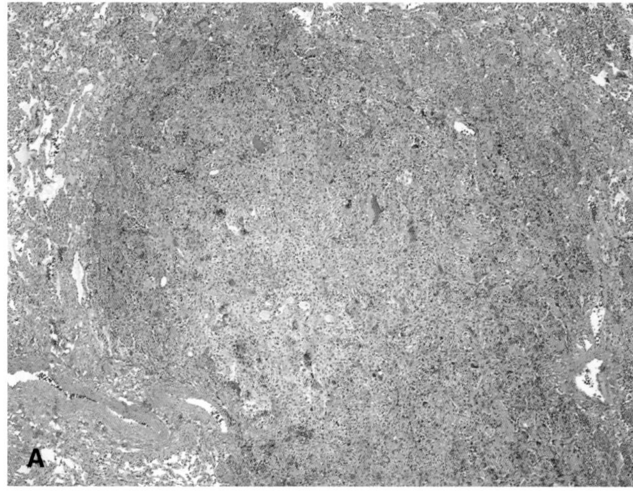

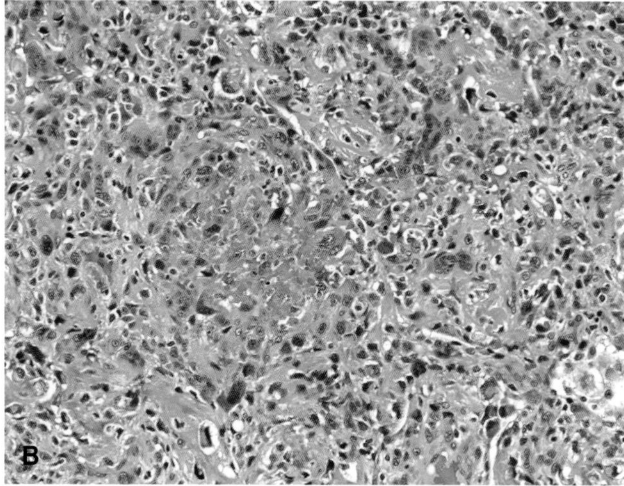

Figure 182.1 This metastatic osteosarcoma is a well-circumscribed nodule (**A**) composed of markedly atypical cells with focal lacy bone formation (**B**).

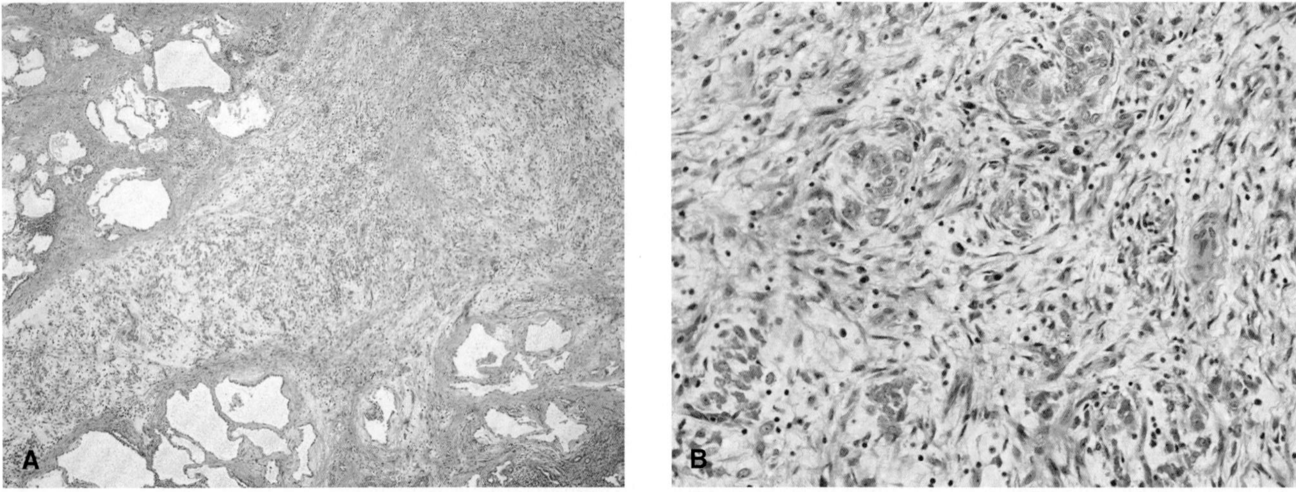

Figure 182.2 A and B: This posttreatment osteosarcoma shows extensive cartilaginous differentiation.

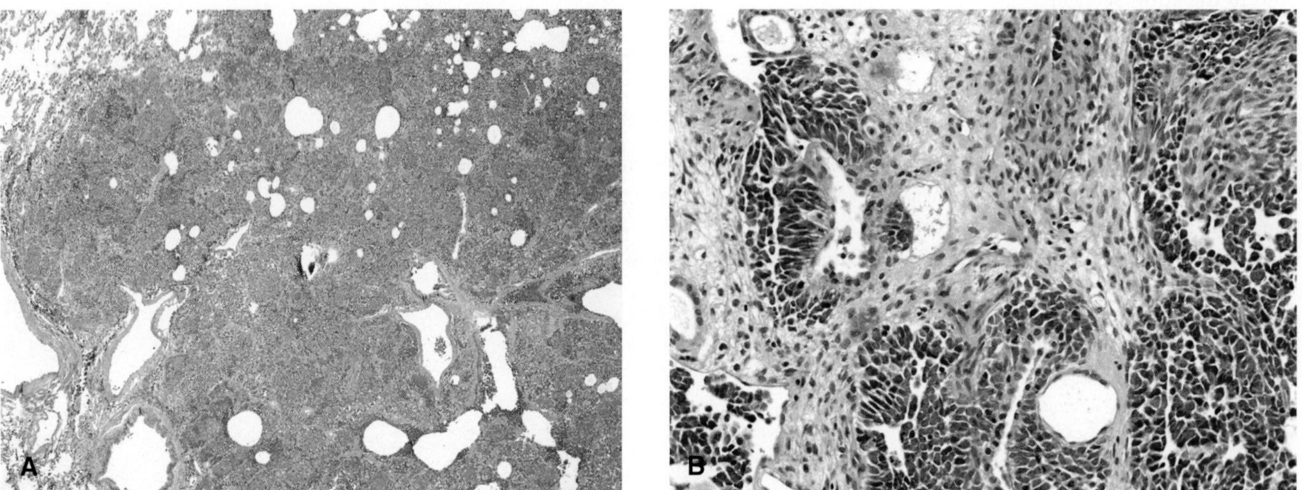

Figure 182.3 This metastatic Wilms tumor has predominantly blastemal cells filling alveolar spaces (**A**); however, foci of epithelial and stromal differentiation are present (**B**).

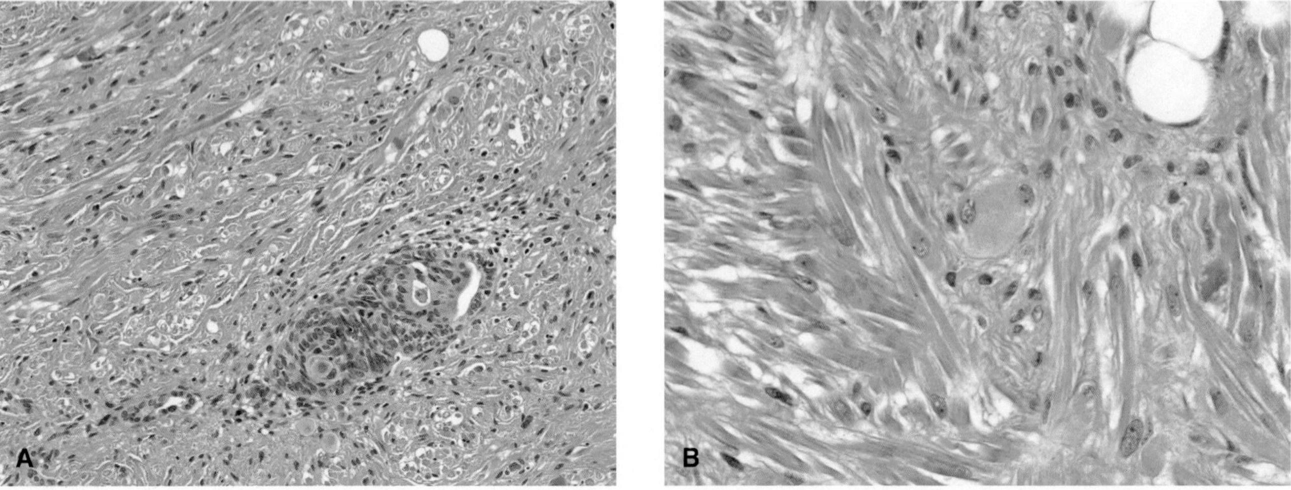

Figure 182.4 This posttreatment metastatic Wilms tumor has only small foci of blastemal tumor (**A**) and extensive rhabdomyoblastic differentiation (**B**).

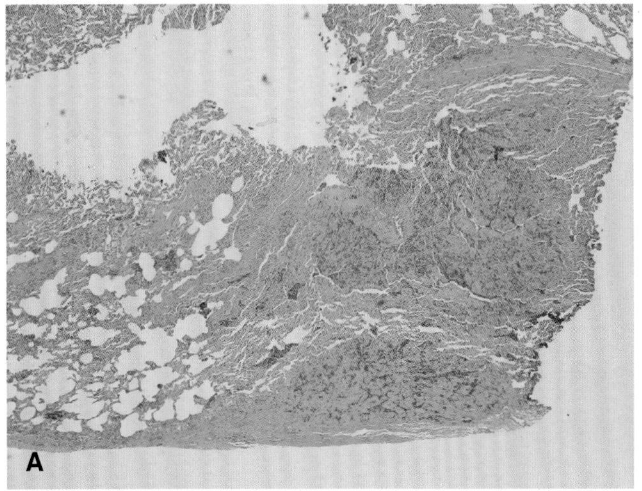

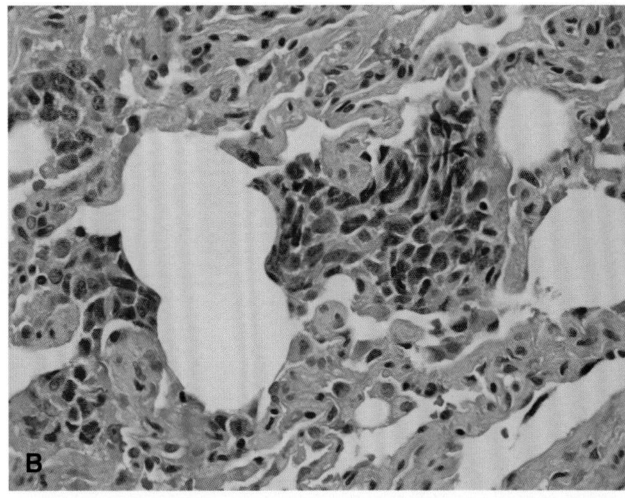

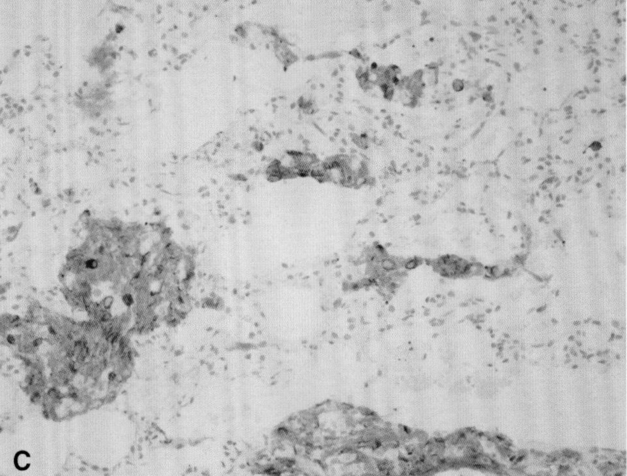

Figure 182.5 A and B: This focus of metastatic neuroblastoma has extensive crush artifact without definitive rosettes or neuropil. Immunohistochemistry for synaptophysin (**C**) is positive. (Images courtesy of Dr. Bruce Pawel, The Children's Hospital of Philadelphia.)

Bibliography

Section 1: Normal Cytology and Histology

Colby TV, Yousem SA. Lungs. In: Sternberg SS, ed. *Histology for Pathologists*. 2nd ed. Philadelphia: Lippincott Williams & Wilkins; 1997:433–435.

Gartner LP, Hiatt JL, eds. *Color Atlas of Histology*. 3rd ed. Philadelphia: Lippincott Williams & Wilkins; 2000.

Junqueira LC, Carneiro J, Kelley RO, eds. *Basic Histology*. 9th ed. New York: McGraw-Hill; 1998.

Kuhn III C. Normal anatomy and histology. In: Thurlbeck WM, Churg A, eds. *Pathology of the Lung*. 2nd ed. New York: Thieme; 1995:4–10.

Silverman JF, Atkinson BF. Respiratory cytology. In: Atkinson B, ed. *Atlas of Diagnostic Cytopathology*. Philadelphia: Saunders; 1992:137–193.

Wang NS. Anatomy. In: Dail DH, Hammar SP, eds. *Pulmonary Pathology*. 2nd ed. New York: Springer-Verlag; 1994:21–44.

Section 2: Artifacts and Age-Related Changes

Anton R, Cagle PT. Intracellular and extracellular structures. In: Cagle PT, Allen TC, Beasley MB, eds. *Diagnostic Pulmonary Pathology*. 2nd ed. New York: Informa; 2008:465–482.

Raparia K, Cagle PT. Endobronchial and transbronchial biopsies. In: Cagle PT, Allen TC, Beasley MB, eds. *Diagnostic Pulmonary Pathology*. 2nd ed. New York: Informa; 2008:11–18.

Section 3: Malignant Neoplasms

Antonescu CR, Argani P, Erlandson RA, Healey JH, Ladanyi M, Huvos AG. Skeletal and extraskeletal myxoid chondrosarcoma: a comparative clinicopathologic, ultrastructural, and molecular study. *Cancer*. 1998;83(8):1504–1521.

Antonescu CR, Tschernyavsky SJ, Woodruff JM, Jungbluth AA, Brennan MF, Ladanyi M. Molecular diagnosis of clear cell sarcoma: detection of EWS-ATF1 and MITF-M transcripts and histopathological and ultrastructural analysis of 12 cases. *J Mol Diagn*. 2002;4(1):44–52.

Antonescu CR, Le Loarer F, Mosquera JM, et al. Novel YAP1-TFE3 fusion defines a distinct subset of epithelioid hemangioendothelioma. *Genes Chromosom Cancer*. 2013;52(8):775–784. doi:10.1002/gcc.22073.

Antonescu CR, Suurmeijer AJ, Zhang L, et al. Molecular characterization of inflammatory myofibroblastic tumors with frequent ALK and ROS1 gene fusions and rare novel RET rearrangement. *Am J Surg Pathol*. 2015. doi:10.1097/PAS.0000000000000404.

Bode-Lesniewska B, Zhao J, Speel EJ, et al. Gains of 12q13-14 and overexpression of mdm2 are frequent findings in intimal sarcomas of the pulmonary artery. *Virchows Arch*. 2001;438(1):57–65. doi:10.1007/s004280000313.

Borczuk AC. Prognostic considerations of the new World Health Organization classification of lung adenocarcinoma. *Eur Respir Rev*. December 2016;25(142):364–371.

Boucher LD, Swanson PE, Stanley MW, Silverman JF, Raab SS, Geisinger KR. Cytology of angiosarcoma: findings in fourteen fine-needle aspiration biopsy specimens and one pleural fluid specimen. *Am J Clin Pathol*. 2000;114(2):210–219.

Broehm CJ, Wu J, Gullapalli RR, Bocklage T. Extraskeletal myxoid chondrosarcoma with a t(9;16)(q22;p11.2) resulting in a NR4A3-FUS fusion. *Cancer Genet*. 2014;207(6):276–280.

Burke AP, Yi ES. Pulmonary artery intimal sarcoma. In: Travis WD, Brambilla E, Burke AP, Marx A, Nicholson AG, eds. *WHO Classification of Tumours of the Lung, Pleura, Thymus, and Heart*. 4th ed. Lyon: IARC; 2015:128–129.

Cagle P, Dacic S. Epithelioid hemangioendothelioma. In: Travis WD, Brambilla E, Burke AP, Marx A, Nicholson AG, eds. *WHO Classification of Tumours of the Lung, Pleura, Thymus, and Heart*. 4th ed. Lyon: IARC; 2015:123–124.

Cai S, Zhao W, Nie X, et al. Multimorbidity and genetic characteristics of DICER1 syndrome based on systematic review. *J Pediatr Hematol Oncol.* July 2017;39(5):355–361. doi:10.1097/MPH.0000000000000715.

Chamberlain BK, McClain CM, Gonzalez RS, Coffin CM, Cates JMM. Alveolar soft part sarcoma and granular cell tumor: an immunohistochemical comparison study. *Hum Pathol.* 2014;45(5):1039–1044.

Choi E-YK, Gardner JM, Lucas DR, McHugh JB, Patel RM. Ewing sarcoma. *Semin Diagn Pathol.* 2014;31(1):39–47. Available from: http://www.sciencedirect.com/science/article/pii/S0740257014000033.

Choong PFM, Broadhead ML, Clark JCM, Myers DE, Dass CR. The molecular pathogenesis of osteosarcoma: a review. *Sarcoma.* 2011;2011.

Cleven AHG, Sannaa GA, Briaire-de Bruijn I, et al. Loss of H3K27 tri-methylation is a diagnostic marker for malignant peripheral nerve sheath tumors and an indicator for an inferior survival. *Mod Pathol.* 2016;29(6):582–590.

Coindre JM, Pédeutour F, Aurias A. Well-differentiated and dedifferentiated liposarcomas. *Virchows Archiv.* 2010;456:167–179.

Dacic S, Franks TJ, Ladanyi M. Synovial sarcoma. In: Travis WD, Brambilla E, Burke AP, Marx A, Nicholson AG, eds. *WHO Classification of Tumours of the Lung, Pleura, Thymus, and Heart.* 4th ed. Lyon: IARC; 2015:127–128.

de Alava E, Ladanyi M, Rosai J, Gerald WL. Detection of chimeric transcripts in desmoplastic small round cell tumor and related developmental tumors by reverse transcriptase polymerase chain reaction. A specific diagnostic assay. *Am J Pathol.* 1995;147(6):1584–1591.

De Giovanni C, Landuzzi L, Nicoletti G, Lollini P-L, Nanni P. Molecular and cellular biology of rhabdomyosarcoma. *Futur Oncol.* 2009;5(9):1449–1475. Available from: http://www.futuremedicine.com/doi/10.2217/fon.09.97.

Dehner LP, Messinger YH, Schultz KA, Williams GM, Wikenheiser-Brokamp K, Hill DA. Pleuropulmonary blastoma: evolution of an entity as an entry into a familial tumor predisposition syndrome. *Pediatr Dev Pathol.* 2015;18(6):504–511. doi:10.2350/15-10-1732-OA.1.

Dim DC, Cooley LD, Miranda RN. Clear cell sarcoma of tendons and aponeuroses: a review. *Arch Pathol Lab Med.* 2007;131:152–156.

Dodd LG. Fine-needle aspiration of chondrosarcoma. *Diagn Cytopathol.* 2006;34:413–418.

Domanski HA, Åkerman M. Fine-needle aspiration of primary osteosarcoma: a cytological-histological study. *Diagn Cytopathol.* 2005;32:269–275.

Douglass EC, Shapiro DN, Valentine M, et al. Alveolar rhabdomyosarcoma with the t(2;13): cytogenetic findings and clinicopathologic correlations. *Med Pediatr Oncol.* 1993;21(2):83–87.

Doyle LA, Vivero M, Fletcher CD, Mertens F, Hornick JL. Nuclear expression of STAT6 distinguishes solitary fibrous tumor from histologic mimics. *Mod Pathol.* March 2014;27(3):390–395. doi:10.1038/modpathol.2013.164.

Doyle LA, Fletcher CD, Hornick JL. Nuclear expression of CAMTA1 distinguishes epithelioid hemangioendothelioma from histologic mimics. *Am J Surg Pathol.* 2016;40(1):94–102. doi:10.1097/PAS.0000000000000511.

England DM, Hochholzer L, McCarthy MJ. Localized benign and malignant fibrous tumors of the pleura. A clinicopathologic review of 223 cases. *Am J Surg Pathol.* 1989;13(8).

Flanagan A, Yamaguchi T. Chordoma. In: Fletcher C, Bridge J, Hogendoorn P, Mertens F, eds. *WHO Classification of Tumours of Soft Tissue and Bone.* 4th ed. Lyon: IARC; 2013:228–229.

Fletcher CDM, Gibbs A. Solitary fibrous tumor. In: Fletcher CDM, Bridge JA, Hogendoorn PCW, Mertens F, eds. *WHO Classification of Tumours of Soft Tissue and Bone.* 4th ed. Lyon: IARC; 2013.

Fletcher C, Bridge J, Hogendoorn P, Mertens F, eds. Malignant peripheral nerve sheath tumor. In: *WHO Classification of Tumours of Soft Tissue and Bone.* 4th ed. Lyon: IARC; 2013: 187–189.

Fletcher C, Chibon F, Mertens F. Undifferentiated/unclassified sarcomas. In: Fletcher C, Bridge J, Hogendoorn P, Mertens F, eds. *WHO Classification of Tumours of Soft Tissue and Bone.* 4th ed. Lyon: IARC; 2013:236–238.

Ginter PS, Mosquera JM, Macdonald TY, D'Alfonso TM, Rubin MA, Shin SJ. Diagnostic utility of MYC amplification and anti-MYC immunohistochemistry in atypical vascular lesions, primary or radiation-induced mammary angiosarcomas, and primary angiosarcomas of other sites. *Hum Pathol.* 2014;45(4):709–716.

Huo L, Moran CA, Fuller GN, Gladish G, Suster S. Pulmonary artery sarcoma: a clinicopathologic and immunohistochemical study of 12 cases. *Am J Clin Pathol.* 2006;125(3):419–424. doi:10.1309/9H8R-HUV1-JL1W-E0QF.

Hart J, Mandavilli S. Epithelioid angiosarcoma: a brief diagnostic review and differential diagnosis. *Arch Pathol Lab Med.* 2011;135:268–272.

Hisaoka M, Ishida T, Kuo T-T, et al. Clear cell sarcoma of soft tissue: a clinicopathologic, immunohistochemical, and molecular analysis of 33 cases. 2008;32(3):452–460.

Hornick JL, Sholl LM, Dal Cin P, Childress MA, Lovly CM. Expression of ROS1 predicts ROS1 gene rearrangement in inflammatory myofibroblastic tumors. *Mod Pathol.* 2015;28(5): 732–739. doi:10.1038/modpathol.2014.165.

Jaber OI, Kirby PA. Alveolar soft part sarcoma. *Am J Surg Pathol.* 2015;139:1459–1462.

Jakowski JD, Wakely PE. Cytopathology of extraskeletal myxoid chondrosarcoma: report of 8 cases. *Cancer.* 2007;111(5):298–305.

Jeon YK, Moon KC, Park SH, Chung DH. Primary pulmonary myxoid sarcomas with EWSR1-CREB1 translocation might originate from primitive peribronchial mesenchymal cells undergoing (myo)fibroblastic differentiation. *Virchows Arch.* 2014;465(4):453–461. doi:10.1007/s00428-014-1645-z.

Errani C, Zhang L, Sung YS, et al. A novel WWTR1-CAMTA1 gene fusion is a consistent abnormality in epithelioid hemangioendothelioma of different anatomic sites. *Genes Chromosom Cancer.* 2011;50(8):644–653. doi:10.1002/gcc.20886.

Kerr DA, Lopez HU, Deshpande V, et al. Molecular distinction of chondrosarcoma from chondroblastic osteosarcoma through IDH1/2 mutations. *Am J Surg Pathol.* 2013;37(6):787–795.

Khin T, Fisher C. Tumors with EWSR1-CREB1 and EWSR1-ATF1 fusions. *Am J Surg Pathol.* 2012;36(7):e1–e11. doi:10.1097/PAS.0b013e31825485c5.

Khin T, Jones RL, Noujaim J, Zaidi S, Miah AB, Fisher C. Dedifferentiated liposarcoma. *Adv Anat Pathol.* 2016;23(1):30–40. doi:10.1097/PAP.0000000000000101.

Kim KH, Roberts CWM. Mechanisms by which SMARCB1 loss drives rhabdoid tumor growth. *Cancer Genet.* 2014;207:365–372.

Klein MJ, Siegal GP. Osteosarcoma. *Am J Clin Pathol.* 2006;125(4):555–581.

Klijanienko J, Caillaud JM, Lagac R. Fine-Needle aspiration in liposarcoma: cytohistologic correlative study including well-differentiated, myxoid, and pleomorphic variants. *Diagn Cytopathol.* 2004;30:307–312.

Klijanienko J, Couturier J, Bourdeaut F, et al. Fine-needle aspiration as a diagnostic technique in 50 cases of primary Ewing sarcoma/peripheral neuroectodermal tumor. Institut Curie's experience. *Diagn Cytopathol.* 2012;40(1):19–25.

Koelsche C, Schweizer L, Renner M, et al. Nuclear relocation of STAT6 reliably predicts NAB2-STAT6 fusion for the diagnosis of solitary fibrous tumour. *Histopathology.* 2014;65(5):613–622. doi:10.1111/his.12431.

Koss MN. Malignant and benign lymphoid lesions of the lung. *Ann Diagn Pathol.* 2004;8:167–187.

Lae ME, Roche PC, Jin L, Lloyd RV, Nascimento AG. Desmoplastic small round cell tumor: a clinicopathologic, immunohistochemical, and molecular study of 32 tumors. *Am J Surg Pathol.* 2002;26(7):823–835.

Lindeman NI, Cagle PT, Aisner D, et al. Updated molecular testing guideline for the selection of lung cancer patients for treatment with targeted tyrosine kinase inhibitors: guideline from the College of American Pathologists, International Association for the Study of Lung Cancer, and the Association for Molecular Pathology. *Arch Pathol Lab Med.* 2018 (in press).

Le Loarer F, Watson S, Pierron G, et al. SMARCA4 inactivation defines a group of undifferentiated thoracic malignancies transcriptionally related to BAF-deficient sarcomas. *Nat Genet.* 2015;47(10):1200–1205. doi:10.1038/ng.3399.

Lovly CM, Gupta A, Lipson D, et al. Inflammatory myofibroblastic tumors harbor multiple potentially actionable kinase fusions. *Cancer Discov.* 2014. doi:10.1158/2159-8290.CD-14-0377.

Machado I, Navarro S, Llombart-Bosch A. Ewing sarcoma and the new emerging Ewing-like sarcomas: (CIC and BCOR-rearranged-sarcomas). A systematic review. *Histol Histopathol.* 2016;31:1169–1181.

Mandong BM, Ngbea JA. Childhood rhabdomyosarcoma: a review of 35 cases and literature. *Niger J Med.* 2011;20(4):466–469.

Messinger YH, Stewart DR, Priest JR, et al. Pleuropulmonary blastoma: a report on 350 central pathology-confirmed pleuropulmonary blastoma cases by the international pleuropulmonary blastoma registry. *Cancer.* 2015;121(2):276–285. doi:10.1002/cncr.29032.

Miettinen M. Smooth muscle tumors of soft tissue and non-uterine viscera: biology and prognosis. *Mod Pathol.* 2014;27:S17–S29. Available from: http://www.nature.com/doifinder/10.1038/modpathol.2013.178.

Montgomery E, Barr F. Pleomorphic rhabdomyosarcoma. In: Fletcher C, Bridge J, Hogendoorn P, Mertens F, eds. *WHO Classification of Tumours of Soft Tissue and Bone.* 4th ed. Lyon: IARC; 2013:132–133.

Murphy AJ, Bishop K, Pereira C, et al. A new molecular variant of desmoplastic small round cell tumor: significance of WT1 immunostaining in this entity. *Hum Pathol.* 2008;39(12):1763–1770.

Naka N, Ohsawa M, Tomita Y, Kanno H, Aozasa K, Uchida A. Angiosarcoma in Japan. A review of 99 cases. *Cancer*. 1995;75(4):989–996.

Nascimento A, FG B. Spindle cell/sclerosing rhabdomyosarcoma. In: Fletcher C, Bridge J, Hogendoorn P, Mertens F, eds. *WHO Classification of Tumours of Soft Tissue and Bone*. 4th ed. Lyon: IARC; 2013:134–135.

Nicholson AG. Pulmonary myxoid sarcoma with EWSR1-CREB1 translocation. In: Travis WD, Brambilla E, Burke AP, Marx A, Nicholson AG, eds. *WHO Classification of Tumours of the Lung, Pleura, Thymus, and Heart*. 4th ed. Lyon: IARC; 2015:129–130.

Oda Y, Biegel J. Extrarenal rhabdoid tumor. In: Fletcher C, Bridge J, Hogendoorn P, Mertens F, eds. *WHO Classification of Tumours of Soft Tissue and Bone*. 4th ed. Lyon: IARC; 2013:228–229.

Ottaviani G, Jaffe N. The epidemiology of osteosarcoma. *Cancer Treat Res*. 2009;152:3–13.

Parham D, Barr F. Embryonal rhabdomyosarcoma. In: Fletcher C, Bridge J, Hogendoorn P, Mertens F, eds. *WHO Classification of Tumours of Soft Tissue and Bone*. 4th ed. Lyon: IARC; 2013:178–179.

Pina-Oviedo S, Weissferdt A, Kalhor N, Moran CA. Primary pulmonary lymphomas. *Adv Anat Pathol*. 2015;22:355–375.

Pritchard DJ, Lunke RJ, Taylor WF, Dahlin DC, Medley BE. Chondrosarcoma: a clinicopathologic and statistical analysis. *Cancer*. 1980;45(1):149–157.

Purgina B, Rao UNM, Miettinen M, Pantanowitz L. Aids-Related EBV-associated smooth muscle tumors: a review of 64 published cases. *Patholog Res Int*. 2011;2011:1–10.

Radu O, Pantanowitz L. Kaposi sarcoma. *Arch Pathol Lab Med*. 2013;137(2):289–294. doi:10.5858/arpa.2012-0101-RS.

Raparia K, Sirajuddin A. Chapter 8. Lymphomas. In: Cagle PT, Allen TC, eds. *Lung and Pleural Pathology*. New York: McGraw-Hill; 2016:141–157.

Robinson DR, Wu YM, Kalyana-Sundaram S, et al. Identification of recurrent NAB2-STAT6 gene fusions in solitary fibrous tumor by integrative sequencing. *Nat Genet*. 2013;45(2):180–185. doi:10.1038/ng.2509.

Schaefer I-M, Fletcher CD, Hornick JL. Loss of H3K27 trimethylation distinguishes malignant peripheral nerve sheath tumors from histologic mimics. *Mod Pathol*. 2016;29(1):4–13.

Sharma A, Bhutoria B, Guha D, Bhattacharya S, Wasim NA. Fine needle aspiration cytology of metastatic alveolar rhabdomyosarcoma. *J Cytol*. 2011;28(3):121–123.

Smith SC, Palanisamy N, Betz BL, et al. At the intersection of primary pulmonary myxoid sarcoma and pulmonary angiomatoid fibrous histiocytoma: observations from three new cases. *Histopathology*. 2014;65(1):144–146. doi:10.1111/his.12354.

Speetjens FM, de Jong Y, Gelderblom H, Bovée JVMG. Molecular oncogenesis of chondrosarcoma. *Curr Opin Oncol*. 2016;28(4):314–322.

Suster S, Moran CA. Lung neoplasms, malignant, primary: lymphoproliferative disorders. In: Thoracic. Suster S, Moran CA, eds. *Diagnostic Pathology Series*. Manitoba: Amirsys, 2012: Part 1, Section 2, 152–183.

Thomas DM, Conyers R, Young S. Liposarcoma: molecular genetics and therapeutics. *Sarcoma*. 2011;2011.

Thway K, Nicholson AG, Lawson K, et al. Primary pulmonary myxoid sarcoma with EWSR1-CREB1 fusion: a new tumor entity. *Am J Surg Pathol*. 2011;35(11):1722–1732. doi:10.1097/PAS.0b013e318227e4d2.

Thway K, Jones RL, Noujaim J, Zaidi S, Miah AB, Fisher C. Dedifferentiated liposarcoma. *Adv Anat Pathol*. 2016;23(1):30–40.

Travis WD, Brambilla E, Noguchi M, et al. International Association for the Study of Lung Cancer/American Thoracic Society/European Respiratory Society international multidisciplinary classification of lung adenocarcinoma. *J Thorac Oncol*. 2011;6(2):244–285.

Travis WD, Brambilla E, Noguchi M, et al. Diagnosis of lung cancer in small biopsies and cytology: implications of the 2011 International Association for the Study of Lung Cancer/American Thoracic Society/European Respiratory Society classification. *Arch Pathol Lab Med*. May 2013;137(5):668–684.

Travis WD, Brambilla E, Burke AP, Marx A, Nicholson AG, eds. *WHO Classification of Tumours of the Lung, Pleura, Thymus and Heart*. 4th ed. Lyon, France: IARC Press; 2015. *World Health Organization Classification of Tumours*; vol. 7.

Truini A, Santos Pereira P, Cavazza A, et al. Classification of different patterns of pulmonary adenocarcinomas. *Expert Rev Respir Med*. October 2015;9(5):571–586.

Vujovic S, Henderson S, Presneau N, et al. Brachyury, a crucial regulator of notochordal development, is a novel biomarker for chordomas. *J Pathol*. 2006;209(2):157–165.

Wakely PE, McDermott JE, Ali SZ. Cytopathology of alveolar soft part sarcoma. *Cancer Cytopathol*. 2009;117(6):500–507.

Wakely PEJ, Ali SZ, Bishop JA. The cytopathology of malignant peripheral nerve sheath tumor: a report of 55 fine-needle aspiration cases. *Cancer Cytopathol.* 2012;120(5):334–341.

Weiss S, Antonescu C, Deyrup A. Angiosarcoma of soft tissue. In: Fletcher C, Bridge J, Hogendoorn P, Mertens F, eds. *WHO Classification of Tumours of Soft Tissue and Bone.* 4th ed. Lyon: IARC; 2013:156–158.

Yang J, Du X, Chen K, et al. Genetic aberrations in soft tissue leiomyosarcoma. *Cancer Letters.* 2009;275:1–8.

Yoshida A, Kobayashi E, Kubo T, et al. 2017. Clinicopathological and molecular characterization of SMARCA4-deficient thoracic sarcomas with comparison to potentially related entities. *Mod Pathol.* doi:10.1038/modpathol.2017.11.

Section 4: Benign Neoplasms

Borczuk AC. Neoplastic and nonneoplastic benign mass lesions of the lung. *Arch Pathol Lab Med.* 2012;136(10):1227–1233.

Fletcher CDM, Cagle P, Desmoid-type fibromatosis. In: Travis WD, Brambilla E, Burke A, Marx A, Nicholson A, eds. *WHO Classification of Tumours of the Lung, Pleura, Thymus and Heart.* 4th ed. Lyon, France: International Agency for Research on Cancer, World Health Organization; 2015.

Laskin WB, Villa C, Golden K, Yeldandi A. Benign lung neoplasms. In: Cagle PT, Allen TC, eds. *Lung and Pleural Pathology.* New York, NY: McGraw Hill; 2015:159–194.

Ohori P. Uncommon endobronchial neoplasms. In: Cagle PT, Allen TC, Beasley MB, eds. *Diagnostic Pulmonary Pathology.* 2nd ed. New York: Informa; 2008:705–730.

Satoh Y, Tsuchiya E, Weng SY, et al. Pulmonary sclerosing hemangioma of the lung. A type II pneumocytoma by immunohistochemical and immunoelectron microscopic studies. *Cancer.* 1989;64(6):1310–1317.

Weissferdt A, Moran CA. Primary vascular tumors of the lungs: a review. *Ann Diagn Pathol.* 2010;14(4):296–308.

Section 5: Pulmonary Histiocytic Proliferations

Alayed K, Medeiros LJ, Patel KP, et al. BRAF and MAP2K1 mutations in Langerhans cell histiocytosis: a study of 50 cases. *Hum Patho.* 2016;52:61–67.

Bubolz AM, Weissinger SE, Stenzinger A, et al. Potential clinical implications of BRAF mutations in histiocytic proliferations. *Oncotarget.* 2014;5:4060–4070.

Cives M, Simone V, Rizzo FM, et al. Erdheim-Chester disease: a systematic review. *Crit Rev Oncol Hematol.* 2015;95:1–11.

DeMartino E, Go RS, Vassallo R. Langerhans cell histiocytosis and other histiocytic diseases of the lung. *Clin Chest Med.* 2016;37:421–430.

Dimmler A, Geddert H, Werner M, Faller G. Molecular analysis of BRAF V600E mutation in multiple nodules of pulmonary Langerhans cell histiocytosis. *Virchows Arch.* 2017;470:429–435.

Elia D, Torre O, Cassandro R, Caminati A, Harari S. Pulmonary Langerhans cell histiocytosis: a comprehensive analysis of 40 patients and literature review. *Eur J Intern Med.* 2015;26:351–356.

Emile JF, Abla O, Fraitag S, et al. Revised classification of histiocytoses and neoplasms of the macrophage-dendritic cell lineages. *Blood.* 2016;127:2672–2681.

Emile JF, Diamond EL, Helias-Rodzewicz Z, et al. Recurrent RAS and PIK3CA mutations in Erdheim-Chester disease. *Blood.* 2014;124:3016–3019.

Haroche J, Arnaud L, Cohen-Aubart F, et al. Erdheim-Chester disease. *Curr Rheumatol Rep.* 2014;16:412.

Haroche J, Charlotte F, Arnaud L, et al. High prevalence of BRAF V600E mutations in Erdheim-Chester disease but not in other non-Langerhans cell histiocytoses. *Blood.* 2012;120:2700–2703.

Hervier B, Haroche J, Arnaud L, et al. Association of both Langerhans cell histiocytosis and Erdheim-Chester disease linked to the BRAFV600E mutation. *Blood.* 2014;124:1119–1126.

Hollingsworth J, Cooper WA, Nicoll KD, et al. Follicular dendritic cell sarcoma of the lung: a report of two cases highlighting its pathological features and diagnostic pitfalls. *Pathology.* 2011;43:67–70.

Kamionek M, Ahmadi Moghaddam P, Sakhdari A, et al. Mutually exclusive extracellular signal-regulated kinase pathway mutations are present in different stages of multi-focal pulmonary Langerhans cell histiocytosis supporting clonal nature of the disease. *Histopathology.* 2016;69:499–509.

Lin L, Salisbury EL, Gardiner I, Varikatt W. Solitary juvenile xanthogranuloma in the lung of a young adult. *Pathology.* 2011;43:503–507.

Mendez JL, Nadrous HF, Vassallo R, Decker PA, Ryu JH. Pneumothorax in pulmonary Langerhans cell histiocytosis. *Chest.* 2004;125:1028–1032.

Menon MP, Evbuomwan MO, Rosai J, Jaffe ES, Pittaluga S. A subset of Rosai-Dorfman disease cases show increased IgG4-positive plasma cells: another red herring or a true association with IgG4-related disease? *Histopathology.* 2014;64:455–459.

Roden AC, Hu X, Kip S, et al. BRAF V600E expression in Langerhans cell histiocytosis: clinical and immunohistochemical study on 25 pulmonary and 54 extrapulmonary cases. *Am J Surg Pathol.* 2014;38:548–551.

Roden AC, Yi ES. Pulmonary langerhans cell histiocytosis: an update from the pathologists' perspective. *Arch Pathol Lab Med.* 2016;140:230–240.

Techavichit P, Sosothikul D, Chaichana T, Teerapakpinyo C, Thorner PS, Shuangshoti S. BRAF V600E mutation in pediatric intracranial and cranial juvenile xanthogranuloma. *Hum Pathol.* 2017.

Yousem SA, Dacic S, Nikiforov YE, Nikiforova M. Pulmonary langerhans cell histiocytosis: profiling of multifocal tumors using next-generation sequencing identifies concordant occurrence of BRAF V600E mutations. *Chest.* 2013;143:1679–1684.

Section 6: Benign and Borderline Lymphoid Proliferations

Bragg DG, Chor PJ, Murray KA, Kjeldsberg CR. Lymphoproliferative disorders of the lung: histopathology, clinical manifestations, and imaging features. *AJR Am J Roentgenol.* August 1994;163(2):273–281.

Gibson M, Hansell DM. Lymphocytic disorders of the chest: pathology and imaging. *Clin Radiol.* July 1998;53(7):469–480.

Guinee Jr DG, Franks TJ, Gerbino AJ, Murakami SS, Acree SC, Koss MN. Pulmonary nodular lymphoid hyperplasia (pulmonary pseudolymphoma): the significance of increased numbers of IgG4-positive plasma cells. *Am J Surg Pathol.* May 2013;37(5):699–709.

Nicholson AG, Wotherspoon AC, Diss TC, et al. Reactive pulmonary lymphoid disorders. *Histopathology.* May 1995;26(5):405–412.

Sirajuddin A, Raparia K, Lewis VA, et al. Primary pulmonary lymphoid lesions: radiologic and pathologic findings. *Radiographics.* January–February 2016;36(1):53–70.

Swigris JJ, Berry GJ, Raffin TA, Kuschner WG. Lymphoid interstitial pneumonia: a narrative review. *Chest.* December 2002;122(6):2150–2164.

Travis WD, Galvin JR. Non-neoplastic pulmonary lymphoid lesions. *Thorax.* December 2001;56(12):964–971.

Tanaka N, Kim JS, Bates CA, et al. Lung diseases in patients with common variable immunodeficiency: chest radiographic, and computed tomographic findings. *J Comput Assist Tomogr.* September–October 2006;30(5):828–838.

Travis WD, Costabel U, Hansell DM, et al. ATS/ERS Committee on Idiopathic Interstitial Pneumonias. An official American Thoracic Society/European Respiratory Society statement: update of the international multidisciplinary classification of the idiopathic interstitial pneumonias. *Am J Respir Crit Care Med.* September 15, 2013;188(6):733–748.

Section 7: Focal Lesions

Borczuk AC. Neoplastic and nonneoplastic benign mass lesions of the lung. *Arch Pathol Lab Med.* 2012;136(10):1227–1233.

Chapman SJ, Cookson WO, Musk AW, et al. Benign asbestos pleural diseases. *Curr Opin Pulm Med.* 2003;9(4):266–271.

Colby TV, Koss MN, Travis WD. Tumor-like conditions. In: *Tumors of the Lower Respiratory Tract.* Washington, DC: Armed Forces Institute of Pathology; 1994:857–863, 870.

Colby TV, Yousem SA. Lungs. In: Sternberg SS, ed. *Histology for Pathologists.* 2nd ed. Philadelphia: Lippincott Williams & Wilkins; 1997:433–460.

Fletcher CDM. *Diagnostic Histopathology of Tumors.* London: Churchill Livingstone; 2000.

Griffin CA, Hawkins AL, Dvorak C, et al. Recurrent involvement of 2p23 in inflammatory myofibroblastic tumors. *Cancer Res.* 1999;59:2776–2780.

Jones RW, Roggli VL. Dendriform pulmonary ossification: report of two cases with unique findings. *Am J Clin Pathol.* 1989;91:398–402.

Lawrence B, Perez-Atayde A, Hibbard MK, et al. TPM3-ALK and TPM4-ALK oncogenes in inflammatory myofibroblastic tumors. *Am J Pathol.* 2000;157:377–384.

Miyake HY, Kawagoe T, Hori Y, et al. Intrapulmonary lymph nodes: CT and pathological features. *Clin Radiol.* 1999;54:640–643.

Muller KM, Friemann J, Stichnoth E. Dendriform pulmonary ossification. *Pathol Res Pract.* 1980;168:163–172.

Ndimbie OK, Williams CR, Lee MW. Dendriform pulmonary ossification. *Arch Pathol Lab Med.* 1987;111:1062–1064.
Roggli VL, Oury T. Interstitial fibrosis, predominantly mature. In: Cagle PT, ed. *Diagnostic Pulmonary Pathology.* New York: Marcel Dekker; 2000:77–102.
Travis WD, Colby TV, Corrin B, et al. Histological typing of tumors of lung and pleura. In: Sobin LH, ed. *World Health Organization International Classification of Tumors.* 3rd ed. Berlin: Springer-Verlag; 1999:61–66.
Travis WD, Colby TV, Koss MN, et al. Miscellaneous diseases of uncertain etiology. In: King DW, ed. *Non-Neoplastic Disorders of the Lower Respiratory Tract.* Washington, DC: American Registry of Pathology and the Armed Forces Institute of Pathology; 2002:857–900.
Yousem SA. Pulmonary apical cap: a distinctive but poorly recognized lesion in pulmonary surgical pathology. *Am J Surg Pathol.* 2001;25:679–683.

Section 8: Granulomatous Diseases

Antin-Ozerkis D, Evans J, Rubinowitz A, Homer RJ, Matthay RA. Pulmonary manifestations of rheumatoid arthritis. *Clin Chest Med.* September 2010;31(3):451–478.
Barnes TW, Vassallo R, Tazelaar HD, Hartman TE, Ryu JH. Diffuse bronchiolar disease due to chronic occult aspiration. *Mayo Clin Proc.* February 2006;81(2):172–176.
Bosken C, Myers J, Greenberger P, Katzenstein A-L. Pathologic features of allergic bronchopulmonary aspergillosis. *Am J Surg Pathol.* 1988;12:216–222
Caplan A. Certain unusual radiological appearances in the chest of coal-miners suffering from rheumatoid arthritis. *Thorax.* March 1953;8(1):29–37.
El-Zammar OA, Katzenstein AL. Pathological diagnosis of granulomatous lung disease: a review. *Histopathology.* Febraury 2007;50(3):289–310.
Engleman P, Liebow AA, Gmelich J, Friedman PJ. Pulmonary hyalinizing granuloma. *Am Rev Respir Dis.* 1977;115:997–1008.
Flieder DB, Moran CA. Pulmonary dirofilariasis: a clinicopathologic study of 41 lesions in 39 patients. *Hum Pathol.* March 1999;30(3):251–256.
Freiman DG, Hardy HL. Beryllium disease. The relation of pulmonary pathology to clinical course and prognosis based on a study of 130 cases from the U.S. beryllium case registry. *Hum Pathol.* March 1970;1(1):25–44.
Gal AA, Koss MN. The pathology of sarcoidosis. *Curr Opin Pulm Med.* September 2002;8(5):445–451.
Ganesan S, Felo J, Saldana M, Kalasinsky VF, Lewin-Smith MR, Tomashefski Jr JF. Embolized crospovidone (poly[N-vinyl-2-pyrrolidone]) in the lungs of intravenous drug users. *Mod Pathol.* April 2003;16(4):286–292.
Gibbs AR, Williams WJ, Kelland D. Necrotising sarcoidal granulomatosis: a problem of identity. A study of seven cases. *Sarcoidosis.* September 1987;4(2):94–100.
Kashiwabara K, Toyonaga M, Yamaguchi Y, Nakamura H, Hirayama S, Kurano R. Sarcoid reaction in primary tumor of bronchogenic large cell carcinoma accompanied with massive necrosis. *Intern Med.* February 2001;40(2):127–130.
Koss MN, Hochholzer L, Feigin DS, Garancis JC, Ward PA. Necrotizing sarcoid-like granulomatosis: clinical, pathologic, and immunopathologic findings. *Hum Pathol.* September 1980; 11(5 suppl):510–519.
Liebow A. The J. Burns Amberson lecture–pulmonary angiitis and granulomatosis. *Am Rev Respir Dis.* 1973;108:1–18.
Mukhopadhyay S, Farver CF, Vaszar LT et al. Causes of pulmonary granulomas: a retrospective study of 500 cases from seven countries. *J Clin Pathol.* January 2012;65(1):51–57.
Mukhopadhyay S, Gal AA. Granulomatous lung disease: an approach to the differential diagnosis. *Arch Pathol Lab Med.* May 2010;134(5):667–690.
Mukhopadhyay S, Katzenstein AL. Pulmonary disease due to aspiration of food and other particulate matter: a clinicopathologic study of 59 cases diagnosed on biopsy or resection specimens. *Am J Surg Pathol.* May 2007;31(5):752–759.
Myers J, Katzenstein A-L. Granulomatous infection mimicking bronchocentric granulomatosis. *Am J Surg Pathol.* 1986;10:317–322.
Myers JL. Bronchocentric granulomatosis. Disease or diagnosis? *Chest.* July 1989;96(1):3–4.
Occupational Safety and Health Administration (OSHA), Department of Labor. Occupational exposure to beryllium. Final rule. *Fed Regist.* January 9, 2017;82(5):2470–2757.
Ro JY, Luna MA, Mackay B, Ramos O. Yellow-brown (Hamazaki-Wesenberg) bodies mimicking fungal yeasts. *Arch Pathol Lab Med.* June 1987;111(6):555–559.
Rosen Y. Four decades of necrotizing sarcoid granulomatosis: what do we know now? *Arch Pathol Lab Med.* February 2015;139(2):252–262.

Segawa Y, Takigawa N, Okahara M et al. Primary lung cancer associated with diffuse granulomatous lesions in the pulmonary parenchyma. *Intern Med.* September 1996;35(9):728–731.

Sheffield EA. Pathology of sarcoidosis. *Clin Chest Med.* December 1997;18(4):741–754.

Sigdel S, Gemind JT, Tomashefski Jr JF. The Movat pentachrome stain as a means of identifying microcrystalline cellulose among other particulates found in lung tissue. *Arch Pathol Lab Med.* February 2011;135(2):249–254.

Spickard 3rd A, Hirschmann JV. Exogenous lipoid pneumonia. *Arch Intern Med.* March 28, 1994;154(6):686–692.

Tomashefski Jr JF, Hirsch CS. The pulmonary vascular lesions of intravenous drug abuse. *Hum Pathol.* March 1980;11(2):133–145.

Williams WJ. A histological study of the lungs in 52 cases of chronic beryllium disease. *Br J Ind Med.* April 1958;15(2):84–91.

Yi E, Aubry MC. Pulmonary pseudoneoplasms. *Arch Pathol Lab Med.* March 2010;134(3): 417–426.

Yousem SA, Colby TV, Carrington CB. Lung biopsy in rheumatoid arthritis. *Am Rev Respir Dis.* May 1985;131(5):770–777.

Yousem SA, Hochholzer L. Pulmonary hyalinizing granuloma. *Am J Clin Pathol.* 1987;87:1–6.

Yuoh G, Hove MG, Wen J, Haque AK. Pulmonary malakoplakia in acquired immunodeficiency syndrome: an ultrastructural study of morphogenesis of Michaelis-Gutmann bodies. *Mod Pathol.* May 1996;9(5):476–483.

Section 9: Diffuse Pulmonary Hemorrhage

Alba MA, Flores-Suarez LF, Henderson AG, et al. Interstital lung disease in ANCA vasculitis. *Autoimmun Rev.* 2017;16(7):722–729.

Andrade C, Mendonca T, Farinha F, et al. Alveolar hemorrhage in systemic lupus erythematosus: a cohort review. *Lupus.* 2016;25(1):75–80.

Appel GB. Thrombotic microangiopathies: similar presentations, different therapies. *Cleve Clin J Med.* 2017;84(2):114–130.

Aubry MC. Necrotizing granulomatous inflammation: what does it mean if your special stains are negative? *Mod Pathol.* 2012;(25 suppl 1):31.

Cordier JF, Cottin V. Alveolar hemorrhage in vasculitis: primary and secondary. *Semin Respir Crit Care Med.* 2011;32(3):310–321.

Cornec D, Cornec-Le Gall E, Fervenza FC, Specks U. ANCA-associated vasculitis – clinical utility of using ANCA specificity to classify patients. *Nat Rev Rheumatol.* 2016;12(10):570–579.

Greco A, Rizzo MI, De Virgilio A, et al. Goodpasture's syndrome: a clinical update. *Autoimmun Rev.* 2015;14(3):246–253.

Katzenstein AL, Bloor CM, Leibow AA. Diffuse alveolar damage–the role of oxygen, shock, and related factors. A review. *Am J Pathol.* 1976;85(1):209–228.

Khorashadi L, Wu CC, Betancourt SL, Carter BW. Idiopathic pulmonary haemosiderosis: spectrum of thoracic imaging findings in the adult patient. *Clin Radiol.* 2015;70(5):459–465.

Krause ML, Cartin-Ceba R, Specks U, Peikert T. Update on diffuse alveolar hemorrhage and pulmonary vasculitis. *Immunol Allergy Clin North Am.* 2012;32(4):587–600.

Krexi D, Sheppard MN. Pulmonary hypertensive vascular changes in lungs of patients with sudden unexpected death. emphasis on congenital heart disease, eisenmenger syndrome, postoperative deaths and death during pregnancy and postpartum. *J Clin Pathol.* 2015;68(1):18–21.

Lesca G, Olivieri C, Burnichon N, et al. Genotype-phenotype correlations in hereditary hemorrhagic telangiectasia: data from the French-Italian HHT network. *Genet Med.* 2007;9(1):14–22.

Mahr A, Moosig F, Neumann T, et al. Eosinophilic granulomatosis with polyangiitis (Churg-Strauss): evolutions in classification, etiopathogenesis, assessment and management. *Curr Opin Rheumatol.* 2014;26(1):16–23.

Martinez-Martinez MU, Oostdam DAH, Abud-Mendoza C. Diffuse alveolar hemorrhage in autoimmune diseases. *Curr Rheumatol Rep.* 2017;19(5):27.

Pagnoux C. Updates in ANCA-associated vasculitis. *Eur J Rheumatol.* 2016;3(3):122–133.

Pedchenko V, Bondar O, Fogo AB, et al. Molecular architecture of the goodpasture autoantigen in anti-GBM nephritis. *N Engl J Med.* 2010;363(4):343–354.

Razazi K, Parrot A, Khalil A, et al. Severe haemoptysis in patients with nonsmall cell lung carcinoma. *Eur Respir J.* 2015;45(3):756–764.

Sabba C, Pasculli G, Lenato GM, et al. Hereditary hemorrhagic telangiectasia: clinical features in ENG and ALK1 mutation carriers. *J Thromb Haemost.* 2007;5(6):1149–1157.

Schwarz MI, Zamora MR, Hodges TN, Chan ED, Bowler RP, Tuder RM. Isolated pulmonary capillaritis and diffuse alveolar hemorrhage in rheumatoid arthritis and mixed connective tissue disease. *Chest.* 1998;113(6):1609–1615.

Susarla SC, Fan LL. Diffuse alveolar hemorrhage syndromes in children. *Curr Opin Pediatr.* 2007;19(3):314–320.

Taytard J, Nathan N, de Blic J, et al. New insights into pediatric idiopathic pulmonary hemosiderosis: the French RespiRare(®) cohort. *Orphanet J Rare Dis.* 2013;8:161.

Villiger PM, Guillevin L. Microscopic polyangiitis: clinical presentation. *Autoimmun Rev.* 2010;9(12):812–819.

von Ranke FM, Zanetti G, Hochhegger B, Marchiori E. Infectious diseases causing diffuse alveolar hemorrhage in immunocompetent patients: a state-of-the-art review. *Lung.* 2013;191(1):9–18.

West JB, Mathieu-Costello O. Structure, strength, failure, and remodeling of the pulmonary blood-gas barrier. *Annu Rev Physiol.* 1999;61:543–572.

Yachoui R, Sehgal R, Amlani B, Goldberg JW. Antiphospholipid antibodies-associated diffuse alveolar hemorrhage. *Semin Arthritis Rheum.* 2015;44(6):652–657.

Section 10: Pulmonary Hypertension and Embolic Disease

Haque AK, Duarte AG. Pulmonary hypertension, emboli, and other vascular diseases. In: Cagle PT, Allen TC, eds. *Lung and Pleural Pathology.* New York, NY: McGraw Hill; 2015:375–398.

Husain AN. Diseases of vascular origin. In: Husain AN, ed. *Thoracic Pathology.* Philadelphia, PA: Saunders; 2012:125–149.

Simonneau G, Galie N, Rubin LJ, et al. Clinical classification of pulmonary hypertension. *J Am Coll Cardiol.* 2004;43(12 suppl S):5S–12S.

Simonneau G, Robbins IM, Beghetti M, et al. Updated clinical classification of pulmonary hypertension. *J Am Coll Cardiol.* 2009;54(1 suppl):S43–S54.

Wagenvoort CA. Pathology of pulmonary thromboembolism. *Chest.* 1995;107(1 suppl):10S–17S.

Section 11: Large Airways

Barker AF. Bronchiectasis. *N Engl J Med.* 2002;346(18):1383–1393.

Decramer M, Janssens W, Miravitlles M. Chronic obstructive pulmonary disease. *Lancet.* 2012;379(9823):1341–1351.

Kwon KY, Myers JL, Swensen SJ, Colby TV. Middle lobe syndrome: a clinicopathological study of 21 patients. *Hum Pathol.* 1995;26(3):302–307.

Sedrak MP, Koshy JT, Allen TC. Large airway diseases. In: Cagle PT, Allen TC, eds. *Lung and Pleural Pathology.* New York, NY: McGraw Hill; 2015:611–620.

Sethi S, Murphy TF. Infection in the pathogenesis and course of chronic obstructive pulmonary disease. *N Engl J Med.* 2008;359(22):2355–2365.

Section 12: Small Airways

Allen TC. Pathology of small airways disease. *Arch Pathol Lab Med.* 2010;134(5):702–718.

Cordier JF. Cryptogenic organising pneumonia. *Eur Respir J.* 2006;28(2):422–446.

Fukuoka J, Franks TJ, Colby TV, et al. Peribronchiolar metaplasia: a common histologic lesion in diffuse lung disease and a rare cause of interstitial lung disease: clinicopathologic features of 15 cases. *Am J Surg Pathol.* 2005;29(7):948–954.

Myers JL, Colby TV. Pathologic manifestations of bronchiolitis, constrictive bronchiolitis, cryptogenic organizing pneumonia, and diffuse panbronchiolitis. *Clin Chest Med.* 1993;14(4):611–622.

Travis WD, Costabel U, Hansell DM, et al. An official american thoracic society/european respiratory society statement: update of the international multidisciplinary classification of the idiopathic interstitial pneumonias. *Am J Respir Crit Care Med.* 2013;188(6):733–748.

Urisman A, Jones K. Small airway disease. In: Cagle PT, Allen TC, eds. *Lung and Pleural Pathology.* New York, NY: McGraw Hill; 2015:521–534.

Wang CW, Muhm JR, Colby TV, Leslie KO. Small airway lesions. In: Cagle PT, Allen TC, Beasley MB, eds. *Diagnostic Pulmonary Pathology.* 2nd ed. New York: Informa; 2008:229–249.

Yousem SA, Dacic S. Idiopathic bronchiolocentric interstitial pneumonia. *Mod Pathol.* 2002;15(11):1148–1153.

Section 13: Alveolar Infiltrates

Allen TC, Bois MC. Acute lung injury. In: Cagle PT, Allen TC, eds. *Lung and Pleural Pathology.* New York, NY: McGraw Hill; 2015:511–520.

Beasley MB. Intra-alveolar exudates and infiltrates. In: Cagle PT, Allen TC, Beasley MB, eds. *Diagnostic Pulmonary Pathology.* 2nd ed. New York: Informa; 2008:155–164.

Capelozzi VL, Allen TC, Beasley MB, et al. Molecular and immune biomarkers in acute respiratory distress syndrome: a perspective from members of the pulmonary pathology society. *Arch Pathol Lab Med.* 2017;141(12):1719–1727.

Guinee D. Pulmonary eosinophilia. In: Cagle PT, Allen TC, Beasley MB, eds. *Diagnostic Pulmonary Pathology.* 2nd ed. New York: Informa; 2008:182–216.

Marchevsky AM. Alveolar infiltrates. In: Cagle PT, Allen TC, eds. *Lung and Pleural Pathology.* New York, NY: McGraw Hill; 2015:557–578.

Section 14: Tobacco-Related Diseases

Berg K, Wright JL. The pathology of chronic obstructive pulmonary disease: progress in the 20th and 21st centuries. *Arch Pathol Lab Med.* 2016;140(12):1423–1428.

Cavazza A, Lantuejoul S, Sartori G, et al. Placental transmogrification of the lung: clinicopathologic, immunohistochemical and molecular study of two cases, with particular emphasis on the interstitial clear cells. *Hum Pathol.* 2004;35(4):517–521.

Churg A, Muller NL, Wright JL. Respiratory bronchiolitis/interstitial lung disease: fibrosis, pulmonary function, and evolving concepts. *Arch Pathol Lab Med.* 2010;134(1):27–32.

Fidler ME, Koomen M, Sebek B, Greco MA, Rizk CC, Askin FB. Placental transmogrification of the lung, a histologic variant of giant bullous emphysema. Clinicopathological study of three further cases. *Am J Surg Pathol.* 1995;19(5):563–570.

Fraig M, Shreesha U, Savici D, Katzenstein AL. Respiratory bronchiolitis: a clinicopathologic study in current smokers, ex-smokers, and never-smokers. *Am J Surg Pathol.* 2002;26(5):647–653.

Katzenstein AL, Mukhopadhyay S, Zanardi C, Dexter E. Clinically occult interstitial fibrosis in smokers: classification and significance of a surprisingly common finding in lobectomy specimens. *Hum Pathol.* 2010;41(3):316–325.

Katzenstein AL. Smoking-related interstitial fibrosis (SRIF), pathogenesis and treatment of usual interstitial pneumonia (UIP), and transbronchial biopsy in UIP. *Mod Pathol.* 2012;(25 suppl 1):68.

Kawabata Y, Hoshi E, Murai K, et al. Smoking-related changes in the background lung of specimens resected for lung cancer: a semiquantitative study with correlation to postoperative course. *Histopathology.* 2008;53(6):707–714.

Kligerman S, Franks TJ, Galvin JR. Clinical-radiologic-pathologic correlation of smoking-related diffuse parenchymal lung disease. *Radiol Clin North Am.* 2016;54(6):1047–1063.

Mirza S, Benzo R. Chronic obstructive pulmonary disease phenotypes: implications for care. *Mayo Clin Proc.* 2017;92(7):1104–1112.

Moran CA, Suster S. Unusual non-neoplastic lesions of the lung. *Semin Diagn Pathol.* 2007;24(3):199–208.

Myers JL, Veal CF, Shin MS, Katzenstein AL. Respiratory bronchiolitis causing interstitial lung disease. A clinicopathologic study of six cases. *Am Rev Respir Dis.* 1987;135(4):880–884.

Tazelaar HD, Wright JL, Churg A. Desquamative interstitial pneumonia. *Histopathology.* 2011;58(4):509–516.

Vassallo R, Harari S, Tazi A. Current understanding and management of pulmonary langerhans cell histiocytosis. *Thorax.* 2017;72(10).

Washko GR, Hunninghake GM, Fernandez IE, et al. Lung volumes and emphysema in smokers with interstitial lung abnormalities. *N Engl J Med.* 2011;364(10):897–906.

Yousem SA. Respiratory bronchiolitis-associated interstitial lung disease with fibrosis is a lesion distinct from fibrotic nonspecific interstitial pneumonia: a proposal. *Mod Pathol.* 2006;19(11):1474–1479.

Section 15: Diffuse Interstitial Lung Diseases

Barnes TW, Vassallo R, Tazelaar HD, Hartman TE, Ryu JH. Diffuse bronchiolar disease due to chronic occult aspiration. *Mayo Clin Proc.* 2006;81(2):172–176.

Bates C, Ellison MC, Lynch DA, Cool CD, Brown KK, Routes JM. Granulomatous-lymphocytic lung disease shortens survival in common variable immunodeficiency. *J Allergy Clin Immunol* 2004;114:415–421.

Camus P, Colby TV. The lung in inflammatory bowel disease. *Eur Respir J.* January 2000;15(1):5–10. PMID:10678613.

Camus P, Piard F, Ashcroft T, Gal AA, Colby TV. The lung in inflammatory bowel disease. *Medicine (Baltimore).* May 1993;72(3):151–183. PMID:8502168.

Casey MB, Tazelaar HD, Myers JL, et al. Noninfectious lung pathology in patients with Crohn's disease. *Am J Surg Pathol.* February 2003;27(2):213–219. PMID:12548168.

Churg A, et al. Airway-centered interstitial fibrosis: a distinct form of aggressive diffuse lung disease. *Am J Surg Pathol.* January 2004;28(1):62–68.

de Carvalho ME, Kairalla RA, Capelozzi VL, et al. Centrilobular fibrosis: a novel histological pattern of idiopathic interstitial pneumonia. *Pathol Res Pract.* August 2002;198(9):577–583.

Deshpande V, Zen Y, Chan JK, et al. Consensus statement on the pathology of IgG4-related disease. *Mod Pathol.* September 2012;25(9):1181–1192. doi:10.1038/modpathol.2012.72. Epub 2012 May 18. PMID:22596100.

Embil J, Warren P, Yakrus M, et al. Pulmonary illness associated with exposure to Mycobacterium-avium complex in hot tub water. Hypersensitivity pneumonitis or infection? *Chest.* March 1997;111(3):813–816.

Eschenbacher WL, et al. Nylon flock-associated interstitial lung disease. *Am J Respir Crit Care Med.* June 1999;159(6):2003–2008.

Fukuoka J, et al. Peribronchiolar metaplasia: a common histologic lesion in diffuse lung disease and a rare cause of interstitial lung disease: clinicopathologic features of 15 cases. *Am J Surg Pathol.* July 2005;29(7):948–954.

Hansell DM, Bankier AA, MacMahon H, McLoud TC, Müller NL, Remy J. Fleischner Society: glossary of terms for thoracic imaging. *Radiology.* March 2008;246(3):697–722. doi:10.1148/radiol.2462070712. PMID:18195376.

Hartono S, Motosue MS, Khan S, et al. Predictors of granulomatous lymphocytic interstitial lung disease in common variable immunodeficiency. *Ann Allergy Asthma Immunol.* 2017;118(5):614–620.

Hu X, Lee JS, Pianosi PT, Ryu JH. Aspiration related pulmonary syndromes. *Chest.* 2015;147:815–823.

Kahana LM, Kay JM, Yakrus MA, Waserman S. Mycobacterium avium complex infection in an immunocompetent young adult related to hot tub exposure. *Chest.* January 1997;111(1):242–245.

Kern DG, Kuhn 3rd C, Ely EW, et al. Flock worker's lung. Broadening the spectrum of clinicopathology, narrowing the spectrum of suspected etiologies. *Chest.* January 2000;117(1):251–259.

Khoor A, Leslie KO, Tazelaar HD, Helmers RA, Colby TV. Diffuse pulmonary disease caused by nontuberculous mycobacteria in immunocompetent people (hot tub lung). *Am J Clin Pathol.* May 2001;115(5):755–762.

Khoor A, Colby TV. Amyloidosis of the lung. *Arch Pathol Lab Med.* 2017;141(2), 247–254. doi:10.5858/arpa.2016-0102-RA.

Kuranishi LT, Leslie KO, Ferreira RG, et al. Airway-centered interstitial fibrosis: etiology, clinical findings and prognosis. *Respir Res.* May 9, 2015;16:55.

Lantuejoul S, Colby TV, Ferretti GR, Brichon PY, Brambilla C, Brambilla E. Adenocarcinoma of the lung mimicking inflammatory lung disease with honeycombing. *Eur Respir J.* September 2004;24(3):502–505. PMID:15358712.

Mannina A, Chung JH, Swigris JJ, et al. Clinical predictors of a diagnosis of common variable immunodeficiency-related granulomatous-lymphocytic interstitial lung disease. *Ann Am Thorac Soc.* 2016;13(7):1042–1049.

Marchevsky A, Damsker B, Gribetz A, Tepper S, Geller SA. The spectrum of pathology of nontuberculous mycobacterial infections in open-lung biopsy specimens. *Am J Clin Pathol.* November 1982;78(5):695–700.

Matsuse T, Oka T, Kida K, Fukuchi Y. Importance of diffuse aspiration bronchiolitis caused by chronic occult aspiration in the elderly. *Chest.* 1996;110(5):1289–1293.

Mukhopadhyay S, El-Zammar OA, Katzenstein AL. Pulmonary meningothelial-like nodules: new insights into a common but poorly understood entity. *Am J Surg Pathol.* April 2009;33(4): 487–495. doi:10.1097/PAS.0b013e31818b1de7. PMID:19047895.

Mukhopadhyay S, Katzenstein AL. Pulmonary disease due to aspiration of food and other particulate matter: a clinicopathologic study of 59 cases diagnosed on biopsy or resection specimens. *Am J Surg Pathol.* 2007;31:752–759.

Myers JL. Hypersensitivity pneumonia: the role of lung biopsy in diagnosis and management. *Mod Pathol.* January 2012;(25 suppl 1) S58–S67. doi:10.1038/modpathol.2011.152. PMID:22214971.

Park J, Levinson AI. Granulomatous-lymphocytic interstitial lung disease (GLILD) in common variable immunodeficiency (CVID). *Clin Immunol.* 2010;134:97–103.

Rao N, Mackinnon AC, Routes JM. Granulomatous and lymphocytic interstitial lung disease: a spectrum of pulmonary histopathologic lesions in common variable immunodeficiency – histologic and immunohistochemical analysis of 16 cases. *Human Pathol.* 2015;46:1306–1314.

Smith M. Update on pulmonary fibrosis: not all fibrosis is created equally. *Arch Pathol Lab Med.* 2016;140:221–229. doi:10.5858/arpa.2015-0288-SA. PMID:26927716.

Smith ML, Gotway MB, Larsen BT, Colby TV, Tazelaar HD, Leslie KO. Pathologic approach to cystic lung disease. *AJSP: Review & Reports.* 2017;22(1):36–45.

Stone JH, Zen Y, Deshpande V. IgG4-related disease. *N Engl J Med.* February 9, 2012;366(6): 539–551. doi:10.1056/NEJMra1104650. PMID:22316447.

Suster S, Moran CA. Diffuse pulmonary meningotheliomatosis. *Am J Surg Pathol.* April 2007;31(4):624–631. doi:10.1097/01.pas.0000213385.25042.cf. PMID:17414111.

Takemura T, Akashi T, Kamiya H, et al. Pathological differentiation of chronic hypersensitivity pneumonitis from idiopathic pulmonary fibrosis/usual interstitial pneumonia. *Histopathology.* December 2012;61(6):1026–1035. doi:10.1111/j.1365-2559.2012.04322.x. Epub August 8, 2012. PMID:22882269.

Utz JP, Swensen SJ, Gertz MA. Pulmonary amyloidosis. The Mayo Clinic experience from 1980 to 1993. *Ann Intern Med.* 1996;124(4):407–413.

Vrana JA, Gamez JD, Madden BJ, Theis JD, Bergen 3rd HR, Dogan A. Classification of amyloidosis by laser microdissection and mass spectrometry-based proteomic analysis in clinical biopsy specimens. *Blood.* 2009;114(24):4957–4959. doi:10.1182/blood-2009-07-230722.

Weissferdt A, Tang X, Suster S, Wistuba II, Moran CA. Pleuropulmonary meningothelial proliferations: evidence for a common histogenesis. *Am J Surg Pathol.* December 2015;39(12): 1673–1678. doi:10.1097/PAS.0000000000000489. PMID:26291511.

Yi ES, Sekiguchi H, Peikert T, Ryu JH, Colby TV. Pathologic manifestations of Immunoglobulin(Ig) G4-related lung disease. *Semin Diagn Pathol.* November 2012;29(4):219–225. doi:10.1053/j.semdp.2012.07.002. PMID:23068301.

Yousem SA, Dadic S. Idiopathic bronchiolocentric interstitial pneumonia. *Mod Pathol.* November 2002;15(11):1148–1153.

Yousem SA, Faber C. Histopathology of aspiration pneumonia not associated with food or other particulate matter: a clinicopathologic study of 10 cases diagnosed on biopsy. *Am J Surg Pathol.* 2011;35:426–431.

Zen Y, Inoue D, Kitao A, et al. IgG4-related lung and pleural disease: a clinicopathologic study of 21 cases. *Am J Surg Pathol.* December 2009;33(12):1886–1893. doi:10.1097/PAS.0b013e3181bd535b. PMID:19898222.

Section 16: Idiopathic Interstitial Pneumonias

Amitani R, Kuse F. Idiopathic pulmonary upper lobe fibrosis (IPFU). *Kokyu.* 1992;11:693–699.

Churg A, Bilawich A. Confluent fibrosis and fibroblast foci in fibrotic non-specific interstitial pneumonia. *Histopathology.* July 2016;69(1):128–135.

Churg A, Muller NL, Silva CIS, Wright JL. Acute exacerbation (acute lung injury of unknown cause) in UIP and other forms of fibrotic interstitial pneumonias. *Am J Surg Pathol.* 2007;31:277–284.

Colby TV. Pathologic aspects of bronchiolitis obliterans organizing pneumonia. *Chest.* July 1992;102(1 suppl):38S–43S.

English JC, Mayo JR, Levy R et al. Pleuroparenchymal fibroelastosis: a rare interstitial lung disease. *Respirol Case Rep.* 2015;3(2):82–84

Frankel SK, Cool CD, Lynch DA, et al. Idiopathic pleuroparenchymal fibroelastosis: description of a novel clinicopathologic entity. *Chest.* 2004; 126:2007–2013.

Hamman L, Rich AR. Acute diffuse interstitial fibrosis of the lungs. *Bull Johns Hopkins Hosp.* 1944;74:177.

Ichikado K, Johkoh T, Ikezoe J, et al. Acute interstitial pneumonia: high-resolution CT findings correlated with pathology. *AJR Am J Roentgenol.* February 1997;168(2):333–338.

Idiopathic Pulmonary Fibrosis Clinical Research Network, Raghu G, Anstrom KJ, King Jr TE, Lasky JA, Martinez FJ. Prednisone, azathioprine, and N-acetylcysteine for pulmonary fibrosis. *N Engl J Med.* May 24, 2012;366(21):1968–1977.

Katzenstein AL, Fiorelli RF. Nonspecific interstitial pneumonia/fibrosis. Histologic features and clinical significance. *Am J Surg Pathol.* February 1994;18(2):136–147.

Katzenstein AL, Myers JL, Mazur MT. Acute interstitial pneumonia. A clinicopathologic, ultrastructural, and cell kinetic study. *Am J Surg Pathol.* 1986;10:256–267.

King Jr TE, Bradford WZ, Castro-Bernardini S, et al. A phase 3 trial of pirfenidone in patients with idiopathic pulmonary fibrosis. *N Engl J Med.* May 29, 2014;370(22):2083–2092. doi:10.1056/NEJMoa1402582. Epub May 18, 2014.

Nicholson AG, Colby TV, du Bois RM, Hansell DM, Wells AU. The prognostic significance of the histologic pattern of interstitial pneumonia in patients presenting with the clinical entity of cryptogenic fibrosing alveolitis. *Am J Respir Crit Care Med.* 2000;162:2213–2217.

Ofek E, Sato M, Saito T, et al. Restrictive allograft syndrome post lung transplantation is characterized by pleuroparenchymal fibroelastosis. *Mod Pathol.* 2013;26:350–356.

Popper HH. Bronchiolitis obliterans. Organizing pneumonia. *Verh Dtsch Ges Pathol.* 2002;86:101–106.

Raghu G, Collard HR, Egan JJ, et al. An official ATS/ERS/JRS/ALAT statement: idiopathic pulmonary fibrosis: evidence-based guidelines for diagnosis and management. *Am J Respir Crit Care Med.* March 15, 2011;183(6):788–824.

Richeldi L, du Bois RM, Raghu G, et al. Efficacy and safety of nintedanib in idiopathic pulmonary fibrosis. *N Engl J Med.* May 29, 2014;370(22):2071–2082.

Travis WD, Costabel U, Hansell DM, et al. An official American Thoracic Society/European Respiratory Society statement: update of the international multidisciplinary classification of the idiopathic interstitial pneumonias. *Am J Respir Crit Care Med.* 2013;188:733–748.

von der Thusen JH, Hansell DM, Tominaga M, et al. Pleuroparenchymal fibroelastosis in patients with pulmonary disease secondary to bone marrow transplantation. *Mod Pathol.* 2011;24:1633–1639.

Section 17: Specific Infectious Agents

Bains SN, Judson MA: Allergic bronchopulmonary aspergillosis. *Clin Chest Med.* 2012;33(2):265.

Bartlett JG. The role of anaerobic bacteria in lung abscess. *Clin Infect Dis.* 2005;40(7):923–925. doi:10.1086/428586.

Carmona EM, Limper AH. Update on the diagnosis and treatment of pneumocystis pneumonia. *Ther Adv Resp Dis.* 2011;5(1):41.

Chiche L, Forel JM, Papazian L. The role of viruses in nosocomial pneumonia. *Curr Opin Infect Dis.* 2011;24(2):152–156.

Davies SF, Sarosi GA. Fungal infections. In: Murray JF, Nadel JA, Mason RJ, Boushey Jr HA, eds. *Textbook of Respiratory Medicine.* 3rd ed. Philadelphia, PA: WB Saunders; 2000:1107–1141.

DelBono V, Mikulska M, Viscoli C. Invasive aspergillosis: diagnosis, prophylaxis and treatment. *Curr Opin Hematol.* 2008;15(6):586.

Husain AN. Pulmonary infections. In: Husain AN, ed. *Thoracic Pathology.* Philadelphia, PA: Saunders; 2012:150–198.

Johansson N, Kalin M, Tiveljung-Lindell A, Giske CG, Hedlund J. Etiology of community-acquired pneumonia: increased microbiological yield with new diagnostic methods. *Clin Infect Dis.* 2010;50(2):202–209. doi:10.1086/648678.

Kim EA, Lee KS, Primack SL, et al. Viral pneumonias in adults: radiologic and pathologic findings. *Radiographics.* 2002;(22 Spec No):S137–S149.

Mukhopadhyay S, Gal AA. Granulomatous lung disease: an approach to the differential diagnosis. *Arch Pathol Lab Med.* 2010;134(5):667–690.

Pina-Oviedo S, Gorman BK. Viral, parasitic, and other infectious diseases. In: Cagle PT, Allen TC, eds. *Lung and Pleural Pathology.* New York, NY: McGraw Hill; 2015:325–374.

Puligandla PS, Laberge JM. Respiratory infections: pneumonia, lung abscess, and empyema. *Semin Pediatr Surg.* 2008;17:42–52.

Roden AC, Schuetz AN. Histopathology of fungal diseases of the lung. *Semin Diagn Pathol.* 2017;34(6):530–549.

Shah RD, Wunderink RG. Viral pneumonia and acute respiratory distress syndrome. *Clin Chest Med.* 2017;38(1):113–125.

Shamsuzzaman SM, Hashiguchi Y. Thoracic amebiasis. *Clin Chest Med.* 2002;23(2):479–492.

Siddiqui AA, Berk SL. Diagnosis of strongyloides stercoralis infection. *Clin Infect Dis.* 2001;33(7):1040–1047.

Suster S, Moran CA. Viral lung infections. In: Epstein JI, ed. *Biopsy Interpretation of the Lung.* 1st ed. Philadelphia: Lippincott Williams & Wilkins; 2013:155–174.

Thibodeau KP, Viera AJ. Atypical pathogens and challenges in community-acquired pneumonia. *Am Fam Physician* 2004;69(7):1699–1706.

Section 18: Transplant-Related Pathology

Ge Y. Transplant-related conditions. In: Cagle PT, Allen TC, eds. *Lung and Pleural Pathology.* New York, NY: McGraw Hill; 2015:425–448.

Takei H, Allen TC, Al-Ibraheemi A, Janssen B, Lee N, Cagle PT. Chronic lung transplant rejection. In: Cagle PT, Yerian L, Truong LD, eds. *Atlas of Transplant Pathology.* Northfield, IL: CAP Press; 2015 [Section 4, Chapter 6].

Husain S, Singh N. Bronchiolitis obliterans and lung transplantation: evidence for an infectious etiology. *Semin Respir Infect.* 2002;17(4):310–314.

Barrios RJ, Allen TC, Seethamraju H, Burns KM, Land GA, Cagle PT. Antibody-mediated (humoral) lung transplant ejection. In: Cagle PT, Yerian L, Truong LD, eds. *Atlas of Transplant Pathology.* Northfield, IL: CAP Press; 2015 [Section 4. Chapter 4].

Roden AC, Aisner DL, Allen TC, et al. Diagnosis of acute cellular rejection and antibody-mediated rejection on lung transplant biopsies: a perspective from members of the pulmonary pathology society. *Arch Pathol Lab Med.* 2017;141(3):437–444.

Allen TC, Consamus E, Lee N, Haque A, Cagle PT. Acute cellular rejection. In: Cagle PT, Yerian L, Truong LD, eds. *Atlas of Transplant Pathology.* Northfield, IL: CAP Press; 2015 [Section 4. Chapter 5].

Section 19: Lung Pathology in Collagen Vascular Diseases

Corte TJ, Copley SJ, Desai SR, et al. Significance of connective tissue disease features in idiopathic interstitial pneumonia. *Eur Respir J.* 2012;39(3):661–668.

Doyle TJ, Dellaripa PF. Lung manifestations in the rheumatic diseases. *Chest.* 2017.

Kim HC, Ji W, Kim MY, et al. Interstitial pneumonia related to undifferentiated connective tissue disease: pathologic pattern and prognosis. *Chest.* 2015;147(1):165–172.

Nakamura Y, Suda T, Kaida Y, et al. Rheumatoid lung disease: prognostic analysis of 54 biopsy-proven cases. *Respir Med.* 2012;106(8):1164–1169.

Omote N, Taniguchi H, Kondoh Y, et al. Lung-dominant connective tissue disease: clinical, radiologic, and histologic features. *Chest.* 2015;148(6):1438–1446.

Tansey D, Wells AU, Colby TV, et al. Variations in histological patterns of interstitial pneumonia between connective tissue disorders and their relationship to prognosis. *Histopathology.* 2004;44(6):585–596.

Tazelaar HD, Wright JL, Churg A. Desquamative interstitial pneumonia. *Histopathology.* 2011;58(4):509–516.

Travis WD, Costabel U, Hansell DM, et al. An official american thoracic society/european respiratory society statement: update of the international multidisciplinary classification of the idiopathic interstitial pneumonias. *Am J Respir Crit Care Med.* 2013;188(6):733–748.

Section 20: Therapeutic Drug Reactions and Radiation Effects

Abratt RP, Morgan GW. Lung toxicity following chest irradiation in patients with lung cancer. *Lung Cancer.* 2002;35:103–109.

Bedrossian CW, Miller WC, Luna MA. Methotrexate-induced diffuse interstitial pulmonary fibrosis. *South Med J.* 1979;72:313–318.

Bennett DE, Million RR, Ackerman LV. Bilateral radiation pneumonitis, a complication of the radiotherapy of bronchogenic carcinoma. (Report and analysis of seven cases with autopsy). *Cancer.* 1969;23:1001–1018.

Chin KM, Channick RN, Rubin LJ. Is methamphetamine use associated with idiopathic pulmonary arterial hypertension? *Chest.* 2006;130:1657–1663.

Coggle JE, Lambert BE, Moores SR. Radiation effects in the lung. *Environ Health Perspect.* 1986;70:261–291.

Connolly HM, Crary JL, McGoon MD, et al. Valvular heart disease associated with fenfluramine-phentermine. *N Engl J Med.* 1997;337:581–588.

Fajardo LF, Berthrong M. Radiation injury in surgical pathology. Part I. *Am J Surg Pathol.* 1978;2:159–199.

Fukuoka J, Leslie KO. Chronic diffuse lung diseases. In: Leslie KO, Wick MR, eds. *Practical Pulmonary Pathology: A Diagnostic Approach.* 2nd ed. Philadelphia, PA: Elsevier Saunders; 2011:241–248.

Gal AA. Drug and radiation toxicity. In: Tomashefski JF, Cagle PT, Farver CF, Fraire AE, eds. *Dail and Hammar's Pulmonary Pathology;* vol. 1: Non-neoplastic Lung Disease. 3rd ed. New York, NY: Springer; 2008:807–830.

Garg L, Akbar G, Agrawal S, et al. Drug-induced pulmonary arterial hypertension: a review. *Heart Fail Rev.* 2017;22:289–297.

Geller M, Dickie HA, Kass DA, Hafez GR, Gillespie JJ. The histopathology of acute nitrofurantoin-associated pneumonitis. *Ann Allergy.* 1976;37:275–279.

Imokawa S, Colby TV, Leslie KO, Helmers RA. Methotrexate pneumonitis: review of the literature and histopathological findings in nine patients. *Eur Respir J.* 2000;15:373–381.

Kennedy JI, Myers JL, Plumb VJ, Fulmer JD. Amiodarone pulmonary toxicity. Clinical, radiologic, and pathologic correlations. *Arch Intern Med.* January 1987;147:50–55.

Larsen BT, Vaszar LT, Colby TV, Tazelaar HD. Lymphoid hyperplasia and eosinophilic pneumonia as histologic manifestations of amiodarone-induced lung toxicity. *Am J Surg Pathol.* April 2012;36:509–516.

Liu V, White DA, Zakowski MF, et al. Pulmonary toxicity associated with erlotinib. *Chest.* 2007;132:1042–1044.

Mark EJ, Patalas ED, Chang HT, Evans RJ, Kessler SC. Fatal pulmonary hypertension associated with short-term use of fenfluramine and phentermine. *N Engl J Med.* 1997;337:602–606.

Myers JL, Kennedy JI, Plumb VJ. Amiodarone lung: pathologic findings in clinically toxic patients. *Hum Pathol.* April 1987;18:349–354.

Ostör AJ, Chilvers ER, Somerville MF, et al. Pulmonary complications of infliximab therapy in patients with rheumatoid arthritis. *J Rheumatol.* 2006;33:622–628.

Rossi SE, Erasmus JJ, McAdams HP, Sporn TA, Goodman PC. Pulmonary drug toxicity: radiologic and pathologic manifestations. *Radiographics.* 2000;20:1245–1259.

Sakata KK, Larsen BT, Boland JM, et al. Nitrofurantoin-induced granulomatous interstitial pneumonia. *Int J Surg Pathol.* 2014;22:352–357.

Sovijarvi AR, Lemola M, Stenius B, Idänpään-Heikkilä J. Nitrofurantoin-induced acute, subacute and chronic pulmonary reactions. *Scand J Respir Dis.* 1977;58:41–50.

Strother J, Fedullo P, Yi ES, et al. Complex vascular lesions at autopsy in a patient with phentermine-fenfluramine use and rapidly progressing pulmonary hypertension. *Arch Pathol Lab Med.* 1999;123:539–540.

The Drug-Induced Respiratory Disease Website. http://www.pneumotox.com.

Zisman DA, McCune WJ, Tino G, Lynch 3rd JP. Drug-induced pneumonitis: the role of methotrexate. *Sarcoidosis Vasc Diffuse Lung Dis.* 2001;18:243–252.

Section 21: Pneumoconioses

Champlin J, Edwards R, Pipavath S. Imaging of occupational lung disease. *Radiol Clin North Am.* 2016;54(6):1077–1096.

Cullinan P, Reid P. Pneumocon. *Prim Care Respir J.* 2013;22(2):249–252.

Laga AC, Allen TC, Cagle PT. Mixed pneumoconiosis and mixed-dust pneumoconiosis. In: Cagle PT, ed. *Color Atlas and Textbook of Pulmonary Pathology.* 2nd ed. New York: Lippincott Williams and Wilkins; 2008:376–377.

Seaman DM, Meyer CA, Kanne JP. Occupational and environmental lung disease. *Clin Chest Med.* 2015;36(2):249–268, viii–ix.

Sheikh UN, Allen TC. Asbestosis and pneumoconiosis. In: Cagle PT, Allen TC, eds. *Lung and Pleural Pathology.* New York: McGraw Hill; 2016.

Section 22: Metabolic Disorders/Storage Diseases

Allen TC, Ostrowski ML, Kerr KM. Pulmonary langerhans-cell histiocytosis. In: Cagle PT, ed. *Color Atlas and Textbook of Pulmonary Pathology.* 2nd ed. New York: Lippincott Williams and Wilkins; 2008:207–209.

Allen TC. Pulmonary langerhans cell histiocytosis and other pulmonary histiocytic diseases: a review. *Arch Pathol Lab Med.* 2008;132(7):1171–1181.

Chung MJ, Lee KS, Franquet T, Müller NL, Han J, Kwon OJ. Metabolic lung disease: imaging and histopathologic findings. *Eur J Radiol.* 2005;54(2):233–245.

Hammar SP, Allen TC. Pulmonary histiocytosis. In: Dail DH, Hammar SP, eds. *Pulmonary Pathology.* 3rd ed. New York: Springer-Verlag; 2008:600–649.

Wang CW, Colby TV. Histiocytic lesions and proliferations in the lung. *Semin Diagn Pathol.* 2007;24(3):162–182.

Section 23: Nonneoplastic Lesions of the Pleura

Cagle PT, Allen TC. *Pleural Histology in Textbook of Pleural Diseases.* Light RW, Lee YCG, eds. 3rd ed. Boca Raton: CRC Press, 2016:243–250.

Borczuk AC. Pleura. In: Cagle PT, Allen TC, eds. *Lung and Pleural Pathology.* New York, NY: McGraw Hill; 2015:229–254.

Bowman RR, Rosenblatt R, Myers LG. Pleural endometriosis. *BUMC Proc.* 1999;12:193–197.

Chapman SJ, Cookson WO, Musk AW, et al. Benign asbestos pleural diseases. *Curr Opin Pulm Med.* 2003;4:266–271.

Corrin B. Pleura and chest wall. In: Corrin B, ed. *Pathology of the Lungs.* London: Churchill Livingstone; 2000:607–642.

Madjar S, Weissberg D. Thoracic splenosis. *Thorax.* 1994;49:1020–1022.

Sarda R, Sproat I, Kurtycz DF, Hafez R. Pulmonary parenchymal splenosis. *Diagn Cytopathol.* 2001;24:352–355.

Syed S, Zaharopoulos P. Thoracic splenosis diagnosed by fine-needle aspiration cytology: a case report. *Diagn Cytopathol.* 2001;25:321–324.

Section 24: Pediatric Pulmonary Pathology

Dehner LP, Stocker JT, Mani H, Hill A, Husain AN. The respiratory tract. In: Husain, AN, Stocker, JT, Dehner LP, eds. *Stocker & Dehner's Pediatric Pathology*. 4th ed. Philadelphia, PA: Lippincott Williams & Wilkins; 2016:441–523.

Dishop MK, Kuruvilla S. Primary and metastatic lung tumors in the pediatric population: a review and 25-year experience at a large children's hospital. *Arch Pathol Lab Med.* 2008;132(7):1079.

Husain AN, Hessel RG. Neonatal pulmonary hypoplasia: an autopsy study of 25 cases. *Pediatr Pathol.* 1993;13(4):475.

Langston C, Dishop MK. Diffuse lung disease in infancy: a proposed classification applied to 259 diagnostic biopsies. *Pediatr Dev Pathol.* 2009;12(6):421.

Langston C. New concepts in the pathology of congenital lung malformations. *Semin Pediatr Surg.* 2003;12(1):17.

Pogoriler J, Husain AN. Pediatric pulmonary diseases. In: Cagle PT, Allen TC, eds. *Lung and Pleural Pathology*. New York, NY: McGraw Hill; 2015:9–40.

Pogoriler JE, Husain AN. The lung. In: Husain AN, ed. *Biopsy Interpretation of Pediatric Lesions (Biopsy Interpretation Series).* 1st ed. Philadelphia, PA: Wolters Kluwer; 2014:271–288.

Yu DC, Grabowski MJ, Kozakewich HP, et al. Primary lung tumors in children and adolescents: a 90-year experience. *J Pediatr Surg.* 2010;45(6):1090.

Index

Note: Page numbers followed by *f* indicate figures and *t* indicate tables.

M

N

O

P